Recent Advances in
MEDICINE

A. M. DAWSON MD FRCP
Physician, St Bartholomew's Hospital and
King Edward VII Hospital for Officers, London;
Physician to the Royal Household

NIGEL COMPSTON MA MD FRCP
Physician, The Royal Free Hospital,
The Royal Masonic Hospital and
King Edward VII Hospital for Officers,
London

G. M. BESSER MD FRCP
Professor of Endocrinology and
Physician, St Bartholomew's Hospital,
London

Recent Advances in
MEDICINE

EDITED BY

A. M. DAWSON
NIGEL COMPSTON
G. M. BESSER

NUMBER EIGHTEEN

CHURCHILL LIVINGSTONE
EDINBURGH LONDON MELBOURNE AND NEW YORK 1981

CHURCHILL LIVINGSTONE
Medical Division of Longman Group Limited

Distributed in the United States of America by
Churchill Livingston Inc., 19 West 44th Street, New York,
N.Y. 10036, and by associated companies,
branches and representatives throughout
the world.

First published 1981

ISBN 0 443 020779 (cased)
ISBN 0 443 02078 7 (limp)
ISSN 0143–6791

British Library Cataloguing in Publication Data

Recent advances in medicine.
  No. 18
  1. Medicine—Periodicals
  I. Dawson, Anthony Michael
  II. Compston, Nigel Deal
  III. Besser, G.M.
  610   R31   80–41912

Printed in Great Britain at The Pitman Press, Bath

Preface

It is a pleasure to introduce the 18th volume of Recent Advances in Medicine but we are sorry to announce Professor D. N. Baron's resignation as one of the co-editors. The new team's policy has not changed and the intention of this volume is once again to highlight various subjects in which advances have been made and to invite contributors to review these for the general reader rather than the specialist in the individual field. The many advances in diagnostic techniques have inevitably meant that in this edition contributions have weighed heavily towards diagnosis but we hope that the net has been cast wide enough to satisfy most tastes.

We would like to thank Churchill Livingstone for their help and cooperation in the preparation of this volume.

London, 1981

A.M.D.
G.M.B.
N.D.C.

Contributors

A. BRECKENRIDGE MD MSc FRCP
Professor of Clinical Pharmacology, University of Liverpool

P. M. BROWN MBBS MRCP(UK)
Lecturer in Medicine, Department of Medicine, St Thomas's Hospital Medical
School, London

R. Y. CALNE MA MS FRCS FRS
Professor of Surgery and Honorary Consultant Surgeon, Department of Surgery,
University of Cambridge, Unit E9, Addenbrookes's Hospital, Cambridge

STEWART W. CLARKE MD FRCP
Consultant Physician, The Royal Free Hospital, The Brompton Hospital and King
Edward VII Hospital for Officers, London

PETER B. COTTON MD FRCP
Consultant Physician, The Middlesex Hospital, London

HEATHER M. DICK MB ChB MRCP MRCPath
Consultant in Clinical Immunology, Tissue Typing/Clinical Immunology
Laboratory, Royal Infirmary, Glasgow

RONALD T. D. EMOND MB ChB FRCP DTM & H
Consultant in Infectious Diseases, The Royal Free Hospital, London

JOHN GRIMLEY EVANS FRCP MFCM
Professor of Medicine (Geriatrics), University of Newcastle Upon Tyne
Consultant Physician in Geriatric and General Medicine, Newcastle University
Hospital

I. KELSEY FRY DM FRCP FRCR
Consultant Radiologist, St Bartholomew's Hospital, London. Director, X-ray
Department, BUPA Medical Centre, London

J. S. GARROW MD PhD FRCP
Consultant Physician and MRC Scientific Staff, Division of Clinical Sciences, Clinical
Research Centre, Harrow, Middlesex

JEFFREY GAWLER MD FRCP
Consultant Neurologist, St Bartholomew's Hospital, London

J. E. HUSBAND MB MRCP FRCR
Consultant Radiologist, Royal Marsden Hospital. Radiologist, BUPA Medical
Centre, London

HYLTON B. MEIRE MBBS FRCR
Consultant in Ultrasound, Clinical Research Centre, Harrow, Middlesex

D. P. O'DONOGHUE MD MRCP
Consultant Physician, St Vincent's Hospital, Dublin

M. L'E. ORME MD MRCP
Senior Lecturer, Department of Pharmacology and Therapeutics, University of
Liverpool, Liverpool

A. J. PINCHING MA DPhil MRCP BM BCh
Senior Registrar, Department of Medicine, Hammersmith Hospital, London

H. GRANT PRENTICE MBBS MRCP(UK) MRCPath
Senior Lecturer and Honorary Consultant, Academic Department of Haematology,
Royal Free Hospital Medical School and Royal Free Hospital, London

B. A. PUSSELL MBBS FRACP
Research Fellow Department of Medicine, Royal Postgraduate Medical School.
Honorary Senior Registrar, Hammersmith Hospital, London

LESLEY H. REES MSc MD MRCPath FRCP
Professor of Chemical Endocrinology and Honorary Consultant Physician, St
Bartholomew's Hospital, London

PHILIP A. ROUTLEDGE MD MRCP
Research Assistant Professor Medicine, Duke University Medical Centre, Durham,
North Carolina, U.S.A.

R. W. ROSS RUSSELL MD FRCP
Consultant Neurologist, St Thomas's Hospital, London

DAVID G. SHAND PhD MB MRCP
Chief of Clinical Pharmacology and Professor of Medicine, Duke University Medical
Centre, Durham, North Carolina.

J. S. SHILLING FRCS DO
Consultant Ophthalamic Surgeon, St Thomas's Hospital and Greenwich District
Hospital, London

P. H. SÖNKSEN MD FRCP
Professor of Endocrinology, Department of Medicine, St Thomas's Hospital Medical School, London

CHRISTOPHER B. WILLIAMS BM FRCP
Consultant Physician, St Mark's and St Bartholomew's Hospitals. Honorary Consultant Physician, Hospital for Sick Children, Great Ormond Street, and Queen Elizabeth's, Hackney, London

H. F. WOODS DPhil FRCP
Professor, University Department of Therapeutics, The Royal Hallamshire Hospital, Sheffield

Contents

1. HLA and disease

Heather M. Dick

The <u>H</u>uman <u>L</u>eucocyte <u>A</u>ntigen (HLA) system is made up of several series of glycoprotein molecules, which can be detected on the surface of most nucleated cells and on platelets. HLA antigens form part of a group of molecules which are involved in the recognition and response mechanisms of graft rejection — hence the general title 'histocompatibility antigens'. These molecules, and several others which are important in the production of an immunological response, are the products of a series of genes, situated in one region of the human genome, on chromosome 6 (an autosomal chromosome). The contribution made by the genes in this region is often recognised by the use of the collective term, major histocompatibility complex (MHC). Most mammalian species possess such a MHC 'region' and these have been shown to have similar properties and functions to the human system. The best understood of these systems is the H-2 system in the experimental mouse, but MHC products have also been defined in the rat, guinea pig, dog, rabbit, pig, various monkey species and chimpanzees.

Interest in histocompatibility antigens first developed from the study of the rejection of transplantable tumours in mice and of skin graft survival when tissue was exchanged between different in-bred strains of mice. The product of an intensive inbreeding programme with strains of laboratory mice (brother-sister and parent-offspring matings) was a wide range of strains which differed from each other by defined genetic markers. Experiments revealed that one system (named H-2) was peculiarly relevant to graft survival. The system was recognisable by simple serological tests (using RBC's, and in later work, lymphocytes) and was shown to include several possible antigens, because of the existence of different alleles for the H-2 gene (Gorer & O'Gorman, 1956; Snell, 1968). The H-2 system in the mouse was recognised as polymorphic (= many shapes) and the presence of specific types of H-2 was important in many aspects of both recognition (of foreign histocompatibility antigens) and response to these molecules.

HLA SYSTEM IN MAN

The HLA system in man was first recognised from experiments to detect possible antibodies against leucocytes in the serum of patients who were suffering from unexplained leucopenia, or who had adverse reactions to blood transfusion which could not be explained on the basis of the development of anti-red cell antibodies (Dausset, 1954; Payne, 1957). It was found that antileucocyte antibodies were present in the serum of such patients. The antibodies were not autoreactive, but did react with the leucocytes of some, but not all, of a panel of selected normal individuals. The antileucocyte antibodies were thus iso-antibodies, recognising antigens on the surface of leucocytes of members of the same species, and revealing specific differences between individuals of the species. Unlike the mouse H-system, human antigens were most readily defined using leucocytes, not red cells. The antileucocyte antibodies were further recognised to be the result of therapeutic blood transfusion, when the transfused leucocytes were of different HLA specificity from that of the recipient. Anti-HLA antibodies were also detected in the sera of parous women, as a result of feto-maternal immunisation during pregnancy (Payne & Rolfs, 1958; van Rood, Eernisse & van Leeuwen, 1958). As with the Rh system, fetal cells bearing paternally derived HLA antigens could, if introduced into the maternal circulation, stimulate antibody production. Unlike Rh antibodies, HLA antibodies were found to have no adverse effect on the fetal cells, although the reason for this crucial difference in behaviour is not clear.

The classification of leucocyte antigens as histocompatibility antigens followed a series of crucial experiments which were designed to study the effect of various degrees of incompatibility on survival times of skin grafts exchanged between volunteers (Amos et al, 1966; Dausset et al, 1969).

The possibility that some of the formed elements of the blood were relevant to graft rejection had been recognised many years before (Landsteiner, 1931) and was foreshadowed by the work of Medawar using skin graft rejection in rabbits (Medawar, 1946) where he demonstrated that red cells were probably not the source of incompatibility, and suggested the leucocytes as the probable cause.

The development of kidney transplantation in man stimulated interest in the use of leucocyte antigens as a means of 'matching' donor and recipient, to minimise the destructive rejection processes which were otherwise the inevitable result of grafts exchanged between individuals other than identical twins. The results of using HLA matching in kidney transplants are encouraging, with increased survival of grafts exchanged between HLA identical pairs, but there are still disappointing failures, pointing to an inadequate knowledge of ideal matching conditions. The extent of knowledge gained about the HLA system and its role in cell behaviour is still increasing and it is now appreciated that the system has a more fundamental biological role than was at first envisaged when it was viewed solely in the context of graft rejection.

HLA antigens

The HLA antigens are the product of at least 5 separate loci closely linked and situated on chromosome 6 of the autosomal chromosomes within the MHC region (see Fig. 1.1). The HLA-A and B series of antigens are well defined, with many known possible alleles. The HLA-A, B and C antigens are all detected by using relatively simple serological procedures (see below). The HLA-D antigens are recognisable only in mixed leucocyte culture, and do not lend themselves to serological tests. Antibodies directed against the HLA-DR antigens (= <u>D</u>-<u>R</u>elated) are reactive mainly with the B-lymphocyte subpopulation on which the DR antigens are predominantly expressed. The possible relationship between HLA-D and DR antigens which is reflected in the name DR, is suggested by the finding that antisera which will detect DR specificities on B-cells will also block the recognition of foreign histocompatibility antigens (HLA-D) in mixed leucocyte culture. If HLA-D and DR antigens are not actually

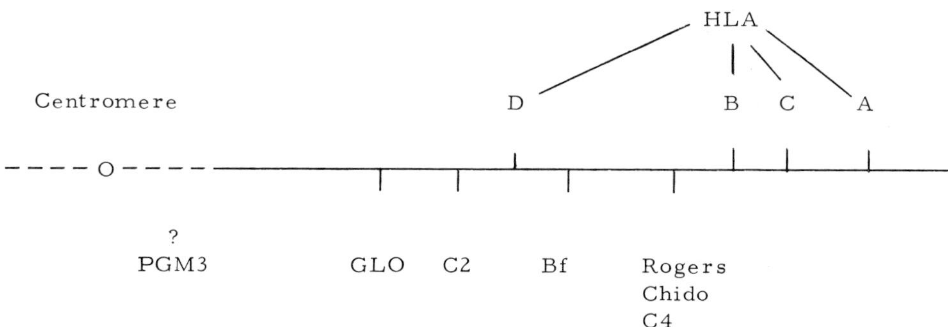

Fig. 1.1 The MHC region in man: diagram of genes in this region (not to scale)
Key:
PGM3 = Phosphoglucomutase 3
GLO = Glyoxylase
C2, C4 = Complement components
Bf = Factor B (complement component)
Rogers = red cell group = C4F
Chido = red cell group = C4S

identical molecules, they must certainly have many similarities as antigenic determinants.

Inheritance of HLA

The polymorphism of the HLA system is very great. The number of different allelic products which coexist is large (Table 1.1). The inheritance of HLA antigens follows simple Mendelian patterns. All alleles are codominant, with no dominance or recessiveness. Each antigen is expressed separately on the cell surface, demonstrable by using separate fluorescent-labelled antibodies, with different emission wavelengths for HLA-A and B products for example. In standardised conditions of temperature etc., the HLA and B molecules can be seen to move separately on the cell membrane, after antigen-antibody interaction, coalescing into separate patches in the process known as 'capping'. Similarly B and C, and A and C molecules have been shown to exist separately in the cell membrane.

Each constituent of the pair of chromosomes (contributed by the two parents) carries its own complement of HLA genes, and an individual will express all the HLA antigens for each series on his or her cells. It is possible to have 2A, 2B, 2C etc. antigens, when the cell is heterozygous, or perhaps one or more genes may give rise to the identical allelic products, when homozygosity is present. Heterozygosity seems to be much commoner than homozygosity, except in rare highly inbred populations.

It can be calculated from the known polymorphism that several million possible combinations of HLA antigens may exist in a population. Within the family group, however, Mendelian inheritance is followed and the children inherit the HLA antigens of their parents in a recognisable way (Fig. 1.2). Family studies reveal that HLA inheritance is remarkably stable; the whole HLA complex (A, B, C, D and DR) is generally handed on from parent to child as a 'package deal'. Breakage and reassortment of DNA in the MHC region is a rare event; recombination occurs

Table 1.1   Listing of recognised HLA specificities, 1980

HLA-A	HLA-B		HLA-C	HLA-D	HLA-DR
HLA-A1	HLA-B5	HLA-Bw42	HLA-Cw1	HLA-Dw1	HLA-DR1
HLA-A2	HLA-B7	HLA-Bw44	HLA-Cw2	HLA-Dw2	HLA-DR2
HLA-A3	HLA-B8	HLA-Bw45	HLA-Cw3	HLA-Dw3	HLA-DR3
HLA-A9	HLA-B12	HLA-Bw46	HLA-Cw4	HLA-Dw4	HLA-DR4
HLA-A10	HLA-B13	HLA-Bw47	HLA-Cw5	HLA-Dw5	HLA-DR5
HLA-A11	HLA-B14	HLA-Bw48	HLA-Cw6	HLA-Dw6	HLA-DRw6
HLA-Aw19	HLA-B15	HLA-Bw49	HLA-Cw7	HLA-Dw7	HLA-DR7
HLA-Aw23	HLA-Bw16	HLA-Bw50	HLA-Cw8	HLA-Dw8	HLA-DRw8
HLA-Aw24	HLA-B17	HLA-Bw51		HLA-Dw9	HLA-DRw9
HLA-A25	HLA-B18	HLA-Bw52		HLA-Dw10	HLA-DRw10
HLA-A26	HLA-Bw21	HLA-Bw53		HLA-Dw11	
HLA-A28	HLA-Bw22	HLA-Bw54		HLA-Dw12	
HLA-A29	HLA-B27	HLA-Bw55			
HLA-Aw30	HLA-Bw35	HLA-Bw56			
HLA-Aw31	HLA-B37	HLA-Bw57			
HLA-Aw32	HLA-Bw38	HLA-Bw58			
HLA-Aw33	HLA-Bw39	HLA-Bw59			
HLA-Aw34	HLA-B40	HLA-Bw60			
HLA-Aw36	HLA-Bw41	HLA-Bw61			
HLA-Aw43	HLA-Bw4	HLA-Bw62			
	HLA-Bw6	HLA-Bw63			

The following is a list of those specificities which have arisen as clear cut splits of other specificities:

HLA-A9	into HLA-Aw23, HLA-Aw24
HLA-A10	into HLA-A25, HLA-A26
HLA-B5	into HLA-Bw51, HLA-Bw52
HLA-B12	into HLA-Bw44, HLA-Bw45
HLA-Bw16	into HLA-Bw49, HLA-Bw50

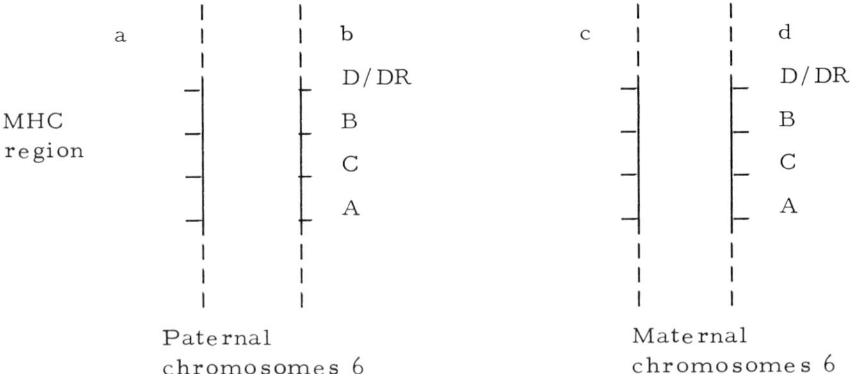

Fig. 1.2   Inheritance of MHC

infrequently (< 1 per cent of meioses) and is only rarely detected. The inheritance of the HLA system and also of closely associated genes of the MHC may be reliably defined in family groups forming a series of useful genetic markers when live donor-recipient matching or disease association studies are performed.

The detection of HLA antigens
HLA-A, B, C antigens are detected most easily on peripheral blood lymphocytes, which are readily available from fresh anti-coagulated blood samples. The method most widely applied requires relatively pure lymphocyte preparations, free of contaminating red cells, granulocytes and platelets. Such material is prepared from fresh venous blood by differential centrifugation techniques which utilise the different size and shape of the formed elements and employ solutions of precise specific gravity. The isolated viable (> 90 per cent) lymphocytes are then incubated with antisera selected to define the HLA-A, B and C antigens. In the presence of fresh rabbit serum as a source of complement components, a positive cytotoxic test indicates the presence of specific HLA antigens on the cells under test. Because of the large number of HLA antigens, an extensive panel of antisera must necessarily be employed, and to conserve material, microtechniques are used. The antibodies used for 'tissue typing' are derived from sera from pregnant or parous women. To ensure accuracy and sensitivity in microcytotoxicity tests, these test sera have to be preselected by lengthy screening and characterisation programmes using lymphocytes of known HLA type.

The detection of HLA-D antigens is complicated by the apparent lack of antibodies which will define this series. Instead, mixed lymphocyte culture (MLC) is necessary, necessitating the incubation of viable lymphocytes in tissue culture for periods of 5–7 days. When lymphocytes from two individuals, X and Y are cultured together, recognition of foreign histocompatibility determinants of the HLA-D series will result in stimulation and proliferation. Thus, cells of individual X, recognising HLA-D determinants on cell Y which are foreign, will proliferate, and vice versa. By careful manipulation of the test cell preparations it is possible to use MLC techniques to recognise HLA-D specificities.

The HLA-DR series of antigens is a relatively recent discovery. DR antigens occur predominantly on B-lymphocytes, monocytes and on a few other cell types, but are apparently not expressed by the majority of T-cells. Selective procedures are required to prepare B-lymphocyte preparations suitable for typing, and a separate panel of selected DR typing sera is required.

Biochemistry of HLA antigens
(For fuller details, see Crumpton & Snary, 1977).

Using isolated cell surface membrane or purified plasma membrane material, it has been possible to determine that the HLA antigens are made up of two chain polypeptides; the A, B and C antigens have chains of molecular weight 43 000 and 12 000. The larger chain carries the specificity and is glycosylated. The light chain is a β2-microglobulin molecule and is the separate product of a gene located in chromosome 15. HLA-DR molecules also have two chains (molecular weight 28 000 and 33 000) both of which have carbohydrate side chains. There is a remarkable resemblance between the molecular structures of A, B and C gene products, suggesting that they have arisen in the distant (evolutionary) past by duplication of a single original gene. There are also some resemblances in amino-acid sequence between human β2-microglobulin and part of the heavy chain of immunoglobulins, but the precise homology between these two kinds of molecule will require determination of the full amino-acid sequence of HLA products.

Other products of MHC

Several other genes which are relevant to cell membrane structures and to immuno-logical responses have been identified in the MHC in close juxtaposition to the HLA loci, in particular the genes defining the C_2 and C_4 components of the complement system and for Factor B (Bf). In addition, congenital deficiencies of these components have been identified and some of these have been noted to show an association with the HLA system. Complement defects are frequently accompanied by auto-immune disorders, and there is presumed to be some basic relationship between the functions of complement, HLA antigens and certain diseases.

Linkage disequilibrium

(For fuller details and references see Bodmer & Bodmer, 1978).

One special feature of the HLA system and its genetics requires examination when a study of HLA and disease associations is contemplated. Despite the polymorphism of the alleles of the HLA loci, the distribution of individual A, B, C, D and DR antigens in the population is not entirely random. Certain pairs of A and B, or B and C or D and DR antigens occur together more often than would be expected in a random (outbred) mating population. In Northern European Caucasoids, for example, the genes for HLA-A1 and B8 are found together (on the same chromosome) more frequently than would be expected, given their individual gene frequencies. The mechanisms by which such close associations are maintained over generations have been the subject of close scrutiny and are further discussed in the literature. In the case of HLA, however, it would seem that the likeliest explanation for linkage disequilibrium must be some form of natural selection, operating on HLA genes or genes so closely linked to HLA that the selective survival effect is indistinguishable from one affecting HLA. Whether the selective process involves susceptibility or resistance to disease, e.g. killing infections, or some more subtle process, is not yet clear. However, it is important to an understanding of HLA and disease associations to recognise that linkage disequilibrium effects are present within the MHC. We can presently identify those affecting HLA gene products; it remains to be seen whether similar effects exist for other genes in the MHC.

Immune response genes

During the course of experiments on the response of inbred mouse strains to a variety of antigens it was discovered that the magnitude and type of response elicited was genetically determined (McDevitt & Chinitz, 1969). Further, the genes responsible were shown to be linked to the genes for the H-2 system, and were mapped, by selective breeding, to a region of the mouse MHC in close juxtaposition to the sites for the major histocompatibility loci. Subsequently, a series of Immune response (Ir) genes, with defined functional activity in immunological reactions, has been identified. The functions controlled by these genes include cell-cell interactions (between macrophage and T-cell, and between T and B cells, for example) as well as MLR activity and delayed hypersensitivity responses. (For a review of Ir genes and their function, see Benacerraf & Germain, 1978.)

In addition to the Ir genes, a further series of I region genes has been detected by the expression of cell membrane antigens, using serological techniques. Because of their close genetic relationship to the Ir region, these surface antigens are known as 'Immune associated' (Ia) antigens. The Ia antigens are present on B cells, macrophages, epithelial cells and sperm, and have marked similarities to the DR antigens of the human HLA system. The mouse MHC therefore includes many genes which are specifically concerned with immunological responsiveness. The practical outcome of this arrangement is seen in the close association of the mouse MHC (identified by H-2 products) with certain disease states. The susceptibility of some mouse strains to autoimmune thyroiditis after injection of thyroglobulin, or to encephalomyelitis (experimental autoimmune form — EAE) after injection of basic myelin protein is linked to specific H-2 types. In addition, susceptibility or resistance to some oncogenic viruses (e.g. Friend leukaemia virus) is also associated with certain H-2 types.

After many years when the functions of cell-membrane antigens such as H-2 and HLA were entirely unknown, it is now evident that these and other products of the MHC have crucial roles in the response to antigen, in cell–cell recognition and interaction, and probably as a result of these basic functions, in the capacity to develop or resist certain immunologically determined diseases.

HLA AND DISEASE

The search for associations between the HLA antigens and human diseases was a natural outcome of the findings in experimental mice of associations between H-2 and disease. What was not so predictable was the plethora of significant associations between HLA and disease states, including many disorders where there was little evidence of involvement of immunological defence mechanisms. The number of disorders with significant associations with the HLA system were so numerous that a complete symposium on the subject was held in 1976 (Dausset & Svejgaard, 1977). An international 'Registry' of studies on HLA and disease now exists (Svejgaard & Ryder, 1977) where positive and negative findings are filed, and a computerised retrieval system provides a ready access to the multiplicity of facts. It is important to examine the results of studies to date, to evaluate their significance and to attempt a synthesis of the relevant findings. A proper understanding of the mechanisms which produce associations between HLA and disease is desperately needed, so that the precise significance of these results may be determined. In particular, some idea of the practical value of HLA typing to the practising clinician and his patient, e.g. in diagnosis or prognosis, is needed.

Certain major disorders have provided the bulk of information upon which we might base our hypotheses of mechanisms, and can be used to illustrate the problems inherent in HLA and disease association work. For details of many other HLA and disease studies, see Dausset & Svejgaard, 1977; Bodmer, 1978; Svejgaard et al, 1979.

Selected diseases are discussed here as illustrative examples of the types of study and analyses which may be performed.

Multiple sclerosis (MS)

The first reported association of MS with the antigen HLA-A3 was soon superseded by reports that the strongest association was with HLA-B7 (Naito et al, 1972; Jersild, Svejgaard and Fog, 1972). Many of the patients typed were of European Caucasoid origin; HLA-A3 and B7 are in strong disequilibrium in this population group, hence the initial reports implicating A3. The HLA antigen implicated is not the same in all racial groups, nor do all affected patients have the relevant antigen(s). In other populations, it would appear that the B7 association is not remarkable, but that other antigens are involved, e.g. Bw22 in Japanese, A10 in Southern Italy.

In subsequent studies of European cases, the antigens HLA-Dw2 and DRw2 have been shown to occur at an even higher frequency in MS patients than either A3 or B7 (for references, see Batchelor, Compston & McDonald, 1978), e.g. HLA-A3 occurs in 21 per cent of normals, and 32 per cent of MS patients, B7 in 20 per cent of normals and 34 per cent of MS patients, Dw2 in 21 per cent of normals and 53 per cent of MS patients, with DRw2 in 22 per cent of normals and over 40 per cent of MS cases. Optic neuritis shows similar associations, with DRw2 occurring in approximately 40 per cent of cases. In some studies, association with DRw2 has occurred in over 50 per cent of cases, and Dw2 has been detected in up to 70 per cent of known MS patients in one carefully documented study (Jersild et al, 1973). Studies where there is more than one case of MS in a family have only rarely been reported. In some studies the HLA-A3, B7, Dw2 association has occurred in all the affected relatives, but is also present in family members unaffected by the disease. The association between MS and HLA is strong but not absolute: the presence or absence of a specific HLA antigen cannot be the sole determining factor in the development of demyelinating lesions. It has been suggested that MS is the result of an interaction between an external agent, e.g. a virus of the measles group, and a disease susceptibility gene linked to HLA. There is conflicting evidence about the association between the development of immunity to measles virus and HLA. In some groups, high antibody titres to measles virus occurred in the A3, B7 positive patients but not in patients lacking these antigens, but other workers have failed to confirm this finding. Even if measles virus were implicated in the development of MS, circulating antibody titres may not represent the most accurate picture of the body's ability or failure to make an appropriate immune response; it may well be that the existing HLA antigen associations are only reflections of a more specific genetic linkage, between unknown genes in the MHC (Ir region?) and an unidentified virus (Jersild, 1978). Batchelor and his colleagues (Batchelor et al, 1978) have suggested that the influence of HLA may occur at two separate points, depending on the biological role which HLA antigens play. HLA could influence the proportion of individuals infected with virus in late childhood who fail to make a full recovery with immunity, but instead, develop modified disease (either persistent, latent virus infection or sensitisation against brain constituents). Subsequently, these individuals may relapse with secondary responses which are triggered by extraneous events, but which ultimately depend on immuno-logical memory generated during the primary phase of infection. The presence of specific Ir genes might be influential in the development of this second phase by determining high or low responsiveness to viral or brain antigen, or by predisposing the individual to sustained cellular immune responses.

Juvenile onset diabetes

Diabetes provides an example of a condition in which genetic factors were long believed to be important but until the advent of HLA typing, simple pedigree analysis failed to show straightforward Mendelian type of inheritance. The disorders collectively known as 'diabetes mellitus' are a heterogenous group of diseases, which can be classified into at least 4 types, only one of which is HLA associated (Cudworth & Woodrow, 1975; Cudworth & Festenstein, 1978), i.e. type 1 or juvenile onset, insulin dependent diabetes. In studies of HLA association, juvenile onset (insulin-dependent) diabetes has shown a marked increase in susceptibility to disease in individuals who are Dw3 and/or DRw3, with a secondary (linked) association with the antigens B8, B18 and A1. A1 and B8 have a high linkage disequilibrium in Northern European Caucasoids, as do B8 and Dw3 and probably DRw3. A second 'predisposing haplotype' has been described, with A2, B15 or B40, Dw4 and DRw4. There is a suggestion that the risk of disease in individuals who carry both types, e.g. B8/B15 is increased compared to that for individuals with only one of these which makes it possible that two (separate) genetic factors can predispose to the disorder.

Juvenile onset diabetes has been studied in great detail in family groups, and provides an excellent example of the value of examining the pedigrees of affected families for both the disease and the inheritance of HLA antigens. Population studies of this condition do show an increase in frequency of HLA-B8, B15, B40 etc., but the association with disease is not absolute. The increased risk of developing type 1 diabetes is about two to three times greater in individuals who are HLA-B8 positive than in those who do not have that antigen. (This increase in risk is often referred to as 'relative risk'). For B8, B15 positive individuals, the risk is calculated to be around six or seven times more than that for B8, B15 negative individuals. If susceptibility to disease is the result of a genetic factor which is linked to HLA, then family studies would be expected to show a very high correlation between the disease state and a given HLA type or haplotype. Thus, two affected children in the same family would be expected to have at least one parental haplotype in common, and in diabetic children this has proved to be the case. Almost all families with more than one affected child show that the diabetic children (and other affected relatives) have at least one HLA haplotype in common; in nearly 60 per cent of affected sibling pairs, the two children share both haplotypes. There are exceptional families where this pattern of inheritance of disease susceptibility and HLA does not occur, emphasising the need to appreciate the lack of a simple 'one gene — one disease' explanation for HLA and disease association.

Additional 'negative' evidence for the importance of the HLA region in disease processes may be deduced from the finding in studies of type 1 diabetics of a relative deficiency of the B7, Dw2 haplotype in diseased patients. It is possible that this HLA type carries with it a factor or factors which increase resistance to whatever aetiological agent precipitates the onset of insulin dependent diabetes.

Type I diabetes is an example of an HLA associated disease, where immune system involvement is not obviously predominant and where some external agent is believed to play an initiating role. In these respects it resembles multiple sclerosis, and it is interesting to speculate on possible mechanisms involving the MHC (or the HLA components of the complex) which might operate in such disorders. It has been suggested that the central lesion in type I diabetes is destruction of β-cells in the pancreas, perhaps as a result of a cytopathic virus infection. Although the evidence is not substantial, Coxsackie B virus infection has been suggested as the initial event. There is a little support for the link between this group of viruses, HLA and type I diabetes in the finding that HLA-B8, B15 positive individuals seem to produce higher titres of Coxsackie B neutralising antibodies after infection than do individuals who are negative for these two antigens. Islet cell antibodies, as evidence of auto-immune processes, occur in about 80 per cent of children with type I diabetes, and appear early in the disease state (Christy et al, 1976; Morris et al, 1976). Persistence of these antibodies is commoner in B8, and B8, B40 positive children, a finding which is in accord with reports of auto-antibody titres in several other disorders which show an association with HLA-B8, e.g. coeliac disease, thyroiditis, suggesting an immunological imbalance which predisposes to the production of auto-immune reactions.

Ankylosing spondylitis and the associated arthritides

The association between HLA-B27 and ankylosing spondylitis (AS) is more dramatic than any of the other HLA associations so far detected. The frequency of B27 in AS patients (over 90 per cent in most published series, compared to 8–10 per cent for this antigen in the healthy population) most nearly approaches an absolute link between an HLA antigen and the disease process (for extensive list of references, see Ryder, Andersen & Svejgaard, 1979). Indeed, the number of AS patients who are B27 negative is so small that there is a strong case for postulating that it is the B27 antigen product itself which is central to the development of the disease. Ankylosing spondylitis is thus an appropriate disease on which to base a hypothesis in which the presence of the B27 molecule on the cell membrane is responsible for a cross-reaction between antibodies directed against antigen(s) closely resembling B27 in structure, the likeliest source of which is thought to be a bacterial or viral product. Thus, infection of a B27 positive individual by an appropriate micro-organism could trigger an immune response, with production of antimicrobial antibodies which would also be capable of combining with B27 molecules. It has been suggested that organisms of the Klebsiella group, common in the gut contents, have antigenic structures similar to the cell membrane products of HLA-B27, and it has been claimed that antisera developed in rabbits against Klebsiella sp., will react preferentially in a cytotoxic test with B27 positive lymphocytes (Ebringer et al, 1978; Seager et al, 1979; Gezcy & Yap, 1979). There is preliminary information on the detailed biochemical structure of HLA antigen molecules, and it should be possible to prove or disprove this relationship. In view of the rarity of AS and the wide distribution of Klebsiella sp. it would be surprising if such a simple explanation were sufficient, but in any case, it is still necessary to explain the arthritic lesions of AS in terms of reactions at the lymphocyte surface.

The high correlation between B27 and AS is also unusual in one aspect (cf. multiple sclerosis for example) in that the same association occurs in all the racial groups so far studied. In Negroes and Japanese, where B27 is a very rare antigen in the population, the presence of AS still correlates very strongly with the B27 antigen. Despite the occurrence of some families where the disease and B27 are not always inherited together, the HLA association for AS is still remarkably consistent, more so than for any other HLA association reported. In disorders which bear strong clinical and pathological similarities to AS, the correlation with B27 is also strong, e.g. Reiter's syndrome, where 65–80 per cent of patients are B27 positive, or the arthritis subsequent to Salmonella or Yersinia infection, where the frequency of B27 is around 60–70 per cent (Brewerton et al, 1973; Aho et al, 1973).

Unfortunately, it is not yet possible to suggest a convincing mechanism to explain this association. Relatively little is known about the pathogenesis of these disorders, apart from the marked familial tendency of AS, and the post-infectious nature of some types of B27-associated joint disease. The precise lesion in the tissues remains unexplained. If an immune response gene predisposing to the development of arthropathy is postulated, then this gene must show a remarkable high degree of linkage disequilibrium with the gene for B27, and this linkage must persist in all populations. This is a phenomenon which does not appear to occur with any of the other diseases which have been reported with HLA associations. It may be that AS and its associated group of disorders are linked with HLA-B27 by a mechanism which is basically different from that occurring in other HLA associated diseases, where the antigen correlation is less firm and it may be wrong to try to fit all HLA-disease associations in a single pathogenic concept.

Other HLA associations
A further complicating factor is introduced by the report of an unduly high frequency of one allelic product of a locus close to that for HLA-B, namely the locus for Bf (properdin factor B of the alternate pathway of complement activation). In an Icelandic study, 19 patients with AS and HLA-B27 were also found to have the Bf^s allele (which occurred in 50 per cent of the controls who were B27 positive but AS negative) (Arnason, Thorsteinsson & Sigurbergsson, 1978). A similar study in Italy failed to confirm this finding (Migone et al, 1978). A detailed study of patients in an American (white) population has recently revealed a significantly high frequency of one rare genetic type of Bf, known as Bf F1, in insulin-dependent diabetics (22.6 per cent as compared to 1.9 per cent in the general population). Further family studies confirmed the association, which provides a genetic marker on chromosome 6, in close juxtaposition to the HLA loci, for nearly 1 in 4 insulin-dependent diabetics.

HLA-B8
Several clinical disorders have been reported to show associations with the presence of HLA-B8. These disorders include coeliac disease, thyroiditis, myasthenia gravis, dermatitis herpetiformis, and chronic active hepatitis (the Hb$_s$Ag negative form). The frequency of HLA-B8 in these conditions ranges from 60–80 per cent in patients (mainly European Caucasoids) with a normal population frequency of around 24 per cent for B8. Many HLA-B8 positive individuals do not develop any of these conditions, and conversely many patients with these disorders are B8 negative. In family studies, patients who are B8 positive frequently have close relatives who are disease free, even when B8 positive (either haplotype or genotype identical with the patient). Thus, it is necessary to envisage a separate factor or more than one such factor, genetically determined, and in linkage disequilibrium with the gene for B8 to

account for the coexistence of disease plus B8, disease without B8, and of healthy individuals with B8.

Most, if not all, B8-associated diseases are characterised by the presence of auto-immunity. This is most readily detected by finding serum autoantibodies directed against one or more 'self' constituents of the tissues but is also characterised by the presence of circulating lymphocytes capable of mediating destruction of autologous tissue, and most probably playing an important role in the lesions of auto-immune disorders. Current views on the development of such autodestructive immunological processes include hypotheses which suggest that there are disturbances in normal regulatory processes which stimulate or suppress the immune response. Several different subpopulations of lymphocytes are suggested, including cells which are cytotoxic, those which co-operate with other cells to stimulate antibody production and still others, whose primary function is to suppress the immune response. Lymphocyte sub-populations recognise and respond to the appropriate stimuli by means of cell membrane markers which are the receptors or recognition signals for antigen or other cells. Some of these membrane proteins are coded for by genes in the MHC, and in experimental studies it has been shown that H-2 (in mouse) and HLA (in man) both function in this way.

HLA-DR

The development of techniques which are suitable for the detection of the HLA-DR antigens has stimulated the study of this new group of B-lymphocyte alloantigens in relation to disease. The HLA-DR antigens are predominantly represented on B-lymphocytes, monocytes and spermatozoa. They appear to be very similar to the 'Ia' antigens identified on the same kinds of cell in the mouse, where they have also been demonstrated on epithelial cells. There is a close relationship between HLA-DR and HLA-D antigens (the latter being identified by MLC techniques, and not apparently by serological methods). Sera which contain HLA-DR antibodies will block MLC reactions, indicating that these antibodies are directed against sites on the cell membrane close to, or identical with the HLA-D antigens.

The parallel between HLA-DR and mouse Ia may indicate that the DR genes are more closely related to immune response genes, because the mouse Ia antigens are coded for by genes in part of the Ir region of the MHC. Do human DR antigens have a substantial association with disease processes? It would appear from preliminary work that this may be so; however, the HLA-DR system has only recently been described, and detailed knowledge of the antigens and the full serological analysis of this series is still awaited.

A small range of allelic products is known, (HLA-DR 1–7 plus a few less well defined antigens) but further collaborative work is proceeding to determine whether this series is indeed small, or whether it has the same degree of polymorphism as HLA-A and B products.

Reported associations for HLA-DR2 include multiple sclerosis and Goodpasture's syndrome. In MS the study of DR frequencies followed the discovery that HLA-Dw2 was increased in frequency in patients, who had an increase in the haplotype HLA-A3, B7, Dw2, DR2, suggesting marked linkage disequilibrium for this genotype in MS sufferers. In another study, HLA-DR3 has been shown to be increased (35 per cent compared with 12 per cent in controls) which is interesting in view of an early report that in addition to the A3, B7 increase, A1, B8 was increased in MS (two antigens known to be in linkage disequilibrium with Dw3 and DR3) (de Moerloose et al, 1979; Bertrams & Kuwert, 1976). Although most studies in European Caucasoids now point to the A3, B7, Dw2, DR2 haplotype being implicated, the association is still not absolute, and it is necessary to explain the incidence of disease in patients who do not have this particular combination of antigens.

Renal disease is now receiving attention of HLA workers and in addition to the Goodpasture's syndrome (Rees et al, 1978) and DR2 association, a new study has shown an association between HLA-DR3 and idiopathic membranous nephropathy (Klouda et al, 1979). Both types of lesion are thought to have a marked immunological component, in particular, abnormal or unusual antibody production. In membranous nephropathy, it is suggested that immune complex deposition causes the glomerular damage. Goodpasture's glomerular basement membrane nephritis is thought to have a hereditary element, and relapse in this disorder is frequently precipitated by infection, a finding remarkably similar to that in the other DR2 associated condition, multiple sclerosis.

HLA-DR4 has been shown to be increased in two rather disparate conditions. The first clear-cut association for DR4 was reported with rheumatoid arthritis (Stastny, 1978), following the initial finding of an increase in frequency of HLA-Dw4 in this condition (Stastny, 1975). DR4 has now been reported in 91 per cent of Jewish patients with pemphigus vulgaris (Park et al, 1979) and it has been suggested that the hypothesis which most closely fits this is that of the cross-reactive antigen, i.e. that microbial infection with an unspecified pathogen is abnormal in DR4 individuals (who are Jewish) because of resemblances between the HLA antigen molecule and the microbial antigens. The authors admit that the same pattern of association was not found in DR4 non-Jewish white patients, and tentatively suggests that there may be more than one 'form' of the DR4 molecule — a substantially new hypothesis which would require specific biochemical confirmation.

Studies of HLA-DR antigen frequencies in disease are still very new and relatively unexplored territory. It remains to be seen whether DR antigens will prove to be the ultimate answer to the mechanisms which produce a multiplicity of disorders of unexplained aetiology and poorly understood pathogenesis.

General conclusions
Given that linkage disequilibrium is a prominent feature of the inheritance of genes within the MHC, it is likely that this disequilibrium might also encompass genes which function in the control of immunological responses. The MHC region may be of major importance for the direct and indirect modulation of the immune response. The HLA associations may have arisen fortuitously, because of linkage disequilibrium between Ir genes and HLA genes, or may be directly produced because of the part played by HLA antigens as cell membrane components. In the latter case, it seems probable that the actual antigen product e.g. HLA-B8 protein, is not the deciding factor, since there are many healthy individuals with HLA-B8 (and disease patients without). In populations other than European Caucasoids, the HLA association for the autoimmune disorders is often with antigens other than B8, e.g. HLA-B5 in Japanese with coeliac disease, and Bw35 with thyroiditis. Since HLA-B8

is relatively rare in Japanese, and B5 and Bw35 relatively common, the latter two antigens represent the Japanese MHC 'equivalent' of the Caucasoid B8 gene, with linkage disequilibrium present between the genes for B5 and Bw35 and the Ir region genes, in this different racial group.

Why should this 'pairing' of genes within the MHC have arisen, and why should it persist? Bodmer (1978) has suggested that natural selection is the most likely explanation for the persistence of linkage disequilibrium within the MHC. The exact selective mechanism, namely the factors which favour the survival of certain pairs of alleles at different loci, is unknown, but it could be postulated that these may represent advantageous genotypes with survival value in serious bacterial or viral epidemics in man's distant past. Whilst having a favourable effect in this situation, the selected combination of genes may also have included those which now predispose to the disorders of immunological response which are expressed as auto-immune diseases. Since most of these conditions appear relatively late in life, and very few of them affect reproductive capacity, there would be no tendency for these selected genotypes to disappear from the population, or any selective effect may not yet have had sufficient time (in evolutionary terms) to become manifest.

None of the recognised HLA associations with disease is absolute. The HLA-B27/arthropathy association comes nearest to this, but even here there are some patients with AS who are not B27 positive. Any hypothesis which attempts to explain HLA association must allow for this, and it should be recognised that external events and non-MHC genes can be relevant to the development of disease. If the disease state depends on an abnormal response to antigen, then the chance of exposure to that antigen must be a significant feature of the acquisition of disease. The precise function of HLA molecules on the cell surface is not yet understood: we are well aware of the presence of HLA on lymphocytes, because we use these cells in the process of HLA typing, but it should be remembered that these antigens are present on many other cells. It has been suggested that HLA molecules may be able to bind certain hormones or enzymes, perhaps because of molecular similarities (mimicry), thus acting competitively with the normal target or substrate for these products and interfering with their functions (Svejgaard & Ryder, 1976). Molecular mimicry of bacterial or viral antigens has also been postulated, so that infection is not followed by the normal development of immunity but by persistent infection (see above, section on arthropathies and B27). Unfortunately, there is only suggestive evidence of microbial infection in a few HLA-associated disorders (e.g. in rheumatoid arthritis, with its Dw4/DR4 association, or in juvenile diabetes) and substantive proof is missing in most others.

Much attention has been focused on positive HLA and disease associations, i.e. those in which there is a significant increase in an HLA antigen frequency. This has had the inevitable result of concentrating attention on susceptibility to disease, while the concept of relative resistance has been largely neglected. Only in the malignant disorders has there been some attempt to recognise survival rather than susceptibility in relation to HLA. In the experimental mouse, resistance to leukaemia virus infection was one of the early observations which was linked to H-2 type. In man, HLA type has been shown to have some association with survival in Hodgkin's disease (Falk & Osoba, 1971) and in acute leukaemia (Lawler et al, 1974). It is probable that clinical heterogeneity in many malignant diseases will mask any HLA association. The improvement in the classification of leukaemias in recent years may help to identify specific types of disease which can be accurately analysed for their relationship to HLA and other genes within the MHC (for details, see Harris, Lawler & Oliver, 1978).

The study of HLA and disease associations has opened up a wide area of intense interest, both for laboratory workers and clinicians. The prospect of elucidating the precise pathogenesis of diseases which are but imperfectly understood at present, is an exciting possibility. It is much too early to predict how useful HLA typing will be as an addition to the existing range of diagnostic tests; it would appear that there are too many false positive and false negative results with our current knowledge. It may be that we are merely touching the edge of the relevant genetic region with our present techniques. Prognosis is an even more dubious area in which to apply HLA typing and until we understand the precise biological function of the products of the MHC region, it is neither feasible nor wise to place too much reliance on incomplete knowledge.

REFERENCES

Aho K, Ahvonen P, Lassus A, Sievers K, Tiilikainen Anja 1973 HL-A antigen 27 and reactive arthritis. Lancet ii: 157

Amos D B, Hattler B G, Hutchin P, McCloskey R, Zmijewski C M 1966 Skin donor selection by leucocyte typing. Lancet i: 300–302

Arnason A, Thorsteinsson J, Sigurbergsson K 1978 Ankylosing spondylitis, HLA-B27 and Bf. Lancet i: 339–340

Batchelor J R, Compston A, McDonald W I 1978 The significance of the association between HLA and multiple sclerosis. British Medical Bulletin 34: 279–284

Benacerraf B, Germain R N 1978 The immune response genes of the major histocompatibility complex. In: Moller G (ed) Immunological reviews. Munksgaard, Copenhagen, vol 38: p 70–119

Bertrams H J, Kuwert E K 1976 Association of histocompatibility haplotype HLA-A3-B7 with multiple sclerosis. Journal of Immunology 117: 1906–1912

Bodmer W F (ed) 1978 The HLA sytem. British Medical Bulletin 34: no 3, British Council

Bodmer W F, Bodmer J G 1978 Evolution and function of the HLA system. British Medical Bulletin 34: 309–316

Brewerton D A, Caffrey Maeve, Nicholls Anne, Walters D, Oates J K, James D C O 1973 Reiter's disease and HL-A27. Lancet ii: 996–998

Christy M, Nerup J, Bottazzo G F, Doniach O, Platz P, Svejgaard A, Ryder L P, Thomsen M 1976 Association between HLA-B8 and auto-immunity in juvenile diabetes mellitus. Lancet ii: 142–143

Crumpton M J, Snary D 1977 Isolation and structure of human histocompatibility (HLA) antigens. In: Porter R R, Ada G L (eds) Contemporary topics in molecular immunology. Plenum Press, New York & London, vol 6: p 58–81

Cudworth A G, Festenstein H 1978 HLA genetic heterogeneity in diabetes mellitus. British Medical Bulletin 34: 285–289

Cudworth A G, Woodrow J C 1975 Evidence for HLA-A-linked genes in 'Juvenile' diabetes mellitus. British Medical Journal 3: 133–135

Dausset J 1954 Leuco-agglutinins. Leuco-agglutinins and blood transfusion. Vox sanguinis 4: 190–198

Dausset J, Rapaport F T, Legrand L, Colombani J, Barge A, Feingold N 1969 Les Antigenès de Transplantation (HLA-A). Etudiés par Greffes de Peau de 90 Enfants sur leurs pères. Nouvelle Revue Francaise d'Haematologie 9: 215–230

Dausset J, Svejgaard A (eds) 1977 HLA and disease. Munksgaard, Copenhagen

Ebringer R W, Cawdell D R, Cowling P, Ebringer A 1978 Sequential studies in ankylosing spondylitis. Annals of the Rheumatic Diseases, 37: 146–151

Falk J, Osoba D 1971 HL-A antigens and survival in Hodgkin's disease. Lancet ii: 1118–1120

Geczy A F, Yap J 1979 HLA-B27, Klebsiella and ankylosing spondylitis. Lancet i: 719–720

Gorer P A, O'Gorman P 1956 The cytotoxic activity of isoantibodies in mice. Transplantation Bulletin 3: 142–143

Harris R, Lawler S D, Oliver R T D 1978 The HLA system in acute leukaemia and Hodgkin's disease. British Medical Bulletin 34: 301–304

Jersild C 1978 In: Birth defects (original article series). A R Liss for The National Foundation, vol XIV, no 5: p 123–170

Jersild C, Fog T, Hansen Grete S, Thomsen M, Svejgaard A, Dupont B 1973 Histocompatibility determinants in multiple sclerosis, with special reference to clinical course. Lancet ii: 1221–1225

Jersild C, Svejgaard A, Fog T 1972 HL-A antigens and multiple sclerosis. Lancet i: 1240–1241

Klouda P T, Manos J, Acheson E J, Dyer P A, Goldby F S, Harris R, Lawler W, Mallick N P, Williams G 1979 A strong association between idiopathic membranous nephropathy and HLA-DRw3. Lancet, In press

Landsteiner K 1931 Individual differences in human blood. Science 73: 403–409

Lawler Sylvia D, Klouda P T, Smith P G, Till Morwenna M, Hardisty R M 1974 Survival and the HL-A system in acute lymphoblastic leukaemia. British Medical Journal 1: 547–548

Medawar P B 1946 Immunity to homologous grafted skin: II The relationship between the antigens of blood and skin. British Journal of Experimental Pathology 27: 15–24

Migone N, Malavasi F, Boschis D, Modena V 1978 Bf polymorphism and ankylosing spondylitis. Lancet ii: 163

de Moerloose Ph, Jeannet M, Martins-da-Silva B, Werner-Fauve Ch, Rohr J, Gauthier G 1979 Increased frequency of HLA-DRw2 and DRw3 in multiple sclerosis. Tissue Antigens 13: 357–360

Morris P J, Vaughan H, Irvine W J, McCallum F J, Gray R S, Campbell C J, Duncan, L J P, Farquhar J W 1976 HLA and pancreatic islet cell antibodies in diabetes. Lancet ii: 652–653

McDevitt H O, Chinitz A 1969 Genetic control of the antibody response: Relationship between immune response and histocompatibility (H-2) type. Science (Wash.) 163: 1207–1208

Naito S, Namerow N, Mickey M R, Terasaki P I 1972 Multiple sclerosis: association with HL-A3. Tissue Antigens 2: 1–4

Park M S, Terasaki P I, Ahmead A R, Tiwari J L 1978 HLA-DRw4 in 91 per cent of Jewish pemphigus vulgaris patients. Lancet ii: 441–442

Payne R 1957 Leukocyte agglutinins in human sera. Archives of Internal Medicine 99: 587–606

Payne R, Rolfs M R 1958 Foeto-maternal leukocyte incompatibility. Journal of Clinical Investigation 37: 1756–1763

Raum D, Stein R, Alper C A, Gabbay K H 1979 Genetic marker for insulin-dependent diabetes mellitus. Lancet i: 1208–1210

Rees A J, Peters D K, Compston D A S, Batchelor J R 1978 Strong association between HLA-DRw2 and antibody-mediated Goodpasture's syndrome. Lancet i: 966–968

Roitt I M, Corbett M, Festenstein H, Jaraquemada D, Papasteriadis C, Hay F C, Nineham L J 1978 HLA-DRw4 and prognosis in rheumatoid arthritis. Lancet i: 990

van Rood J J, Eernisse J G, van van Leeuwen A 1958 Leucocyte antibodies in sera from pregnant women. Nature (Lond.) 181: 1735–1736

Ryder L P, Andersen E, Svejgaard A 1979 HLA and disease registry. 3rd report. Munksgaard, Copenhagen

Seager K, Bashir H V, Geczy A F, Edmonds J, de Vere-Tyndall A 1979 Evidence of a specific B27-associated cell surface marker on lymphocytes of patients with ankylosing spondylitis. Nature 277: 68–70

Snell G D 1968 The H-2 locus of the mouse. Observations and speculations concerning its component genetics and its polymorphism. Folia Biologica, Prague 14: 335–358

Stastny P 1975 MLC determinants associated with rheumatoid arthritis. In: Kissmeyer-Nielsen F (ed) Histocompatibility testing 1975, Munksgaard, Copenhagen, p 797–802

Stastny P 1978 Association of the B-cell alloantigen DRw4 with rheumatoid arthritis. New England Medical Journal 298: 868–871

Svejgaard A, Hauge M, Jersild C, Platz P, Ryder L P, Staub Nielsen K, Thomsen M 1979 The HLA system. An introductory survey. In: Karger, Basel, Monographs in human genetics, vol 7, 2nd revised ed

Svejgaard A, Ryder L P 1976 Interaction of HLA molecules with non-immunological ligands as an explanation of HLA and disease associations. Lancet ii: 547–549

Svejgaard A, Ryder L P 1977 Associations between HLA and disease. Notes on methodology and a report from the HLA and disease registry. In: Dausset J, Svejgaard A (ed) HLA and disease. Munksgaard, Copenhagen, pp 46–71

2.   The biology of human ageing

John Grimley Evans

The proportion of elderly people in an economically developed community such as the United Kingdom is growing and various factors are reducing the family support available to them (Evans, 1977). These demographic and social trends will dominate the demand for medical care until the end of the present century and detailed knowledge of age-associated changes in the structure and function of the human body will be needed by doctors in most specialties. This chapter is primarily concerned with the broader issues of human ageing as a biological phenomenon. The theme is to consider whether the multitudinous aspects of senescence can be related to definable underlying processes or categorised in other ways that might lead to more constructive approaches to the problems raised by human ageing than are at present available to us.

WHAT IS AGEING?

Mortality as an index of ageing

The central concept of ageing is loss of adaptability of an individual organism with time so that on average the old are more vulnerable to environmental challenge than the young. Vulnerability is demonstrable in animal experiments in which fatality rates in response to thermal or other stresses increase with the age. It is apparent clinically in the increase with age in the fatality of disease, including trauma, surgical operations and infections (Phair, 1979), although in epidemic infections specific immunity may be a modifying factor. In the influenza pandemic of 1918 death rates in Britain were higher in younger than in older persons, presumably because the latter had encountered an immunologically similar virus at some time around 1890.

Provided that environmental conditions are not so harsh that ageing effects are totally obscured by deaths due to accidents or predation increasing vulnerability will manifest itself in population statistics in mortality rates that rise with age. If environmental hazards are very high few individuals will survive long enough for the functional decrement due to ageing to be apparent and natural selection may result in the older members of a group being as fit on average as the younger. Typically such a population will show constant age-specific mortality rates over adult life and a survival curve which falls as a negative exponential function of age. This is sometimes referred to as the 'ecological' survival curve. In more benign circumstances ageing manifests itself in mortality rates that increase with age and the survival curve is convex upwards in a form sometimes called 'physiological' because it reflects the age-associated changes in functional capacity of individuals. At different times and places the human species has exhibited both these types of survival. In 16th century York, for example, the townsfolk showed survival curves close to the ecological form while their aristocratic contemporaries were already showing the physiological curve of survival which is characteristic of economically advanced cultures (Cowgill, 1970).

In 20th century Britain age-specific mortality rates fall from birth to a nadir around the age of 12. After perturbations in adolescence and early adult life due to accidents and complications of reproduction, rates rise as an exponential function of age. These properties of the age-specific mortality curve have not altered in the last 70 years despite overall reductions in mortality rates. On a statistical definition, therefore, human ageing begins near the onset of puberty and is a continuous process thereafter without any discontinuity which might provide a rational basis for separating off a particular age group of adults as 'the elderly'. The present policy of regarding 65 as a demarcation age merely reflects political and economic history in that 65 was the qualifying age for retirement pensions chosen by Bismarck's administration for the world's first social security system a hundred years ago.

A number of general theories of ageing reviewed by Strehler (1977) have been advanced which attempt to deduce in mathematical terms the properties of the underlying processes generating the exponential increase in mortality with age. These theories provide a stimulating conceptual background to gerontological studies but are unlikely to identify directly the physical nature of ageing processes.

Ageing reflected in function

Most measures of human function show on average an increase through childhood and early adult life followed by a decline at later ages. The age at which maximal average function is attained and the degree and timing of subsequent decline varies between individuals and also with the specific function being measured. In general, functions requiring the integrated actions of several body systems show greater decline than functions of single systems. The age-associated decline in mean function is usually associated with an increase in variance. This is partly due to increasing differences between individuals in whom age-associated changes are taking place at different rates and partly due to increasing within-individual variability reflecting impairment of homeostatic mechanisms. These points are exemplified in the changes of blood pressure with age. An additional factor may be increasing errors in measurement with age. Again taking blood pressure as an example, Spence, Sibbald & Cape (1978) have shown that the differences between direct and indirect measurements of blood pressure are greater in old than in young subjects.

Homeostatic mechanisms tend to become slower, less sensitive and less accurate with age and these trends may be associated with secondary, partly compensatory, changes in body function. Helderman et al (1978) have found evidence that osmoreceptor sensitivity increases with age possibly as an adaptive response to the age-associated diminution in the ability of the kidney to conserve salt and water (McLachlan, 1978). The increase in osmoreceptor sensitivity restores homeostasis for minor disturbances in salt and water balance but at the cost of a greater liability to hypo- and hypernatraemic syndromes.

One factor underlying changes in the sensitivity, speed and accuracy of homeostatic mechanisms may be an increase in informational 'noise' in the body's communications system. Gregory (1974) has suggested that many of the perceptual changes character-istic of ageing are compatible with an increase in neural 'noise'. This is an important concept with many implications for the care of old people varying from the lower suspension of their room lights (Gilkes, 1979) to the benefits of talking more slowly and tautologically to them than would be necessary for younger people of similar intelligence. These manoeuvres counteract the effects of neural noise by, respectively, improving the signal/noise ratio, facilitating temporal summation and increasing informational redundancy.

Ageing in vitro
Although cells derived from malignant tissue or which have undergone viral transformation or chromosomal aberration may produce immortal cell lines in tissue culture clones of normal differentiated cells die out after a limited number of population doublings and death is preceded by a phase of reduced or disordered function (Hayflick, 1976). This finding does not necessarily imply that all cells in the culture undergo ageing changes in unison. More probably, cells undergo 'commitment' to senescence and ultimate death of their progeny as a more or less random event and the ultimate demise of the culture occurs because the process of successive subculturing dilutes out the uncommitted, still potentially immortal, cells (Holliday, et al, 1977). The immortality of malignant or transformed cells could come about by a reduction in the risk of commitment or by a reduction in the number of generations between commitment and death which would reduce the dilutional effects of subculturing. Study of transplanted mammary tissue and of immunocyte clones in mice suggest that the potential number of divisions of clones of differentiated cells is limited in vivo as well as in vitro (Daniel, 1977) although the trauma of serial transplantation is an unavoidable interfering factor.

In all these experiments the lifespan of the tissue in terms of cell doublings is in excess of that necessary to sustain the maximum lifespan of the species studied. For human embryonic fibroblasts the limit is approximately 50 doublings and Kay (1965) has shown that by a system of asynchronous divisions this amount of reproductive capacity is enough to maintain the cell output for even such active tissues as bone marrow over a human life time. Evidence that the reproductive capacity of fibroblasts is used up in the course of life is a report that the doubling capacity of fibroblasts varies inversely with the age of the donor (Martin, Sprague & Epstein, 1970) but there are wide variations between samples from the same donor. Hayflick (1976) has suggested that doubling capacity of embryonic fibroblasts may be directly correlated with the maximum lifespan of the donor or species but in a more extensive review of available data Lints (1978) concludes that this is probably not so. Because the doubling capacity of cells in vitro is larger than that required for the characteristic lifespan of the species the relevance of the Hayflick Limit to ageing of the organism is dubious although Burnet (1974) implies that it might lead to exhaustion of frequently stimulated immunocyte clones and could therefore be the reason for very old people succumbing to infection from commonplace organisms. There is no direct evidence to support this at present. It is possible that the various changes in cell metabolism which precedes the terminal phase may have more relevance to the ageing of organisms than clonal death itself.

Hayflick (1976) summarises studies by his group into the effect of fusing nuclei and cytoplasms from clones of cultured fibroblasts that have undergone different numbers of divisions. Their results indicate that the 'clock' determining the cell's replicative capacity lies in the nucleus.

THE COMPONENTS OF HUMAN AGEING

Some differences in average function between old and young people are not due to ageing but to *pseudo-ageing* or *aggravated ageing*.

Pseudo-ageing

Ideally, human ageing should be studied longitudinally by following the changes occurring in individuals as they grow older. Studies of this type are expensive and present several methodological problems including difficulties in maintaining standardised methods over time, practice effects as the participants undertake the same tests repeatedly and bias through selective loss from the cohort by death, migration or non-cooperation. Most available evidence on the effects of human ageing is derived from cross-sectional study. This method also has problems of sampling and differential non-cooperation but the most serious hazard is the intrusion of cohort effects. In developing societies people aged 20 and people aged 70 are from very different cultural backgrounds. Cultural effects have been well recognised in the interpretation of the association between tests of mental function and race but have been widely overlooked in the interpretation of age-associated changes.

Schaie & Strother (1968) compared age-associated changes in mental abilities found by cross-sectional methods with those revealed in a longitudinal study based on a follow-up of the same subjects. For most aspects of mental function the longitudinal study indicated smaller and later decrements with age than those suggested by the cross-sectional data. Figure 2.1, for example, shows the findings relating to a measure of reasoning ability. A problem with the method is to ensure that the subjects available for follow-up are representative of those taking part in the cross-sectional phase of the study but longer-term studies have in general confirmed the original findings (Schaie & Labouvie-Vief, 1974). An important part of what appears as ageing

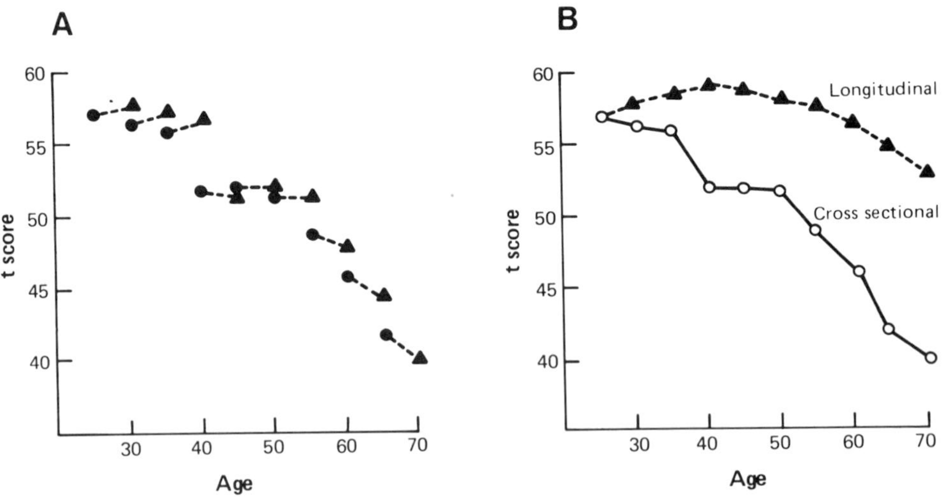

Fig 2.1 Mean standardised scores for reasoning ability among individuals followed over seven years. Figure 2.1A shows observed changes in mean scores in separate age groups; Figure 2.1B presents observed cross-sectional and deduced longitudinal trends from the same data. (Redrawn with permission of the authors and the editor of Psychological Bulletin from Schaie & Strother, 1968.)

in cross-sectional studies of mental function is due to the differences in cultural backgrounds of successive generations in a developing society.

The measure of reasoning ability shown in Figure 2.1 was one component of a validated index of educational aptitude which showed similar differences between longitudinal and cross-sectional analysis. In the longitudinal study this index showed very little decline up to retirement age suggesting that the assumption that older workers cannot be retrained for new technologies, a view that is urged to justify age-related industrial redundancy programmes, is false. Later studies have demonstrated the considerable ability of older adults to learn new skills and improve mental performance if appropriate methods of education are used (Plemons, Willis & Baltes, 1978).

As Schaie & Labouvie-Vief (1974) point out much (though not all) of their data support the general distinction between 'crystallised' and 'fluid' abilities in mental function. The first set of abilities are dependent on learnt skills and patterns of response reflecting educational opportunities and experience throughout life and may be expected to show little decline due to ageing in the individual. 'Fluid' abilities require attributes of speed and fluency which may be more affected by truly age-associated changes in physiological function. There will be considerable individual variation in the changes in these two components with age and different tasks will require different mixtures of the two types of ability. Although the effects of pseudo-ageing due to generation differences are particularly insidious in the area of mental function similar influences are to be expected in aspects of physical structure and function.

Aggravated ageing
Since ageing is indicated by the organism's ability to respond optimally to environmental challenge its effect may be amplified if environmental challenges are greater for older people than for younger. The high incidence of hypothermia in older people is only partly explained by the age-associated autonomic dysfunction described by Collins et al (1977). A further cause is that older people are more likely to be in cold domestic environments than are younger (Fox et al, 1973). The homes of older people are less likely to have central heating and older people are less able to afford fuel to keep warm than are younger people. Poor housing and lack of social resources also contribute to the increases with age in hospital admission rates and mean length of hospital stay and, presumably, in mortality.

True ageing
The changes shown by individuals studied over periods of time and representing true ageing trends also have complex origins which include some factors that may not have analogues among the laboratory animals and fibroblast cultures used for gerontological research. Many textbooks attempt to draw a distinction between 'normal' and 'abnormal' ageing or between 'normal ageing' and 'disease'.This approach is unhelpful as apart from possible confusion between the implications of at least three entirely different meanings of the word 'normal' there is no rational basis at present for defining normality and attempts to specify it empirically may be seriously misleading. There is no reason to assume that what is normal (i.e. healthy) will be found normally (i.e. most commonly) or that it will necessarily lie within so many standard deviations

of a normal (i.e. Gaussian) distribution around the population mean. A preferable model is to regard human ageing as arising from *intrinsic* and *extrinsic* factors and from the interaction between them. The advantages of this model are that it leads directly to empirical study using established methods and that it provides a constructive approach to the clinical and other problems associated with human ageing.

Intrinsic ageing

Although improvements in public health over the last century and a half in Britain have greatly extended average lifespan there has been no change in maximum lifespan. Observation and breeding experiments show that every species of animal has a characteristic maximum lifespan, sometimes referred to as specific lifespan, which is inherited in natural populations as a polygenic characteristic. The genetically controlled processes which place this upper limit on the lifespan of an individual comprise intrinsic ageing.

A simple model of intrinsic ageing might see it as a process analogous to the wearing out of components of a motor car, but a basic property of living matter is a capacity for self-repair so a problem remains in why the body does not repair the ravages of age. Various theories of ageing have attempted to answer this question from a pathophysiological consideration of the mechanisms of age-associated decline in adaptability or from the standpoint of evolutionary biology. These two approaches are complementary and attempt respectively to answer the 'how' and the 'why' of ageing. With a maximum lifespan of about 110 years Homo sapiens is the longest living mammal and one of the longest living vertebrates. Sacher (1975) has shown that in mammals characteristic maximum lifespan correlates with the ratio of brain weight to total body weight. Although this might suggest that the brain is the site of some biological clock the explanation is more likely to lie in the effect of large brain size in prolonging gestation and so reducing reproduction rate and in the probability that biological advantages of a large brain will not be apparent unless individuals live long enough. (We assume here that one of the significant advantages of a large brain is a greater capacity for learned as distinct from innate behaviour.) Thus the genes for large brain weight and the genes for long life are likely to become associated through selection.

There have been many theories proposed to account for the biological origin and significance of the genes coding for intrinsic ageing processes and maximum lifespan. Broadly these theories fall into three groups. The first group propose that the genes represent a 'self-destruct' system specifically developed to prevent older organisms competing with younger ones. At first sight one reason why such competition might be undesirable is that if ageing did not exist old organisms would be highly adapted by learning and natural selection to a particular environment and so would compete successfully with the younger more variable individuals and this would render the species vulnerable to changes in environmental conditions. This proposal contains the implicit assumption that natural selection can act for the survival of the species as well as of the gene and this is a doubtful, possibly untenable, hypothesis (Dawkins, 1976). Furthermore, Medawar (1952) and others have pointed out that even without ageing, deaths from disease, accidents and predation will always result in there being fewer older than younger organisms in competition for reproductive and other resources so there would be no biological need for older organisms to be further handicapped by the evolution of ageing processes. The idea that ageing may include a specifically evolved self-destruct element is still advanced from time to time but is generally considered improbable.

The second group of theories takes an opposite view and suggests that the general trend of evolution within a species is to lengthen lifespan and that intrinsic ageing processes represent uneradicated determinants of non-adaptive metabolism (Cutler, 1972). In relation to human ageing Medawar (1952) and others have proposed that the genetic component of ageing represents the actions of deleterious genes whose effects have been postponed until later life through selection. This idea has been mathematically evaluated by Hamilton (1966). A deleterious gene which acts near puberty will be at a reproductive disadvantage compared with a gene producing the same effect later in life when the organism carrying it will have had more chance to reproduce. Through successive generations of evolution the effects of deleterious genes will therefore tend to accumulate in later life.

The third group of theories suggest that intrinsic ageing represents 'side-effects' of genes which have other beneficial effects that have been favoured by evolution. One type of theory in this group is to regard ageing as a direct consequence of the cessation of growth or of cellular differentiation. It is suggested that both these states involve switching-off genes which would be required to replace cell components damaged by heat, radiation or accident. Calow (1978) & Kirkwood (1977) have recently produced theories of this type. Kirkwood (1977) contrasts the inevitable senescence of somatic cells with the apparent immortality of germ-line cells. He suggests that accurate repair of cellular damage is 'expensive' in terms of the energy and metabolic materials required so that although high accuracy of repair is essential in the germ-line there has been little selection pressure to prevent damage accumulating in somatic cells after the age of reproductive maturity.

'Side-effect' theories have been proposed at an organismic as well as at a cellular level. Williams (1957) has pointed out that a gene which has a beneficial effect early in reproductive life may be selected for, even though it has a deleterious effect later in life. So far with the doubtful exception of Huntington's chorea no pleiotropic genes of this type have been definitely identified. It may also be relevant that human evolution took place under environmental conditions very different from today's world so that the early beneficial effect of Williams's postulated pleiomorphic genes may no longer be apparent. Neel (1962) suggested the existence of a 'thrifty' gene which enables individuals possessing it to survive periods of famine by storing excess food energy as fat but which in times of overadequate food supply leads to obesity, diabetes and arterial disease later in life. The recently demonstrated lower thermogenesis of obese subjects compared with the non-obese may reveal the thrifty gene at work (Jung et al, 1979).

Burnet (1974) has also proposed what is essentially a 'side-effect' theory of intrinsic ageing. He suggests that ageing is due to accumulating errors in cellular DNA generating somatic mutations. The errors come about because of inaccuracies in the DNA repair system and the rate of inaccuracy is a genetically determined characteristic. Burnet suggests that the beneficial effects of this inaccuracy, which have led to its persistence, include the genesis of germ-line mutations making evolution possible, and a contribution through somatic mutations to immunocyte variability broadening an individual organism's range of immune responses.

FEW OR MANY GENES?

It is of interest to know whether ageing and maximum lifespan are under the control of many or few genes, for if only few genes are involved the modification of ageing rate or pattern is a more realistic possibility. Walford (1974) has commented that when a viral infection renders a tissue culture immortal, the amount of genetic information entering the cell from the virus must be small and that therefore the mortality of the cultured cells may be determined by a small number of genes, possibly only four to six. Clearly, however, the control of senescence in isolated fibroblasts may be an inadequate model of ageing in whole organisms.

Cutler (1975) has argued from current knowledge of higher primate evolution that the maximum lifespan of the direct-line ancestors of Homo sapiens increased so rapidly over a period about 100 000 years ago that given reasonable estimates of mutation rates relatively few genetic loci must have been involved. He suggests approximately 250 which is equivalent to about 0.6 per cent of the genome. The estimates of maximum lifespan of man's primate ancestors is inevitably somewhat speculative but the agreement of the estimate based on the age of death of individual fossils with the prediction derived from Sacher's (1975) formula relating lifespan to brain and body size is encouragingly close. It is conceivable however that mutation rates were higher during the evolution of the early Hominids than they are now.

King & Wilson (1975) have drawn attention to the very close correspondence in peptide sequences between the proteins of man (maximum lifespan 110 years) and the corresponding proteins of the chimpanzee (maximum lifespan 45 years). On average, human polypeptides are more than 99 per cent identical with those of the chimpanzee. The implication is that a relatively small number of changes in systems controlling expression of genes coding for structured proteins may explain the difference between man and the lower primates. In this we may be witnessing the sophisticated rebirth of an old idea that man is merely an overgrown fetal ape.

IDENTIFYING THE GENES CONTROLLING AGEING

The three lines of reasoning in the last section suggest that lifespan may be under the control of relatively few genetic loci. If this is so we might anticipate that mutations or some alleles at relevant loci may have clinically discernible effects as partial premature ageing syndromes. Martin (1978) has reviewed the many genetic syndromes in man which produce changes in early life that are apparently similar to those of ageing. He concludes that no single syndrome, even Progeria or Werner's syndrome is an exact copy of senescence but such conditions may identify genetic loci which play a part in the control of ageing.

Another approach is to capitalise on the differential survival effect in cross-sectional studies to compare the characteristics of individuals attaining healthy old age with those of younger persons in order to identify phenotypes favouring longevity. Such studies require large samples of very elderly subjects and are fraught with problems of sampling bias.

There is no convincing evidence at present of any association of the ABO or other major blood groups with longevity. Smith & Walford (1977) have found evidence in mice that the main histocompatability complex, the H-2 system, is one of the gene systems involved in the control of maximum lifespan. In view of this finding and the known association of the corresponding HL-A system or closely linked genes in man with certain disease states (Bodmer, 1980) there is considerable interest in the possible association of HL-A alleles with longevity. Data so far available are scanty and contradictory (Yarnell, et al, 1979). Bender et al (1973) have suggested that heterozygosity in HL-A antigens will have survival advantage through facilitating immune surveillance. They postulate that chromosomal abnormalities involving duplication or deletion of segments are more likely to produce recognisable alterations in the histocompatability phenotype of the affected if there is a high degree of heterozygosity. Alternatively, a high degree of heterozygosity in HL-A antigens may be associated with longevity simply because it indicates high heterozygosity in other loci. A survival advantage in possessing a wide repertoire of cell proteins is one postulated basis for the phenomenon of hybrid vigour (heterosis) found in breeding experiments in animals although Comfort (1979) has commented that hybrid vigour probably reflects factors additional to heterozygosity.

Greenberg and Yunis (1978) compared the immune responses and HL-A types of groups of young and old subjects. They found a significantly reduced prevalence of the A1-B8 haplotype in old women but not in old men and also that women with B8 showed evidence of significantly poorer cell mediated immune responses.

Glueck and colleagues (1977) have extended the method to study the kindreds of subjects who have reached healthy old age. They found higher prevalences of hypobeta- and hyperalphaproteinaemias than would be expected from the frequencies in the general population and suggest that this reflects the protective effect of these phenotypes against vascular disease.

The search for genetically determined partial ageing syndromes could in principle be extended beyond a study of clearly established single gene effects. The association of age-associated diseases within individuals or kindreds in order to identify genetically determined groupings might repay study. Albert, Child & Bell (1978) have demonstrated an excess of early deaths from non-cancer causes in the kindred of cancer patients. Clearly environmental factors will contribute but a genetic link of susceptibility to carcinogenesis with other age-associated diseases could provide a clue to the control of intrinsic ageing processes. Comfort (1979) has devised a battery of tests to measure the rate of ageing in various human body systems. Although primarily aimed at the evaluation of methods of intervention in ageing the battery might also be used in the search for clustering of age-associated effects.

MECHANISMS OF INTRINSIC AGEING

There is a wide range of theories on the mechanisms of intrinsic ageing and extensive reviews can be found in Comfort (1979) & Strehler (1977). It has become conventional to divide these theories into those which propose 'programmed' ageing and those which are based on 'random error' mechanisms.

PROGRAMMED AGEING

This concept implies that ageing comes about through the action of an orderly sequence of genes acting essentially without error. Programmed decline in function and death of cells is seen during embryonic development and the deaths of some insects and fish after reproduction appears to be the direct result of genetically programmed metabolism or behaviour, but there is no direct evidence for programmed death of this type in higher mammals.

The original programmed ageing theories envisaged senescence and death as being coded directly in the gene sequence. Such theories then propose mechanisms of senescence such as chalones (Bullough, 1977) or the permanent locking of cells into a non-cycling phase (Gelfant & Grove, 1974). Comfort (1979) has proposed a variant in suggesting that ageing occurs when the cell runs out of programme so that the orderly sequence of gene action associated with development is succeeded by random repression and derepression of genes. Apart from leading to general impairment of function this process could create specific correlates of ageing such as malignancy, reappearance of foetal antigens and autoimmunity. It might also explain such bizarre features of ageing as the occasional appearance of cellulose fibres in subcutaneous tissue of aged persons. In the animal kingdom cellulose only occurs in the silkworm and in the adult sedentary Tunicata (sea-squirts) the free-living larval form of which are related to the early chordate ancestors of the vertebrates. The idea that old age might involve the derepression of genes that have been dormant through 550 million years of evolution has something of the quality of science-fiction (Hall, 1976).

Many programmed ageing theories propose the existence of a biological clock in the organism which paces the changes of senescence. An early fashion for placing this clock in the endocrine system (e.g. Dilman, 1971) has been overtaken by increasing attention to the immune system (Burch, 1968; Walford, 1969; Burnet, 1974). Age-associated changes in the human immune system are complex but in general are dominated by a decline in T-cell function with relatively well preserved B-cell function (Makinodan, Good & Kay, 1976). The onset of T-cell decline begins at sexual maturity with the involution of the thymus which is therefore seen by some as the main pacer for senescence. Roberts-Thomson et al (1974) showed that evidence of reduced T-cell function in elderly persons was associated with subsequent mortality but whether impaired T-cell function is a cause of death or merely a sign of its imminence remains an open question. Mackay, Whittingham & Matthews (1976) demonstrated an increase with age in various auto-antibodies and data from the Busselton Survey suggest an association of auto-antibodies with vascular disease and subsequent mortality in men though not in women. The authors point out that the appearance of auto-antibodies may be a manifestation of suppressor T-cell dysfunction. There seems little doubt that changes in the immune system are an idex of ageing but their causative role remains to be established.

RANDOM-ERROR THEORIES

These propose that ageing is a consequence of damage to cell components and particularly to those components concerned with control and repair. A number of specific mechanisms of damage have been proposed including thermal denaturation, radiation and free radical reactions. The last, which are probably involved in radiation-induced damage, have received considerable attention because of the possibility of modifying their effects by chemical means (Packer & Smith, 1974). Two particular types of free-radical reactions have been proposed as having fundamental significance for ageing processes, the autoxidation of fats (Dormandy, 1969) and cross-linkage of complex molecules (Bjorksten, 1974). Cross-linkage of collagen fibres contributes to age-associated changes in connective tissue (Hall, 1976) and within the cell cross-linkage might lead to inactivation of enzymes and to chromosomal damage.

Much random-error damage to the complex molecules of the cell will presumably be detected and made good by specific repair systems or by functional feedback and turnover mechanisms. Orgel (1970) has drawn attention to the particular significance of damage to molecules involved in information transfer in the cell. Damage to a single molecule of RNA or a synthetase might lead to the creation of many molecules of mis-specified protein of aberrant function. Accumulation of informational errors over time might then lead to accelerating dysfunction of the cell which would eventually die of an 'error catastrophe'. Error catastrophe will not be an inevitable consequence of damage to information molecules; if the cellular feedback systems have particular properties a stable function state may be achieved despite errors in the information system.

A number of studies, though not all, have found evidence that in ageing cells the ratio of biochemically measured enzyme to immuno-reactive measures of the same enzyme may diminish which would be compatible with the accumulation of mis-specified protein in the old (Holliday & Tarrant, 1972; Gershon & Gershon, 1973). An important question is whether the inactive enzyme has arisen through errors in transcription and translation as required by Orgel's hypothesis or through post-translational changes. Rubinson et al (1976) found no evidence of lower specific molecular activity of seven enzymes in the granulocytes of older persons suggesting that there had been no accumulation of errors in the protein-specification of systems of stem cells in older persons. There is, however, evidence of impaired accuracy of DNA polymerase activity among ageing human fibroblasts in culture (Linn, Kairis & Holliday, 1976).

Somatic mutation is a specific random-error mechanism postulated as a basis of ageing and there is evidence for the accumulation of somatic mutations in human fibroblasts in tissue culture (Fulder, 1979). The theories of Walford (1969) and Burnet (1974) draw attention to the wide range of effects that somatic mutation might lead to through the immune system. Somatic mutation may prove to be the basis of malignancies and of some diseases of later life that appear to be due to clones of cells with disordered function such as Paget's disease of bone and primary acquired sideroblastic anaemia. The suggestion by Burnet (1974) that atherosclerotic lesions start as mutated clones of cells depended on the observation of Benditt & Benditt (1973) that cells in atherosclerotic plaques of Negresses heterozygous for glucose-6-phosphate dehydrogenase were all of one haplotype. However, this uniformity of haplotypes in a plaque may come about during the evolution of a plaque from thrombus rather than being present from the beginning (Pearson et al, 1979).

At one time support for a somatic mutation theory of ageing appeared to come from experiments in which age-associated changes in some species were accelerated by radiation. However, the effects of radiation vary considerably between species and with experimental conditions so it is not possible to regard radiation simply as an inducer of accelerated or premature ageing (Storer, 1978). The follow-up studies on the Japanese exposed to irradiation in the atomic bomb explosions have shown increased incidence of some malignancies (Nakamura, 1977) but no consistent evidence of generalised accelerated ageing (Anderson, Yamamoto & Thorslund, 1974). This finding is not crucial to the somatic mutation theory for Burnet (1974) considers that the limiting determinant of mutation rate is the error proneness of the DNA repair system and the increase in DNA damage from sublethal doses of radiation will lead to very few extra mutations.

On the basis of work in plants chromosomal aberrations have been regarded as an indicator of mutation rates. Crowley & Curtis (1963) showed that chromosomal aberrations in the cells of regenerating livers of mice increased with age as it did also, though less steeply, for guinea pigs (Curtis & Miller, 1971). In dogs chromosomal aberrations accumulate with age much more slowly (Curtis, Leith & Tilley, 1966). The rates of accumulation of aberrations in these three species are in an inverse relationship to their lifespans and may reflect differences in the capacity of DNA repair systems. Hart & Setlow (1974) provided evidence that differences in the repair of DNA damage induced by ultraviolet radiation between species correlated with lifespan. However, in the experiments of Curtis and colleagues the proportion of aberrations present by the typical age of death varied from over 70 per cent for mice to probably less than 20 per cent for dogs which does not suggest a direct relationship between mutations and death. In the human hypodiploidy increases with age but its relevance to ageing changes and mortality is dubious since it is more common in females than in males (Schneider, 1978). (The same objection applies to auto-immunity as a single cause of ageing.)

COMBINING PROGRAMMED AND RANDOM-ERROR THEORIES
Programmed and random-error theories of ageing are not incompatible as some authors seem to assume. The suggestion by Burnet (1974) of the genetic specification of the rate of random-error occurrence is one example of the combination of the two concepts. If in addition to a random-error theory of ageing we accept the evidence set out earlier that the evolution of higher animals has been associated with increasing longevity it seems inevitable that the lifespan of each species will tend to be limited by a critical failure in the body systems which have least developed their defences against cumulative error. In other words death will appear to be due to a biological 'clock' but will not reflect genetic programming in the traditional sense.

Extrinsic ageing
An ability to construct genetic models of ageing does not necessarily imply that ageing is entirely under genetic control. There is cogent evidence that many age-associated changes in man are at least partly extrinsic in origin arising from environmental factors and from aspects of a culturally-determined way of life. Evidence for this can be found in transcultural comparisons of ageing trends and from comparing groups of individuals with different life experience within a single culture. Thus the leftward shift in electrocardiographic axis widely thought to be a 'normal' age-associated change in Western populations may not occur in populations at low risk of coronary heart disease (Evans, Prior & Tunbridge, 1981). The age-associated decline in lung function is accelerated by cigarette smoking (Ashley et al, 1975). The effect of obesity in modulating the development of glucose intolerance with age may be seen as an interaction between extrinsic and intrinsic factors. Similarly the rise of mean blood pressure with age in most populations is probably largely environmentally determined and it is increasingly suspected that dietary sodium (Freis, 1976) or the ratio of dietary sodium to potassium (Meneely & Battarbee, 1976) acting on genetically susceptible

individuals may be a responsible factor. The possibility that an age-associated change with such important consequences in morbidity and mortality as high blood pressure may be the result of a ubiquitous environmental factor interacting with genetic susceptibility is of great gerontological interest. There are analogous possibilities in the hypotheses that senile dementia of Alzheimer's type may be a consequence of unusual aluminium metabolism (Crapper, Karlik & De Boni, 1978) or viral infection (Gibbs & Gajdusek, 1978). For sodium intake there is an additional point of interest in that the appetite for salt which determines individual intake is acquired in childhood from parental cooking and this familial effect might be mistakenly included in an estimate of the genetic influence on blood pressure.

Although closely age-associated it seems clear from epidemiological studies that coronary heart disease has extrinsic determinants although Burch (1978) questions the quantitative importance of these. Similarly, there appear to be significant geographical and secular variations in the incidence of cerebrovascular disease (Hansen & Marquardsen, 1977; Garraway et al, 1979).

Most adult cancers, with important exceptions, some of which are discussed below, show a power-law relationship with age and many authors have proposed that carcinogenesis is a consequence of intrinsic ageing processes (Hirsch, 1978). However the age-association could reflect the fact that the longer an individual lives the more likely he is to accumulate a carcinogenic dose of an environmental factor, and variations in incidence and in sex ratio of cancer around the world suggest that most malignancies are partly extrinsically caused (Boyland, 1980).

In an attempt to identify a specific age effect on liability to neoplasm Peto et al (1975) applied benzpyrene to the skin of mice of different ages. They found that incidence of malignant epithelial tumours increased approximately as a power of the duration of exposure to benzpyrene and there was no independent effect of age. In so far as this animal model is relevant to human disease the finding suggests that adult cancers are extrinsically age-associated.

The decline in cardiorespiratory reserve with age includes a component due to a way of life that discourages physical exertion after the early 20s (Bassey, 1978). The incidence of fractured proximal femur increases exponentially with age but varies between different parts of the United Kingdom to a degree that suggests the effect of extrinsic factors (Evans, Prudham & Wandless, 1979). Studies of indices of bone mass in pairs of monozygotic and dizygotic twins suggest an important genetic influence but the degree of concordance within monozygotic twin pairs declines with age (Smith et al, 1973) indicating that extrinsic factors are probably also involved. A similar pattern of age changes has been observed in measures of psychological function in a longitudinal study of twins indicating that in this area too both intrinsic and extrinsic factors are active (Bank & Jarvik, 1978).

If, to oversimplify somewhat, intrinsic ageing determines maximum lifespan and extrinsic factors determine how close to maximum lifespan an individual reaches it is to be expected that the relative importance of extrinsic factors in determining differences in morbidity and mortality between individuals of the same age will decline in old age. This may partly explain such findings as age-associated changes in the pattern of risk factors for vascular disease (Burch, 1978; Evans, Prudham & Wandless, 1980) but the greater variability and inaccuracy of some measurements in old age described earlier will also contribute.

Inheritance of longevity in man

There have been several studies on the familial distribution of longevity in man. There are many methodological pitfalls in such studies but there seems little doubt that longevity is a familial trait. Twin studies suggest that genetic factors are partly responsible (Kallman, 1957) but data on wider family relationships indicate that a simple genetic model is not tenable and that extrinsic factors are involved. The study reported by Abbott et al (1974) on the lifespan of offspring of nonagenarians examined the age at death of children, one of whose parents had reached 90, according to the age at death of the other parent. There was significant evidence of a positive relationship but this was more obvious for male children and was more apparent in mother-child relationships than in father-child relationships. This latter finding raises the possibilities of X-linked genetic factors and of cytoplasmic or mitochondrial inheritance but is probably explicable by environmental influences because human children inherit more than cell components from their parents. From the father children inherit social class with its associated aspirations and lifestyle and from the mother dietary habits and tastes. In the past these inherited but non-genetic influences probably underwent more modification in adult life in females than in males because of the female's lifestyle was more determined by whom she married than would be the case for the male.

Sex and longevity

Greater longevity in the female of the species than in the male is a widespread but not universal phenomenon in higher animals. Where the female has the task of bearing and rearing the young there may be a genetic advantage in the female being more durable than the male who becomes somewhat superfluous after copulation. In modern societies female mortality rates are lower than male at all ages. One mechanism of such superiority may be associated with Lyonisation of the X-chromosome so that the female is phenotypically a mosaic expressing more genes than the male and therefore having a greater 'library' of immune responses. However, historical and archaeological evidence suggest that greater longevity in the female is a fairly recent phenomenon. As late as the 16th century males outlived females on average in the lower socioeconomic groups although the aristocracy showed the greater survival in the female that is characteristic of modern societies (Cowgill, 1970).

Even in advanced societies extrinsic factors are also involved in the sex difference in longevity. It is an established epidemiological axiom that since men and women differ more in their environments than in their genes variation in the sex ratio of mortality or disease incidence from place to place, or *a fortiori* from time to time in the same place, indicates environmental influence. Figure 2.2 shows the sex ratio of total mortality rates at different ages in England and Wales over this century. In 1900 the ratio was approximately constant at around 1.3 over adult life. Since then two prominent peaks have appeared centred on ages 20 and 65 when the ratio rises to over 2.0. The younger peak is easily explicable in terms of deaths from accident and trauma, mostly road traffic accidents, and vanishes if such deaths are removed from the calculations. The causes of the later peak are less clear. Removal of deaths from coronary heart disease and other major cigarette-associated diseases bronchitis and bronchial carcinoma reduces but does not remove the rise in sex ratio after middle-age. There may be other environmental determinants of excess male mortality over the ages 65 to 74 apart from cigarette smoking. Lewis & Lewis (1977) have drawn attention to the possible effect that the Women's Liberation Movement may have in equalising the environmental hazards to which men and women are exposed and it will be of great interest to see the impact of this on sex differences in mortality.

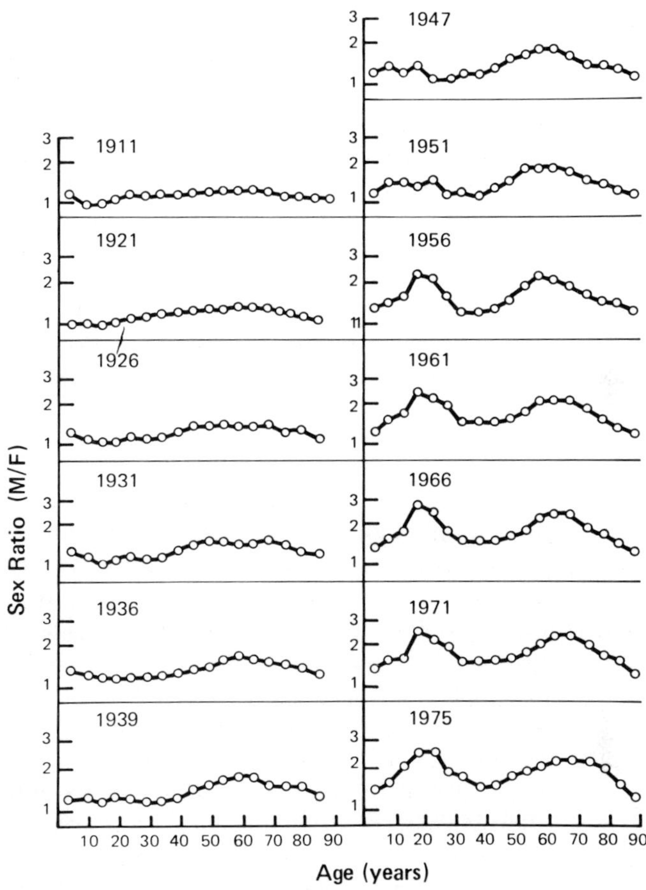

Fig. 2.2   Ratio of male to female age-specific mortality rates — England and Wales, 1911–1975. Note logarithmic scale.

The reasoning set out above presupposes that purely genetically-determined difference in mortality between the sexes would be similar at all ages otherwise one might argue that the constant ratio with age seen in 1900 was due to an environmentally increased mortality in females at ages under 55 and over 75 obscuring the true genetic pattern which has now emerged. Although implausible on evolutionary grounds there is no definite evidence to refute this view except for some inadequate animal data suggesting that the sex ratio of mortality rates does not alter significantly with age (Comfort, 1959).

The menopause
At first sight the menopause has some of the characteristics of programmed ageing in that it is a genetically determined characteristic universal to the human species and which occurs with remarkably little variation around a median age of about 50. It is commonly supposed that the menopause is associated with an acceleration of age-associated disease but this is by no means established. There is no change in the slope of age-specific rates of total mortality in females around the age of the menopause and the relative advantage of the female over the male in terms of total mortality rate is enhanced rather than diminished after middle-age (Fig. 2.2).

The supposed relationship of the menopause with mental illness appears to be without foundation (Wood, 1979) although for social and cultural reasons psychologically vulnerable women may react to the menopause as to a stressful event (Ballinger, 1976). In contrast the menopause does seem to be associated with accelerated bone loss which can be successfully retarded with oestrogens (Lindsay et al, 1978). There is a sharp steplike rise in the incidence of fractured distal forearm in females at the time of the menopause perhaps reflecting this accelerated bone loss (Alffram & Bauer, 1962). Although loss of bone mass occurs throughout adult life changes at the menopause suggest the intrusion of a new pathogenic factor, presumably oestrogen withdrawal, rather than an acceleration of established age-associated changes.

The Framingham workers (Gordon et al, 1978) have presented evidence that both surgical and natural menopause are associated with increase in risk of coronary heart disease independent of age. Several, but not all, case/control studies have also found evidence for this. Clearly, in all studies on this subject validation of ages is crucial since some women with 'premature' menopause or coronary heart disease may actually be older than they claim. The sex ratio of mortality rates from coronary heart disease is lower after the age of 50 than at younger ages but as Heller & Jacobs (1978) demonstrated this is due to a relative diminution in the rate of increase with age in the death rate of men rather than to a disproportionate increase in women. Unless, therefore, the menopause increases only non-fatal coronary heart disease, and the Framingham figures do not suggest this, there is an apparent conflict of evidence if it is postulated that the menopause causes an increase in coronary heart disease risk. On the other hand the anomaly between the Framingham data and national mortality data can be reconciled if the menopause is not a primary even but is a consequence of underlying ageing changes some of which are also antecedents of coronary heart disease. This would also explain why oestrogen therapy fails to reduce the incidence of coronary heart disease in postmenopausal women (Rosenberg, Armstrong & Jick, 1976).

It is almost a universal finding in population studies that mean blood pressure in women is lower than that of men in younger adult life and higher in late middle life and beyond, the cross-over occurring typically at ages 40 to 54. The trends seen in cross-sectional data do not suggest a sudden increase in blood pressure in women in the menopause (e.g. Johnson, Epstein & Kjelsberg, 1965). Longitudinal data from the Framingham study also provide no evidence for a menopausal effect on blood pressure but the trends observed in this particular set of data do not follow those expected from cross-sectional analysis and may not be typical (Kannel, 1976). Mean serum cholesterol levels are higher in women than in men after middle-age, having been lower in early adult life but this reflects the continuous increase in women into the seventh decade while levels in men decline after middle-age (Johnson, Epstein & Kjelsberg, 1965).

In its relation to cancer incidence the menopause appears to have, if anything, a beneficial effect. Most adult cancers increase in incidence in a power-law relationship with age until late in life. Exceptions include cancers of the female breast, ovary, cervix uteri and other uterine cancer. The incidence of breast and endometrial cancer show an abrupt deceleration in the rate of increase with age around the menopause. Cervical cancer shows a similar pattern even when adjusted for known cohort effects. These relationships give serious concern that the use of hormone 'replacement' therapy after the menopause may increase the incidence of some of these cancers. There seems little reasonable doubt on present evidence that this occurs for endometrial cancer (Editorial, 1979) but there is no satisfactory evidence on the numerically more important, and more fatal, cancer of the breast (Hoover et al, 1976).

It may be that the menopause is an adaptive response to ageing other than a primary ageing event. Although many animals show a decline in reproductive function and efficiency with age the menopause as a more or less abrupt and irrevocable cessation of reproductive ability appears to be unique to women (Finn, 1976). We may postulate that if reproductive efficiency declines with age and if family structure and the development, through speech, of a cumulative culture have led to grandparents having a significant role in raising their grandchildren, there may come a point in a woman's life when in terms of gene propagation it is biologically more appropriate for her to cease increasingly unsuccessful attempts to produce more children of her own and to devote her energies to caring for her grandchildren. For animals which do not make a significant contribution to the rearing of grandchildren and for the male, whose biological investment in unsuccessful pregnancies is so much less than the female's, this point would be reached much later in life if at all. This view of the menopause as a biological adaptation to an age-associated decline in reproductive efficiency has also been advanced by Dawkins (1976). Perhaps if this view were more widely publicised women's attitudes to the menopause might become more positive.

If this theory is correct one would predict that the menopause will fall earlier in groups where reproductive efficiency declines more steeply with age but the data on this are difficult to evaluate because of uncertainty about the degree to which menopause is directly affected by the environmental factors that also determine reproductive efficiency. Although the age of the menarche appears to be controlled by a hypothalamic mechanism sensitive to body size and so to malnutrition there is no direct evidence for a similar mechanism for the menopause. A lowering of the age of the median menarchal age in the last hundred years, compatible with improving nutrition, has almost certainly occurred but there is no satisfactory evidence of any change in menopausal age (Burch & Grunz, 1967).

Conclusion

At present there appear to be almost as many theories of intrinsic ageing as there are gerontologists. In the interpretation of available evidence a great deal depends on how appropriate studies of tissue culture or laboratory animals are to human ageing. It seems likely that no single mechanism will be sufficient explanation for intrinsic ageing and that many of the proposed mechanisms may contribute.

Evolutionary pressure will tend to lengthen the lifespan of higher species and in man a relatively small number of mutations has probably been responsible for an important increase in maximum lifespan. Species will tend to have characteristic modes of death in old age which reflect failure in the least evolved body system and even if intrinsic ageing processes are essentially random in nature a limiting system of this kind may appear to be functioning as a biological clock. The immune system may prove to have this critical role in the human but there is no reason to assume that the same will be found in other species.

For the medical gerontologist and for the clinician the most immediate challenge is to identify extrinsic factors in human ageing both at the population and individual level. This approach will be more successful if it concerns itself with function as well as with 'disease' since the latter may have been defined with reference to an implicit and inappropriate model of 'normal' ageing. Modification of extrinsic ageing processes may be expected to extend the average lifespan and to improve the levels of morbidity in later life but not to extend maximum lifespan. Limited extension of maximum lifespan may prove to be possible at some time in the future if some of the current hypotheses about the origins of intrinsic ageing prove to be correct but the primary reason for research into intrinsic ageing processes at present is to elucidate mechanisms of morbidity in later life rather than to extend lifespan.

REFERENCES

Abbott M H, Murphy E A, Bolling D R, Abbey H 1974 The familial component in longevity: a study of offspring of nonagenarians II. Preliminary analysis of the completed study. Hopkins Medical Journal 134: 1–16

Albert S, Child M A, Belle S 1978 Non-cancer deaths in cancer and non-cancer lineages. American Journal of Epidemiology 108: 373–376

Alffram P A, Bauer G C H 1962 Epidemiology of fracture of the forearm. Journal of Bone and Joint Surgery 44A: 105–114

Anderson R E, Yamamoto T, Thorslund T 1974 Ageing in Hiroshima and Nagasaki atomic bomb survivors: Soluble-insoluble collagen ratio. Journal of Gerontology 29: 153–156

Ashley F, Kannel W B, Sorlie P D, Masson R 1975 Pulmonary function: relation to ageing, cigarette habit and mortality. Annals of Internal Medicine 82: 739–745

Ballinger C B 1976 Psychiatric morbidity and the menopause: clinical features. British Medical Journal 1: 1183–1185

Bank L, Jarvik L F 1978 A longitudinal study of ageing human twins. In: Schneider E L (ed) The genetics of ageing, Plenum, New York p 303–333

Bassey E J 1978 Age, inactivity and some physiological responses to exercise. Gerontology, 24: 66–77

Bender K, Rüter G, Mayerova A, Hiller C 1973 Studies on the heterozygosity at the HL-A gene loci in children and old people. Symposium Series Immunobiological Standardisation 18: 287–290

Benditt E P, Benditt J M 1973 Evidence for a monoclonal origin of human atherosclerotic plaques. Proceedings of the National Academy of Sciences, USA 70: 1753–1756

Bjorksten J 1974 Cross-linkage and the ageing process. In: Rockstein M, Sussman M L, Chesky J (eds) Theoretical aspects of ageing. Academic Press, New York, p 43–59

Bodmer W F 1980 The HLA system and disease. Journal of the Royal College of Physicians of London 14: 43–50

Boyland E 1980 The history and future of chemical carcinogenesis. British Medical Bulletin 36: 5–10

Bullough W S 1977 Ageing of mammals. Nature 229: 608–610

Burch P R J 1968 An inquiry concerning growth, disease and ageing. Oliver & Boyd, Edinburgh

Burch P R J 1978 Coronary heart disease: risk factors and ageing. Gerontology 24: 123–155

Burch P R J, Gunz F W 1967 The distribution of menopausal age in New Zealand. New Zealand Medical Journal 66: 6–10

Burnett M 1974 Intrinsic mutagenesis. MTP, Lancaster

Calow P 1978 Bidder's hypothesis revisited. Gerontology 24: 448–458

Collins K J, Dore C, Exton-Smith A N, Fox R H, MacDonald I C, Woodward P M 1977 Accidental hypothermia and impaired temperature homeostasis in the elderly. British Medical Journal 1: 353–356

Comfort A 1959 Studies in the longevity and mortality of English thoroughbred horses. In: Wolstenholme G E W, O'Connor M (eds) The lifespan of animals, Ciba Foundation Colloquia on Ageing. Churchill, London, Vol. 5, p 35–54

Comfort A 1979 The biology of senescence, 3rd ed. Churchill Livingstone, Edinburgh

Cowgill U M 1970 The people of York 1538–1812. Scientific American 222: (1) 104–112

Crapper D R, Karlik S, De Boni U 1978 Aluminium and other metals in senile (Alzheimer) dementia. In: Katzman R, Terry R D, Bick K C (eds) Alzheimer's disease: senile dementia and related disorder. Raven Press, New York, p 471–485

Crowley C, Curtis H J 1963 The development of somatic mutations in mice with age. Proceedings of the National Academy of Sciences, USA 49: 626–628

Curtis H J, Leith J, Tilley J 1966 Chromosome aberrations in liver cells of dogs of different ages. Journal of Gerontology 21: 268–270

Curtis H J, Miller K 1971 Chromosome abberations in liver cells of guinea pigs. *Journal of Gerontology* 26: 292–293

Cutler R G 1972 A working hypothesis of senescence. In: Strehler B L (ed) Advances in gerontological research. Academic Press, New York vol. 4, p 220–321

Cutler R G 1975 Evolution of human longevity and the genetic complexity governing ageing rate. Proceedings of the National Academy of Sciences, USA 72: 4664–4668

Daniel C W 1977 Cell longevity in vivo. In: Finch C E, Hayflick L Handbook of the biology of ageing. Van Nostrand, New York p 122–158

Dawkins R 1976 The selfish gene. University Press, Oxford

Dilman V M 1971 Age-associated elevation of hypothalamic threshold to feedback control and its role in development, ageing and disease. Lancet 1: 1211–1219

Dormandy T L 1969 Biological rancidification. Lancet 2: 684–688

Editorial 1979 Oestrogen therapy and endometrial cancer. Lancet 1: 1121–1122

Evans J Grimley 1977 Issues in institutional care in the United Kingdom. In: Exton-Smith A N, Evans J Grimley (eds) Care of the elderly: meeting the challenge of dependence. Academic Press, London 128–146

Evans J Grimley, Prudham D, Wandless I 1979 A prospective study of fractured proximal femur: incidence and outcome. Public Health, London 93: 235–241

Evans J Grimley, Prior I A M, Tunbridge W M G 1981 Age-associated changes in QRS axis: intrinsic or extrinsic ageing? In preparation

Evans J Grimley, Prudham D, Wandless I 1980 Risk factors for stroke in the elderly. In: Barbagallo-Sangiorgi G, Exton-Smith A N (eds) The ageing brain: neurological and mental disturbances. Plenum Press, London. In press

Finn C A 1976 Investigations into reproductive ageing in experimental animals. In Beard R J (ed) The menopause: a guide to current research and practice. MTP, Lancaster p 1–24

Fox R H, Woodward P M, Exton-Smith A N, Green M F, Donnison D V, Wilks M H 1973 Body temperatures in the elderly: a national study of physiological, social and environmental conditions. British Medical Journal, 1: 200–206

Freis E D 1976 Salt, volume and the prevention of hypertension. Circulation 53: 589–595

Fulder S J 1979 Evidence for an increase in presumed somatic mutation during the ageing of human cells in culture. Mechanisms of Ageing and Development 10: 101–115

Garraway W M, Whisnant J P, Furlan A J, Phillips L M, Kurland L T, O'Fallon W M 1979 The declining incidence of stroke. New England Journal of Medicine 300: 449–452

Gelfant S, Grove G C 1974 Cycling, non-cycling cells as an explanation for the ageing process. In: Rockstein M, Sussman M L, Chesling J (eds) Theoretical aspects of ageing. Academic Press, New York p 105–117

Gershon H, Gershon D 1973 Inactive enzyme molecules in ageing mice: liver aldolase. Proceedings of the National Academy of Sciences, USA 70: 909–913

Gibbs C J, Gajdusek D C 1978 Subacute spongiform virus encephalopathies: the transmissible virus dementias. In: Kalzman R, Terry R D, Bick K L (eds) Alzheimer's Disease: Senile Dementia and Related Disorders. Raven Press, New York

Gilkes M J 1979 Eyes run on light. British Medical Journal 1: 1681–1683

Glueck C J, Gartside P S, Steiner P M, Miller M, Todhunter T, Haaf, J, Pucke M, Terrawa M, Fallat R W, Kashyap M L 1977 Hyperalpha- and hypobeta-lipoproteinaemia in octogenarian kindreds. Atherosclerosis 27: 387–406

Gordon T, Kannel W B, Hjortland M C, McNamara P M 1978 Menopause and coronary heart disease. The Framingham study. Annals of Internal Medicine 89: 157–161

Greenberg L J, Yunis E J 1978 Genetic control of auto-immune disease and immune responsiveness and the relationship to ageing. In: Bergsma D, Harrison D E, Paul N W (eds) Genetic effects on ageing. Liss, New York p 249–260

Gregory R L 1974 Concepts and Mechanisms of Perception. Duckworth, London p 167–227

Hall D A 1976 The ageing of connective tissue. Experimental Gerontology 3: 77–89
Hamilton W D 1966 The moulding of senescence by natural selection. Journal of Theoretical Biology 12: 12–45
Hansen B S, Marquardsen J 1977 Incidence of stroke in Fredericksberg, Denmark. Stroke 8: 663–665
Hart R W, Setlow R B 1974 Correlation between deoxyribonucleic acid excision-repair and lifespan in a number of mammalian species. Proceedings of the National Academy of Sciences, USA 71: 2169–2173
Hayflick L 1976 The cell biology of human ageing. New England Journal of Medicine 295: 1302–1308
Helderman J H, Vestal R E, Rowe J W, Tobin J D, Andres R, Robertson G L 1978 The response of arginine vasopressin to intravenous ethanol and hypertonic saline in man: the impact of ageing. Journal of Gerontology 33: 39–47
Heller R F, Jacobs H S 1978 Coronary heart disease in relation to age, sex and the menopause. British Medical Journal 1: 472–474
Hirsch G P 1978 Somatic mutations and ageing. In: Schneider E L (ed) The Genetics of Ageing. Plenum, New York p 91–136
Holliday R, Tarrant G M 1972 Altered enzymes in ageing human fibroblasts. Nature 238: 26–30
Holliday R, Huschtscha L I, Tarrant G M, Kirkwood T B L 1977 Testing the commitment theory of cellular ageing. Science 198: 366–372
Hoover R, Gray L A, Cole P, MacMahon B 1976 Menopausal estrogens and breast cancer. New England Journal of Medicine 295: 401–405
Johnson B C, Epstein F H, Kjelsberg M O 1965 Distribution and familial studies of blood pressure and serum cholesterol levels in a total community — Tecumseh Michigan. Journal of Chronic Diseases 18: 147–160
Jung R T, Shetty P S, James W P T, Barrand M A, Callingham B A 1979 Reduced thermogenesis in obesity. Nature 279: 322–323
Kallman F J 1957 Twin data on the genetics of ageing. In: Methodology of the study of ageing, Ciba Foundation Colloquia on Ageing. Churchill, London vol. 3, p 131–143
Kannel W B 1976 Blood pressure and the development of cardiovascular disease in the aged. In Caird F I, Dall J L C, Kennedy R D (eds) Cardiology in old age. Plenum, New York, p 143–175
Kay H E M 1965 How many cell generations? Lancet 2: 418–419
King M C, Wilson A C 1975 Evolution at two levels in humans and chimpanzees. Science 188: 107–116
Kirkwood T B L 1977 Evolution of ageing. Nature 270: 301–304
Lewis C E, Lewis M A 1977 The potential impact of sexual equality on health. New England Journal of Medicine 297: 863–869
Lindsay R, Hart D M, MacLean A, Garwood J, Aitken J M, Clark A C, Coutts J R T 1978 Pathogenesis and prevention of post-menopausal osteoporosis. In: Cooke I (ed) Estrogen and progestogen in the management of the menopause. MTP, Lancaster p 9–25
Linn S, Kairis M, Holliday R 1976 Decreased fidelity of DNA polylerase activity isolated from ageing human fibroblasts. Proceedings of the National Academy of Science, USA 73: 2818–2822
Lints F A 1978 Genetics and ageing. Karger, Basel
MacKay I R, Whittingham S F, Mathews J D 1976 The immunoepidemiology of ageing. In: Makinodan T, Yunis E (eds) Immunology and ageing. Plenum, New York, p 35–50
Makinodan T, Good R A, Kay M B M 1976 Cellular basis of immunosenescence. In: Makinodan T, Yunis E (eds) Immunology and Ageing. Plenum, New York, p 9–22
Martin G M 1978 Genetic syndromes in man with potential relevance to the pathobiology of ageing. In: Bergsma D, Harrison D E, Paul N W (eds) Genetic effects on ageing. Liss, New York, p 5–39
Martin G M, Sprague C A, Epstein C J 1970 Replicative lifespan of cultivated human cells. Effects of donor's age, tissue and genotype. Laboratory Investigation 23: 86–92
McLachlan M S F 1978 The ageing kidney. Lancet 2: 143–146
Medawar P 1952 An unsolved problem in biology. Lewis, London
Meneely G R, Battarbee H D 1976 High sodium — low potassium environment and hypertension. American Journal of Cardiology 38: 768–785
Nakamura K 1977 Stomach cancer in atomic-bomb survivors. Lancet 2: 866–867
Neel J V 1962 Diabetes mellitus: a 'thrifty' genotype rendered detrimental by 'progress'? American Journal of Human Genetics 14: 353–362
Orgel L E 1970 The maintenance of the accuracy of protein synthesis and its relevance to ageing: a correction. Proceedings of the National Academy of Sciences, USA 67: 1426–1429
Packer L, Smith J R 1974 Extension of the lifespan of cultured normal human diploid cells by vitamin E. Proceedings of the National Academy of Sciences, USA 71: 4763–4767
Pearson T A, Dillman J, Solez K, Heptinstall R H 1979 Monoclonal characteristics of organising arterial thrombi: significance in the origin and growth of human artherosclerotic plaques. Lancet 1: 7–11
Peto R, Roe F J L, Lee P N, Levy L, Clack J 1975 Cancer and ageing in mice and men. British Journal of Cancer 32: 411–426

Phair J P 1979 Ageing and infection: a review. Journal of Chronic Diseases 32: 535–540

Plemons J K, Willis S C, Baltes P B 1978 Modifiability of fluid intelligence in ageing: a short-term longitudinal training approach. Journal of Gerontology 33: 224–231

Roberts-Thomson I C, Whittingham S, Youngchaiyud, U, Mackay I R 1974 Ageing, immune response and mortality. Lancet 2: 368–370

Rosenberg L, Armstrong B, Jick H 1976 Myocardial infarction and estrogen therapy in post-menopausal women. New England Journal of Medicine 294: 1256–1259

Rubinson H, Kahn A, Boivin P, Schapira F, Gregori C, Dreyfus J-C 1976 Ageing and accuracy of protein synthesis in man: search for inactive enzymatic cross-reacting material in granulocytes of aged people. Gerontology 22: 438–448

Sacher G A 1975 Maturation and longevity in relation to cranial capacity in hominid evolution. In: Tuttle R H (ed) Primate functional morphology and evolution. Mouton, The Hague, p 417–441

Schaie K W, Strother C R 1968 A cross-sequential study of age changes in cognitive behaviour. Psychological Bulletin 70: 671–680

Schaie K W, Labouvie-Vief G 1974 Generational versus ontogenetic components of change in adult cognitive behaviour: a fourteen-year cross-sectional study. Developmental Psychology 10: 305–320

Schneider E L 1978 Cytogenetics of ageing. In: Schneider E L (ed) The genetics of ageing. Plenum, New York, p 27–52

Smith D M, Nance W C, Kang K W, Christian J C, Johnston C C 1973 Genetic factors in determining bone mass. Journal of Clinical Investigation 52: 2800–2808

Smith G S, Walford R L 1977 Influence of the main histocompatibility complex on ageing in mice. Nature 270: 727–729

Spence J D, Sibbald W J, Cape R D 1978 Pseudohypertension in the elderly. Clinical Science & Molecular Medicine 55: 399s–402s

Storer J B 1978 Effect of ageing and radiation in mice of different genotypes In: Bergsma D, Harrison D E (eds) Genetic effects on ageing. Liss, New York, p 55–70

Strehler B L 1977 Time cells and ageing, 2nd ed. Academic Press, New York

Walford R L 1969 The immunologic theory of ageing. Munksgaard, Copenhagen

Walford R L 1974 Immunologic theory of ageing: current status. Federation Proceedings 33: 2020–2027

Williams G C 1957 Pleiotropy, natural selection and the evolution of senescence. Evolution 11: 398–411

Wood C 1979 Menopausal myths. Medical Journal of Australia 1: 496–499

Yarnell J W G, St Leger A S, Balfour I C, Russell R B (1979) The distribution, age-effects and disease associations of HLA antigens and other blood group markers in a random sample of an elderly population. Journal of Chronic Diseases 32: 555–561

3. Drug interactions

Philip A. Routledge   David G. Shand

INTRODUCTION

Interactions between drugs have been observed for the better part of a century and have been described under the classical headings of antagonism, synergism and potentiation. Indeed many interactions have been, and still are being deliberately used with beneficial effect in therapeutics. Adverse interactions, however, are becoming an increasingly important problem for several reasons. Newly introduced drugs are much more potent than their predecessors and their pharmacology is not always completely understood. This problem is reflected by the continuing habit of polypharmacy whereby hospitalised patients may be prescribed an average of 6 to 10 drugs simultaneously (May, Stewart & Cluff, 1974). The frequency of adverse reactions to drugs and the chance of interactions increases disproportionately with the increase in number of drugs administered concomitantly (Smith, Seidl, & Cluff, 1966; May, Stewart & Cluff, 1977). It has been observed that the number of drugs prescribed by medical house staff to individual patients increased, rather than the reverse, as they gained medical experience, so that the potential for adverse interactions remains high.

Drug interactions have been estimated to account for 6.9 per cent (Boston Collaborative Drug Surveillance Program, 1972) to 22 per cent (Borda, Slone & Jick, 1968) of all adverse drug reactions. Since adverse reactions are relatively common (Smith et al, 1966), and interactions involve many different types of drugs it may appear at first sight an almost impossible task for any physician to retain a perspective on the subject. Fortunately, although perhaps 1000 drug interactions have been described (Stockley, 1973), the number of clinically important ones is much smaller and involves a relatively small number of pharmacological groups of drugs. Several excellent monographs detailing these clinically important interactions have been published (Cohen & Armstrong, 1974; Hansen, 1975; Avery, 1976, 1977) and it is not the purpose of this chapter to duplicate this information. Rather, we intend to use interactions to illustrate the general mechanisms involved and to discuss the ways in which unwanted interactions may be avoided.

MECHANISMS OF DRUG INTERACTIONS

Interactions may occur outside or inside the body. The former are referred to as pharmaceutical incompatibilities and generally occur when two or more agents are mixed in infusions or in the same syringe, or when a drug reacts with the infusion fluid itself. Guides to intravenous admixture incompatibility exist but the possibility of their occurrence can be minimised by taking the following precautions. Never add a drug to an infusion fluid unless absolutely necessary. Never add more than one drug to the syringe or infusion fluid and do not add drugs to whole blood or blood products, amino-acid or lipid solutions, mannitol or sodium bicarbonate.

Interactions occurring within the body result either from an alteration in the delivery of the drug to its site of action (pharmacokinetic interactions) or from a drug-induced alteration in receptor or organ response to another agent (pharmaco-dynamic interactions). The principles governing the pharmacokinetics and pharmaco-dynamics of drugs given on their own are discussed in Chapter 4. Often these characteristics are altered when other drugs are given and both types of interaction are equally important. Pharmacokinetic interactions will be discussed first however, because in the elucidation of mechanisms of interaction, this group must generally first be excluded before the possibility of a pharmacodynamic interaction is explored (Table 3.1).

Table 3.1   Mechanisms of drug interactions

Pharmaceutical incompatibility

Pharmacokinetic interactions
    A. Absorption interactions
    B. Altered drug elimination
       (i) hepatic metabolism
       (ii) renal excretion
    C. Changes in drug distribution

Pharmacodynamic interactions
    Drugs acting at the same receptor sites
    Drugs acting at different sites

PHARMACOKINETIC INTERACTIONS

These may occur during any one or more of the processes whereby drug reaches its site of action and then is eliminated, i.e. absorption, distribution and elmination. Such interactions may result either in enhanced or decreased delivery to the site of action and although the former may result in drug toxicity, decreased effectiveness will expose the patient to an increased risk from the disease process itself.

Absorption interactions

For most drugs, absorption is a passive process dependent on the properties of the drug and its particular formulation, the pH of the absorption media and the length of time the drug remains at the site of absorption. Drugs may interact with each other during all of these processes as well as directly with each other by formation of poorly absorbed complexes. It is important to distinguish in this context between changes in the rate and extent of drug absorption. Alteration of the rate of absorption alone will change the shape of the concentration/time curve after oral administration but will not alter the average or steady state drug concentration. Such changes may be important however in the case of drugs given in single doses and in which a threshold concentration for drug effect exists (e.g. analgesics). A delay in absorption under these circumstances, especially if the rate of elimination of the drug is high, may result in an inability to reach a drug concentration associated with drug effectiveness. In contrast, a change in extent of absorption will result in a change in delivery of drug to its site of action both after a single and repeated doses.

Drug-induced changes in the pH of the gastrointestinal media may increase or decrease the rate and extent of drug absorption. Alkalis may aid dissolution of poorly soluble acidic drugs and stimulate gastric emptying. It is probably for these reasons that aspirin is more rapidly and completely absorbed when administered in buffered alkaline rather than buffered acidic solutions (Cooke & Hunt, 1970). Sodium bicarbonate may decrease the dissolution rate of tetracycline tablets however and result in reduced drug absorption (Barr, Adir & Garrettson, 1971). These changes are different from the effects of aluminium, calcium, or magnesium antacids on the absorption of several drugs including tetracycline and iron, with which insoluble complexes are formed.

Alterations in gut motility induced by one drug may alter the rate and/or extent of absorption of another. Sparingly soluble drugs, e.g. digoxin, may be unable to undergo complete disintegration and dissolution when gastric emptying and intestinal transit rates are increased by such drugs as metoclopramide (Manninen et al, 1973) and their extent of absorption may therefore be reduced. In contrast, since the greatest proportion of drug absorption occurs in the small intestine, the rate limiting step for absorption of well absorbed drugs is the rate of gastric emptying. Metoclopramide therefore increases the absorption rate of paracetamol (Heading, et al, 1973), in relation to the increase in gastric emptying rate. Opposite effects are seen with anticholinergic and opiate drugs. Propantheline increased the extent of absorption of one brand of digoxin tablets, presumably by allowing greater time for dissolution, since when digoxin was taken in solution, propantheline had no effect (Manninen et al, 1973). The rate, but not extent, of paracetamol absorption was however reduced both by propantheline (Heading et al, 1973) and pentazocine, pethidine and diamorphine (Nimmo, Wilson & Prescott, 1975).

The formation of chelates, ion pairs and complexes has already been alluded to. The majority of these resultant products are less soluble than the original drug and result in a reduced extent of absorption. Ion exchange resins such as cholestyramine and colestipol have been shown to decrease the extent of absorption of warfarin, thyroxine and triiodothyronine, and digitalis glycosides (Robinson, Benjamin & McCormack, 1970; Northcutt et al, 1969; Bazzano & Bazzano 1972). Para-aminosalicylic acid (PAS) may impair absorption of rifampicin presumably due to bentonite present in PAS granules. Antacids and kaolin-pectin mixtures may decrease the bioavailability of digoxin also (Brown & Juhl, 1976). There are occasions when the complex formed by an interaction is more soluble than the drug and this mechanism has been cited for the increased absorption of dicoumarol in the presence of magnesium hydroxide (Ambre & Fischer, 1973).

Drugs may interfere with absorption of other drugs more indirectly by causing malabsorption syndromes. Colchicine, neomycin and PAS may thus impair the absorption of folate, iron and vitamin B_{12} (Faloon, 1970), and neomycin can reduce the extent of digoxin absorption (Lindenbaum, Maulit & Butler, 1976).

The causes of drug absorption interactions are therefore numerous. Their importance may have been underestimated since physicians are more likely to attribute inadequate response to other factors such as poor compliance with prescribed therapy.

It would seem wise however, to advise patients who take antacids or ion-exchange resins to separate the time of administration of other drugs as much as possible, preferably up 4 to 6 hours, and in the case of PAS and rifampicin up to 8 to 12 hours (Boman et al, 1974).

Interactions due to altered drug elimination

Drugs are either excreted directly in the urine or are first metabolized by other organs (e.g. gut, liver) to more water soluble products which can be more easily excreted by the kidney. Interactions may occur during any of these processes and result in enhancement or diminution of drug effect.

Hepatic metabolism

The chemical reactions involved in drug metabolism are generally classified as phase I (oxidation, reduction or hydrolysis) or phase II reactions (conjugation with glucuronic acid, sulphates or acetates). Any drug may undergo one or more of these types of reaction before being excreted by the kidney but the most important of these are oxidation and glucuronic acid conjugation. Because of its size, enzyme content and plentiful blood supply, the liver is the major site of drug metabolism, although the intestine, lung and kidney have been shown to be other minor sites of metabolism.

The major group of drug metabolising enzymes, the cytochrome P-450 system, is extremely versatile and is responsible for the biotransformation of a large number of drugs as well as endogenous compounds. Because of its relative non-specificity, however, several interactions can take place between drugs using this route of metabolism. Before these can be discussed, it is necessary to define the quantitative aspects of drug elimination by the liver as they relate to drug clearance and half-life.

Drug clearance is a measure of the efficiency of removal of the compound and unlike half-life of elimination $(T_{\frac{1}{2}})$, is unaffected by drug distribution. Systemic clearance (Cl_s) of a drug after i.v. administration can be described by

$$Cl_s = Q\left(\frac{Cl_i}{Q + Cl_i}\right) = QE \tag{1}$$

where Q is organ blood flow and E (the extraction efficiency), is expressed in terms of intrinsic clearance Cl_i (i.e. when organ blood flow is non-limiting). For those drugs in which intrinsic clearance, and therefore extraction efficiency, is high, systemic (i.v.) clearance is rate limited by blood flow to the organ. In contrast, the systemic clearance of poorly extracted compounds is limited predominantly by the intrinsic clearance of the organ. The lower the initial extraction ratio, the more a given change in enzyme activity will alter systemic clearance (Table 3.2).

After oral administration however, changes in intrinsic clearance will equally affect the clearance of drugs both poorly and well extracted by the liver. This occurs despite the fact that the systemic clearance of the oral dose of a highly extracted drug will be much less affected by any change in intrinsic clearance analagous to after i.v. administration. The reason for this phenomenon is that increasing intrinsic clearance will increase the hepatic extraction ratio, described by a rearrangement of formula (1)

$$E = \frac{Cl_i}{Q + Cl_i} = 1\text{-}F \tag{2}$$

Table 3.2 The effect of increasing intrinsic clearance twofold on the kinetic parameters of three drugs of varying initial clearance. $T_{\frac{1}{2}}$ was calculated assuming an apparent volume of distribution of 100 litres. Liver blood flow was assumed to remain constant at 1.5 l/min

		Intrinsic (apparent oral) clearance Cl_i (l/min)	Percentage change in Cl_i (%)	Bioavailability F $(1 - E)$	Percentage change in F (%)	Systemic (intravenous) clearance Cl_s (l/min)	Percentage change in Cl_s (%)	Elimination half-life $T_{\frac{1}{2}}$ (hrs)	Percentage change in $T_{\frac{1}{2}}$ (%)
Low intrinsic clearance	A	0.1		0.94		0.09		12.8	
		0.2	+ 100	0.88	− 6	0.18	+ 100	6.4	− 50
	B	1.0		0.60		0.60		1.9	
		2.0	+ 100	0.43	− 28	0.86	+ 43	1.3	− 32
High intrinsic clearance	C	10.0		0.13		1.30		0.9	
		20.0	+ 100	0.07	− 46	1.40	+ 8	0.8	− 11

so that a much smaller proportion (F) of the highly extracted drug will reach the systemic circulation even for the first time. Thus for all drugs completely absorbed from the gut, and metabolised by the liver the area under the plasma concentration/ time curve (AUC) is described by

$$AUC = \frac{D}{Cl_i} \tag{3}$$

(where D is the dose of the drug administered) and thus independent of changes in blood flow. Two important consequences emerge from these theoretical considerations. In contrast to poorly extracted drugs, changes in enzyme activity caused by other compounds will affect plasma levels of highly extracted drugs much more after oral administration than after the intravenous route. Poorly extracted drugs will be affected approximately equally, whatever the route of administration. Table 3.2 illustrates the changes in these parameters calculated to be seen when the intrinsic clearance of three theoretical drugs of varying initial clearance is doubled. Whereas the apparent oral clearance of each is equally affected, the systemic (i.v.) clearance of the highly extracted compound is affected to a varying extent. These changes are shown in Figures 3.1 and 3.2 which also illustrate the second important consideration. The half-life of drug elimination ($T_{\frac{1}{2}}$) of orally administered highly extracted drugs will be much less affected by changes in intrinsic clerance than the half life of poorly extracted compounds. A recent example is the difference in lidocaine kinetics between six epileptic patients and six normal subjects all given an oral and intravenous dose of lidocaine on separate occasions (Perucca & Richens, 1979). The epileptic patients who were receiving chronic doses of one or more of the enzyme inducing agents phenytoin, phenobarbitone or primidone, did not differ significantly from controls in $T_{\frac{1}{2}}$ or systemic clearance. Despite this, intrinsic (apparent oral) clearance was increased by 196 per cent in the epileptics resulting in much lower plasma lidocaine concentrations than the controls after equivalent oral doses. A more clinically important interaction

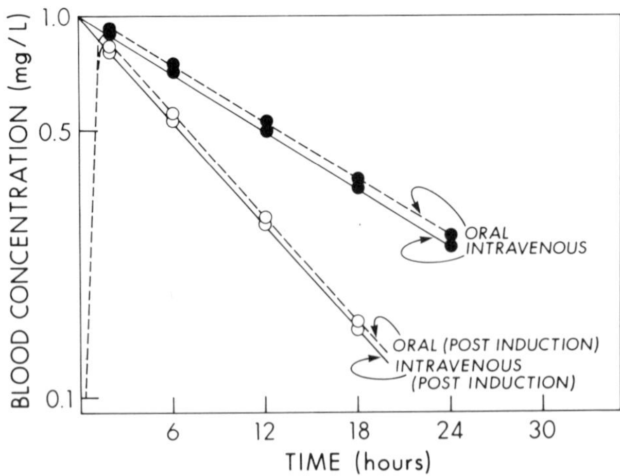

Fig. 3.1   The effect of increasing hepatic total intrinsic clearance (Cl_i) twofold on the total blood/time concentration curves of the poorly cleared drug A (in Table 3.2) after oral and intravenous administration of an equal dose (100 mg).

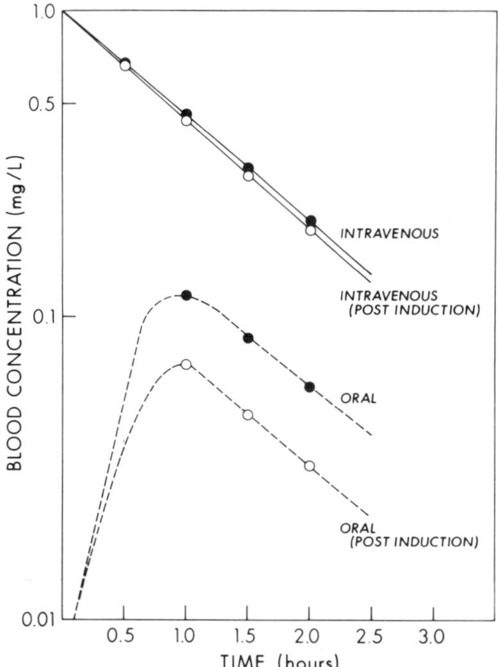

Fig. 3.2   The effect of increasing hepatic total intrinsic clearance (Cl_i) twofold on total blood concentration/time curves of the highly cleared drug C (in Table 3.2) after an oral and intravenous administration of an equal dose (100 mg).

due to enzyme induction, was reported by Alvan et al (1977). Alprenolol was administered orally and intravenously to 5 subjects before and after 10 to 14 daily doses of pentobarbitone (0.1 g). The apparent oral clearance was increased by 360 per cent yet the $T_{\frac{1}{2}}$ was reduced by only 4 per cent. Half-life of elimination ($T_{\frac{1}{2}}$) may therefore be a poorer indicator than clearance of changes in hepatic drug metabolism particularly for already highly extracted compounds.

Several agents had been implicated as inducers of hepatic drug metabolism. The more important ones are listed in Table 3.3. It is important to remember that not all patients receiving these agents will necessarily be affected since wide interindividual variation exists. There is also a lag period of approximately one to two weeks before maximum induction occurs. When the drug is stopped, there is a lag period of similar length for enzyme activity to return to preinduction levels and these phenomena may tend to disguise the causative relationship between the drug interaction and adminis-tration of the inducing agent. Although interactions involving induction usually result in decreased drug action, toxicity may occur if the production of toxic metabolites is increased. Phenobarbitone increases the demethylation of pethidine to norpethidine which may cause c.n.s. depression and prolonged sedation (Stambaugh et al, 1977).

Inhibition of drug metabolism is also a well established and potentially more serious phenomenon since it may lead directly to toxic concentrations of some drugs. Because in many cases, inhibition is of the competitive type, two simultaneously administered drugs may inhibit the metabolism of each other. Several of the compounds which have

Table 3.3   Some drugs causing enzyme induction

Group	Compound
Barbiturates	e.g. Phenobarbitone pentobarbitone
Hypnotics	Dichloralphenazone Glutethimide Ethchlorvynol
Anticonvulsants	Phenytoin Carbamazepine
Analgesics	Phenylbutazone
Antibiotics	Rifampicin
Environmental and miscellaneous agents	Lindane DDT Ethanol

been observed to cause inhibition of metabolism are listed in Table 3.4. One important interaction illustrating both inhibition and induction of drug metabolism is that between phenylbutazone and warfarin. Warfarin consists of a racemic mixture of equal parts of dextro-warfarin and laevo-warfarin. Phenylbutazone increases the clearance of dextro-warfarin and simultaneously decreases the clearance of laevo-warfarin (Lewis et al, 1974). Phenylbutazone does not therefore affect the clearance or $T_{\frac{1}{2}}$ of warfarin when it is measured as the racemate. Since laevo-warfarin is

Table 3.4   Some interactions occurring by enzyme inhibition

Drug	Metabolism inhibited by	Reference
Warfarin	phenylbutazone d-propoxyphene cimetidine metronidazole disulfiram	Lewis et al, 1974 Orme & Breckenridge, 1976; Silver et al, 1979 O'Reilly, 1976 O'Reilly, 1973
Nortriptyline	perphenazine	Gram & Overø, 1972
Phenytoin	disulfiram (Antabuse) isoniazid sulthiame chloramphenicol	Olesen, 1964 Murray, 1962 Richens & Houghton, 1973 Christensen & Skovsred, 1969
Tolbutamide	chloramphenicol phenylbutazone	Christensen & Skovsted, 1969 Tannebaum, 1974
6-mercaptopurine	allopurinol	Coffey et al, 1972
Propranolol	chlorpromazine	Vestal et al, 1979
Ketamine	diazepam secobarbital	Lo & Cumming, 1975 Domino, Domino & Zsigmond, 1979

approximately five times more potent as an anticoagulant compared with dextro-warfarin however, the overall effect of the interaction is to augment the hypo-prothrombinaemia produced by the racemic drug.

It can be seen from equation (1) that liver blood flow is an important determinant of hepatic systemic clearance of drugs. Whereas changes in intrinsic clearance will have more effect on the systemic clearance of poorly cleared drugs, and changes in liver blood flow will have little effect, the converse is true for highly cleared agents. When intrinsic clearance is high compared with liver blood flow the term

$$\frac{Cl_i}{Q + Cl_i}$$

approaches unity so that systemic (intravenous) clearance is directly proportional to liver blood flow. Estimates of liver blood flow have varied from approximately 0.8 to 2.2 litres/minute (Kornhauser et al, 1978). Therefore changes in drug clearance by this mechanism in excess of two-to threefold are unlikely and no clinically important interactions of this type have yet been described in man. The hepatic elimination of intravenous lignocaine was reduced by propranolol, which reduces liver blood flow as a result of beta-adrenergic blockade, but not by the pharmacologically inactive isomer d-propranolol, in dogs (Branch et al, 1973). The possibility of haemodynamic drug interactions in man awaits further investigation.

Renal excretion

Drugs are excreted by the kidney both by glomerular filtration and tubular secretion. They may then be reabsorbed by the process of active tubular reabsorption. Changes in any of these processes induced by one agent may result in altered excretion of another compound.

Frusemide in low doses may reduce the renal clearance of cephaloridine and gentamicin and this has been attributed to a frusemide induced reduction in glomerular filtration rate (GFR) (Tilstone et al, 1977). Other work has indicated, however, that frusemide may increase GFR so although frusemide may increase the nephrotoxicity of cephalosporins and the ototoxicity of gentamicin the role of altered GFR in these interactions is unclear.

Tubular secretion is an active process by which some acids and bases are transported into tubular fluid against a concentration gradient. Competition for this relatively non-specific process between two acidic or two basic drugs may lead to diminished excretion of one or both of the agents. Clinically significant interactions will only occur, however, if this process is responsible for major proportion of the total excretion of the drug(s). Probenecid and salicylates can reduce the elimination of methotrexate by this mechanism and may lead to severe toxicity if methotrexate dosage is not adjusted accordingly (Aherne et al, 1978; Liegler et al, 1969). No clinically significant interactions occurring by this mechanism involving basic drugs have yet been described.

Recent data suggest that quinidine can reduce the renal clearance of digoxin (Doering, 1979; Hager et al, 1979). Displacement of the glycoside from tissues also occurs leading to a reduced volume of distribution. As a result of these offsetting changes, $T_{\frac{1}{2}}$ changes little (see also below). Weak bases are less ionised when the urine is alkalinised by other agents. Acetazolamide and antacids, which render urine alkaline, have thus caused toxicity due to impaired excretion of the basic compound, amphetamine (Davis et al, 1971) and also reduce quinidine excretion by the kidney (Gerhardt et al, 1969).

Conversely alkalinisation of urine may increase the excretion of acidic drugs such as salicylate and phenobarbitone and this interaction has been put to clinical use in the treatment of poisoning by these agents with forced alkaline diuresis. It has recently been appreciated however that the so-called 'non-systemic' antacids such as aluminium and magnesium hydroxide may increase urine pH significantly (Gibaldi, Grunhofer & Levy, 1974). This mechanism has been implicated in the reduced serum salicylate concentrations seen in children with rheumatic fever who received aspirin and antacids concomitantly (Levy, Lampman & Kamath, 1975).

Changes in drug distribution

Most drugs do not merely distribute throughout body fluids but are bound or in some cases actively transported into blood and tissue elements. Interactions involving redistribution have been little studied because of the limitations of available methodologies for measuring unbound and bound concentrations in tissue compartments. The paucity of clinical examples of these interactions may therefore reflect this limited knowledge rather than the unimportance of these mechanisms. Changes in drug binding in the circulation may also affect the clearance of many drugs and may have different effects on highly cleared and poorly-cleared compounds. These effects will first be discussed and their clinical significance evaluated.

Poorly cleared compounds have been termed restrictively-eliminated compounds since their clearance, either by glomerular filtration or by the liver metabolism, is limited by their degree of binding in the blood. This occurs when the extraction ratio of the drug is less than the free fraction of that drug in blood. Displacement of such compounds from plasma protein binding sites will cause an immediate rise in free drug concentration. This increase will only be temporary however, since the increase in free fraction will allow more of the drug to be eliminated until a new steady state is reached when the unbound (free) concentration returns to its original level (Fig. 3.3). Permanent changes will be seen in the total plasma concentration since total clearance of the drug has been increased.

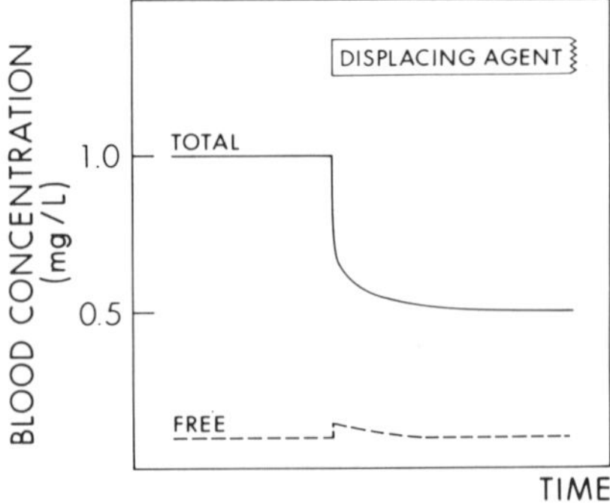

Fig. 3.3   The effects of doubling the free fraction in blood of compound poorly cleared by the liver. The drug is assumed to be initially 90 per cent bound to albumin in blood but not to tissues and to be distributed in total body water.

The magnitude of the temporary increase of unbound drug will depend on the original volume of distribution of the displaced drug, the original degree of binding in the blood, and the degree of binding to tissues. Thus it is likely that only when poorly cleared drugs have a high degree of binding in blood and poor binding to tissues, will plasma protein displacement interactions cause, albeit temporarily, a significant increase in free drug concentration. Warfarin fulfils these criteria. Unfortunately several drugs which have been shown to displace warfarin from plasma binding sites such as clofibrate (Bjornsson et al, 1979) and phenylbutazone (Aggeler et al, 1967), or increase plasma binding such as heparin (Nilsen, Storstein and Jacobsen, 1977; Routledge et al, 1979) also interact in other ways with warfarin. It is therefore difficult to quantitate the effect produced by the transient increase in free drug concentration. Chloral hydrate's metabolite trichloracetic acid can displace warfarin from its plasma protein binding sites and this may be responsible for the temporary increase in warfarin's anticoagulant effect (Sellers & Koch-Weser, 1970).

Many drugs are effectively cleared by the body so that the extraction ratio of the eliminating organ(s) is greater than, and therefore not limited by, the fraction of drug free in the blood (Routledge & Shand, 1979). Displacement of these compounds from plasma binding sites will theoretically result in a permanent increase in *free* drug concentration but only a temporary increase in *total* drug concentration in blood (Fig. 3.4). The magnitude of the permanent increase in free drug concentration will also depend on the relative degrees of initial binding in blood and tissues, being greatest for drugs with high binding in blood and poor tissue binding. To date, no clinically important interactions involving this mechanism alone have been described for highly cleared drugs.

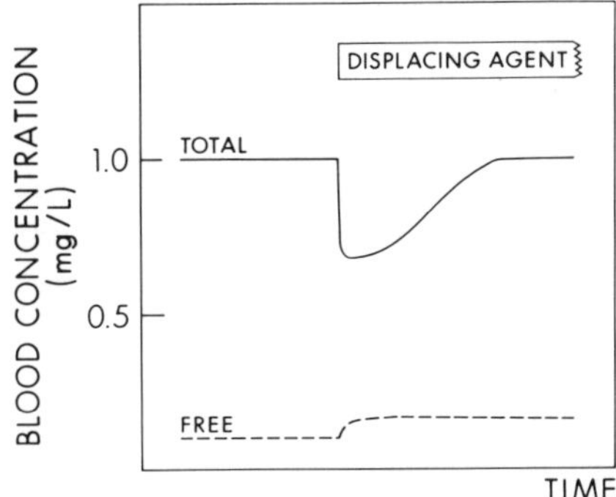

Fig. 3.4   The effects of doubling the free fraction in blood of a compound highly cleared by the liver and with the same distribution parameters as the drug described in Figure 3.3.

Drugs are also bound or taken up by extravascular tissue sites and alterations in tissue binding are likely to have marked effects on drug disposition (Gillette, 1971). It has been calculated by Gillette (1971) that even when 90 per cent of drug in plasma is bound to albumin, the amount of bound drug would only represent about 50 per cent of the total drug in the body. In contrast, if 90 per cent of drug in muscle were bound, this would represent 85 per cent of the total amount of drug in the body because of the size of this tissue compartment. Clearly, therefore, even small changes in tissue binding would markedly alter the amount of drug in the unbound form. The time course of these changes should, as with changes in plasma protein binding, depend on whether the drug is highly cleared or poorly cleared. Thus the free blood concentration of poorly cleared drugs should be only transiently altered by changes in tissue binding although total blood concentration will be permanently affected. Conversely the free blood concentration of highly cleared drugs should theoretically remain altered after tissue displacement occurs. Total blood concentration will however return to control values. We have recently observed that a bolus dose of heparin (1000 units i.v.) can temporarily increase the unbound concentration of diazepam in blood by 92 per cent and of propranolol by 20 per cent after oral administration of single doses of these agents (unpublished observations). This effect is presumed to be due to displacement of these compounds from their binding sites on albumin by non-esterified fatty acid (NEFA) formation after heparin induced lipolysis. The temporary nature of this interaction is also related in time to a return of NEFA to control levels. The magnitude of the changes in free drug concentration strongly suggest that displacement of drug from extravascular binding sites is taking place and it is known that 60 per cent of the albumin in the body lies outside the vascular compartment (Jusko & Gretch, 1976). The clinical significance of these interactions again is presently unknown.

A clinically important interaction thought to involve tissue displacement has been observed between digoxin and quinidine (Ejvinsson, 1978; Reiffel et al, 1978). Total serum digoxin concentrations were approximately 2.5-fold higher when quinidine was prescribed to 38 patients (Doering, 1979). Tissue displacement of digoxin by quinidine is suggested by a 36 per cent reduction in the volume of distribution of digoxin during quinidine administration (Hager et al, 1979). There is evidence however that renal clearance of digoxin is also reduced by quinidine so that this may be the most important mechanism of the interaction between these two drugs (Hager et al, 1979, Doering, 1979).

The interaction between digoxin and quinidine illustrates the fact that all classifications of drug interactions by mechanism are somewhat arbitrary, since many interactions occur by multiple mechanisms. Several examples (e.g. phenylbutazone and warfarin) have already been given. Inhibition of active transport of one drug into or out of a tissue compartment by another agent is another important mechanism of redistributional interactions. The adrenergic neurone blocking drugs guanethidine, bethanidine and debrisoquine are all substrates for the amine pump which normally takes up noradrenaline into the adrenergic nerve ending. Inhibitors of this pump such as imipramine, amitriptyline and even chlorpromazine prevent uptake of these neurone blocking drugs and thus antagonise their antihypertensive effect. Blockade of the noradrenaline pump also potentiates the pressor effects of directly acting sympathomimetics such as noradrenaline and may result in severe hypertension (Mitchell et al, 1970). Amphetamines also antagonise guanethidine's effect but in this case, amphetamines may directly displace guanethidine from the adrenergic neurone (Oates et al, 1971).

Recent work in animals has shown that in addition to its effect on active renal tubular secretion, probenecid can inhibit the excretion of methotrexate out of cerebrospinal fluid by a similar mechanism (Ramu et al, 1978). This mechanism may be clinically significant in man and further study of its importance is necessary.

PHARMACODYNAMIC INTERACTIONS

Pharmacodynamic interactions occur when one drug alters the response of another by interaction at the receptor site or acts at a different site to enhance or diminish the primary drug's effects.

The interactions which were first recognised are those in which drugs act at the same receptor site. Some of the important receptors, their function and the drugs which act on them are shown in Table 3.5. Drugs which combine with the receptor to

Table 3.5   Some interactions occurring at the receptor site

Receptor type	Some effects mediated by agonist	Typical agonists	Typical antagonists
Adrenergic: α	Väsoconstriction of skin & coronary vessels	Phenylephrine Methoxamine Noradrenaline	Phentolamine Phenoxybenzamine
β₁	Bronchoconstriction Increased intropic and chronotripic effect on heart	Dobutamine	Atenolol Metoprolol Propranolol
β₂	Vasodilatation of skin and coronary vessels Bronchodilatation	Salbutomol Terbutaline	Propranolol
Dopaminergic	Renal vasodilation Central nervous neurotransmission	Dopamine Bromocriptine	Haloperidol Chlorpromazine
Cholinergic (nicotinic)	Neuromuscular transmission	Acetycholine	d-tubocurarine gallamine
Cholinergic (muscarinic)	Decreased heart rate	Actylcholine	Atropine Benzhexol
Histaminergic: H₁	Bronchoconstriction *v.c.* vasodilatation	Histamine	Chlorpheniramine
H₂	Stimulation of gastric acid secretion	Histamine	Cimetidine
Opiate receptors	Regulation of pain perception	Morphine	Naloxone

initiate a response are termed agonists. Drugs which interact with the receptor to inhibit the action of an agonist but which do not initiate a response themselves are termed antagonists. Antagonism may be competitive when increasing the agonist concentration restores its effects completely, or it may be non-competitive (irreversible). Partial agonists act on the same receptor as the agonist to initiate a minor response but by occupying a significant fraction of the receptors, they antagonise the action of more potent agonists. Thus naloxone is a potent antagonist of the agonist action of morphine. Nalorphine however, although possessing antagonist activity, is also a partial agonist and may add to respiratory depression produced by morphine. Many of the interactions at the receptor site are used to advantage clinically, either to antagonise or augment the effect of endogenous mediators or to counteract toxicity due to overdose of administered agents. Unwanted interactions most commonly occur when one fails to realise that a drug which acts at one receptor may also act at another receptor. Antihistamines, which block H_1 receptors also have muscarinic anticholinergic activity, for example, as do some phenothiazines and tricyclic antidepressants and co-administration of two or more of these agents may lead to excessive anticholinergic activity. Conversely some tricyclic antidepressants, particularly the tertiary amines doxepin and amitriptyline, are potent H_1 receptor blockers, although the clinical significance of this property is still unclear (Richelson, 1979).

Pharmacodynamic interactions may also occur when two drugs act at separate sites to cause potentiation, summation or antagonism of their normal actions. Such interactions are often used clinically in therapy of angina (e.g. beta blockers and vasodilators), hypertension (beta blockers and diuretics) and malignant disease (combined cytotoxic chemotherapy). They may also occur inadvertently however. Several drugs, including anabolic steroids, clofibrate, quinidine and salicylates an act on the synthesis of vitamin K dependent clotting factors or the normal coagulation mechanism to potentiate the anticoagulant action of warfarin. Another long-recognised example is the ability of diuretic-induced hypokalaemia to potentiate digitalis toxicity.

AVOIDANCE OF ADVERSE DRUG INTERACTIONS

An inordinate proportion of serious adverse interaction occurs with a relatively small number of therapeutic agents. These are generally drugs in which the therapeutic ratio, i.e. difference between effective and toxic concentrations, is small, such as oral anticoagulants, cytotoxic drugs, anticonvulsants, hypotensive and hypoglycaemic agents. The co-administration of barbiturates and warfarin remains the commonest potential anticoagulant interaction by far, despite wide publicity of the problems involved (Hull et al, 1978). Special care should be taken when these groups of drugs are prescribed, particularly to sick patients who are also receiving several other agents. The number of drugs precribed and changes in drug therapy should be kept to an absolute minimum and the patient warned of the possible dangers of suddenly changing his own therapy or taking non-prescription remedies.

On a broader front, more sensitive and reliable parameters of drug effect are needed. It is reassuring to note that when physicians have a reliable and simple measure of drug effect as in the case of anticoagulants and the one-stage prothrombin time, drug interactions are often quickly recognised and appropriate adjustment of therapy is made.

REFERENCES

Aggeler P M, O'Reilly R A, Leong L, Kowitz P E 1967 Potentiation of anticoagulant effect of warfarin by phenylbutazone. New England Journal of Medicine 276: 496–501

Aherne G W, Piall E, Marks V, Mould G, White W F 1978 Prolongation and enhancement of serum methotrexate concentration by probenecid. British Medical Journal 1: 1097–1099

Alvan G, Piafsky K, Lind M, Bahr C 1977 Effect of pentobarbital on the disposition of alprenolol. Clinical Pharmacology and Therapeutics 22: 316–321

Ambre J J, Fischer L F 1973 Effect of coadministration of aluminum and magnesium hydroxides on absorption of anticoagulants in man. Clinical Pharmacology and Therapeutics 14: 231–237

Avery G S (ed) 1976 Drug Treatment: Principles and practice of clinical pharmacology and therapeutics. Sydney ADIS Press

Avery G S 1977 Drug interactions that really matter: A guide to major importance drug interactions. Drugs 14: 132–146

Barr W H, Adir J, Garrettson L 1971 Decrease of tetracycline absorption in man by sodium bicarbonate. Clinical Pharmacology and Therapeutics 12: 779–784

Bazzano G, Bazzano G S 1972 Digitalis intoxication. Treatment with a new steroid-binding resin. Journal of the American Medical Assocation 220: 828–830

Bjornsson T D, Meffin P J, Swezey S, Blaschke T F 1979 Clofibrate displaces warfarin from plasma proteins in man: An example of a pure displacement interaction. Journal of Pharmacology and Experimental Therapeutics 210: 316–321

Boman G, Morselli P L, Garattini S, Cohen S N (eds) 1974 Drug interactions. Raven Press, New York

Borda I T, Slone D, Jick H 1968 Assessment of adverse reactions within a drug surveillance program. Journal of the American Medical Association 205: 645–647

Boston Collaborative Drug Surveillance Program 1977 Adverse drug interactions. Journal of the American Medical Association 220: 1238–1239

Branch R A, Shand D G, Wilkinson G R, Nies A S 1973 The reduction of lidocaine clearance by dl-propranolol: an example of hemodynamic drug interaction. Journal of Pharmacology and Experimental Therapeutics 184: 515–519

Brown D D, Juhl R D 1976 Decreased bioavailability of digoxin due to antacids and kaolin-pectin. New England Journal of Medicine 295: 1034–1937

Christensen L K, Skovsted L 1969 Inhibition of drug metabolism by chloramphenicol. Lancet 2: 1397–1399

Coffey J J, White C A, Lesk A B, Rogers W I, Serpick A A 1972 Effect of allopurinol on the pharmacokinetics of 6-mercaptopurine (NSC 755) in cancer patients. Cancer Research 32: 1283–1289

Cohen S N, Armstrong M F 1974 Drug interactions: A handbook for clinical use. Williams & Wilkins, Baltimore

Cooke A R, Hunt J N, 1970 Absorption of acetylsalicylic acid from unbuffered and buffered gastric contents. American Journal of Digestive Diseases 15: 95–102

Davis J M, Kopin I J, Lemberger L, Axelrod J 1971 Effects of urinary pH on amphetamine metabolism. Annals of the New York Academy of Science 179: 493–501

Doering W 1979 Quinidine-digoxin interaction pharmacokinetics, underlying mechanism and clinical implications. New England Journal of Medicine 301: 400–404

Domino L E, Domino E. F, Zsigmond E K 1979 Enhancement of ketamine plasma levels by diazepam in man. Clinical Research 27: 716A

Ejvinsson G 1978 Effect of quinidine on plasma concentrations of digoxin. British Medical Journal 1: 279–280

Faloon W W 1970 Drug production of intestinal malabsorption. New York State Journal of Medicine 70: 2189–2191

Gerhardt R E, Knouss R P, Thyrum P T, Luchi R J, Morris J J 1969 Quinidine excretion in aciduria and alkaluria. Annals of Internal Medicine 71: 927–933

Gibaldi M, Grundhofer B, Levy G 1974 Effect of antacids on pH of urine. Clinical Pharmacology and Therapeutics 16: 520–525

Gillette J R 1971 Factors affecting drug metabolism. Annals of the New York Academy of Science 179: 43–66

Gram L F, Overø K F, 1972 Drug interaction: Inhibitory effect of neuroleptics on metabolism of tricyclic antidepressants in man. British Medical Journal 1: 463–465

Hager W D, Fenster P E, Mayersohn M, Perrier D G, Graves P E, Marcus F I 1979 Digoxin-quinidine interaction: pharmacokinetic evaluation. Clinical Research 27: 233A

Hansen P D 1975 Drug interactions 3rd edn Lea and Febiger, Philadelphia

Heading R C, Nimmo J, Prescott L F, Tothill P 1973 The dependence of paracetamol absorption on the rate of gastric emptying British Journal of Pharmacology 47: 415–421

Hull J H, Murray W J, Brown H S, Williams B O, Chi S L, Koch G G 1978 Potential anticoagulant drug interactions in ambulatory patients. Clinical Pharmacology and Therapeutics 24: 644–649

Jusko W J, Gretch M 1976 Plasma and tissue protein binding of drugs in pharmacokinetics. Drug Metabolism Reviews 5: 43–140

Kornhauser D M, Wood A J J, Vestal R E, Wilkinson G R, Branch R A, Shand D G 1978 Biological determinants of propranolol disposition in man. Clinical Pharmacology and Therapeutics 23: 165–174

Levy G, Lampman T, Kamath B L 1975 Decreased serum salicylate concentrations in children with rheumatic fever treated with antacid. New England Journal of Medicine 293: 323–325

Lewis R J, Trager W, Chan K, Breckenridge A, Orme M, Rowland M, Schary M 1974 Warfarin — stereochemical aspects of its metabolism and the interaction with phenylbutazone. Journal of Clinical Investigation 53: 1607–1617

Liegler D G, Henderson E S, Hahn M A, Oliveria V T 1969 The effect of organic acids on renal clearance of methotrexate in man. Clinical Pharmacology and Therapeutics 10: 849

Lindenbaum J, Maulitz M, Butler V P, Jr 1976 Inhibition of digoxin absorption by neomycin. Gastroenterology 71: 399–404

Lo J N, Cumming J F 1975 Interaction between sedative premedicants and ketamine in man and in isolated perfused rat livers. Anesthesiology 43: 307–312

Manninen V, Apajalathi A, Melin J, Karesoja M 1973 Altered absorption of digoxin in patients given propantheline and metoclopramide. Lancet 1: 398–401

May F E, Stewart R B, Cluff L E 1974 Drug use in the hospital. Evaluation of determinants. Clinical Pharmacology and Therapeutics 16: 834–835

May F E, Stewart R B, Cluff L E 1977 Drug interactions and multiple drug administration. Clinical Pharmacology and Therapeutics 22: 322–328

Mitchell J R, Cavanaugh J H, Arias L, Oates J A 1970 Guanethidine and related agents III. Antagonism by drugs which inhibit the norepinephrine pump in man. Journal of Clinical Investigation 49: 1596–1604

Murray F J 1962 Outbreak of unexpected reactions among epileptics taking isoniazid. American Review of Respiratory Diseases 86: 729–732

Nilsen O G, Storstein L, Jacobsen S 1977 Effect of heparin and fatty acids on the binding of quinidine and warfarin in plasma. Biochemical Pharmacology 26: 229–235

Nimmo W S, Wilson, J, Prescott L F 1975 Narcotic analgesics and delayed gastric emptying during labour. Lancet 1: 890–893

Northcutt R C, Stiel J N, Hollified J W, Stant E G 1969 The influence of cholestyramine on thyroxine absorption. Journal of the American Medical Association 208: 1857–1861

Oates J A, Mitchell J R, Feagin O T, Kaufmann J S, Shand D G 1971 Distribution of guanidinium anitihypertensives-mechanism of their selective action. Annals of the New York Academy of Science 179: 302–308

Olesen O V 1966 Disulfiram (Antabuse) as an inhibitor of phenytoin metabolism. Acta Pharmacologica et Toxicologica 24: 317–322

O'Reilly R A 1973 Interaction of sodium warfarin and disulfiram (Antabuse) in man. Annals of Internal Medicine 78: 73–76

O'Reilly R A 1976A The stereoselective interaction of warfarin and metronidazole in man. New England Journal of Medicine 295: 354–357

Orme M, Breckenridge A 1976 Warfarin and distalgesic interaction. British Medical Journal 1: 200

Perucca E, Richens A 1979 Reduction of oral bioavailability of lignocaine by induction of first pass metabolism in epileptic patients. British Journal of Clinical Pharmacology 8: 21–31

Ramu A, Glaubiger D, Ramu N P, Eldridge N, Blaschke T F 1978 Probenecid inhibition of methotrexate excretion from cerebrospinal fluid in dogs. Journal of Pharmacokinetics and Biopharmaceutics 6: 389–397

Reiffel A, Leahey E B, Drusin R E 1978 A digoxin/quinidine adverse drug interaction. American Journal of Cardiology 41: 368

Richelson E 1979 Tricyclic antidepressants and histamine H_1 receptors. Mayo Clinic Proceedings 54: 669–674

Richens A, Houghton G W 1973 Phenytoin intoxication caused by sulthiame. Lancet 2: 1442–1443

Robinson D S, Benjamin D M, McCormack J J 1970 Interaction of warfarin and non-systemic gastrointestinal drugs. Clinical Pharmacology and Therapeutics 12: 491–495

Routledge P A, Bjornsson T D, Kitchell B B, Shand D G 1979 Heparin administration increases plasma warfarin binding in man. British Journal of Clinical Pharmacology 8: 281–282

Routledge P A, Shand D G, 1979 Presystemic drug elimination. Annual Review of Pharmacology and Toxicology 19: 447–468

Sellers E M, Koch-Weser J 1970 Potentiation of warfarin-induced hypoprothrombinemia by chloral hydrate. New England Journal of Medicine 283: 827–831

Silver B A, Bell W R 1979 Cimetidine potentiation of the hypoprothrombinemic effect of warfarin. Annals of Internal Medicine 90: 348–349

Smith J W, Seidl L G, Cluff L E 1966 Studies on the epidemiology of adverse drug reactions. V. Clinical factors influencing susceptibility. Annals of Internal Medicine 65: 629–640

Stambugh J E, Wainer I W, Hemphill D M, Schwartz I 1977 A potentially toxic drug interaction between pethidine (meperidine) and phenobarbitone. Lancet 1: 398–399

Stockley I 1973 Drug interactions. Pharmaceutical press, London p 78

Tannenbaum H, Anderson L G, Soeldner J S 1974 Phenylbutazone-tolbutamide drug interaction. New England Journal of Medicine 290: 344

Tilstone W J, Semple P F, Lawson D H, Boyle J A 1977 Effects of furosemide on glomerular filtration rate and clearance of practolol, digoxin, cephaloridine, and gentamicin. Clinical Pharmacology and Therapeutics 22: 389–394

Vestal R E, Kornhauser D M, Hollified J W, Shand D G 1979 Inhibition of propranolol metabolism by chlorpromazine. Clinical Pharmacology and Therapeutics 25: 19–24

4. Pharmacokinetics

A. Breckenridge   M. L'E. Orme

Pharmacology is a hybrid discipline and clinical pharmacology, the scientific study of drugs in man, especially so. Clinical pharmacology is first concerned with the investigation of how drugs affect the body to produce both therapeutic and toxic effects, i.e. pharmacodynamics. Second, it addresses itself to the investigation of what the body does to drugs both in health and disease; the mathematical description of the processes of drug absorption, distribution, metabolism and excretion is collectively known as pharmacokinetics. This topic has made significant advances over the past few years for two main reasons. First, methods for drug analysis have improved in terms of innovation, specificity and sensitivity, so that there are few drugs in therapeutic use whose concentration in biological fluids cannot now be measured. Second, the mathematical approach to pharmacology by producing a variety of models of varying complexity which envisage the body as a series of compartments has given great insight into the biological problems of drug handling. Thus, if a drug cannot reach a specified site in the body, e.g. the brain, it is unlikely that it will exert an effect in that area.

Many drugs act by forming reversible bonds with receptors, and the effect of the drug is related to its concentration in the fluid surrounding the receptor. Further, concentration of drug in tissue may depend on its plasma concentration because in most instances drug is conveyed to tissues via the blood. Thus, the onset, duration and intensity of the pharmacological effect should be reflected by the concentration of drug in plasma; Figure 4.1 illustrates some of the factors that influence the amount and persistence of drug in the body and thus pharmacological effects.

PHYSICOCHEMICAL CONSIDERATIONS

There are three important physicochemical properties of a drug molecule which will largely influence its behaviour in the body: (a) lipid solubility, (b) extent to which it is ionized, and (c) molecular size. Many therapeutic agents are highly soluble in lipids and this property allows them to cross the gastrointestinal wall, to gain access to their sites of action, to cross the placenta or the blood brain barrier. Having been filtered through the glomerulus, lipid soluble drugs will be almost completely reabsorbed during their passage through the nephron. Such drugs would remain in the body for an indefinite period unless they were metabolised to more water soluble metabolites which can be excreted in the urine. Drug molecules are transferred across cell membranes mainly by passive diffusion — the movement of drug molecules down a concentration gradient. Many drugs can be considered as weak electrolytes and exist in two forms, ionized or unionized. It is widely and reasonably assumed that only unionized drug is sufficiently lipid soluble to diffuse across most biological mem-

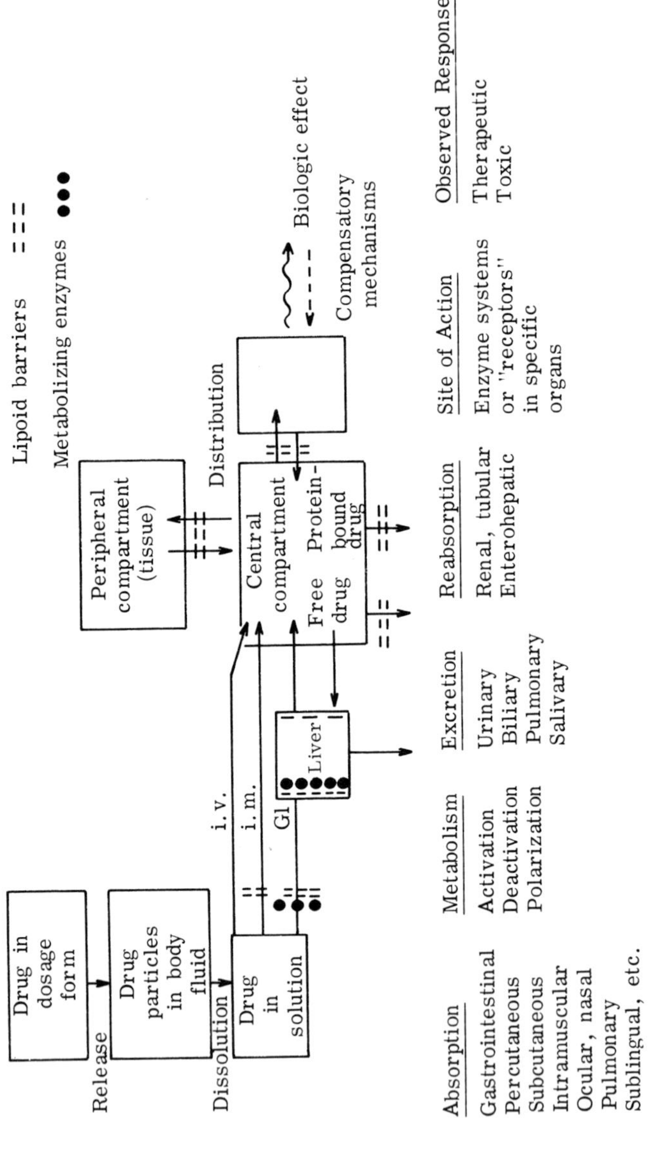

Fig. 4.1 Factors influencing amount and persistence of drug in the body. (From Barr W H 1968 American Journal of Pharmaceutical Education 52: 958.)

branes. A highly ionized water soluble drug will pass through the pores of the biological membrane if it is of small molecular size and the limit for this is usually considered as a molecular weight of less than 100. Almost all drugs have a molecular weight considerably in excess of 100 and thus cannot pass through pores, a notable exception being lithium carbonate.

The extent to which a drug is ionized depends on the pH of the medium and the pKa of the drug. The pKa of a drug is defined as the pH at which the drug is 50 per cent ionized. The relationship between a weak acidic drug, its pKa and the pH of the solution is defined mathematically in the Henderson-Hasselbalch equation

$$pH = pKa + \log\frac{A^-}{HA}$$

where HA is the concentration of unionized acidic drug and A^- represents the concentration of the ionized drug. If the equation is rearranged such that

$$\log\frac{A^-}{HA} = pH - pKa$$

it can be seen that small changes in pH near the pKa of a weak acidic drug will markedly affect its degree of ionization in the body. An example of this is phenobarbitone, a weakly acidic drug with a pKa of 7.2. This information is used in 'forced alkaline diuresis', whereby in an alkaline urine most of the phenobarbitone will be ionized and thus not reabsorbed from the renal tubule. Warfarin, an acidic drug with a pKa of 5.1 is unionized at gastric pH (1.4) which will aid its absorption. On the other hand, basic drugs will tend to be excreted in the stomach since they will be ionized at gastric pH and unable to cross back through the gastric mucosa.

KINETIC CONSIDERATIONS

One-compartment model (Fig. 4.2)

Pharmacokinetics deals with the mathematical description of the biological processes which affect the time course of the absorption and fate of drugs. The simplest description is to consider the body as a single compartment. In this model it is assumed that drugs are homogeneously and instantly distributed throughout the fluids and tissues of the body.

The one compartment has a defined volume V and this is referred to as the apparent volume of distribution (Vd) of the drug. The apparent volume of distribution is really a proportionality constant which describes the amount of drug in the body relative to

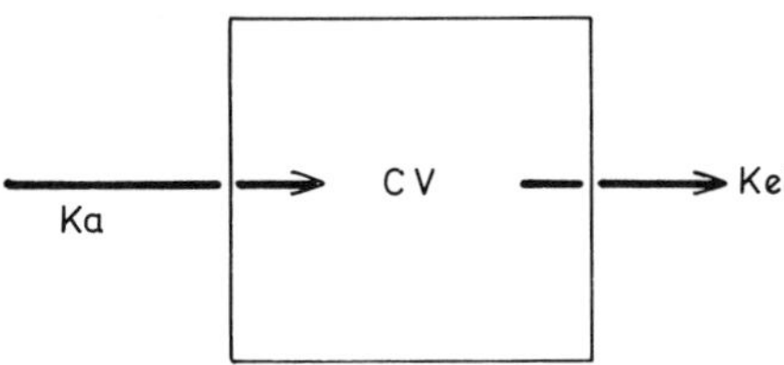

Fig. 4.2   Representation of the one compartment model where Ka is the absorption rate constant, V is the volume of the compartment, C the drug concentration and Kel is the elimination rate constant.

that in plasma at any one time, and as such has no direct physiological meaning. The term Ka represents a rate constant of absorption of drug into the body and Kel is the rate constant for elimination of the drug from the body. Most processes in pharmacokinetics can be described satisfactorily by first order kinetics. Thus the rate at which a drug enters or leaves a compartment is proportional to the concentration of drug in it and the higher the concentration the more drug enters or leaves it in any given time. This can be illustrated in Figure 4.3 in which the plasma concentration of antipyrine is plotted over 50 hours after a single oral dose of 600 mg. Note that the plasma concentration scale is logarithmic, which converts the usual exponential decay slope into a straight line, and the slope of the line gives the rate constant in terms of half-life $(T_{\frac{1}{2}})$, the time required for any given drug concentration to decrease by half. In the case of Figure 4.3 the plasma half life of antipyrine is 10.5 hours.

In a one-compartment model proposed for antipyrine the plasma concentration (Cp) is directly proportional to the amount of drug in the compartment. Thus

$$\frac{d}{dt}Cp = KCp \tag{1}$$

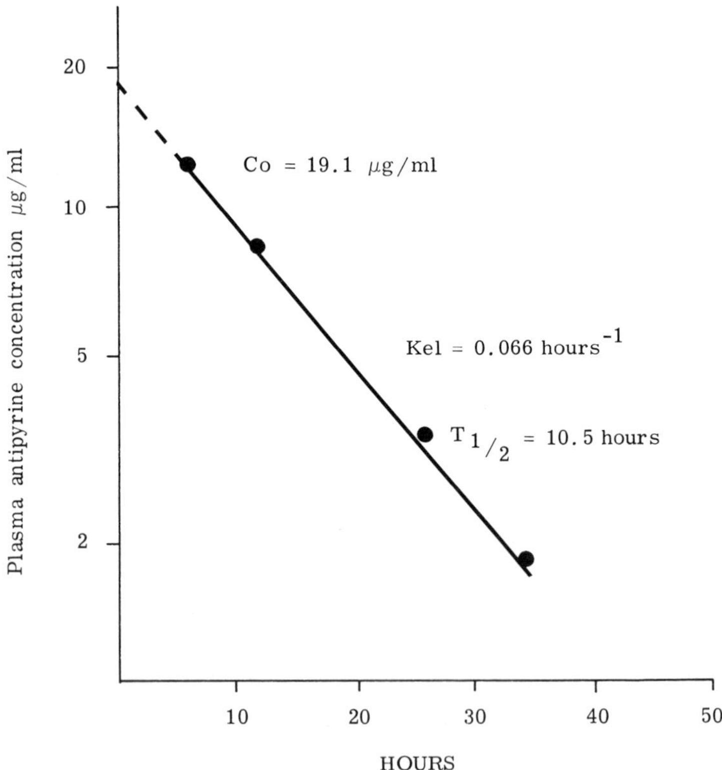

Fig. 4.3 An illustration of the one compartment model. Plasma concentration curve of antipyrine after a single oral dose of 600 mg to a healthy volunteer. The drug is eliminated by first order processes and thus the disappearance curve becomes linear if plotted as above on log-linear paper. [From Avery (ed) 1976 Drug therapy. Adis Press, Sydney, p 6.]

which, upon integration with respect to t(time) gives

$$Cp = Cp_0 e^{-kt} \qquad (2)$$

where Cp_0 is the concentration at time zero.

To calculate the half life of antipyrine

$$Cp = \frac{Cp_0}{2}$$

thus $\qquad Cp_0 = Cp_0 e^{-kt_{\frac{1}{2}}} \qquad\qquad (3)$

or $\qquad \log_e \frac{1}{2} = Kt_{\frac{1}{2}} \qquad\qquad (4)$

or $\qquad t_{\frac{1}{2}} = \frac{0.693}{K} \qquad\qquad (5)$

If we extrapolate the decay slope back to zero time, we get a value for this plasma concentration at zero time (Co) of 19.1 μg/ml. This concentration enables us to give a figure for the apparent volume of distribution by dividing the dose 600 mg (or 600 000 μg) by the value for Co (19.1 μg/ml). The result gives a figure of 31 413 ml (31.4 litres) which for a 60 kg man in fact equates with total body water.

The rate of elimination of a drug varies among individuals to a considerable extent. If a drug is excreted unchanged in the urine (e.g. digoxin, gentamicin) the elimination rate will depend upon renal function. Many drugs depend for their elimination on metabolism, usually in the liver, and rates of metabolism can vary 30-fold among individuals. Metabolism, like absorption and elimination, is nearly always a 'first order' process. Zero order metabolism, where the rate proceeds at a constant speed independent of the concentration of the drug in the body, applies to relatively few situations. Examples of drugs whose elimination is zero order are phenytoin, dicoumarol, salicylic acid and perhaps alcohol.

Two-compartment model
It is surprising, given the simplicity of the one compartment model, how often it describes the processes which take place after drug administration to man. However, there are situations when the log plasma concentration versus time yields two linear portions rather than one, and this is illustrated in Figure 4.4. This may be seen after an intravenous injection of a drug such as lignocaine, with an initial rapid decay slope followed by a slower decay. The first phase is considered to represent mainly distribution of the drug into body tissues and the second slower phase represents elimination. The elimination rate constant is calculated from the second or β decay slope and the slope of the first (or α) phase can be calculated by the method of residuals, and the interested reader is referred elsewhere (e.g. Greenblatt & Koch-Weser, 1975) for this methodology.

The two-compartment model likens the body to central and peripheral compartments, which are inter-connected as illustrated in Figure 4.5. It is usual but not obligatory to consider absorption and elimination to occur into and from the central compartment.

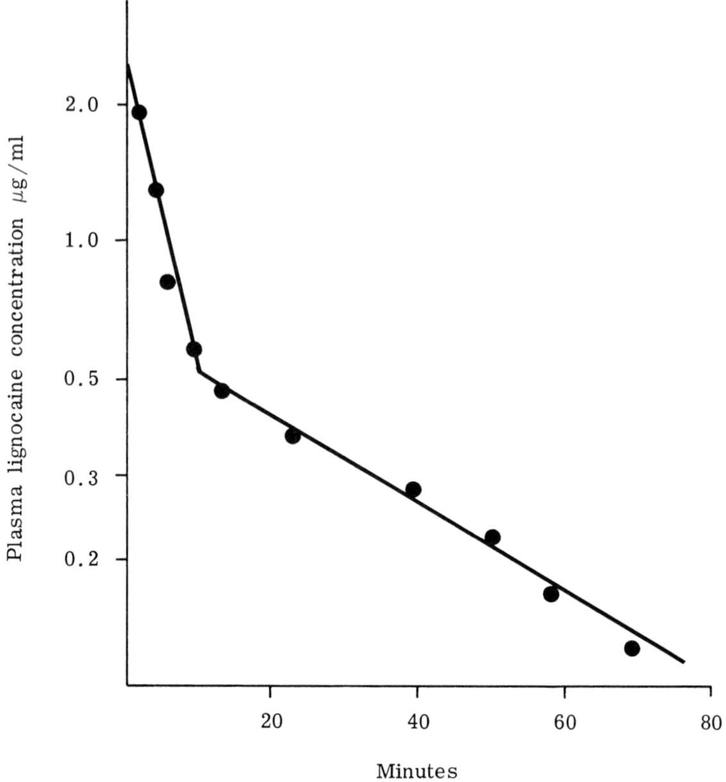

Fig. 4.4 Log plasma lignocaine concentration V time after a single intravenous dose of 50 mg

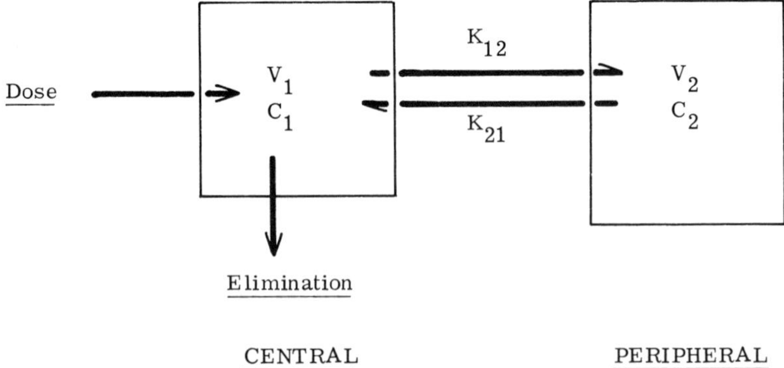

Fig. 4.5 Representation of the two compartment open model where the dose is absorbed into and the drug eliminated from the central compartment (C_1) which is volume V_1. The peripheral compartment (C_2) has a volume of V_2 and the transfer of the drugs between the two compartments is represented by the two rate constant K_{12} and K_{21}

BIOAVAILABILITY

An important application of pharmacokinetics is in the determination of the proportion of unchanged drug that reaches the systemic circulation. This is known as the bioavailability of the drug. The amount of drug in the systemic circulation can be calculated by measuring the area under the plasma concentration versus time curve (A.U.C.) in Figure 4.3 from 0 to 50 hours (the last sampling point). The bioavailable fraction (F) of an oral dose is then simply expressed as

$$F = \frac{\text{A.U.C. after oral dose}}{\text{A.U.C. after i.v. dose}} \tag{6}$$

Low oral bioavailability may not necessarily mean poor absorption from the gut but can be caused by metabolism of the drug in the gut wall or in the liver during the first circulation through these organs. This is known as the 'first pass effect', and drugs like morphine, isoprenaline, ethinyl oestradiol show a first pass effect due to gut wall metabolism. Propranolol and lignocaine show a first pass effect because of uptake and metabolism in the liver (Cleaveland & Shand 1972, DelVilar, Sanchez & Tephly 1974).

The apparent volume of distribution of a drug, whose disposition conforms to the two compartment model system, will have different values in the two compartments. The apparent volume of distribution of the drug can be calculated by dividing the fraction (F) of the dose (D) absorbed by the A.U.C. and by the elimination rate constant Kel.

$$Vd = \frac{F.D.}{\text{A.U.C. Kel}} \tag{7}$$

The apparent volume of distribution of some drugs may seem to be very high, e.g. 1400 litres for some tricyclic antidepressants, but this information indicates that these drugs must reach much higher concentrations in tissues than they do in plasma. On the other hand, a drug like warfarin will have a low apparent volume of distribution (8–10 litres) which indicates that the drug concentration in tissues is much lower than in plasma.

PLASMA CLEARANCE OF DRUGS

Clearance of drugs is of importance because the term is a better index of the efficiency of drug elimination than the more commonly used half life. An important determinant of plasma half life is the apparent volume of distribution, and for a given clearance, the smaller the distribution volume, the shorter the half life of the drug will be. The term clearance is well known in nephrology, where it is used to describe the rate of renal elimination of compounds. Plasma clearance can be calculated by a simplification of the previous equation: (7)

$$\text{Plasma clearance} = \frac{F.D.}{\text{A.U.C.}} \tag{8}$$

$$= Vd. \, Kel \tag{9}$$

By definition, clearance is also the product of blood flow and the extraction ratio. For many drugs the most important organ of elimination is the liver. Drugs metabolized by the liver can be divided into two main types with respect to their hepatic clearance (Wilkinson & Shand, 1975). First, those drugs whose extraction ratio by the liver is high (e.g. propranolol, lignocaine). These drugs have a high hepatic clearance and their clearance is limited by the hepatic flow (usually about 1.5 l/min). The rate of metabolism of these drugs by the liver is dependent, therefore, on the rate of transport of the drug to the liver.

For low extraction drugs, hepatic clearance is dependent on the capacity of the liver cells to take up and metabolize the drug and liver blood flow is of little or no importance. Drug binding to protein in plasma may be of importance. For drugs whose clearance is limited by liver blood flow, binding to plasma proteins will serve to increase the concentration of drug delivered to the liver for elimination. For drugs whose elimination is not dependent on liver blood flow, protein binding is of less importance.

STEADY STATE CONCENTRATIONS

We have so far considered pharmacokinetic processes as they apply after single dose administration. In practice, many drugs are given on a regular basis. Let us consider a drug whose plasma half life is 12 hours and which is given every 8 hours (Fig. 4.6). By the time the second dose is given, the plasma concentration of the drug will still be more than half its peak concentration and so the peak concentration after the second dose will rise to higher levels than before. This process will be repeated until the

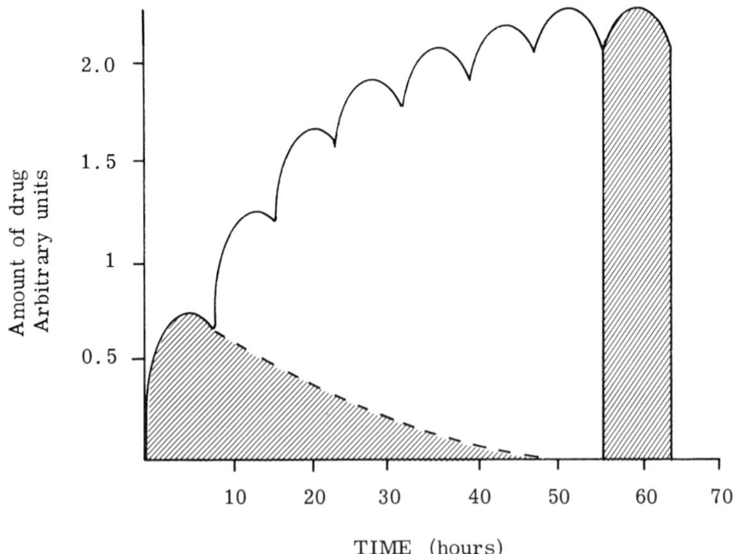

Fig. 4.6   Schematic representation of the accumulation of drug in the body (or plasma) after oral dosing. The drug is given every 8 hours and has a half life of 12 hours. The area under plasma concentration versus time curve after the first dose is equal to the area under the curve during the dosage interval, provided that plateau (steady-state) concentrations have been reached. [From Avery 1976 (ed) Drug therapy. Adis Press, Sydney, 19 (p 8).]

plateau is reached at which time the net input of drug every 8 hours is balanced by its elimination. Of course, at 'steady state' the area under the plasma concentration curve during a dosage interval will be the same as the A.U.C. after the first dose (Sjoqvist, Borga & Orme, 1980). The time taken to achieve 'steady state' is entirely dependent on the plasma half life of the drug as is shown in Table 4.1. Thus for imipramine with a half life of 30 hours 97 per cent of the final concentration will be achieved by 150 hours if given regularly. This partly helps to explain the delay in achieving a therapeutic response with this drug. Clearly, if a drug has a plasma half life of over 30 hours (e.g. phenytoin, phenobarbitone, tricyclic antidepressants) once daily dosing is quite sufficient to maintain adequate plasma (and tissue) concentrations.

Table 4.1.   The plasma concentration at different time points as a percentage of the steady state concentration (C_{ss})

Number of half-lives	Plasma conc. as % of steady state
1	50
2	75
3	88
4	94
5	97
6	98
7	99

The time points are expressed as the number of half lives elapsed from starting therapy.

The same principles apply to the intravenous dosage of a drug. If an intravenous infusion is started it will take a defined time to reach plateau concentrations in blood. This time can be shortened by giving an initial loading dose of the drug. The required loading dose can be calculated if the apparent volume of distribution (see Table 4.2) and required plasma concentrations are known, by multiplying these.

$$\text{Loading dose} = C_{ss} \times Vd \tag{10}$$

The maintenance dose is then half the loading dose given every half life.

Table 4.2   Apparent volume of distribution (Vd) of various commonly used drugs

Drug	Vd l/kg body weight
Frusemide, warfarin	0.1
Tolbutamide	0.14
Valproic acid	0.15
Glybenclamide, nalidixic acid penicillin G	0.3
Phenytoin	0.6
Indomethacin	0.9
Lignocaine	1.3
Digoxin, methaqualone	6
Nortriptyline, chlorpromazine	20
Diazepam	0.7
Antipyrine	0.6

A number of concepts follow from these observations of the steady state situation. Firstly, the shorter the half life of the drug the sooner will the steady state concentration (C_{ss}) be reached. However, for drugs with a very short half life the plasma concentration will fluctuate markedly between doses since it is impractical to give doses more frequently than four times daily. One way to overcome these fluctuations is to prepare the drug as a sustained release preparation.

Secondly, if the biological half life is prolonged unduly (e.g. digoxin in renal failure) the time taken to reach steady state will be correspondingly longer and the concentration reached will be considerably higher than under normal circumstances. The dose must, therefore, be decreased. Thirdly, it is possible to predict the steady state concentration of a drug in plasma (Css) if its half life, bioavailability and apparent volume of distribution are known.

$$Css = \frac{F.D.}{Kel\ Vd.\ \triangle t} \tag{11}$$

where Kel is the elimination rate constant, and $\triangle t$ is the dosage interval.

If the value $T_{\frac{1}{2}}$ is preferred the formula is

$$Css = \frac{1.44 . F.D. T_{\frac{1}{2}}}{Vd . \triangle t} \tag{12}$$

This information is often of help in planning therapy where a therapeutic range of drug concentration is known.

SPECIAL PROCESSES IN PHARMACOKINETICS

Drug absorption after various routes of administration

1. Oral administration
Approximately 70 per cent of all drugs prescribed are given by mouth. Some factors governing drug absorption from the gastrointestinal tract are shown in Table 4.3.

Table 4.3   Factors affecting drug absorption from the gastrointestinal tract

(1) Formulation and characteristics of drug product
    (a) tablet disintegration time
    (b) dissolution time
    (c) presence of excipients
    (d) stability in gastrointestinal tract

(2) Patient factors
    (a) pH of lumen
    (b) gastric emptying time
    (c) intestinal transit time
    (d) surface area of gut
    (e) presence of local disease
    (f) blood flow

(3) Presence of other agents
    (a) drugs
    (b) food

(4) Pharmacokinetic characteristics
    (a) drug metabolism by gut wall
    (b) drug metabolism by gut bacteria

Before a drug can be absorbed, the tablet or capsule must disintegrate and the drug dissolved in gastrointestinal fluids. Many studies of drug absorption are carried out with drug in solution, which tends to minimize pharmaceutical factors which may be limiting in drug absorption. Variations in the formulation of the drug product may have dramatic effects on its absorption. Changes in the formulation of phenytoin (Tyrer, Eadie, Sutherland & Hooper, 1970) and digoxin (Lindenbaum, Mellow, Blackstone & Butler, 1971) carried out by changing the excipients used, led to dramatic differences in bioavailability, plasma drug concentration and therapeutic response. The presence of other drugs and excipients, otherwise inert, may alter drug absorption. Cations such as iron and calcium may modify tetracycline absorption by forming large insoluble complexes, and bentonite, a constituent of PAS granules is responsible for a marked impairment of rifampicin absorption when given together with PAS, since rifampicin becomes adsorbed on to bentonite (Boman, Lundgren & Stjernstrom, 1975).

The absorption of drugs from the gut into the body is governed chiefly by the pharmacokinetic factors that were considered early in the chapter, and there are four main processes.

(a) PASSIVE DIFFUSION

This is proportionately the most important; the drug is transferred across the gastrointestinal wall down a concentration gradient with no energy expenditure. The drug must be in aqueous solution at the surface of the cell membrane, then dissolves in lipid membrane to passes into the cell.

(b) ACTIVE TRANSPORT

This involves the utilization of energy to convey a drug across a cell, if necessary against a concentration gradient. It is a highly specific transport system and is used by naturally occurring substances such as amino acids and sugars. Drugs which utilize such a system have a chemical structure similar to a naturally occurring compound absorbed by active transport. This is probably true for both methyldopa and levodopa.

(c) FILTRATION THROUGH PORES

In practice these pores between cells are too small to allow drug absorption (maximum molecular weight of 100). The total area of the pores is very small compared to the total cell membrane area.

(b) PINOCYTOSIS

This process, whereby small particles are engulfed by the cell membrane is not of major importance for the absorption of drugs. It may become of some importance in the future if drugs are given bound to macromolecular structures (e.g. liposomes).

Large intra- and interpatient variability in drug absorption may occur. Among the most important causes are differences in rates of gastric emptying and of gastrointestinal motility, the presence or absence of food, the pathological state of the gastrointestinal tract, the position of the patient, and other drugs taken (Prescott, 1974).

According to the pH partition hypothesis, moderately strong acids, e.g. salicylic acid, will exist in predominantly unionized form in the stomach from there they should be readily absorbed. However, it is now realized that the major determinants of absorption from the gut are blood flow and surface area and thus even acidic drugs will tend to be absorbed more from the duodenum and jejunum than from the stomach. Obviously the rate of gastric emptying is critical in determining drug absorption and subsequent therapeutic effect. The rate of gastric emptying may vary up to ten-fold. It is slowed by emotion, exercise, pain, hot food, peptic ulcer, and speeded by hunger and mild exercise. Thus, in the fasting state, gastric emptying is accelerated. The effect of variations in rate of gastric emptying on plasma concentrations of paracetamol is shown in Figure 4.7 with metoclopramide speeding up gastric

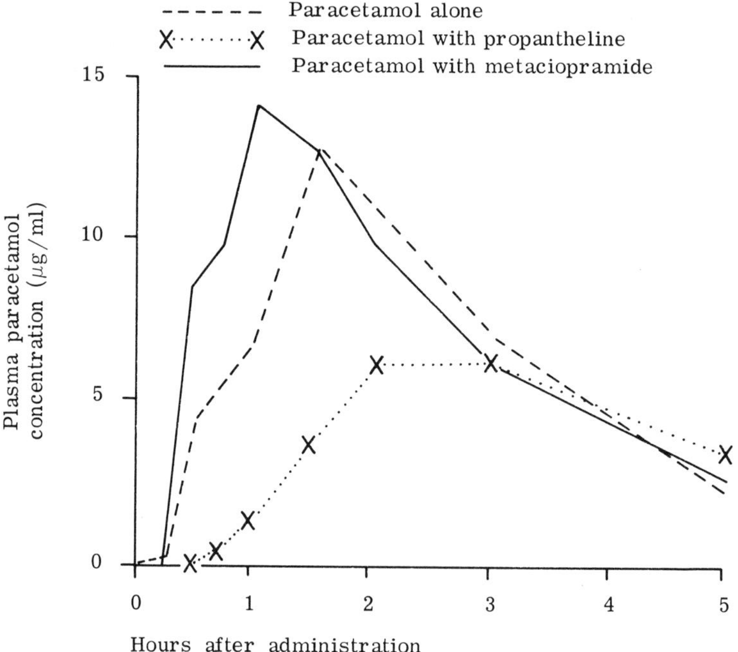

Fig. 4.7 Effects of changes in gastric emptying produced by metoclopramide and propantheline on plasma concentrations of paracetamol. (From Nimmo J, Heading R C, Tothill P, Prescott R 1973. British Medical Journal 1: 587.)

emptying and propantheline delaying it (Nimmo, Heading, Tothill & Prescott, 1973). Food will delay gastric emptying, but while this will slow down the rate of absorption in many cases, the total amount of drug absorbed will not be affected. If the drug is one that has a low bioavailability under normal conditions, the amount of drug absorbed may be actually increased by the presence of food in the stomach. This has been demonstrated for propranolol and hydralazine, perhaps because their first pass effect is decreased.

2. Rectal administration

The purpose of giving drugs by rectum is either to achieve a local effect or to achieve systemic effects especially in patients who are vomiting, or in children. In addition, this route has been used to minimize the gastric irritation caused by drugs given by mouth, but for agents such as indomethacin, gastric irritation may be caused by systemic drug concentrations as well as local effect. If drugs are destroyed by the liver, administration via the rectum rather than by mouth gives some advantage because only part of the venous draining of the rectum (superior haemorrhoidal vein) enters the portal circulation, the middle and lower veins draining directly into the inferior vena caval circulation.

3. Sublingual administration

Administration of drugs by this route also protects them from a first pass effect in the gut wall or liver, since the venous drainage to the territory of the superior vena cava effectively bypasses the hepatic portal system. Further, the drug is not exposed to a high gastric acid concentration, and once the desired therapeutic effect has been obtained, i.e. the relief of angina pectoris by glyceryl trinitrate, the drug can be spat out. Neither rectum nor mouth have been fully exploited as routes for effective drug administration.

4. Intravenous administration

The principal rationale for intravenous drug administration is rapidity of response achieved. Further, a predictable drug concentration can be achieved within the body and the rate of drug administration can be controlled and should vary according to the agent given. For the hypotensive agent diazoxide, current dogma suggests that rapid intravenous administration is required in order to create an instantaneous disequilibrium between bound (inactive) and free (active) drug since diazoxide is highly bound to serum albumen (Mroczek, Leibel, Davidov & Finnerty, 1971). A slow rate of administration is indicated when a drug response must be maintained over long periods (e.g. heparin). The intravenous administration of heparin illustrates two other important indications for this route of administration. First, heparin would be inactivated by gastric acids and cannot be given by mouth, and second, its rate of elimination is rapid (plasma half life one hour). Thus intravenous administration allows precise quantities of heparin to be delivered at defined rates. Too often, however, this route of administration is abused and used merely as a route of convenience. Incompatibilities with other drugs given simultaneously by this route and even with the fluid vehicle may occur. (See Chapter 17.) The hazards of precipitating venous thrombosis and infection must also be taken into consideration when potentially irritant drugs are given intravenously.

5. Intramuscular and subcutaneous administration

Drug response following these routes of administration is neither so rapid nor so predictable as after intravenous administration. Absorption is frequently erratic, especially in the shocked patient or in other conditions where blood flow from the injection site is impaired. In addition, some drugs are not very water soluble at physiological pH and will tend to precipitate out in the muscle after injection (e.g. digoxin, diazepam, phenytoin). Currently, there is considerable interest in the use of subcutaneous depot preparations of drugs such as contraceptive steroids. The success or otherwise of this approach depends on satisfactory technical development for vehicles and solvents.

6. Percutaneous absorption
As with sublingual administration the potential of the percutaneous route has not yet been fully realized. The large area of skin available, its accessibility, the ability to bypass sites of hepatic and gut wall metabolism and to remove excess drug once the desired response has been achieved, are all advantages. Drugs are now given percutaneously not only to evoke a local response (e.g. in eczema) but also for systemic effects (e.g. antihistamines in motion sickness or glyceryl trinitrate in angina). Rates of percutaneous drug absorption are not the same for all areas. Local rates of blood flow, thickness of epidermis and other factors are important. On the obverse side, of course, it is now appreciated that many toxins may be absorbed percutaneously when the same principles apply as those agents which may be put to therapeutic advantage.

7. Pulmonary absorption
Many drugs can be readily absorbed from the lungs. This applies not only to anaesthetic gases but to drugs delivered in aerosol or particulate inhalations. Many drugs, initially given by inhalation for their local effects on the lungs, are in fact absorbed into the body via this route. Most inhaled drug is, in fact, swallowed so dosage levels absorbed through the lung are likely to be small. Repetitive inhalation of isoprenaline aerosols was probably responsible for a number of deaths from cardiac arrhythmias in the 1960s (Speizer, Doll, Heaf & Strang, 1968). Particle sizes of 2μ or less are likely to reach the narrowest bronchioles and be absorbed.

Distribution of drugs
After absorption of the drug into the body, the drug will then be distributed to its sites of action, metabolism, and excretion, as well as to storage sites.

Three principal factors govern drug distribution:

1. The first is the chosen route of drug administration, discussed above. Clearly, if a drug is given by intravenous infusion it will initially be distributed to organs with high blood flow, e.g. brain, heart, liver and kidneys. Thus, agents used for achieving rapid anaesthesia, or for emergency treatment of convulsions or arrhythmias, are given intravenously.

2. The second factor is the inherent physiochemical property of the drug, i.e. its pKa. Basic drugs (e.g. tricyclic antidepressants, phenothiazines) tend to be distributed to the tissues rather than to plasma, that is, their apparent volume of distribution is high. For similar reasons, beta-adrenoceptor blocking agents are found in high concentrations in lung tissue. Acidic drugs, on the other hand (e.g. oral anticoagulants, antiinflammatory drugs), tend to distribute to plasma where they are tightly bound and thus their apparent volume of distribution is small.

3. The third factor is protein binding. The degree of protein binding will affect the apparent volume of distribution of the drug. It can be calculated that if a drug is 90 per cent bound to plasma proteins, then 88 per cent of the drug in the body will be in the plasma. However, if the drug is 50 per cent bound to albumin then only 12 per cent of the drug will be in plasma (Gillette, 1974). It might be more appropriate to calculate the apparent volume of distribution of a drug on the basis of its free concentration in plasma rather than its total concentration. Table 4.2 gives a list of the apparent volume of distribution of some commonly used drugs.

Under steady state conditions, rather than those of instantaneous disequilibrium discussed above, protein binding is an important determinant of drug distribution and response. For example, the concentrations of anticonvulsants reaching the c.s.f. and the brain are determined by the free (i.e. non protein bound) fraction in plasma (Vajda, Williams, Davidson, Falconer & Breckenridge, 1974).

Displacement of protein bound drugs

The pharmacological consequences of displacement of a drug from plasma protein binding are relatively clear if that drug has negligible binding to tissues. These consequences are:

1. Decreased concentration of total drug in plasma.
2. Increased unbound concentration in plasma and tissues.
3. Increased pharmacological effects, provided that the initial plasma binding is high and the concentration-effect curve is steep.
4. Increased rate of metabolism, as a consequence of more drug being available to metabolic sites.

If, however, the drug is bound in the tissues as well as plasma, these consequences are less well defined. Manifestly, the apparent volume of drug distribution, higher to begin with, is increased even further by displacement, and thus the sequence of events described above is less evident. Thus, from a pharmacokinetic point of view, changes in plasma protein binding are important only when the initial volume of drug distribution is low (0.15 l/kg) as at higher values, it can be calculated that only some 30 per cent of the total body drug store exists in plasma (Gillette, 1974). For drugs with an initial high apparent volume of distribution a displacement interaction at plasma protein level may lead to:

1. Decreased total drug concentration in plasma.
2. Little or no increase in unbound concentration in plasma.
3. Few pharmacological sequelae.
4. Possibly a decrease in rate of metabolism, as described above (for drugs with high hepatic extraction).

Disease conditions in which either the quantity of plasma proteins or its nature is disturbed, e.g. cirrhosis, uraemia, impose further constraints on the effects of protein binding. In uraemia, an effective 'displacer' circulates in plasma, the exact nature of which is uncertain. Further, the total number of binding sites is decreased by virtue of hypoalbuminaemia and the same is true in cirrhosis.

Metabolism

As above, lipid soluble drugs will tend to be well absorbed, but in the unchanged form they will tend to be excreted through the glomerulus and then reabsorbed in the distal part of the nephron. Such drugs must, therefore, be metabolized to more water soluble compounds that can be excreted in the urine. The rate of metabolism of such drugs will determine the duration and magnitude of the therapeutic effect as we have seen already. The metabolites formed are usually, but not always, less active than the parent drug. Some drugs are only active through a metabolite while in many others (see Table 4.4) the metabolite is at least as active as the parent drug. The contribution of the metabolite to the therapeutic or toxic effects of a drug will be determined by the activity, the amount produced and the half life of the metabolite. Desmethyldiazepam

Table 4.4 Some drugs with pharmacologically active metabolites

Drug	Active metabolite
Allopurinol	Alloxanthine
Amitriptyline	Nortriptyline
Chlordiazepoxide	Desmethylchlordiazepoxide
Codeine	Morphine
Cyclophosphamide*	Hydroxy-cyclophosphamide
Diazepam	Desmethyldiazepam
Imipramine	Desmethylimipramine
Phenacetin	Paracetamol
Phenylbutazone	Oxyphenbutazone
Prednisone	Prednisolone
Primidone	Phenobarbitone
Procainamide	N-acetyl procainamide
Propranolol	4-hydroxy propranolol
Rifampicin	Desacetyl rifampicin
Spironolactone	Canrenone, canrenoate
Sulphasalazine	Sulphapyridine

* Parent drug is inactive

with a longer half life than diazepam will accumulate in plasma (especially in the elderly) and may cause hangover effects (Schwartz, 1973).

Recently, attention has been paid to the fact that small quantities of metabolites may be produced, which may be responsible for drug toxicity. While these metabolites are very reactive chemically, they may be covalently bound to tissue macromolecules. The hepatotoxicity of large doses of paracetamol is due to a metabolite which, with standard doses of paracetamol, is further metabolized by conjugation with glutathione, but in overdosage causes liver damage (Prescott, Wright, Roscoe & Brown, 1971).

Sites of drug metabolism
Although the liver is the main site of drug metabolism in the body most other tissues have some capacity for drug metabolism. The gut wall is capable of metabolizing drugs during the absorptive process. The lungs, kidney, skin, and blood cells can also metabolize drugs.

Routes of drug metabolism
A wide variety of biochemical reactions can take place during the metabolism of a drug and it is possible here to give only a simple outline of the processes involved. There are two types of reaction. In phase I reactions, polar groups (water soluble groups) are introduced into the molecule (e.g. by oxidation, reduction, hydrolysis). Phase II reactions are synthetic and involve conjunction of the drug with glucuronic acid, sulphate, or glycine or other groups (see Table 4.5). Some drugs may pass through a Phase I reaction and then through a phase II reaction, while other drugs may be involved in only one of the pathways. Phenacetin, for example, is oxidized in the body to paracetamol, an active metabolite, which is then conjugated. The enzymes involved in drug oxidation are located on the smooth endoplasmic reticulum of the

Table 4.5 Examples of important drug metabolic reactions

Reaction	Substances
1. Cytochrome P450 mediated hydroxylation	Many drugs, insecticides, fatty acids and endogenous steroids
2. Oxidation of Purines (Xanthine oxidase)	Allopurinol, azathioprine 6-mercaptopurine
3. Oxidation by monoamine Oxidase (MAO)	Tyramine, catecholamines
4. Hydrolysis	Suxamethonium
5. Reduction	Chloralhydrate
6. Glucuronidation	Indomethacin paracetamol, oxazepam
7. Sulphate conjugation	Isoprenaline, ethinyl oestradiol
8. Glycine conjugation	Salicylic acid
9. Acetylation	Isoniazid, hydralaxine, procainamide, dapsone

cells which, after homogenization and ultracentrifugation, is recovered as the microsomal fraction. Cytochrome P450 serves as the terminal oxidase in this oxidation pathway. It is now clear that P450 is not a homogenous cytochrome, and several separate subfractions have been identified. The subcellular organization of metabolizing enzymes is now reasonably clear. There is evidence that the endoplasmic reticulum is a highly organized structure and enzymic components subserving both oxidation and glucuronidation are asymmetrically distributed in both lateral and transverse planes (Dallner, 1979). At the inner surface, the completion and transport of proteins, glycoproteins and lipoproteins takes place, while most of the metabolic reactions are localized at the cytoplasmic luminal surface.

There are two important features of the cytochrome P450 mediated reaction. Firstly, a large variety of foreign compounds have the ability to increase the rate of drug metabolism by enzyme induction. The induction process involves increased synthesis of cytochrome P450 and increased formation of liver cell membranes containing the enzyme. Enzyme induction may be caused by drug administration and by environmental factors such as cigarette smoking. This is dealt with in the chapter on drug interactions. Secondly, these metabolic steps (particularly drug oxidation) show marked interindividual variation. In a group of say 30 individuals the rate of oxidation of a drug may vary 20- or 30-fold and this will be reflected in the steady state concentration of the drugs. In a group of 15 individuals given nortriptyline 25 mg three times daily the steady state plasma concentration may vary between 10 and 295 ng/ml. This type of variation makes it difficult to treat patients by giving them all the same dose of a drug as is still fairly common practice. Some patients may derive no therapeutic benefit, while others may suffer toxic side effects.

Many factors may alter the rate of drug metabolism and some examples are given in Table 4.6. Genetic influences are probably most important for both oxidation and conjugation, so that for example slow acetylation of drugs (seen in 60 per cent of Causcasians, but only 10 per cent of Japanese) implies that side effects would be more likely to occur if drug toxicity is due to parent drug. Drug induced systemic lupus syndrome following procaine amide or hydralazine is much commoner in slow acetylators of these drugs (La Du, 1972). Age can affect drug metabolism, but apart from the newborn, when the rate of drug oxidation is slow, it is not of great therapeutic importance. In liver disease, such as cirrhosis, drug metabolism may be impaired if the disease is severe. If a drug has high clearance characteristics (e.g. propranolol) liver disease may increase its bioavailability by reducing the extraction of the drug in the liver (Branch & Shand, 1976). Diet has been reported to affect drug metabolism, with a reduced rate of drug metabolism in severe malnutrition. In addition, a high carbohydrate diet will inhibit drug metabolism, while a high protein diet and ingestion of vegetables such as cabbage will enhance drug metabolism (Conney, Pantuck, Pantuck et al, 1979).

Table 4.6   Factors which may affect drug metabolism

Factor	Example
Genetic	Acetylation, e.g. isoniazid Oxidations, e.g. debrisopin
Age	Reduced metabolism in newborn and in old
Pregnancy	Reduced rate of metabolism
Liver disease	Reduced metabolism of some drugs in severe liver disase
Diet	Enhanced rate of metabolism by high protein diet — cabbage, brussels sprouts
Alcohol	Acute intake inhibits metabolism Chronic intake enhances metabolism until liver damage is severe
Other drugs	Can inhibit or enhance drug metabolism

Excretion of drugs

Drugs are excreted from the body by many routes, including the kidney, bowel, bile, milk, saliva and skin.

Renal excretion

Three processes may be involved in renal drug excretion — filtration, active secretion via carrier systems and passive reabsorption by the kidney. Comparatively few drugs are excreted by filtration. Even digoxin, often cited as an example, is influenced by tubular mechanisms and this is important especially in patients with severely compromised glomerular filtration. The antibiotics streptomycin and gentamicin depend primarily upon glomerular filtration for their excretion from the body. If renal function is impaired, the plasma concentration of these drugs will increase to toxic levels, unless the dosage is modified. Similarly, active metabolites of drugs which are normally excreted in the urine will accumulate in plasma if renal function is impaired. The n-acetyl metabolite of procainamide may accumulate in plasma with toxic effects in patients with disturbed renal function (Reidenberg, 1971).

Some organic bases such as mecamylamine and some organic acids such as penicillin and probenecid undergo active tubular secretion. It is envisaged that the organic acid is carried across the tubular cell by a carrier which liberates the drug in the tubule and then returns to carry more drug as in the process of active transport involved in drug absorption. Competition for the carrier may arise and in this way probenecid may impair the renal excretion of penicillin.

The renal clearance of many acidic and basic drugs varies over the urinary pH range (4.8–7.5) in accordance with the principles explained earlier. Strong acids (pKa less than 2) and strong bases (pKa greater than 12) are virtually completely ionized over the physiological range of urinary pH and their clearance cannot be affected by changing the urine pH. Weak organic bases (pKa 7.5–10.0) such as amphetamine, are more ionized at lower pH values and their rates of excretion can be increased by acidifying the urine with ammonium chloride. Phenobarbitone and salicylates as weak organic acids are ionized in alkaline pH and their excretion rate can be increased by the use of sodium bicarbonate to make the urine alkaline.

Biliary excretion

Many drugs are actively transported by hepatic cells from blood to bile. Drugs and their metabolites are likely to be excreted in bile if their molecular weight exceeds 400 (Williams, 1959). Ampicillin and rifampicin are excreted in high concentration into the bile and use is made of this in treating patients with biliary tract infection.

Some drugs are excreted as conjugated metabolites in bile and then undergo an enterohepatic circulation (e.g. digitoxin, indomethacin, ethinyloestradiol). The conjugated metabolite reaches the gastrointestinal tract where it is broken down by enzymes in the gut bacteria to liberate the unchanged drug. This can then be reabsorbed and this cycle will continue. How much this cycle contributes to the overall plasma concentration of the drug is unknown (Williams, 1959).

Alteration of the enterohepatic circulation may cause interactions with broad spectrum antibiotics which kill gut bacteria and may interrupt drug enterohepatic circulation. Biliary excretion may serve as an alternative route of elimination of some polar drugs in patients with renal impairment (e.g. oxazepam) but for other drugs such as digoxin, the reduction in the rate of renal elimination is only partially compensated by biliary excretion.

REFERENCES

Boman G, Lundgren P, Stjernstrom G 1975 Mechanism of the inhibitory effect of PAS granules on the absorption of rifampicin. European Journal of Clinical Pharmacology 8: 293–299
Branch R, Shand D G 1976 Propranolol disposition in chronic liver disease: a physiological approach. Clinical Pharmacokinetics 1: 264–279
Cleaveland C R, Shand D G 1972 Effect of route of administration on the relationship between β adrenergic blockade and plasma propranolol levels. Clinical Pharmacology and Therapeutics 13: 181–189

Conney A H, Pantuck E J, Pantuck C B, Buening M, Jerina D M et al 1979 Role of environment on diet in the regulation of human drug metabolism. In: Estabrook R W, Lindenlaub E, (eds) The induction of drug metabolism. Schattauer Verlag, Berlin p 583–605

Dallner G 1979 Structural organisation of the endoplasmic reticulum. In Eastabrook R W, Lindenlaub E (eds) The induction of drug metabolism. Schattauer Verlag, Berlin p 133–146

Davies D M 1977 Textbook of adverse drug reactions. Oxford University Press

Del Villar E, Sanchez E, Tephly T R 1974 Morphine metabolism. II. Studies on morphine glucuronyl-transferase activity in intestinal microsomes of rats. Drug Metabolism and Disposition 2: 370–374

Gillette J R 1974 Overview of drug-protein binding. Annals of the New York Academy of Sciences 226: 6–17

Greenblatt D J, Koch-Weser J 1975 Clinical pharmacokinetics. New England Journal of Medicine 293: 702–705

La Du B N 1972 Pharmacogenetics: Defective enzymes in relation to reactions to drugs. Annual Review of Medicine 23: 453–468

Lindenbaum J, Mellow M H, Blackstone M O, Butler V P 1971 Variation in biological activity of digoxin from four preparations. New England Journal of Medicine 285: 1344–1347

Mroczek W M, Leibel B A, Davidov M, Finnerty F A 1971 The importance of rapid administration of diazoxide in accelerated hypertension. New England Journal of Medicine 285: 603–606

Nimmo J, Heading R C, Tothill P, Prescott L F (1973) Pharmacological modification of gastric emptying; effects of propantheline and metoclopramide on paracetamol absorption. British Medical Journal 1: 587–589

Prescott L F, Wright N, Roscoe P, Brown S S 1971 Plasma paracetamol half life and hepatic necrosis in patients with paracetamol overdosage. Lancet 1: 519–522

Reidenberg M 1971 Renal function and drug action. Saunders, Philadelphia

Rowland M 1978 In: Melmon K, Morelli H (eds) Clinical pharmacology, basic principles in therapeutics, 2nd ed. Macmillan, London, p 25–70

Schwartz M 1973 Benzodiazepine metabolism In: Garratini S, Mussini E, Randall L O (eds) The benzodiazepines. Raven Press, New York p 53–74

Sjoqvist F, Borga O, Orme M L'E 1980 Fundamentals of clinical pharmacology. In Avery G S (ed) Drug treatment, 2nd edn. Adis Press, Sydney p 1–42

Speizer F E, Doll R, Heaf P, Strang L B (1968) Investigation into use of drugs preceding death from asthma. British Medical Journal 1: 339–343

Tyrer J H, Eadie M J, Sutherland J M, Hooper W D 1970 Outbreak of anticonvulsant intoxication in an Australian city. British Medical Journal 4: 271–273

Vajda F, Williams F M, Davidson S, Falconer M A, Breckenridge A (1974) Human brain, cerebrospinal and plasma concentrations of diphenylhydantoin and phenobarbital. Clinical Pharmacology and Therapeutics 15: 597–603

Wilkinson G R, Shand D G 1975 Commentary: a physiological approach to hepatic drug clearance. Clinical Pharmacology and Therapeutics 18: 377–390

Williams R T 1959 Detoxication Mechanisms. John Wiley, New York

5. Obesity and energy balance

J. S. Garrow

SCOPE OF THIS REVIEW

In the last five years there have been many publications about obesity and energy balance, notably from the first International Congress on Obesity, held in London (Howard, 1975) and the Second International Congress, held in Washington (Bray, 1978a). It would be impossible to give an adequate summary of all this research in the space available here, so the starting point for this review will be a report 'Research on Obesity' by a joint DHSS/MRC Study Group (James, 1976). I will use the conclusions from that report as a background for subsequent advances, but will not reanalyse the evidence on which the 1976 report was based. Almost all the work cited concerns investigations on human subjects. Animal work is largely ignored, partly due to constraints of space, and partly because it takes some time to find out if discoveries about the regulation of energy balance in experimental animals will prove to be a 'recent advance' which is of real value to the practising clinician.

The problems of energy balance in other conditions (for example anorexia nervosa, and in patients undergoing surgery) are clinically important, but have been excluded from this review.

THE INFLUENCE OF OBESITY ON HEALTH

The report (James, 1976) starts with the words: 'We are unanimous in our belief that obesity is a hazard to health and a detriment to well-being. It is common enough to constitute one of the most important medical and public health problems of our time, whether we judge importance by a shorter expectation of life, increased morbidity or cost to the community in terms of both money and anxiety'. Life insurance statistics show that overweight subjects tend to die younger than their contemporaries of normal weight, and there are many diseases which occur more commonly as a cause of death in overweight subjects (Levinson, 1977). However people taking out life insurance are a highly self-selected group, and well-conducted prospective trials may fail to show the anticipated strong correlation between overweight and mortality. Mann (1974) was not convinced by the evidence that obesity in itself shortened life.

The relationship of obesity to the risk of ischaemic heart disease has become much clearer as a result of several recently-published surveys. The data from five surveys (1823 Albany civil servants, 1264 employees of the Chicago Peoples' Gas Company, 1983 from the Chicago Western Electric Company, 2193 from the Framingham study and 1240 from Tecumseh), together with 4013 other subjects, have been pooled (Cook, 1978). So far as overweight is concerned, the risk of a first major coronary event is *increased* only for men in their 40s (the youngest group studied), while at age

50–54 overweight carries no extra risk, and among men aged 55–59 there is a slight, but insignificant *reduction* in risk with increasing weight. Similar conclusions come from the Manitoba study (Rabkin, Mathewson & Hsu, 1977) of 3983 men, who were followed for 26 years. The risk of ischaemic heart disease, and especially of sudden death, was increased in men under the age of 40, but this effect only became evident after a follow-up period of 16 years. Similar age-related effects have emerged concerning the association between overweight and hypertension. Stamler et al (1978) studied the relationship of overweight (self-reported) to high blood pressure (diastolic over 95 mmHg, or current use of antihypertensive medication) in a survey of one million Americans. They found the risk of hypertension among subjects who were 20–39 years old was twice as high in the overweight than the normal weight group, and three times as high compared with underweight subjects. Among subjects aged 40–64 the trend was similar, but less strong: hypertension was $1\frac{1}{2}$ times as common in overweight compared with normal weight, and twice as common in overweight than underweight subjects.

There is still controversy about the role of physical activity in the link between obesity and heart disease: Stern (1978) suggests that overweight leads to inactivity, which leads to an increased risk of heart disease (Chave et al, 1978). There is evidence for the second part of this scheme: in 3686 San Francisco longshoremen (Paffenbarger et al, 1978) and in 8171 Puerto Ricans (Costas et al, 1978) it is inactivity rather than overweight which is associated with heart disease. However, it is not easy to find convincing evidence that obesity is in general associated with inactivity (Warwick & Garrow, 1979). It is a popular myth that obese people are typically gluttonous and slothful, but there are few data to support this idea.

Although cross-sectional surveys (Juustila, 1977) or surveys with a follow-up period of less than five years (Costas et al, 1978; Keys et al, 1972) fail to show a significant association between overweight and coronary heart disease, longer term studies consistently show this association. A very large survey organised by the American Cancer Society (Lew and Garfinkel, 1979) showed that the major factor in the higher relative mortality among overweight people was coronary disease, and this increased risk became more marked in the second six years of the survey than it was in the first six years. Both the American Cancer Society study and life insurance data (Blair and Haines, 1966) show that the excess mortality associated with overweight falls more heavily on young than old people, but that it takes many years for this risk to become manifest. Moderate obesity in men over 55 carries very little excess risk. With so complex a relationship it is not surprising that there has been confusion about the correct interpretation of earlier surveys.

There are still many unanswered questions about the influence of obesity on other aspects of health, for example on complications of surgery. There is good evidence that severely obese patients have poor lung function: they have stiff lungs, reduced functional residual capacity, and poor oxygenation, and after weight loss these parameters improve greatly (Santesson and Nordenström, 1978). Since anaesthetic gases are fat-soluble patients with excess fat require more gas, but apparently not more relaxant (Tsueda et al, 1978). It is generally supposed that obese patients are more liable to wound infection and thromboembolism (Strauss & Wise, 1978). However Printen et al (1978) report the remarkably low incidence of only four fatal pulmonary emboli among 564 grossly obese patients having gastric bypass operations.

There is no doubt that severely obese patients present both surgeons and anaesthetists with difficult problems but, as Strauss and Wise (1978) point out, controlled prospective trials are lacking, so we cannot quantify these hazards, or judge to what extent the situation is improved by preoperative weight loss.

Obesity may bring social and psychological handicaps as well as physical morbidity and mortality, but these handicaps are difficult to measure and there have been no significant recent advances in this field.

DEFINITION AND PREVALENCE OF OBESITY

Obesity is a condition in which there is an excessive amount of fat in the body. This definition is useless unless the amount of fat in an individual can be determined, and then compared with 'ideal' amount of fat. Techniques for measuring body fat in the laboratory have improved considerably in the last five years (Garrow, 1978a). These developments will be discussed in the next section. The most accurate methods are not suitable for field use, so for epidemiological purposes obesity is usually defined, and prevalence is measured, in terms of 'excess weight' compared with some standard.

To define an 'ideal' amount of fat is much more difficult. If Olympic athletes are taken as a reference standard of perfect physique the ideal weight-for-height varies with the event at which they excel. Sprinters are relatively heavily built, and typically weigh about 70 kg at a height of 1.75 m (Khosla, 1978), while longer distance runners ar progressively lighter, so a marathon champion of the same height weighs only about 60 kg. By comparison the average American aged 18–24 years in 1960–62 weighed 72 kg, and in 1971–74 this average weight had increased to 75 kg (Abraham, Johnson and Najgar, 1979).

The ratio W/H^2. where W is body weight in kilogrammes, and H is height in metres, is now generally adopted as a measure of weight-for-height. Thus the Olympic sprinter would have a W/H^2 ratio of 24.5 and the champion marathon runner a ratio of 19.6. In the experience of life insurance companies the range associated with greatest longevity is from about 19–24 for women and from 20–25 for men (Bray, 1978b). To facilitate calculation a nomogram (Bray, 1978b) or a slide rule device (Cole and James, 1978) have been published from which the value of W/H^2 can easily be read.

The epidemiological evidence suggests that obesity is becoming increasingly common in the USA (Abraham et al, 1979) in the UK (James, 1976) and in Denmark (Sonne-Holm & Sorensen, 1977). In 1973 the cost to the National Health Service of drug treatment of obesity was about £2.5m and by 1975 this had increased to £3.5m. It is estimated that treating obesity occupies about 600 000 doctor-hours per year (Mahler, 1978). Social class is inversely related to obesity, but a report by Ashwell, North & Meade (1978a) showed that in men the relationship of smoking to obesity seems to be dependent on social class: among men in social class I and II obesity is positively related to smoking, but in social class IV and V the relationship is negative. Among women this effect is not found: smokers are less obese than non-smokers in all social classes.

RECENT ADVANCES IN THE MEASUREMENT OF BODY COMPOSITION

The chemical composition of a typical male adult is shown diagrammatically in Figure 5.1, based on chemical analyses of six adult human cadavers (Garrow, 1978a). It is obvious that the clinician requires a non-destructive test of the composition of his patients. In this direction there have been several recent advances.

Hill et al (1978) combined the measurement of weight, skinfold thickness and neutron activation to yield an estimate of the composition of ill patients. The principle of the method is that neutron activation of the human body renders the elements K, N, Na, Cl, Ca and P transiently radioactive, so the body content of these elements can be estimated from the intensity of the radiation in the energy bands which are characteristic of these induced isotopes. The measurement takes about 40 minutes and the accuracy claimed (as percentage of body weight) for fat is 4.5 per cent, for protein 1.6 per cent, for mineral 0.8 per cent and for water 4.9 per cent. For students of obesity and energy balance the method has two disadvantages: first, the neutron activation equipment is complex, expensive, and not generally available; and second, the accuracy of measurement for fat, protein and water, is not very good. It is likely that neutron activation will throw new light on the mineral metabolism of the body, and indeed it offers the best method for estimating total body nitrogen, but other methods are cheaper and more accurate for fat and water.

Of all the components shown in Figure 5.1 the largest is water, which typically contributes about 42 kg to a 70 kg man. It is a well-mixed pool, so a tracer reaches equilibrium with virtually all body water in about three hours. In the past the main limitation in the accurate measurement of total body water has been the accurate determination of the dilution of a tracer dose of labelled water, particularly when tritium was used as the tracer isotope (Sheng and Huggins, 1979). However the stable isotope, deuterium, can be measured with accuracy of about 0.5 per cent after a dose of 1–2 g deuterated water (Halliday and Miller, 1977). This is probably the best accuracy which can usefully be achieved.

The components of body weight which are of importance in energy storage are fat, protein and glycogen. Of these fat represents by far the largest energy store: the 12 kg of fat shown in Figure 5.1 represents a store of about 10^5 kcal (400 MJ), while 12 kg of protein is equivalent to about 5×10^4 kcal (200 MJ), and 1 kg of glycogen is only equivalent to about 4×10^3 kcal (14 MJ). In obesity it is chiefly (but not exclusively) the fat store which is increased — often to four times the normal size. An accurate and convenient means of measuring total body fat would therefore be most valuable. Theoretically it should be possible to measure total body fat using a fat-soluble gas as a dilution tracer, using similar mathematics to that for total body water. Unfortunately there has been no progress in this field in the last four years: earlier work is reviewed elsewhere (Garrow, 1978a). It seems that body fat is not uniformly and constantly perfused with blood (Bulow, Hansen & Madsen, 1976), so it is impractical to achieve a reliably uniform saturation of total body fat with marker gas.

Measurement of skinfold thickness with calipers is the most convenient field method. Womersley and Durnin (1977) report that in skilled hands the skinfold measurement at four sites gives an estimate of total body fat with an error of about 3 per cent of body weight (or about 2 kg in normal subjects). However in very obese subjects it is difficult or impossible to obtain skinfold measurements, and the

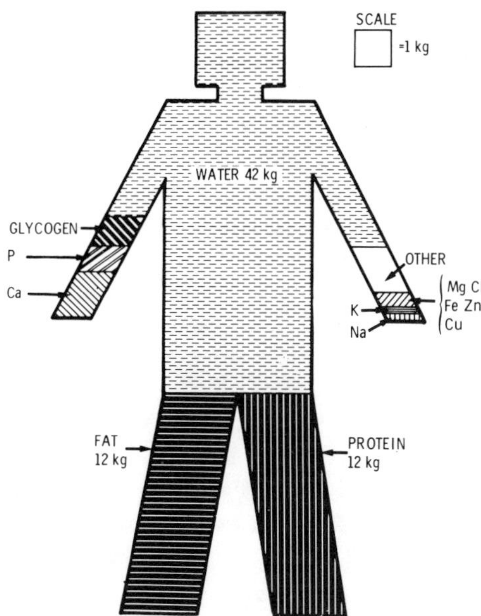

Fig. 5.1 Diagrammatic scheme of body composition in a normal adult male

distribution of fat between subcutaneous and deep sites varies between different ethnic groups (Jones et al, 1976), and between different series (Franklin, Buskirk & Mendez, 1978).

Probably the most accurate method for measuring total body fat is to determine the average density of the body. Human fat at 37°C has a density of $0.900\,\mathrm{g.cm^{-3}}$, and the density of fat-free tissues averages about $1.10\,\mathrm{g.cm^{-3}}$ (Keys & Brozek, 1953). If the average density of a human subject is determined, and these values for the density of the fat, and fat-free, components is assumed, the proportion of fat can readily be calculated. The technical problem is to measure the volume of the subject with sufficient accuracy, especially if the subject is unable or unwilling to submerge totally in water. A recent advance has been the development by Diethelm, Garrow and Stalley (1977) of a whole body plethysmograph with high accuracy which does not require total immersion of the patient. There has been little practical experience of this instrument so far, but a preliminary study (Garrow et al, 1979) suggests that it provides a more reliable estimate of total body fat than methods based on measurements of water or potassium.

A method for predicting total body volume, and hence density and percentage fat, is reported by Weltman and Katch (1978). They measured the circumference of many limb and trunk segments, and derived an equation relating body weight and thigh girth to total body volume. This method is convenient for field use, but since the error in predicting fat is from 4 per cent to 9 per cent it is still less accurate than the skinfold technique.

Lean tissue contains about 60 mmol K/kg (in women, rather more in men), and that potassium has a natural radioactive isotope ^{40}K which emits a characteristic and easily-detected gamma radiation. There have been considerable advances in the construction and calibration of whole body counters to detect potassium radiation

(Smith, Hesp and Mackenzie, 1979). Figure 5.2 shows the relationship of percentage body fat (estimated from ^{40}K measurements) to the obesity index (W/H^2) in women aged 16–64 years (Garrow, 1979). When the obesity index exceeds the 'desirable' range of 19–25 the percentage of body fat usually exceeds 35 per cent, but it is obvious that any given obesity index may indicate very different degrees of obesity. In the sample shown in Figure 5.2 there is one woman with an obesity index of 35 who had only 38 per cent fat, while another of similar obesity index had 54 per cent.

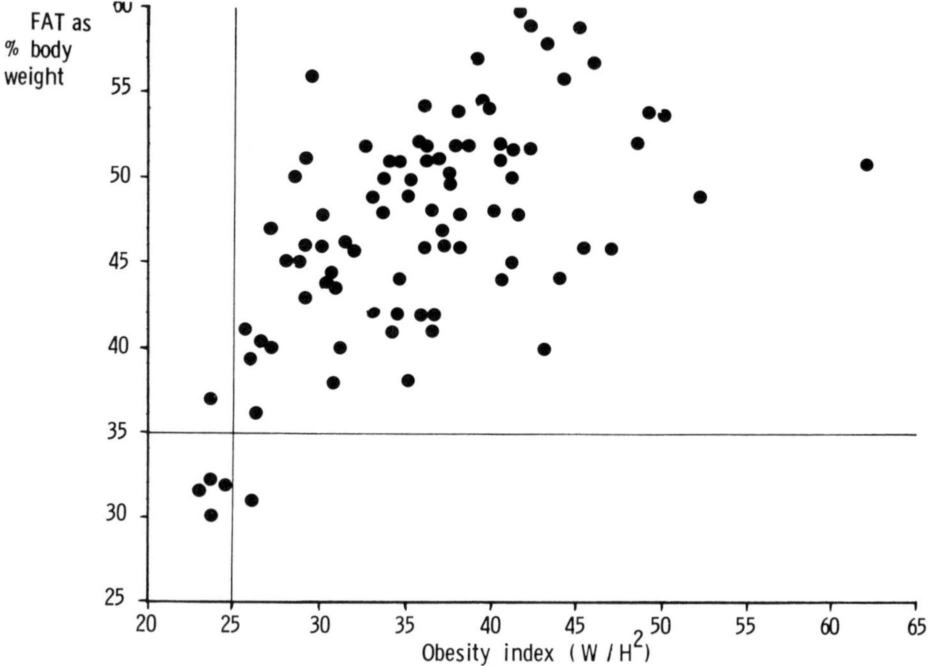

Fig. 5.2   The relationship between the fat content of the body, derived from potassium estimation and the obesity index in adult women (Garrow, 1980).

This section on recent advances in the measurement of body composition may be summarised: techniques are now available for the accurate measurement of total body water, density and total body potassium, but we have no method for measuring total body fat to better than 2 per cent of body weight. An inevitable error derives from the assumption that fat or fat-free tissue bears a constant relationship to some other body component, such as water or potassium or density. Since this assumption is not quite true the estimates are not quite correct. For maximum accuracy a battery of several measurements should be made, since different methods involve different assumptions, and thus the margin of error can be narrowed.

RECENT ADVANCES IN UNDERSTANDING THE AETIOLOGY OF OBESITY

a. Adipocytes

A typical non-obese male human would contain about 12 kg of fat (see Figure 5.1), and a needle biopsy of subcutaneous adipose tissue would show that, on average, each fat cell contained about $0.4\,\mu$g of triglyceride. If it is assumed that this sample of adipose tissue yields an estimate of average fat cell size which is true of all the fat cells in the body the number of these cells can be calculated:

$$\text{Fat cell number} = \frac{\text{total body fat (g)}}{\text{average fat per cell (g)}} = \frac{12 \times 10^3}{4 \times 10^{-7}} = 3 \times 10^{10}$$

It was suggested that this calculation of total fat cell number was useful, in that it permitted the classification of obese patients into 'hyperplastic' or 'hypertrophic' types. For example, if the subject illustrated in Figure 5.1 became obese and trebled his fat stores this could theoretically be done by trebling the fat content of each fat cell (hypertrophic obesity), or by trebling the number of fat cells, but keeping the triglyceride content of each cell at $4\,\mu$g (hyperplastic obesity), or by some combination of hypertrophy and hyperplasia. In recent years there has been controversy about the validity and usefulness of these calculations.

The validity of the calculation obviously depends on the assumption that total body fat can be measured, that the average triglyceride per fat cell in a biopsy can be measured, and that this biopsy sample indicates the size of fat cells elsewhere in the body. Each one of these assumptions is open to attack. The problems of measuring total body fat have been discussed in the previous section. The problems of measuring the fat per cell in a biopsy have been reviewed by Gurr and Kirtland (1978a, b). Here there are technical difficulties concerning the chemical or histological treatment of the biopsy sample, and even more severe difficulties in defining what is, or is not, a fat cell. The boundaries between an obvious fat cell and an obvious connective tissue fibroblast have been blurred, and 'preadipocytes' are now described which are potentially fat cells, but do not contain enough fat to be counted by standard techniques (Ashwell, 1978).

The concept of 'hypercellular obesity' has been vigorously attacked by Jung et al (1978) on the grounds that subcutaneous fat cell size does not accurately reflect the size of fat cells in deep sites, such as the omentum. This is true, and it is also true that the errors in estimating fat cell number are so large that on serial measurement patients may change from apparently hyperplastic to hypertrophic types, or vice versa (Garrow, 1978a). However Björntorp and Sjöström (1979) have rebutted the paper by Jung et al (1978), and the Göteborg group continue to maintain that hypercellular obesity has a worse long-term prognosis than hypertrophic obesity (Krotkiewski et al, 1977; Warnold Carlgren and Krotkiewski, 1978). This effect is not evident in the short term, under controlled metabolic conditions (Ashwell, Durrant and Garrow, 1978b), but it is still possible that the hypercellular obese patient is more liable than the hypertrophic patient to relapse from treatment. The relationship of fat cell number to the age of onset of obesity will be considered in the next section.

An important, but unresolved, question concerns the extent to which the metabolic abnormality in obese patients can be shown to reside in the adipose tissue. It has been repeatedly shown in vitro that large fat cells tend to have a higher rate of lipolysis than small fat cells, so in principle the adipocyte might have a system to control its own fat content, and hence that of the whole body. Bray et al (1977) studied adipose tissue from obese subjects before and after weight loss, and before and after weight gain in non-obese volunteers. They concluded that the in vitro behaviour of these samples of adipose tissue suggested that there were metabolic differences in the adipocytes of lean and obese subjects even when fat cell size and diet were controlled. However these differences were not shown in a series of transplantation experiments conducted by Ashwell et al (1976) and Ashwell and Meade (1978). If the defect in the genetically obese mouse (obob) existed within the fat cell it should be possible to demonstrate that adipose tissue transplanted from an obese mouse into a lean heterozygous littermate, or vice versa, should show the fat cell size characteristic of the genes of the donor mouse. In fact the reverse was found: transplanted adipose tissue tended to show the fat cell size of the host mouse rather than the donor. This work suggests that the factors which cause obesity in this strain of mouse are in the environment of the adipose tissue, rather than in the fat cell itself.

b. Obesity in children

Obesity in children, like obesity in adults, arises because energy intake from the diet is greater than energy expenditure. However, the level of energy intake and expenditure in children is affected by many factors: genetic, biochemical, social and environmental (Weil, 1977).

It is now generally agreed that fat cell number does *not* relate to the age of onset of obesity (Hirsch and Batchelor, 1976; Ashwell, 1979) provided that subjects with equal degree of obesity are compared. However it is still true that the most massively obese patients tend to be those in whom obesity started in childhood, and such patients also have a high fat cell number.

Although it is true that retrospective analyses of obese adults have shown that they were probably overweight children (Garrow, 1978b) prospective surveys have repeatedly failed to show that a study of the weight or diet of an infant can forecast the likelihood that it will be obese at age 4 years (Sveger, 1978), or 5 years (Poskitt and Cole, 1978) or 10 years (Wilkinson et al, 1977). There is a statistically significant association between maternal weight, weight gain in pregnancy, and weight-for-dates of the child (Udall et al, 1978), but the babies of massively obese mothers are not unusually obese at birth, or at the age of 6 months, although they become so by the age of one year (Edwards et al, 1978). Rapid fat gain in infants is not necessarily due to bottle-feeding, since Oakley (1977) found that breast-fed babies increased in skinfold thickness in the first six weeks of life at a greater rate than formula-fed infants.

Obesity in children and adolescents is difficult to treat effectively (Coates and Thorensen, 1978), so it is all the more important to prevent children becoming overweight. However, as the foregoing review shows, we are no nearer identifying a group of children (or adults) who are at particularly high risk to develop obesity. It is true that fat parents tend to have fat children, but this does not necessarily indicate a genetic influence (Garn and Clark, 1976): fat dogs tend to have fat owners, but the link here cannot be genetic (Mason, 1970).

c. Psychological factors affecting food intake

It is very difficult to study spontaneous food intake in man (Garrow, 1978a) but relatively easy in the laboratory rat, so human physiologists tended to argue on the basis of data obtained with rats. Five years ago it was standard teaching (Davidson et al, 1975) that food intake was determined by the relative activity of two 'centres' in the hypothalamus: a lateral 'feeding centre' which initiated feeding, and a ventromedial 'satiety centre' which terminated feeding. Our recent advances have been, first, to realise that the 'dual centre' theory was inadequate to explain eating behaviour in the rat, and second, that the factors affecting the food choice of free-range modern supermarket man extended far beyond the activity of nerve centres in his hypothalamus. The work of Nisbett (1968) and Schachter (1971) seemed to show that obese people were particularly susceptible to 'external' (i.e. non-nutritive) stimuli to eat. Subsequent work has shown that 'external' food cues are potent in both fat and thin people, and recent work has sought reliable differences between obese and non-obese people in this respect (Novin, Wyrwicka and Bray, 1976; Silverstone, 1976).

Energy intake can be manipulated by deceiving the subject, either by using an apparatus which misleads the subject about the amount which he has eaten (Pudel and Oetting, 1977) or by covertly substituting the artificial sweetener aspartame for sucrose in the diet (Porikos, Booth and van Itallie, 1977). However obese patients report greater hunger if their energy intake is covertly reduced (Durrant and Royston, 1979). No difference was found between obese and normal subjects in sensitivity to sweet taste by Grinker (1978), or between anorectic and control patients by Lacey et al (1977). Overweight female students were observed at a University cafeteria to return significantly less of their food uneaten than normal-weight female students, but there was no significant difference with male students (Krassner, Brownell & Stunkard, 1979).

The investigation of psychological factors affecting food intake is proving a fertile field for publications, but many questions remain unanswered. We really do not know how food intake is regulated in either normal or obese human subjects. There is increasing evidence that the sensation of satiety, which stops eating, is a *learned* response (Booth, 1977).

d. Dietary fibre and obesity

It is a plausible hypothesis that, since modern food technology tends to refine carbohydrates and increase the energy density of food, this has increased the risk of overeating, and hence of obesity (Heaton, 1973). Specifically, Hunt, Cash and Newland (1978) suggested that with energy-dense foods, although gastric emptying was slowed, it was slowed enough to control the rate at which energy was available for absorption in the small bowel. Grimes and Goddard (1977) showed that gastric emptying was slower with wholemeal bread than with white bread, so spontaneous food intake should be less if wholemeal bread is offered than if white bread is offered. A trial by Bryson, Doré and Garrow (1979) did not find this effect, and Durrant and Mann (1977) found that obese patients were able to detect differences in the energy content of the diet, even when energy density was manipulated to disguise this difference. A review by van Itallie (1978) concludes that it is uncertain how much a fibre-rich diet would contribute to the prevention of obesity.

e. Thermogenesis

Since it is so difficult to show that the aetiology of obesity lies in some demonstrable disorder of the regulation of energy intake, the alternative explanation must be considered — that the defect lies in regulation of energy expenditure. The question of physical activity, and its bearing on energy expenditure, will be considered in the next section. There has been considerable recent work on resting metabolic rate in obese people, and on the magnitude of thermogenic responses in lean and obese subjects. This work has been made possible by recent advances in techniques for measuring energy expenditure.

Almost all the recent measurements of metabolic rate and energy expenditure in man have been made by indirect calorimetry. Techniques for indirect calorimetry and their limitations have recently been reviewed by Durnin (1978). In certain circumstances, even skilled operators may find errors of 10 per cent or more when measurements made by indirect calorimetry are checked against a direct calorimeter. Probably the most important source of error is the uncertainty about the energy equivalence of the oxygen consumed: this depends on the nature of the fuel (protein, fat, carbohydrate or alcohol) which is being consumed at the time of the measurement. In addition to this there are many technical traps for the inexperienced observer which are reviewed elsewhere (Garrow, 1978a).

A lively correspondence was started by James et al (1978a) on the observation that in general obese subjects had a *higher* absolute resting metabolic rate than normal-weight people of similar age, sex and height. This set off a debate about the way in which metabolic rate should be expressed, because it is possible, by dividing by surface area, to reduce the absolute difference in metabolic rate between fat and thin humans, or indeed between mice and elephants (James et al, 1978b). Figure 5.3 shows the resting metabolic rate of women admitted to our unit at Northwick Park Hospital for investigation of obesity. It is true that, in general, the more grossly obese the patient the higher is her resting metabolic rate, but it is also striking that at any value

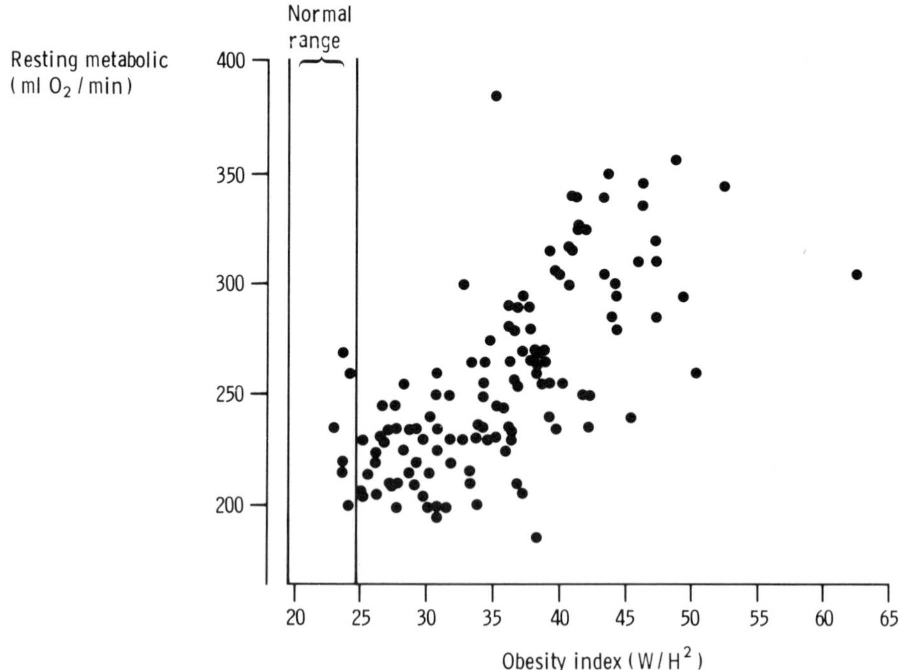

Fig. 5.3   The relationship between the resting metabolic rate and the obesity index in women ranging from normal build to severe obesity (Garrow, 1980).

of obesity index there is a huge range of variation in metabolic rate. Thus although as a group it is true that obese people have raised metabolic rates compared with normal-weight people, it is also true that some obese people have lower metabolic rates than some lean people.

The thermogenic response of fat and thin women to an oral dose of 50 g glucose has been studied by Jéquier, Pitlet and Gygax (1978). They found that in lean subjects metabolic rate rose by 13.0 per cent in the 150 minute period after taking the glucose, but only by 5.2 per cent in obese subjects. This is probably the most convincing evidence that there are differences between fat and thin people in their capacity for thermogenesis, but even so the effect is small compared with the range of individual variation shown in Figure 5.3. It was suggested by Miller and Wise (1975) that physical activity potentiated dietary-induced thermogenesis, but Garby and Lammert (1977) found no difference in the energy cost of a standardised exercise test whether their subjects had been overfed or underfed the previous day.

f. Exercise

It is obvious that physical activity increases energy expenditure, and therefore that the level of physical activity of a person is relevant to that person's state of energy balance. Confusion arises when the contribution of exercise is assessed quantitatively. For example the latest recommended intake tables (DHSS, 1979) suggest that a sedentary man aged 18–34 years requires 2510 kcal (10.5 MJ) per day, whereas moderately active one requires 2900 kcal (12.0 MJ) and a very active man requires 3350 kcal (14.0 MJ) per day. The main determinant of total energy expenditure, even among very active people like soldiers, is resting metabolic rate, so it is unrealistic for a sedentary person, with the physique and resting metabolic rate which goes with a sedentary life, to imagine that he can alter his daily energy expenditure by more than 400 kcal (1 MJ) even if he adopts a quite vigorous exercise programme and keeps to it every day.

It is very difficult to assess the effect of physical activity on disease risk, since those who choose to take exercise are self-selected and not necessarily comparable to those who do not (Milvy, Forbes and Brown, 1977). It is also difficult to obtain reliable data about habitual physical activity in epidemiological research (Taylor et al, 1978; LaPorte et al, 1979), and still more difficult to persuade large groups of people to undertake exercise programmes for more than about three months (Reid and Morgan, 1979). However there is no doubt that exercise increases work capacity and efficiency (Taylor and Jones, 1979), it causes an increase in the protective high-density lipoprotein (Miller et al, 1979), and will reverse involutional bone loss (Aloia et al, 1978). It seems that the effect of physical training is chiefly on the muscle which is exercised, rather than on general cardiopulmonary fitness (Fentem, 1978).

RECENT ADVANCES IN THE TREATMENT OF OBESITY

Since obesity is characterised by excess energy stored as fat, there is no possible effective treatment other than creating a negative energy balance so the excess fat is burned off. However, within these limitations dictated by fundamental thermodynamics, there is scope for developing more effective or more acceptable means by which this negative energy balance can be established.

a. Dietary treatment

Recent publications concern the optimum protein-fat-carbohydrate proportions in a reducing diet. With a diet supplying about 1000 kcal (4 MJ) per day, weight loss in the first 15 days is significantly more rapid if the carbohydrate content of the diet is low (102 kcal) than if it is high (697 kcal), with reciprocal differences in fat to make the diets isoenergetic (Rabast, Kasper & Schöborn, 1978): however over longer period the difference in weight loss ceases to be significant.

There has been much attention to the 'protein-sparing modified fast' diet. The rationale is that, with any reducing diet, there is a tendency to lose lean tissue: with total starvation loss of protein is initially at the rate of about 75 g/day. If protein is added to the diet nitrogen balance becomes less negative, and if this trend is extrapolated one might expect nitrogen balance with an intake of about 1.5 g protein/kg body weight/day (Bistrian, 1978). However, many investigators remain sceptical (Mann, 1977), and the popularity of the diet has elicited warning of the potential dangers of vitamin and mineral deficiency in those taking only protein (Anonymous, 1978). Although the trend line predicts that nitrogen equilibrium should be achieved at an intake of 1.5 g protein/kg body weight there is not much evidence that this actually happens (Garrow, 1978a).

b. Behaviour therapy and drug treatment

Anorectic drugs, such as diethylpropion, fenfluramine and mazindol, consistently produce greater weight loss than placebo drugs, but their effect diminishes with time. When Stuart (1967) reported excellent weight loss in eight patients over a year by the use of behaviour modification techniques there was optimism that behavioural techniques might have a more sustained effect on weight loss. Recent publications do not support this hope. Ashby and Wilson (1977) failed to find any effect of booster sessions after subjects had lost about 4–5 kg in eight weeks of behaviour therapy. Dahms et al (1978) found that subjects treated by behaviour therapy lost rather more than those on either mazindol or diethylpropion, but only 33 of their 120 subjects completed the 14 week study. Obese patients under psychoanalysis tend to lose weight, but only slowly (Rand and Stunkard, 1978): 47 per cent had lost more than 9 kg in 42 months, and 19 per cent had lost more than 18 kg. Behaviour therapists concentrate on identifying the cues to eat and trying to help the patient to avoid them. It is evident that financial incentives are also important (Ferguson, 1978). Jeffery, Thompson & Wing (1978) note that if patients can be induced to enter into contracts by which they have strong monetary incentives to lose weight they tend to do better than those who are not so motivated, but it is not clear if this approach merely selects those who are determined to succeed. Brownell & Stunkard (1978) find no evidence that weight loss is in fact related to behavioural change.

Neither drug treatment nor behaviour therapy has revolutionised the treatment of obesity, and there is no consensus on how these techniques should be applied. Common sense suggests that anorectic drugs should help those obese patients who are driven by hunger to abandon their reducing diet, and behaviour therapy should help those who eat from habit or social pressures even when they are not hungry. However, attempts to identify patients in these categories have so far failed. Far too many reports of treatment trials are rendered useless by high attrition rate, or a short follow-up, or by total absence of any control group. However well-controlled long-term trials with complete follow-up are extremely difficult to arrange.

c. Surgical treatment of obesity

Since advice, drugs and psychotherapy are generally inadequate to produce massive weight loss in severely obese patients, the alternative is some form of surgery. The most commonly performed operation to date has been jejunoileal bypass, so the patient is left with only 45 cm of small bowel in continuity, and consequently develops a malabsorption syndrome. The results of this operation have been reviewed by Iber and Cooper (1977): patients usually lose a lot of weight, but at a high price in long-term morbidity. Since dietary fat is not well absorbed from the shortened gut the fat-soluble vitamins are also not absorbed, and the absorption of calcium and magnesium is also impaired. In the long term, renal damage is an important side effect: oxalate deposits in the kidneys are being discovered several years after the operation. It has also been convincingly shown that the main cause of weight loss in patients after jejunoileal bypass is that they eat less (Pilkington et al, 1976; Bray et al, 1978) although the reason for this decreased intake is not clear: neither depression, nausea, malabsorption, liver disease, decreased appetite or the attempt to avoid diarrhoea can entirely explain it (Robinson, Folstein and McHugh, 1979).

The operation which is now gaining in popularity, and which may replace jejunoileal bypass, is some form of gastric bypass (Mason and Ito, 1969). The principle of the operation is to create a stenosis in the stomach so food enters a small pouch at the fundus which is connected by a small stoma to the rest of the stomach. After the operation it is impossible for the patient to take a large meal without vomiting, but the food which is eaten is normally absorbed, so this operation does not have the serious metabolic consequences of the jejunoileal bypass.

Yet another approach is to immobilise the stomach by vagotomy (Kral, 1978). So far there has been insufficient time to evaluate the long-term results of this technique. Still simpler is the technique of wiring the jaws together to inhibit eating, but this does not solve the problem of weight regain when the fixation is removed. It may be, however, that jaw wiring is a useful prelude to an operation such as gastric bypass (Fordyce et al, 1979), since it is easier to anaesthetise and operate on a patient who is not grossly obese (Kreienbühl, 1978).

FUTURE ADVANCES IN THE FIELD OF ENERGY BALANCE

The most exciting recent developments, and the most likely future advances, concern hormonal influences on energy expenditure. In obesity there is often abnormality in production of sex hormones (Schneider et al, 1979; Glass et al, 1978), although there is no reason to believe that this is the cause of obesity. Abnormalities of prolactin secretion are reported (Kopelman et al, 1979), but the normal function of prolactin is obscure (Editorial, 1979). Cushing's syndrome is often listed in the causes of obesity, but it rarely causes severe obesity (Printen and Blommers, 1977). Metabolic rate decreases when patients are semistarved, and so does the concentration of serum tri-iodothyronine (Vagenakis et al, 1977; Grant et al, 1978), but serum T_3 concentration is not related to body weight (Wilcox, 1977) and thyroid function tests on obese people give a similar range of results to those found in non-obese people (Strata et al, 1978). All these results indicate that there is no obvious endocrine abnormality which characterises, or causes, obesity.

However, recent work suggests that obese and lean human subjects, or rats, may differ in their thermogenic response to catechol amines. Shetty, Jung and James (1979) showed that the fall in metabolic rate which is associated with semistarvation can be prevented by giving a dose of 4 g/day of levodopa, a precursor of catecholamine synthesis. The expected decrease in tri-iodothyronine occurred, so the fall in metabolic rate cannot be due simply to changes in thyroid hormones. This work was extended by Jung et al (1979) who showed that after an infusion of noradrenalin obese women, and those who had previously been obese, showed a smaller thermogenic response than lean controls with no family history of obesity. They suggested that the thermogenic defect in obese subjects might lie in their inability to generate heat in brown adipose tissue, for which there is a convincing animal model. This idea is further strengthened by the observations of Rothwell and Stock (1979) who have blocked the thermogenic response to overeating in rats by injecting propranolol, and shown in a human subject that there are warm patches on the skin one hour after taking an oral dose of ephedrine. These warm patches may well indicate the presence of metabolically active brown adipose tissue.

SUMMARY

Obesity is a major public health problem, especially in young people. Its prevalence is increasing. There have been many recent advances in techniques for measuring energy balance and body composition in man. Both energy intake and energy expenditure are influenced by several factors, and individuals vary greatly in their response to such stimuli. We still do not understand the system which controls energy balance in man well enough to be able to manipulate the factors controlling the system to the advantage of all obese patients, but encouraging progress is being made.

REFERENCES

Abraham S, Johnson C L, Najjar M F 1979 Weight and height of adults 18–74 years of age, United States 1971–74. *DHEW publication* 79–1659, National Center for Health Statistics, Maryland

Aloia J F, Cohn S H, Ostuni J A, Cane R, Ellis K 1978 Prevention of involutional bone loss by exercise. Annals of Internal Medicine 89: 356–358

Anonymous 1978 Statement by the American Dietetic Association on diet protein products. Journal American Dietetic Association 73 547–548

Ashby W A, Wilson G T 1977 Behaviour therapy for obesity: Booster sessions and long term maintenance of weight loss. Behaviour Research and Therapy 15: 451–463

Ashwell M 1978 The 'fat cell pool' concept. International Journal of Obesity 2: 69–72

Ashwell M 1979 How can research into fat cells and fat distribution help the treatment of obesity? International Journal of Obesity 3: 188–189

Ashwell M, North W R, Meade T W 1978a Social class, smoking and obesity. British Medical Journal ii: 1466–1467

Ashwell M, Durrant M & Garrow J S 1978b Does adipose tissue cellularity or the age of onset of obesity influence the response to short-term inpatient treatment of obese women? International Journal of Obesity 2: 449–456.

Ashwell M A, Meade C J 1978 Obesity: do fat cells from genetically obese mice (C57BL/6J ob/ob) have an innate capacity for increased fat storage? Diabetologia 15: 465–470

Ashwell M, Meade C J, Medawar P M, Sowter C 1976 Adipose tissue: contributions of nature and nurture to the obesity of an obese mutant mouse (obob). Proceedings of the Nutrition Society 36: 16A

Bistrian 1978 Clinical use of a protein-sparing modified fast. Journal of the American Medical Association 240: 2299–2302

Björntorp P, Sjöström L 1979 Adipose tissue cellularity. International Journal of Obesity 3: 181–187

Blair B F, Haines L W 1966 Mortality experience according to build at higher durations. Transactions Actuarial Society of America 18: 35–41

Booth D A 1977 Satiety and appetite are conditioned reactions. Psychosomatic Medicine 39: 76–81

Bray G A (ed.) 1978a Recent advances in obesity research: II. Newman Publishing, London, p 419

Bray G A 1978b Definition, measurement and classification of the syndromes of obesity. International Journal of Obesity 2: 99–112

Bray G A, Glennon J A, Salans L B, Horton E S, Danforth E, Sims E A H 1977 Spontaneous and experimental human obesity: Effects of diet and adipose cell size on lipolysis and lipogenesis. Metabolism 26: 739–748

Bray G A, Zachary B, Dahms W T, Atkinson R L, Oddie T H 1978 Eating patterns of massively obese individuals. Journal of the American Dietetic Association 72: 24–27

Brownell K D, Stunkard A J 1978 Behaviour therapy and behaviour change: uncertainties in programs for weight control. Behaviour Research and Therapy 16: 301

Bryson E, Doré C, Garrow J S 1979 Wholemeal bread and satiety. Lancet ii: 260–261

Bulow J M, Hansen M, Madsen J 1976 Variation in human subcutaneous adipose tissue blood flow. Acta Physiologica Scandinavica 96: 30A–31A

Chave S P, Morris J N, Moss S, Semmence A M 1978 Vigorous exercise in leisure time and the death rate: a study of male civil servants. Journal of Epidemiology and Community Health 32: 239–243

Coates T J, Thorensen C E 1978 Treating obesity in children and adolescents: A review. American Journal of Public Health 68: 143–152

Cole T J, James W P T 1978 The slimdicator: a slide rule device for assessing obesity. Practitioner 220: 628–630

Cook L 1978 Relationship of blood pressure, serum cholesterol, smoking habit, relative weight and ECG abnormalities to incidence of major coronary events: final report of the pooling project. The Pooling Project Research Group. Journal of Chronic Diseases 31: 201–306

Costas, P Jr, Garcia-Palmieri M R, Nazario E, Sorlie P D 1978 Relation of lipids, weight and physical activity to incidence of coronary heart disease: the Puerto Rico heart study. American Journal of Cardiology 42: 653–658

Dahms W T, Molitch M E, Bray G A, Greenway F L, Atkinson R L, Hamilton K 1978 Treatment of obesity: cost-benefit assessment of behavioural therapy, placebo, and two anorectic drugs. American Journal of Clinical Nutrition 31: 774–778

Davidson S, Passmore R, Brock J F, Truswell A S 1975 Human nutrition and dietetics. Churchill Livingstone Edinburgh p 36

Department of Health and Social Security 1979 Recommended daily amounts of food energy and nutrients for groups of people in the United Kingdom. Her Majesty's Stationery Office (London), p 27

Diethelm R, Garrow J S, Stalley S F 1977 An apparatus for measuring the density of obese patients. Journal of Physiology 267: 14–15

Durnin J V G A 1978 Indirect calorimetry in man: a critique of practical problems. Proceedings of the Nutrition Society 37: 5–12

Durrant M, Mann S 1977 Investigations into patient responses to feeding low- and high-energy foods. Proceedings of the Nutrition Society 36: 113A

Durrant M L, Royston P 1979 The effect of preloads of varying energy density and methyl cellulose on hunger, appetite and salivation. Proceedings of the Nutrition Society 37: 87A

Editorial 1979 What does prolactin do in man? Lancet ii: 234–235

Edwards L E, Dickes W F, Alton I R, Hakanson E Y 1978 Pregnancy in the massively obese: Course outcome and obesity prognosis of the infant. American Journal of Obstetrics and Gynecology 131: 479–483

Fentem P H 1978 Advice on exercise. British Medical Journal ii: 429

Ferguson J 1978 Dieticians as behaviour-change agents. Journal American Dietetic Association 73: 231–238

Fordyce G L, Garrow J S, Kark A E, Stalley S F 1979 Jaw wiring and gastric bypass in the treatment of severe obesity. Obesity Bariatric Medicine 8: 14–17

Franklin B A, Buskirk E R, Mendez J 1978 Validity of skinfold equations on lean and obese subjects. American Journal of Clinical Nutrition 31: 563–565

Garby L, Lammert O 1977 Effect of the preceding day's energy intake on the total energy cost of light exercise. Acta Physiologica Scandinavica 101: 411–417

Garn S M, Clark D C 1976 Trends in fatness and the origins of obesity. Pediatrics 57: 443–456

Garrow J S 1978a Energy balance and obesity in man (2nd edn). Elsevier, Amsterdam, p 243

Garrow J S 1978b Infant feeding and obesity of adults. Bibliotheca Nutritio et Dieta 26: 29–35

Garrow J S 1980 Combined medical-surgical approaches to treatment of obesity. American Journal of Clinical Nutrition 33: 425–430

Garrow J S, Stalley S, Diethelm R, Pittet P, Hesp R, Halliday D 1979 A new method for measuring the body density of obese adults. British Journal of Nutrition 42: 173–183

Glass A R, Dahms W T, Abraham G, Atkinson R L, Bray G A, Swerdloff R S 1978 Secondary amenorrhea in obesity: etiologic role of weight-related androgen excess. Fertil Steril 30: 243–244

Grant A M, Edwards O M, Howard A N, Challand G S, Wraight E P, Mills I H 1978 Thyroidal hormone metabolism in obesity during semistarvation. Clinical Endocrinology (Oxford) 9: 227–231

Grimes D S, Goddard J 1977 Gastric emptying of wholemeal and white bread. Gut 18: 725–729

Grinker, J 1978 Obesity and sweet taste. American Journal of Clinical Nutrition 31: 1078–1087

Gurr M I, Kirtland J 1978a Adipose tissue cellularity: a review. 1. Techniques for studying cellularity. International Journal of Obesity 2: 401–427

Gurr M I, Kirtland J 1978b Adipose tissue cellularity: a review. 2. The relationship between cellularity and obesity. International Journal of Obesity 3: 15–55

Halliday D, Miller A G 1977 Precise measurement of total body water using trace quantities of deuterium oxide. Biomedical Mass Spectrometry 4: 82–87

Heaton K W 1973 Food fibre as an obstacle to energy intake. Lancet ii: 1418–1421

Hill G L, McCarthy I D, Collins J P, Smith A H 1978 A new method for the rapid measurement of body composition in critically ill surgical patients. British Journal of Surgery 65: 732–735

Hirsch J, Batchelor B 1976 Adipose tissue cellularity in human obesity. Clinics in Endocrinology and Metabolism 5: 299–311

Howard A (ed) 1975 Recent advances in obesity research: I. Newman Publishing, London, p 419

Hunt J N, Cash R, Newland P 1978 Energy density of food, gastric emptying, and obesity. American Journal of Clinical Nutriton 31: (10 Suppl) S259–S260

Iber F L & Cooper M 1977 Jejunoileal bypass for the treatment of massive obesity. Prevalence, morbidity and short- and long-term consequences. American Journal of Clinical Nutrition 30: 4–15

James W P T (Compiler) 1976 Research on obesity: a report of the DHSS/MRC group. Her Majesty's Stationery Office, London, p 94

James W P T, Dauncey M J, Davies H L 1978b Elevated metabolic rates in obesity. Lancet ii: 472

James W P T Davies H L, Bailes J, Dauncey M J 1978a Elevated metabolic rates in obesity. Lancet i: 1122–1125

Jeffery R W, Thompson P D, Wing R R 1978 Effects on weight reduction of strong monetary contracts for calorie restriction or weight loss. Behaviour Research & Therapy 16: 363–369

Jéquier E, Pittet P, Gygax P H 1978 Thermic effect of glucose and thermal body insulation in lean and obese subjects: a calorimetric approach. Proceedings of the Nutrition Society 37: 45–53

Jones P R M, Bharadwaj H, Bhatia M R, Malhotra M S 1976 Differences between ethnic groups in the relationship of skinfold thickness to body density. In: Bhatia B, Chhina G S, Baldev Singh (eds) Selected topics in environmental biology. Interprint Publications, New Delhi

Jung R T, Gurr M I, Robinson M P, James W P T 1978 Does adipocyte hypercellularity in obesity exist? British Medical Journal ii: 319–321

Jung R T, Shetty P S, James W P T, Barrand M A, Callingham B A 1979 Reduced thermogenesis in obesity. Nature 279: 322–323

Juustila H 1977 Overweight and obesity as risk factors of IHD. Acta Medica Scandinavica 613: 17–19

Keys A, Aravanis C, Blackburn H, Buchem F S P, Buzina R, Djordjevic B S, Fidanza F, Karvonen M J, Menotti V, Taylor H L 1972 Coronary heart disease: overweight and obesity as risk factors. Annals of Internal Medicine 77: 15–27

Keys A, Brozek J. 1953 Body fat in adult man. Physiological Reviews 33: 245–325

Khosla T 1978 Standards on age, height and weight in Olympic running events for men. British Journal of Sports Medicine 12: 97–101

Kopelman P G, White N, Pilkington T R, Jeffcoate S L 1979 Impaired hypothalamic control of prolactin secretion in massive obesity. Lancet i: 747–750

Kral J G 1978 Vagotomy for treatment of severe obesity. Lancet i: 307–308

Krassner H A, Brownell K D, Stunkard A J 1979 Cleaning the plate: food left over by overweight and normal weight persons. Behaviour Research Therapy 17: 155–156

Kreienbühl G 1978 Anaesthesie bei extremer adipositas. Anaesthetist 27: 416–420

Krotkiewski M, Sjöström L, Björntorp P, Carlgren G, Garellick G, Smith U 1977 Adipose tissue cellularity in relation to prognosis for weight reduction. International Journal of Obesity 1: 395–416

Lacey J H, Stanley P A, Crutchfield M, Crisp A H 1977 Sucrose sensitivity in anorexia nervosa. Journal of Psychosomatic Research 21: 17–21

LaPorte R E, Kuller L H, Kupfer D J, McPartland R J, Matthews G, Caspersen C 1979 An objective measure of physical activity for epidemiologic research. American Journal of Epidemiology 109: 158–168

Levinson M L 1977 Obesity and health. Preventive Medicine 6: 172–180

Lew E A, Garfinkel L 1979 Variations in mortality by weight among 750,000 men and women. Journal of Chronic Diseases 32: 563–576

Mahler R F 1978 Fat: the good, the bad and the ugly. Journal of the Royal College of Physicians, London 12: 107–121

Mann G V 1974 The influence of obesity on health. New England Journal of Medicine 291: 178–185 and 226–232

Mann G V 1977 Diet and obesity. New England Journal of Medicine 296: 812

Mason E 1970 Obesity in pet dogs. Vetinary Record 86: 612–616

Mason E E, Ito C 1969 Gastric Bypass. Annals of Surgery 170: 329–336

Miller D S, Wise A 1975 Exercise and dietary-induced thermogenesis. Lancet i: 1290

Miller N E, Rao S, Lewis B, Bjørsvik G, Myhre K, Mjøs O D 1979 High density lipoprotein and physical activity. Lancet i: 111

Milvy P, Forbes W F, Brown K S 1977 A critical review of epidemiological studies of physical activity. Annals of New York Academy of Sciences 301: 519–549

Nisbett R E 1968 Determinants of food intake in obesity. Science 159: 1254–1255

Novin D, Wyrwicka W, Bray G (eds) 1976 Hunger: basic mechanisms and clinical applications. Raven Press, New York, p 494

Oakley J R 1977 Differences in subcutaneous fat in breast and formula-fed infants. Archives of Disease in Childhood 52: 79–80

Paffenbarger R S Jr, Brand R J, Sholtz R I, Jung D L 1978 Energy expenditure, cigarette smoking, and blood pressure level as related to death from specific diseases. American Journal of Epidemiology 108: 12–18

Pilkington T R E, Gazet J C, Ang L, Kalvcy R S, Crisp A H, Day S 1976 Explanation for weight loss after ileojejunal bypass in gross obesity. British Medical Journal 1: 1504–1505

Porikos K P, Booth G. van Itallie T B 1977 Effect of covert nutritive dilution on the spontaneous food intake of obese individuals: a pilot study. American Journal Clinical Nutrition 30: 1638–1644

Poskitt E M E, Cole T J 1978 Nature, nurture and childhood overweight. British Medical Journal 1: 603–605

Printen K J, Blommers T J 1977 Morbid obesity in Cushing's syndrome? A Nonentity? American Journal of Surgery 134: 579–580

Printen K J, Miller E V, Mason E E, Barnes R W 1978 Venous thromboembolism in the morbidly obese. Surgery, Gynecology and Obstetrics 147: 63–64

Pudel V E, Oetting M 1977 Eating in the laboratory: behavioural aspects of the positive energy balance. International Journal of Obesity 1: 369–386

Rabast U, Kasper H, Schöborn J 1978 Comparative studies in obese subjects fed carbohydrate-restricted and high-carbohydrate 1000-calorie formula diets. Nutrition and Metabolism 22: 269–277

Rabkin S W, Mathewson F A L, Hsu P-H 1977 Relation of body weight to development of ischaemic heart disease in a cohort of young North American men after a 26 year observation period: the Manitoba study. American Journal of Cardiology 39: 452–458

Rand C, Stunkard A J 1978 Obesity and psychoanalysis. American Journal of Psychiatry 135: 547–551

Reid E L, Morgan R W 1979 Exercise prescription — a clinical trial. American Journal of Public Health 69: 591–595

Robinson R G, Folstein M F, McHugh P R 1979 Reduced caloric intake following small bowel bypass surgery: a systematic study of possible causes. Psychological Medicine 9: 37–53

Rothwell N J, Stock M J 1979 A role for brown adipose tissue in diet-induced thermogenesis. Nature 281: 31–35

Santesson J, Nordentröm J 1978 Pulmonary function in extreme obesity. Influence of weight loss following intestinal shunt operation. Acta Chirurgica Scandinavica (Suppl) 482: 36–40

Schachter S 1971 Some extraordinary facts about obese humans and rats. American Psychologist 26: 129–144

Schneider G, Kirchner M A, Berkowitz R, Ertel N H 1979 Increased estrogen production in obese men. Journal of Clinical Endocrinology and Metabolism 48: 633–638

Sheng H P, Huggins R A 1979 A review of body composition studies with emphasis on total body water and fat. American Journal of Clinical Nutrition 32: 630–647

Shetty P S, Jung R T, James W P 1979 Effect of catecholamine replacement with levodopa on the metabolic response to semistarvation. Lancet 1: 77–79

Silverstone T (ed.) 1976 Appetite and food intake. Dahlem Konferenzen, Berlin, p 498

Smith T, Hesp R, MacKenzie J 1979 Total body potassium calibrations for normal and obese subjects in two types of whole body counter. Physics in Medicine and Biology 24: 171–175

Sonne-Holm S, Sorensen T I A 1977 Post-war course of the prevalence of extreme overweight among Danish young men. Journal of Chronic Diseases 30: 351–358

Stamler R, Stamler J, Reidlinger W F, Algera G, Roberts R H 1978 Weight and blood pressure. Findings in hypertension screening of one million Americans. Journal of the American Medical Association 240: 1607–1610

Stern S 1978 Obesity and ischaemic heart disease. American Journal of Cardiology 41: 622

Strata A, Ugolotti G, Contini C, Magnati G, Pugnoli C, Tirelli F, Zuliani U 1978 Thyroid and obesity: survey of some function tests in a large obese population. International Journal of Obesity 2: 333–340

Strauss R J, Wise L 1978 Operative risks of obesity. Surgery, Gynecology and Obstetrics 146: 286–291

Stuart R B 1967 Behavioural control of overeating. Behaviour Research and Therapy 5: 357–365

Sveger T 1978 Does overnutrition or obesity during the first year affect weight at age four? Acta Paediatrica Scandinavica 67: 465–468

Taylor H L, Jacobs D R, Schucker B, Knudsen J, Leon A S, Debacker G 1978 A questionnaire for the assessment of leisure time physical activities. Journal of Chronic Diseases 31: 741–745

Taylor R, Jones N L 1979 The reduction by training of CO_2 output during exercise. European Journal of Cardiology 9: 53–62

Tsueda K, Warren J E, McCafferty L A, Nagle J P 1978 Pancuronium bromide requirement during anaesthesia for the morbidly obese. Anesthiology 48: 438–439

Udall J N, Garrison G G, Vaucher Y, Walson P D, Morrow G 1978 Interaction of maternal and neonatal obesity. Pediatrics 62: 17–21

Vagenakis A G, Portnay G I, O'Brien J T, Rudolph M, Arky R A, Ingbar S H, Braverman L E 1977 Effect of starvation on the production and metabolism of thyroxine and triiodothyronine in euthyroid obese patients. Journal of Clinical Endocrinology and Metabolism 45: 1305–1309

van Itallie T B 1978 Dietary fibre and obesity. American Journal of Clinical Nutrition 31: (10 suppl) S43–52

Warnold I, Carlgren G, Krotkiewski M 1978 Energy expenditure and body composition during weight reduction in hyperplastic obese women. American Journal of Clinical Nutrition 31: 750–763

Warwick P M, Garrow J S 1979 Diet and activity in obese patients in a metabolic ward. Proceedings of the Nutrition Society 38: 81 A

Weltman A, Katch V L 1978 A non population-specific method for predicting total body volume and percent fat. Human Biology 50: 151–158

Weil W B 1977 Current controversies in obesity. Journal of Pediatrics 91: 175–187

Wilcox R G 1977 Triiodothyronine T S H and prolactin in obese women. Lancet 1: 1027–1029

Wilkinson P W, Parkin J M, Pearlson J, Philips P R, Sykes P 1977 Obesity in childhood: a community study in Newcastle upon Tyne. Lancet i: 350–352

Womersley J, Durnin J V G A 1977 A comparison of the skinfold method with extent of 'overweight' and various weight-height relationships in the assessment of obesity. British Journal of Nutrition 38: 271–284

6. Ultrasound

Hylton B. Meire

THE PRINCIPLES OF ULTRASOUND

Diagnostic ultrasound employs very high frequency sound waves to investigate internal structures. Where blood flow is to be detected the sound is emitted as a continuous beam and the Doppler effect is employed to indicate the presence of a moving target within the area examined. To produce a sectional image of internal structures the sound is emitted in very brief pulses, approximately one millionth of a second in duration, and the echoes reflected from internal structures are collected and electronically processed to form the image. The commonest form of sectional imaging device is the 'B' scanner in which a transducer, which both emits and receives the sound pulses, is manually scanned over the surface of the patient. The transducer is confined by a mechanical gantry to move in a single plane and the resulting image is a representation of the structures within a thin slice of the patient beneath the transducer. In general the slice thickness is of the order of three millimetres and the resolution within the image is usually from one to five millimetres.

Ultrasound has two major limitations. The first is unavoidable and results from its total reflection by bone and gas. The anatomical areas accessible to ultrasound are therefore limited to those regions which can be accessed without the sound beam traversing bone or gas containing structures. Secondly, manually operated B scanners require considerable skill, knowledge and expertise on behalf of the operator and where these are not available a B scanner is likely to be more of a liability than a powerful diagnostic weapon.

The high frequency sound emitted by ultrasound transducers is of exceedingly low power and is also rapidly attenuated as it passes through tissues. Although it is possible to induce biological change and tissue damage by ultrasound radiation, the power levels necessary to achieve this are many orders of magnitude greater than those present in diagnostic ultrasound equipment. A great many research projects have been undertaken in an attempt to confirm the innocuous nature of diagnostic ultrasound and none has yet shown any adverse effects to either patients, their offspring or the equipment operators.

The operation and applications of ultrasound equipment and the potential biological effects of ultrasound have been admirably reviewed recently by Wells (1977) and those readers who wish to study these aspects of the subject are referred to this excellent book.

Over the past few years two major changes have occurred in diagnostic ultrasound equipment. The first of these was the introduction of a stored grey scale image. This form of display enables us to differentiate various soft tissues structures by virtue of the strength of the echoes returning from them. This capability has vastly increased the application of ultrasound both in obstetrics and general medical and surgical practice. The second development, which is still progressing rapidly, is the advent of the 'real-time' scanner. These devices produce live moving images of internal structures by means of an automatic mechanical or electronic device which steers the beam through the patient whilst the transducer assembly is held stationary over the area of interest. They substantially reduce the operator dependence of diagnostic ultrasound, which has been a major limitation to the development and application of conventional 'static' B scanners. At the present time, however, both B scanners and real-time scanners are complementary and both have their particular advantages and limitations.

A further recent technical development is the combination of Doppler detection with pulsed ultrasound scanning to permit non-invasive imaging of blood vessels. The early clinical results with this device are discussed below in the section of vascular imaging.

The applications of all forms of ultrasound scanning in clinical investigation have recently been reviewed (Meire, 1979). In this chapter some of the more recent and important or interesting developments which have occurred will be briefly discussed.

Obstetrics

Whilst ultrasound has been in regular use in obstetrics for nearly 20 years it was primarily used to measure the diameter of the fetal head and determine the placental site. However, with the greatly improved image quality and resolution now available, detailed fetal anatomy can be seen early in pregnancy and a rapidly expanding range of fetal abnormalities have been detected. In many hospitals it is now routine practice to perform ultrasound examination on every pregnant patient during the first trimester. This permits confirmation of the gestational age, exclusion or confirmation of multiple pregnancy and the diagnosis of many of the more severe congenital malformations. For many years it has been possible to diagnose anencephaly in fetuses beyond about the 12th week of gestation but it is now possible to make this diagnosis from about the 9th week, and by 16 weeks the normal fetal spine and spinal canal can be reliably visualised. It is therefore now possible to exclude significant neural tube defects by 16 weeks of pregnancy. In those cases where they are diagnosed or suspected it is possible to perform confirmatory amniocentesis and alfa-feto-protein estimation before proceeding to termination. This perhaps tends to suggest that AFP estimation should be the final arbiter. In my own department in the past two years we have had two cases with abnormally high AFP measurements in whom ultrasound has excluded the presence of neural tube defects and normal fetuses have ultimately been born at term. Conversely ultrasound has correctly diagnosed a closed lumbar neural tube defect in a patient with a strong family history but normal amniotic AFP. In our own experience ultrasound has been more accurate than AFP estimation and these experiences are by no means unique. The application of ultrasound for the examination of neural tube lesions has recently been reviewed by Sample (1978).

Whilst numerous case reports have been published concerning a wide range of fetal abnormalities diagnosed by ultrasound we have in our department been performing a prospective study of nearly 1000 patients per year to assess the ability of ultrasound to diagnose a multitude of fetal abnormalities. During the past two years of this study 25 significant and potentially detectable malformations have occurred in the study group. Ultrasound has correctly diagnosed 24 of these. The lesions include neural tube defect, hydrocephalus, hydranencephalus, urinary and intestinal obstructions and congenital heart disease (Farrant, 1980). Figure 6.1 illustrates an ultrasound scan performed on a 20-week pregnancy. The fetal liver and bowel can be seen surrounded by ascites and the placenta is unusually large. These findings indicate fetal hydrops due either to haemolytic anaemia or cardiac malformation. The fetus was severely affected by rhesus isoimmunisation and died in utero despite early ultrasound guided intrauterine transfusion. Ultrasound is proving to be extremely valuable in the management of the few remaining cases of this disorder.

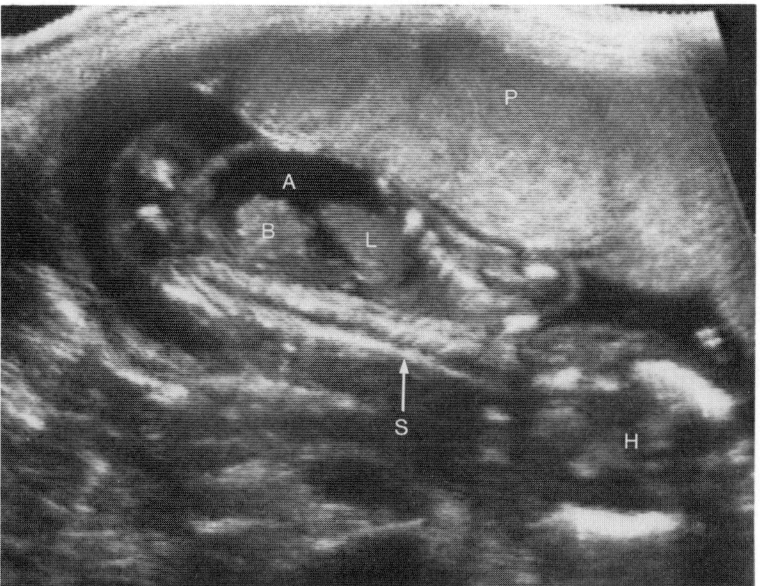

Fig. 6.1   Longitudinal scan of a 20-week fetus with ascites. Fetal spine S, liver L, bowel B, ascites A, head H, placenta P.

Significant advances are also being made in the assessment of intrauterine fetal growth. It is now recognised that the detection of delayed or reduced fetal head growth carries with it almost certain intellectual impairment after birth. Current investigations are therefore aimed at much earlier detection of intrauterine growth retardation by assessing the size of the fetal liver. This is achieved by taking measurements of the upper abdominal circumference of the fetus, as described by Campbell & Wilkin (1975). Our own work on this subject has shown that it is now possible to detect impaired fetal growth 8 to 10 weeks before head growth is affected and, on rare occasions, we have noted the onset of intrauterine growth retardation before 24 weeks of gestation and up to 15 weeks prior to head growth reduction. We therefore now have a technique which should permit the expectant management of this disorder and thereby permit obstetric intervention before the fetus suffers irreversible intellectual impairment.

Gynaecology

The most significant recent advance in the application of ultrasound to gynaecology has been in the management of patients being treated for infertility. In those patients whose infertility results from failed ovulation hormonal stimulation of the ovaries may well prove beneficial. However, the price not infrequently paid by the patient is that of a multiple conception, sometimes with so many fetuses that none have any hope of survival. Since the response of different patients to identical doses of gonadotrophin may vary enormously it is helpful to have some objective measurement of the response.

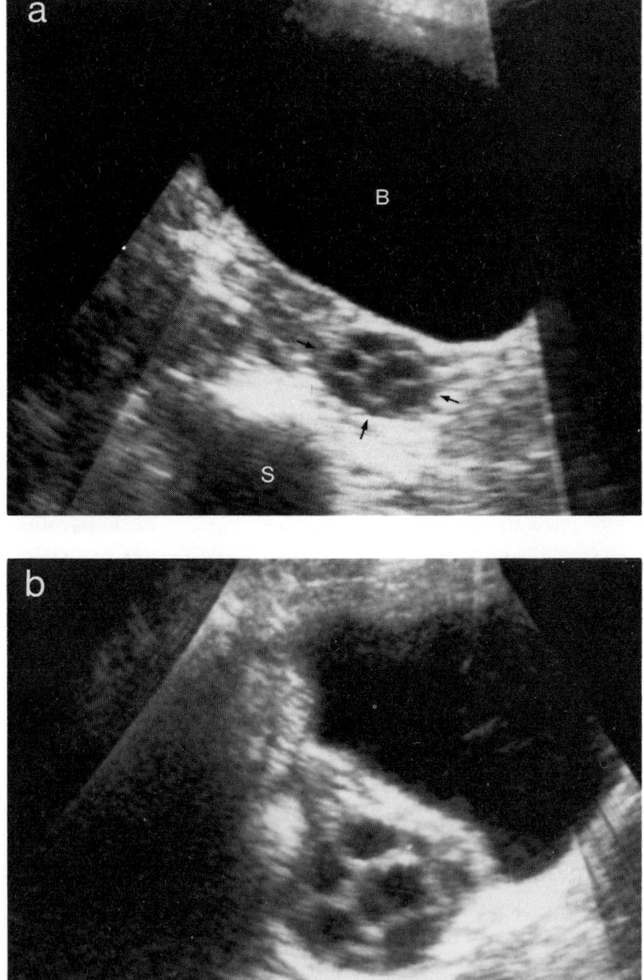

Fig. 6.2   (a) The right ovary (arrowed) of a patient undergoing gonadotrophin therapy. Multiple small follicles are present. Patient's bladder B, spine S.
(b) The same ovary 24 hours later. Overstimulation has occurred, that is multiple large cysts seen in ovary.

Modern grey scale ultrasound has the ability not only to see the normal ovaries but also to identify the developing follicles within them (Hackelöer, 1978). At a very early stage in the patients treatment the formation of multiple follicles can be observed (Fig. 6.2a) and their exceptionally rapid growth can be monitored (Fig. 6.2b). Fortunately even when multiple follicles have developed very few will give rise to viable ova. Experience to date suggests that those follicles with a diameter greater than 18 mm are most likely to produce ova whilst those less than this diameter can safely be ignored. If daily ultrasound scans are performed on these patients and the individual follicles measured, chorionic gonadotrophin can be administered to precipitate ovulation at the optimal time. Similarly if overstimulation and multiple large follicles are detected ovulation should not be stimulated and the patient should be advised to avoid the risk of pregnancy during the current cycle.

Liver disease

Prior to the advent of grey scale display it was virtually impossible to diagnose the majority of liver metastases. However, since this development ultrasound has become the technique of choice for the diagnosis or exclusion of hepatic metastatic disease. Radionuclide imaging will detect filling defects within the liver but will not differentiate benign from malignant or solid from cystic. Similarly, computerised X-ray tomography will also detect many forms of focal liver disease but will often not reliably differentiate between different pathologies. Ultrasound has been shown to be nearly 100 per cent accurate for the differentiation of solid from cystic lesions and a wide range of different appearances has been noted in metastatic disease (Green et al, 1977). The normal liver parenchyma appears as a relatively homogeneous mid-grey structure on ultrasound images. Metastatic disease has the appearance of local disturbances in this pattern which may appear either brighter or darker than the background liver echoes. Brighter echoes (Fig. 6.3) generally indicate metastases from a primary colonic neoplasm, although some other intra abdominal adenocarcinomas may produce a similar appearance. Conversely metastases from carcinoma of the breast reflect a smaller proportion of the ultrasound energy and therefore appear as darker spaces within the liver. Oat cell carcinoma of the lung may occasionally produce a combination of these appearances with concentric rings producing a 'target' appearance. Carcinoma of the oesophagus frequently results in metastases containing irregular fluid filled spaces whilst those lesions arising from the kidney or ovary may exhibit frank cystic change. It is likely that only about three per cent of metastases reflect ultrasound to the same degree as normal liver and are therefore undetectable. In those lesions which are detectable the ultrasound pattern may often give the clinician a vital clue to the possible origin of the disease, if this is not already known.

Diffuse liver disease is generally more difficult to diagnose by all imaging techniques and ultrasound is no exception. It has been known for many years that the strength of echoes returning from the livers of many patients with cirrhosis is substantially greater than from normal livers. However, it has also been noted that there is little if any correlation between the extent of this ultrasound change and the severity of the liver disorder. Conversely many patients with proven cirrhosis have ultrasonically normal livers. During the past year there have been two important developments in our understanding of this confusing situation. Firstly, Joseph, Dewbury & McGuire (1979) have shown that abnormally high echo amplitudes (the

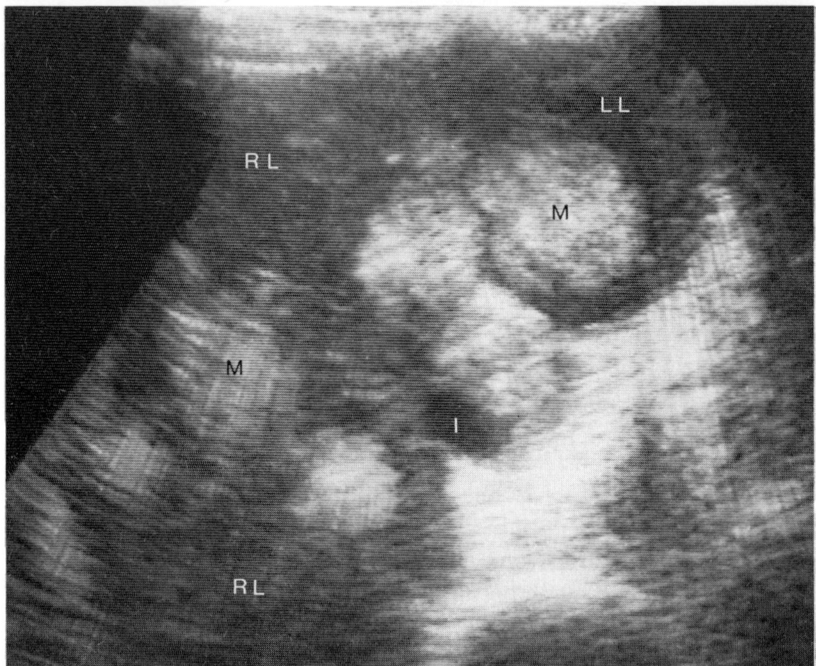

Fig. 6.3   Transverse scan of a liver with multiple 'bright' metastases (M) from a colonic carcinoma. Right lobe of liver RL, left lobe LL, inferior vena cava I.

'bright liver') may result from a range of diseases including cirrhosis, fatty infiltration, portal tract fibrosis, severe hepatitis or longstanding congestive cardiac failure. They noted that although ultrasound appears to be sensitive in the detection of generalised liver disease it is relatively non specific. They also noted that several patients with proven liver disease had no demonstrable ultrasound abnormality. The probable cause for this latter finding has been demonstrated by Dewbury & Clark (1979) who have shown that the typical bright liver pattern is seen in 80 per cent of patients with micronodular cirrhosis whereas macronodular cirrhosis is associated with an abnormal liver ultrasound scan in only 20 per cent of patients. The reasons for these discrepancies remain unproven at present but our understanding of this otherwise perplexing phenomenon is at last progressing.

Jaundice

Jaundice can be either medical or surgical in origin and in the majority of patients the differentiation is clinically or biochemically straight forward. In a significant minority however the differentiation is less clear and in these patients the modern imaging techniques have assumed an important role. Within the past two years ultrasound has become almost mandatory in the examination of this latter group of patients since it has been shown that ultrasound will reliably diagnose or exclude an obstructive cause in virtually 100 per cent of patients (Malini & Sabel, 1977).

Dewbury et al (1979) have emphasised that ultrasound diagnosis in the jaundiced patient can now be taken one stage further. In a review of 111 patients they had technical failures in only 3 and in the remaining 108 had an accuracy of 97 per cent in the differentiation between obstructive and medical jaundice. In 15 of the 41 patients with non-obstructive jaundice a bright liver echo pattern was detected thus indicating the underlying cause for these patients jaundice also. In the obstructive group they were able to determine the level of obstruction in nearly 80 per cent, but more importantly, they emphasise that not only the level but the cause of obstruction can often be identified. They correctly diagnosed the cause of obstruction in 59 per cent of patients, including 12 out of 18 cases of pancreatic carcinoma and 11 out of 19 patients with common bile duct stones.

Ultrasound examination is therefore now capable of supplying the surgeon with all the information he may require before operating upon a patient with obstructive jaundice. We may therefore expect a reduction in the use of percutaneous transhepatic cholangiography and ERCP and, in many hospitals including my own, patients having a satisfactory ultrasound examination with a confident diagnosis of the level and cause of obstruction now proceed to surgery without any further investigation.

Gallbladder

It is now possible to detect the gallbladder by ultrasound scanning in almost 100 per cent of patients (Gonzalez & Johnson 1978). The size and shape of the gallbladder can rapidly be assessed and scanning after a fatty meal allows confirmation of satisfactory gallbladder emptying. The majority of gallbladder calculi can be detected by ultrasound, provided a thorough and systematic examination is performed, and the thickness of the gallbladder wall can also be gauged accurately. It is therefore very likely that diagnostic ultrasound will supply nearly all the information customarily obtained from a conventional oral cholecystogram but without reliance upon hepatic excretion of a contrast medium and without exposure of the patient to ionising radiations. In several radiology departments ultrasound is now being used as the initial technique for evaluation of the gallbladder, particularly if calculus disease is to be confirmed or excluded. The recent developments of medical techniques for the dissolution of gallstones may require repeated assessment of the size and number of calculi present. These assessments should now always be done with ultrasound where this is available.

The development of automatic 'real-time' scanners has further increased the speed with which the gallbladder can be both located and assessed and has also permitted, for the first time, assessment of gallbladder kinetics without recourse to X-ray techniques (Palframan & Meire, 1979).

Pancreas

The pancreas remains one of the most difficult organs to image successfully whatever technique is employed. Whilst modern computed X-ray tomography will demonstrate the pancreas in virtually 100 per cent of patients its ability to differentiate the cause of enlargement has been rather disappointing, and the technique is also expensive and utilises ionising radiation. There has therefore recently been an increased interest in the ability of ultrasound to demonstrate the pancreas (Fig. 6.4) and success rates of 89 per cent (Haber, Freimanis & Asher, 1976) and 82 per cent (Weill et al, 1977) have recently been reported. In a personal communication Professor Weill (University of Besançon, France) now states that he is able to see the pancreas in 100 per cent of patients by use of a 'real-time' scanner with the patient erect. Studies on the diagnostic accuracy of ultrasound compared with other imaging techniques for the diagnosis of pancreatic lesions are becoming very numerous. Their results are very disparate reflecting the high degree of operator dependence of current ultrasound equipment. Where a high degree of operator expertise is available ultrasound generally produces more specific diagnostic results than does CT and there can now be little doubt that ultrasound should be done as the first imaging procedure for investigating the pancreas. In those patients where the examination is technically unsatisfactory or further information is required it is then reasonable to proceed to the more expensive and invasive techniques.

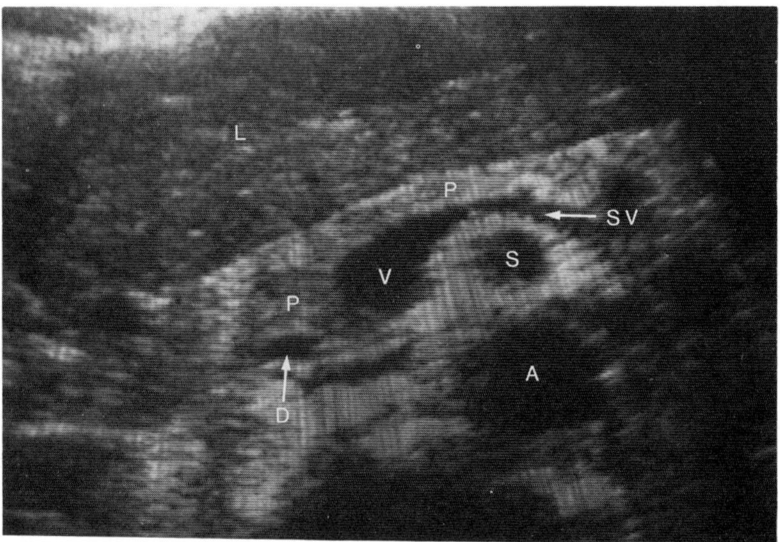

Fig. 6.4   Transverse scan of a normal pancreas (P). Liver L, aorta A, superior mesenteric artery S, superior mesenteric vein V, splenic vein SV, common bile duct D.

The grey scale ultrasound findings in malignant pancreatic tumours have recently been reviewed (Wright, Maklad & Rosenthal 1979) and whilst these are not absolutely specific and may sometimes be confused with the appearances from chronic pancreatitis they are nevertheless sufficiently characteristic to permit the correct diagnosis in a high proportion of patients.

Vascular studies

It has been known for many years that the major blood vessels could be detected by conventional ultrasound scanning, but as equipment has improved we have been able to visualise smaller and smaller vessels in greater detail. The use of a conventional manually operated grey scale B scanner to image the extra cranial carotid arteries has recently been described (Gompels, 1979) and both significant stenosis and atheromatous plaques can apparently be visualised by this technique. High frequency high resolution 'real-time' scanners have also been used in the same application and are beginning to gain wide acceptance as a valid method of investigation in the United

States of America. Both B scan and 'real-time' imaging systems will therefore outline the vascular anatomy but give little or no information concerning the functional integrity of a vessel or the haemodynamic significance of a stenosis. In order to assess these factors it is necessary to use equipment which employs the Doppler principle. The recent introduction of pulsed Doppler ultrasound (Fish, 1975) now permits the production of ultrasound angiograms of both arteries and veins. The clinical applications of this apparatus are still under evaluation but there is little doubt that it will be enormously valuable for the investigation of the extra cranial carotid and vertebral arteries and for the examination of short segments of vessels at many other sites including the femoral and popliteal arteries (Figs 6.5 and 6.6) and veins (Meire &

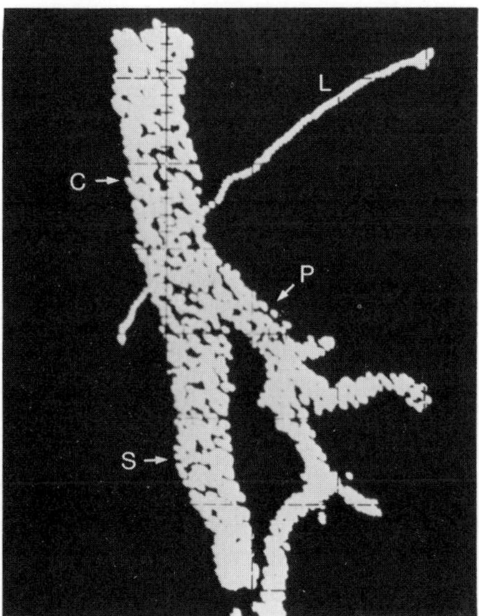

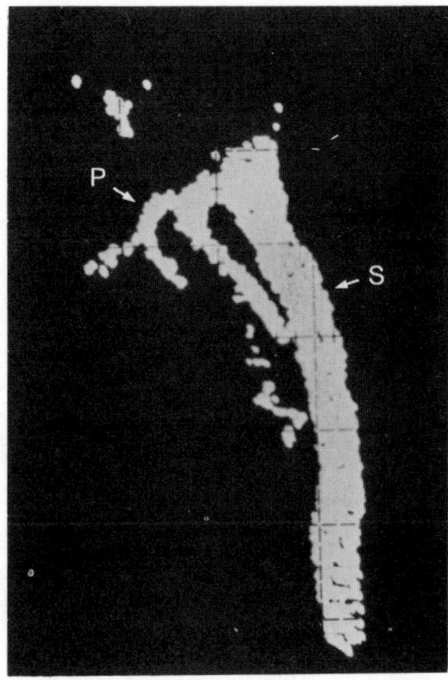

Fig. 6.5   Pulsed Doppler ultrasound angiogram of a normal left femoral artery. Common femoral C, superficial femoral S, profunda femoris P, inguinal ligament L.

Fig. 6.6   Pulsed Doppler ultrasound angiogram of the right groin in a patient with an obstructed common femoral artery. The superficial femoral artery S is filling via the profunda P.

Wood, 1980). The current interest in operative correction of vascular lesions in the extra cranial carotid arteries has increased the importance of vascular imaging techniques in patients with transient cerebral ischaemic attacks and arterial bruits within the neck. It is questionable whether it is clinically and economically justifiable to perform conventional angiography on all these patients and our initial results with a pulsed Doppler vessel imaging system (GEC MAVIS) indicate that haemodynamically significant lesions can be reliably detected with this apparatus. A special technique has also been developed for imaging the origin and proximal few centimetres of the vertebral artery (Wood & Meire, 1980) and has so far seen successful in 93 per cent of patients. This technique represents a significant advance in the investigation of the vertebrobasilar system.

The same apparatus can be used for imaging the deep veins of the lower limb. Preliminary results from a prospective study comparing ultrasound imaging with conventional venography show agreement between the two techniques in 19 of the first 22 patients, the three false negatives occurring in patients with minor thrombosis in the small calf veins.

A further development of this form of vascular imaging is the Hybrid or Duplex scanner. These systems combine conventional real-time imaging with pulsed Doppler apparatus so that the vessel can be rapidly located by virtue of the gross anatomy, and haemodynamic studies can then be performed using the pulsed Doppler mode.

Within the last months sophisticated computer analysis of the Doppler signals has permitted accurate and entirely non invasive ultrasound measurement of the volume blood flow within the carotid vessels. This technique will shortly be applied to other peripheral vessels and will certainly represent a very significant advance in the management of vascular disease.

Ultrasound-guided biopsy and aspiration
For many years the value of ultrasound for guiding biopsy and aspiration needles has been appreciated and many special transducers have now been developed to aid in the accurate placement of needles within cysts and tumours. The procedure has now been applied to renal cyst puncture, amniocentesis, pericardiocentesis, renal, liver and pancreatic biopsy to name only a few (Holm & Gammelgaard, 1978; Goldberg, 1978). The diagnostic and therapeutic importance of this advance is considerable. It seems likely that few if any significant complications occur from fine needle aspiration and that satisfactory cytological specimens can be obtained in a high proportion of cases. This therefore means that when a suspicious mass is detected by ultrasound fine needle biopsy can be performed and the diagnosis rapidly confirmed without recourse to open surgical biopsy. This is particularly important in patients with inoperable primary tumours or in those shown to have hepatic metastases of uncertain origin. Similarly fluid collections at many sites in the body are now both diagnosable by ultrasound and treatable by ultrasound guided aspiration. Whilst blind needle aspiration is unlikely to fail where the fluid collection is large ultrasound will help locate the optimal site of puncture in, for instance, a small pleural effusion. It will also help prevent accidental damage to adjacent structures such as the myocardium, or fetus and placenta in early pregnancy. The incidence of fetal bleeding after early pregnancy amniocentesis is reduced from 80 per cent to 10 per cent when ultrasound guidance is employed.

Conclusion
Very rapid technical developments have taken place in the field of ultrasound imaging over the past few years. This rapid rate of progress will continue for the foreseeable future, especially in the development of automatic scanners and blood vessel imaging and blood flow measurement apparatus. It is pleasing to report that the new technology is being widely applied in clinical medicine and surgery and is leading to genuine reductions in alternative invasive radiological procedures.

REFERENCES

Campbell S, Wilkin D 1975 Ultrasonic measurement of the fetal abdominal circumference in the estimation of fetal weight. British Journal of Obstetrics and Gynaecology 82: 689–697

Dewbury K C, Clark B 1979 The accuracy of ultrasound in the detection of cirrhosis. British Journal of Radiology 52: 945–948

Dewbury K C, Joseph A E A, Hayes S, Murray C 1979 Ultrasound in the evaluation and diagnosis of jaundice. British Journal of Radiology 52: 276–280

Farrant P H 1980 Ultrasound diagnosis of major fetal abnormalities. In: Proceedings of 3rd international symposium on recent advances in ultrasound diagnosis, Dubrovnik, 1st–5th October, 1979. Excerpta Medica, Amsterdam

Fish P J 1975 Multichannel direction-resolving Doppler angiography. In: Kazner et al (ed) Ultrasonics in medicine. Excerpta Medica, Amsterdam, p 153–159

Goldberg B B 1978 Ultrasonic aspiration biopsy techniques. In: de Vlieger et al (ed) Handbook of clinical ultrasound. John Wiley and Sons, New York

Gompels B M 1979 High definition imaging of carotid arteries using a standard commercial ultrasound 'B' scanner. A preliminary report. British Journal of Radiology, 52: 608–619

Gonzalez A C, Johnson J A 1978 Ultrasonic examination of the gallbladder: A review. Clinical Radiology 29: 171–176

Green B, Bree, R L, Goldstein H M, Stanley C 1977 Grey scale ultrasound evaluation of hepatic neoplasms: patterns and correlations. Radiology 124: 203–208

Haber K, Freimanis A K, Asher, W M 1976 Demonstration and dimensional analysis of the normal pancreas with grey scale echography. American Journal of Roentgenology, 126: 624–628

Hackelöer, B J 1978 Ultrasonic demonstration of follicular development. Lancet 1: 941

Holm H H, Gammelgaard, J 1978 Ultrasonically guided biopsy in malignant disease. In: Hill C R, et al (eds) Ultrasound in tumour diagnosis. Pitman Medical, London

Joseph A E A, Dewbury K C, McGuire P G 1979 Ultrasound in the detection of chronic liver disease (the 'bright liver'). British Journal of Radiology 52: 184–188

Malini, S, Sabel J 1977 Ultrasonography in obstructive jaundice. Radiology 123: 429–433

Meire H B 1979 Review article. Diagnostic ultrasound. British Journal of Radiology 52: 685–703

Meire H B, Wood C P L 1980 Pulsed Doppler ultrasound angiography. In: Proceedings of 3rd International Symposium on Recent Advances in Ultrasound Diagnosis, Dubrovnik, 1st–5th October 1979. Excerpta Medica, Amsterdam

Palframan A, Meire H B 1979 Real-time ultrasound. A new method for studying gall bladder kinetics. British Journal of Radiology 52: 801–803

Sample W F 1978 The role of sonography in identifying neural tube defects. UCLA Forum of Medical Science, 20: 123–137

Weill F, Schraub A, Eisencher A, Bourgoin A 1977 Ultrasonography of the normal pancreas. Radiology 123: 417–423

Wells P N T 1977 Biomedical ultrasonics, Academic Press, London

Wood C P L, Meire H B 1980 A technique for imaging the vertebral artery using pulsed Doppler ultrasound. Ultrasound in Medicine and Biology (In press)

Wright C H Maklad F, Rosenthal S J 1979 Grey scale ultrasonic characteristics of carcinoma of the pancreas. British Journal of Radiology 52: 281–288

7.1. Computed axial tomography: Introduction and basic principles

I. Kelsey Fry   Jeffrey Gawler

Computed tomography (CT) is an X-ray technique which uses a computer to reconstruct an image of a thin slice of the body. The images are normally obtained in the cross-sectional axial plane and for this reason the technique may be referred to as computed axial tomography or CAT scanning. The cross-sectional anatomical display avoids the overlap of superimposed structures involved in most conventional radiography. The principal advantage of CT over conventional radiography is however the ablity of CT to record very small variations in tissue density. For instance, cerebrospinal fluid in the ventricles and subarachnoid space is readily distinguished from the brain tissue without the use of contrast medium. The technique is sufficiently sensitive to detect the difference in density between grey and white matter. Although originally applied only to the head CT now provides a non-invasive method of imaging any part of the body. A CT examination consists of a series of scans through the part to be examined, each scan demonstrating a slice which is usually about 1 cm thick (Fig. 7.1).

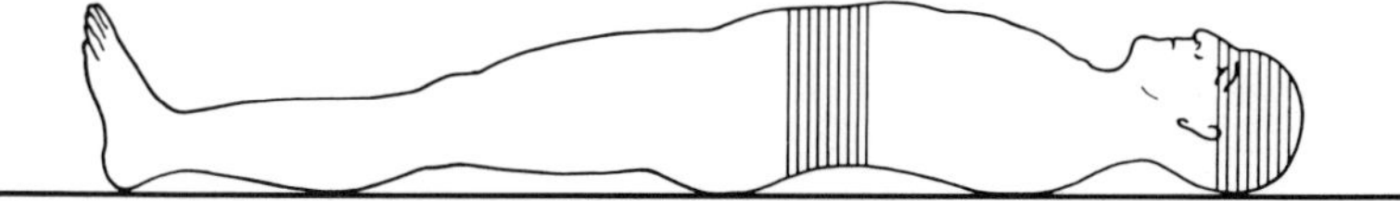

Fig. 7.1   Slices for CT examination of brain and abdomen.

The basic parts of the system are shown diagrammatically in Figure 7.2. An X-ray source is mounted on a gantry opposite to an array of detectors. The gantry rotates round a central tunnel in which the patient lies so that the part to be examined is in the plane of the gantry (Fig. 7.3). As the X-ray tube rotates round the patient the detectors record the amount of X-rays emerging from the patient. Data from the

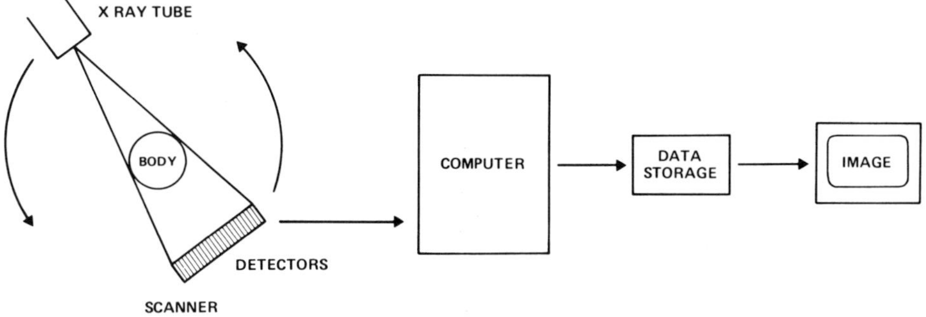

Fig. 7.2   Basic parts of CT system.

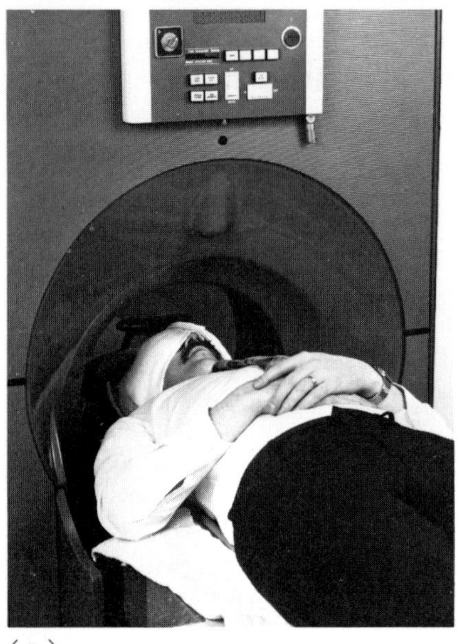
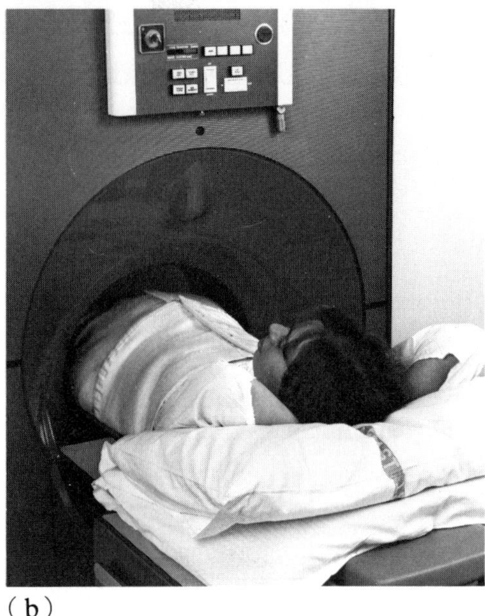

(a)   (b)

Fig. 7.3   Patient in position for scan of (A) brain, (B) upper abdomen.

detectors about the X-ray absorption in different tissues is fed continuously into a computer. The computer calculates an X-ray attenuation value for each point on the cross-section of the body and reconstructs an image. The data is stored on tape or a floppy disc and displayed on a video screen.

The scanner

In the original system developed by Hounsfield (1973) the gantry carrying the X-ray tube and opposing detectors moves across the patient and then rotates through a small angle, these movements being repeated through an arc of at least 180° (Fig. 7.4). All single-purpose brain scanners are of this type, as were the earlier 'body' scanners such as the EMI CT 5005 General Purpose Scanner which is the most widely used 'body' scanner in this country. Almost all machines with this type of movement have scan times of 15–20 seconds or longer. Although relatively long scan times are acceptable for scanning the brain, shorter scan times are highly desirable for body scanning because even minor movements degrade the quality of the image. For this reason scanners have been developed with scan times of the order of 3–5 seconds. This has been achieved by having the X-ray tube rotate round the patient with the detectors and tube moving together or with a ring of stationary detectors (Fig. 7.5). At the same time resolution has improved owing to more efficient use of the X-rays.

With some machines the gantry angles in the vertical plane. This allows, for example, scans to be obtained perpendicular to the axis of a vertebra and facilitates coronal sections of the head. Slice thickness can also be varied.

The term 'body' scanner has sometimes caused confusion. It suggests that the machine is dedicated to scanning the body in the same way as the brain scanner is to

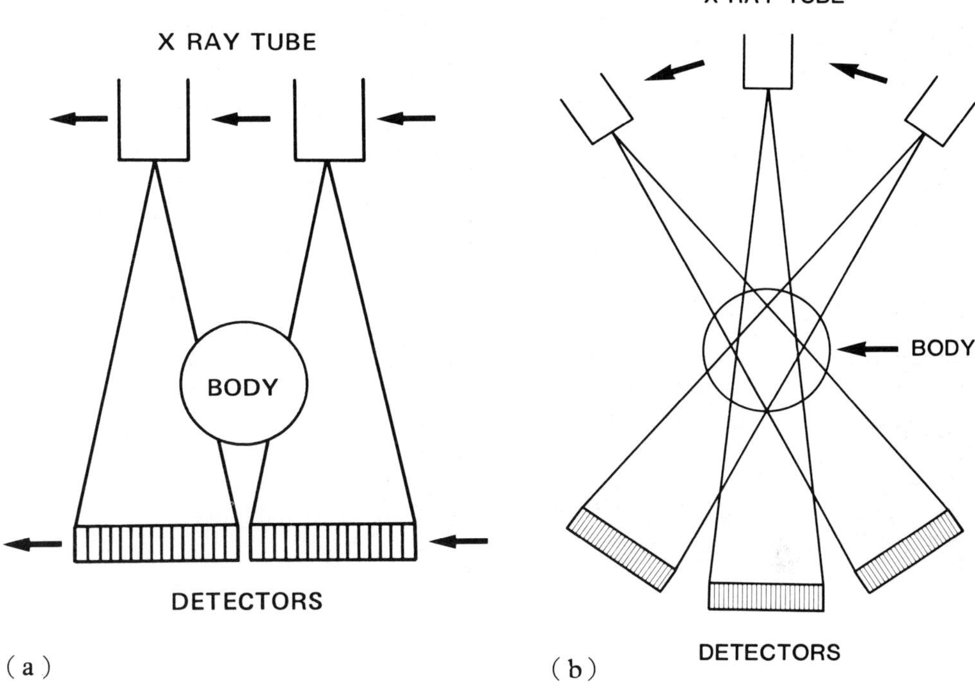

Fig. 7.4   Translate-rotate movement.
(a) The tube and detectors move across the patient.
(b) The transverse movement is repeated at different angles round the patient.

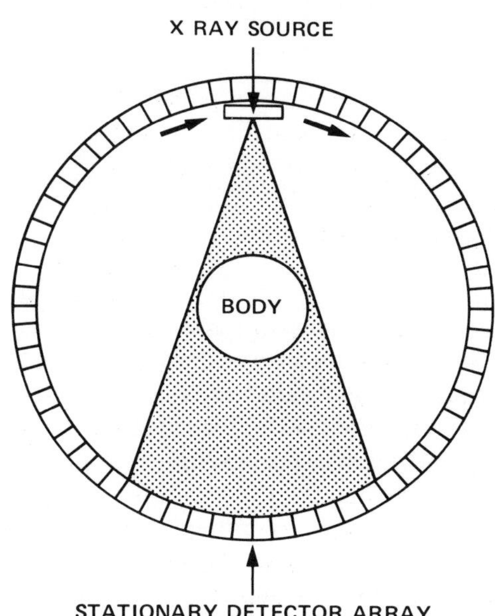

Fig. 7.5   Rotate only movement. The X-ray tube rotates round the patient. The detectors are stationary.

scanning the head. This is not so. 'Body' scanners are general purpose scanners and are expected to be used for brain scanning for which they are as effective as the older single purpose brain scanners. A 'body' scanner is thus likely to be used for brain scanning for a substantial part of the time unless adequate facilities for scanning the brain are already available.

The image
The image consists of a matrix of picture elements (pixels) representing the X-ray attenuation value (CT number) for each point on the cross-section of the body. The image is usually displayed using a grey scale but a colour scale is sometimes available. Each picture element represents the mean X-ray attenuation value from a segment of tissue (the voxel) shaped like a short matchstick, approximately 1 mm × 1 mm × 10 mm (Fig. 7.6). When a coarse matrix is used each picture element will represent a relatively large voxel; with a fine matrix each voxel will be correspondingly smaller. Thus using the EMI 5005 General Purpose Scanner with 320 × 320 matrix the cross-sectional area represented by each picture element is 0.75 mm × 0.75 mm. Using the coarser 160 × 160 matrix the cross-sectional area is 1.5 mm × 1.5 mm.

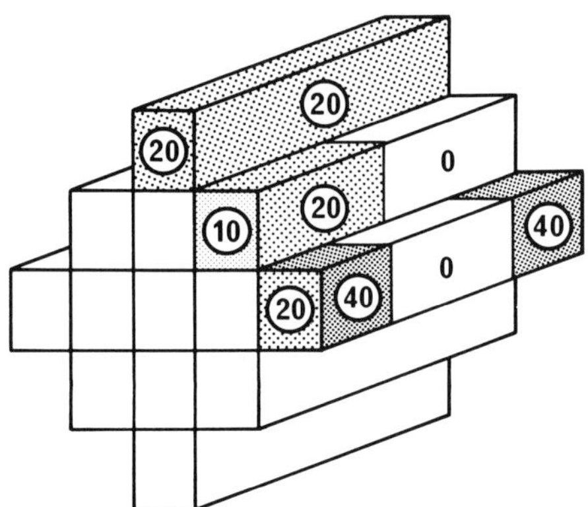

Fig. 7.6 Segments of tissue (voxels) contributing to each picture element. The precise length and cross-sectional area varies with matrix size and slice width. Each element of the CT image represents the mean attenuation value (CT number) of all the structures within a voxel.

CT numbers are determined on a linear scale which assigns a specific value to water and air. Confusingly, two scales are in use. Both assign value zero to water but the Hounsfield scale, which is the most widely used, assigns a value of −1000 to air which is given a value of −500 on the EMI scale. Two Hounsfield units are thus equal to one EMI unit. Irritatingly, EMI themselves have used the Hounsfield scale for the more modern brain scanners while using the EMI scale for some general purpose scanners. The values assigned to different tissues on the Hounsfield scale are shown in Figure 7.7.

One of the great advantages of CT as an imaging technique is the way in which the data can be manipulated to produce the maximum amount of information. The most important manipulation is the ability to vary *window level* and *window width*.

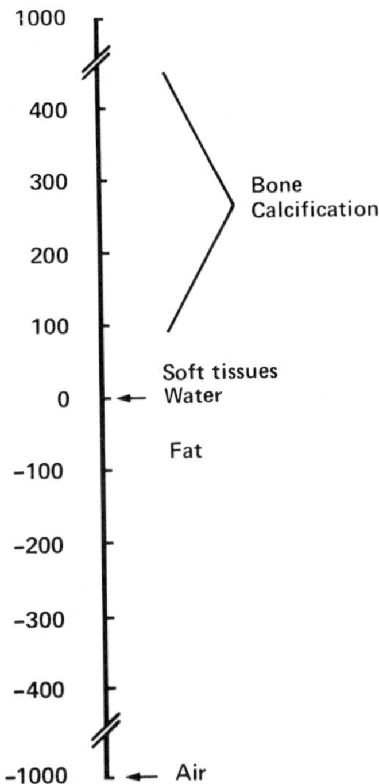

Fig. 7.7 Hounsfield scale.

Because it is not practical to display the whole range of CT values simultaneously, a range of numbers is chosen for display which is appropriate for the tissues being examined. The centre of the range is known as the window level and the range on either side of the window level is the window width. The effect of varying window level and window width is illustrated in Figures 7.8 and 7.9. Figure 7.8 shows the effect of varying window level. The images are from a single scan of the thorax viewed at three different window levels using a relatively wide window (+ 200 EMI units) throughout. At a level appropriate to the lungs, between −300 and −500 EMI units, the pulmonary vascular tree is clearly outlined but the soft tissues and bones are obscured. At a level of +5 EMI units appropriate to soft tissues the mediastinum and muscles of the thoracic cage are shown but the lungs are black and the bones are white. At a level of +99 EMI units bone structure is shown but the other tissues are not seen.

Figure 7.9 shows the effect on a scan of the liver of varying window widths with window level unchanged (+18 EMI units). At a wide window of 400 EMI units each grey scale step represents a wide range of numbers so that there is very little contrast and the liver appears homogenous. At a window width of 50 EMI units each grey scale step represents only a narrow range of numbers so that there is more contrast and metastases are readily seen.

The general anatomy is clearer with the narrower window.

A narrow window is used when examining structures such as the liver or brain in which small differences in density are important. A wide window is commonly used in

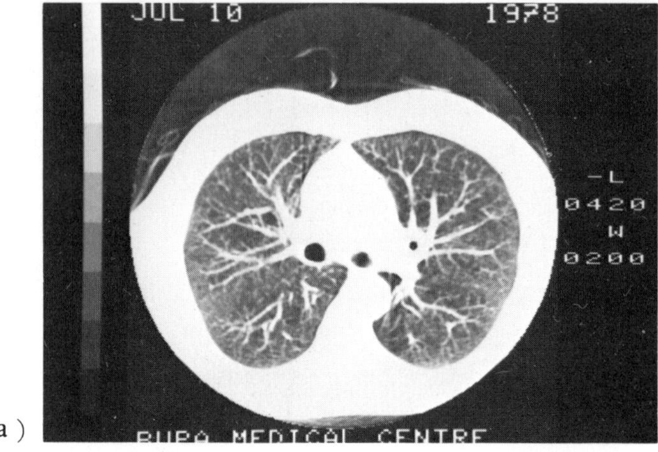

(a)

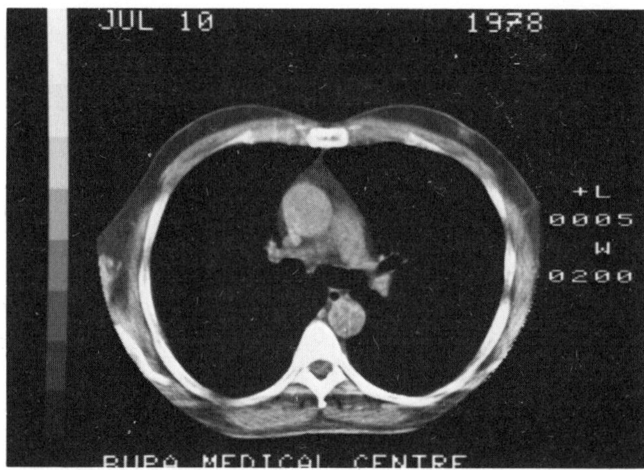

(b)

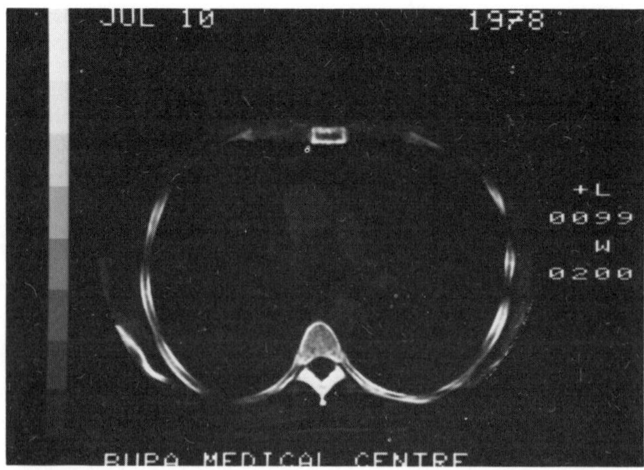

(c)

Fig. 7.8   Effect of varying window level. Scan of thorax with fixed window width (200 EMI units). The level chosen to show (a) the lungs, (b) the soft tissres, (c) bones.

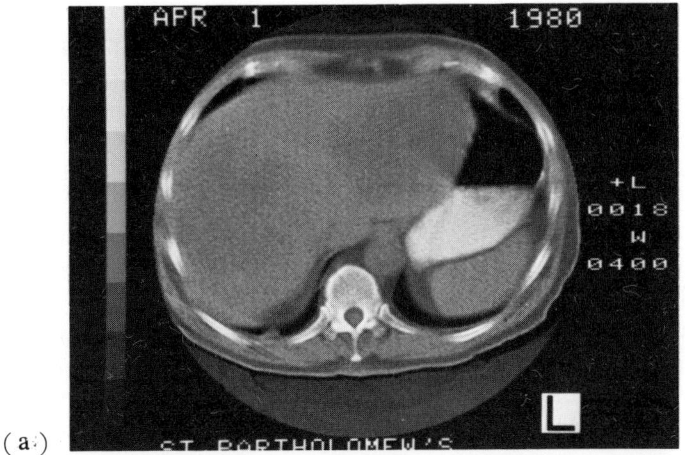

(a)

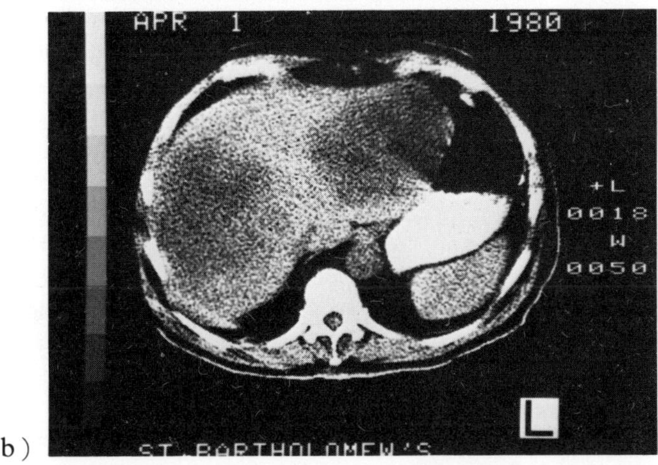

(b)

Fig. 7.9   Effect of varying window widths. CT scan of liver with fixed window level (+18 EMI units) (a) wide window (+400 EMI units) (b) narrow window (+50 EMI units). The metastases are more clearly seen with the narrow window. The general anatomy is clearer with the wider window.

body scanning where there is adequate contrast between different tissues and where the shape and contours of structures are the main criteria for diagnosis.

The viewing console can also have facilities for determining the mean CT number within a region of interest or for measuring the distance between two points. The cross-sectional area of a mass can be calculated. A segment of the image can be enlarged. The computer can reconstruct images in planes other than the axial plane. Such reconstruction, particularly in the sagittal or coronal planes has obvious diagnostic applications. It is becoming an increasingly important part of CT technique now that scanners capable of obtaining thin slices have been developed.

It is essential to recognise that the reporting of scans is based on careful manipulation of the image on the viewing console. Any hard copies that are obtained such as polaroid or X-ray film only illustrate the salient features of a complex examination.

Partial volume effect

Since the CT number of each picture element is the mean of the attenuation values of all the structures throughout the thickness of the slice a structure or lesion which only occupies part of the slice may be falsely represented due to partial volume averaging. This has two effects. Firstly, the shape and size of structures occupying only part of a slice may be misinterpreted. This problem can usually be resolved by examining contiguous slices or, if necessary, by obtaining intermediate slices. Secondly, the composition of a lesion may be misdiagnosed (Fig. 7.6). For instance, a cyst occupying only part of a slice in the kidney or liver may look relatively dense, the CT number approximating to that of the surrounding normal tissue. Such a lesion may be misdiagnosed as a tumour rather than a fluid-containing cyst. Lesions only occupying a small part of the slice may be missed altogether, unless there is a large density difference such as is found with a calculus in the kidney or a small metastasis in the lung.

Resolution

The larger the lesion and the greater the difference in density between it and neighbouring structures the more easy it is to detect. Assuming that there is a detectable difference in density most lesions can be diagnosed provided they occupy the full thickness of the slice. This means that using 1 cm contiguous slices one can expect to diagnose lesions 2 cm or more in diameter. Smaller lesions will be detected if they happen to occupy the full slice thickness or if the density difference is sufficiently great.

Detection of differences in density (contrast resolution) depends on the precision of the CT numbers which in turn depends very largely on the X-ray dose to the patient. The smaller the dose the smaller the number of X-ray photons reaching the detectors and the greater the imprecision of the CT numbers due to statistical variations (noise value). The greater the noise the more difficult it is to distinguish differences in density.

The larger the volume of tissue contributing to one picture element the less the statistical variation, so that noise increases as the matrix becomes finer and the slice becomes thinner. Thus, for a given dose of radiation contrast resolution improves with the use of a relatively coarse matrix and a relatively thick slice. Good spatial resolution is associated with a finer matrix and where applicable a thinner slice. A coarse matrix is therefore used when examining a structure in which small variations in tissue density are important. Brain scans are therefore carried out using a coarse matrix, e.g. 160×160, while most body scans which depend more on spatial resolution than contrast resolution are done with a finer matrix, e.g. 320×320.

Artefacts

Artefacts are seen as linear streaks or as ill-defined areas of falsely low or high density. They not only degrade the image but they also invalidate density measurements. The most common artefacts are caused by movement. Artefacts due to respiration, peristalsis and cardiac pulsation are common when using scanners with scan times of 15–20 seconds or longer. They are largely eliminated using 3–5 second scanners. High density material such as barium, myodil or the metal in clips or hip prostheses cause very dense artefacts even in the absence of movement. The same applies to dense areas of bone which can, for instance, cause artefacts in scans through the base of the skull or through the shoulders.

Enhancement

The term 'enhancement' is used during CT scanning to refer to the increase in density of tissues after the injection of intravenous iodine-containing contrast medium. The contrast medium is the same as that used for urography. There are two types of enhancement:

1. General opacification of the tissues, partly by contrast medium in the vascular tree and partly by contrast medium in the extracellular space (except in the kidney where the contrast medium is concentrated in the tubules). The timing of the scans is not critical for this type of enhancement. The different degrees of opacification observed in normal tissues and different types of tumour and other abnormalities can be of great diagnostic value. It is particularly important when scanning the brain.

2. Opacification of major vessels to show vascular anatomy and pathology, and to distinguish vessels from other structures. To achieve this type of enhancement the plasma level of contrast medium must be high and the scans should be obtained during or immediately after injection when the plasma level is at its peak.

Radiation dose

The radiation dose to the patient during CT scan using X-rays is well within the range associated with other diagnostic X-ray investigations. The skin dose for a single scan varies from approximately 0.5–5 rad according to the type of equipment and the technique used (Hobday & Parker, 1978; McCullough & Payne, 1978; Cohen, 1979). For a series of contiguous scans the dose is higher and may double owing to scattered radiation from neighbouring scans. If scans are repeated as for instance for enhancement of a brain scan the skin dose may reach 12–14 rad. This has to be compared with doses up to 40 rads associated with cerebral angiography (Fitzgerald & White, 1975). A single film of the abdomen gives a skin dose of about one rad and an i.v.p. 5–10 rad.

REFERENCES

Cohen G 1979 Contrast — detail — dose analysis of six different computed tomographic scanners. Journal of Computer Assisted Tomography 3: 197–203
Fitzgerald M, White D R 1975 A survey of patient doses arising from diagnostic X-ray examinations. Proceedings of the Third European Congress of the International Radiation Protection Association. Excerpta Medica, Amsterdam
Hobday P, Parker R P 1975 Radiation exposure to the patient in computerized tomography. British Journal of Radiology 51: 925–926
Hounsfield G N 1973 Computerized transverse axial scanning (tomography). Part 1. Description of system. British Journal of Radiology, 46: 1016–1022
McCullough E C, Payne J T 1978 Patient dosage in computed tomography. Radiology 129: 457–463

7.2. Computed axial tomography of the body

I. Kelsey Fry   J. E. Husband

First reports of the use of computed tomography (CT) of the body did not appear until 1976 (Kreel, 1976a; Sagel, Stanley & Evens, 1976; Sheedy et al, 1976) and only in the last two years has the technique become widely available. Even now access to it is very limited in the United Kingdom. Sufficient evidence has however accumulated to show that CT can have important benefits for both diagnosis and management in many parts of the body.

GENERAL CONSIDERATIONS

Clinical aspects of scanning

CT is potentially applicable to any clinical problem where there might be:
1. A mass large enough to distort the normal tissue outline
2. A mass the density of which differs significantly from that of surrounding tissue
3. A pathological change in the texture of a normal structure leading to detectable abnormality of density such as, for example, fatty change in the liver.

In most parts of the body, except the lungs, the delineation of soft tissues by CT depends on the contrast between the soft tissues and surrounding fat (Fig. 7.10). In

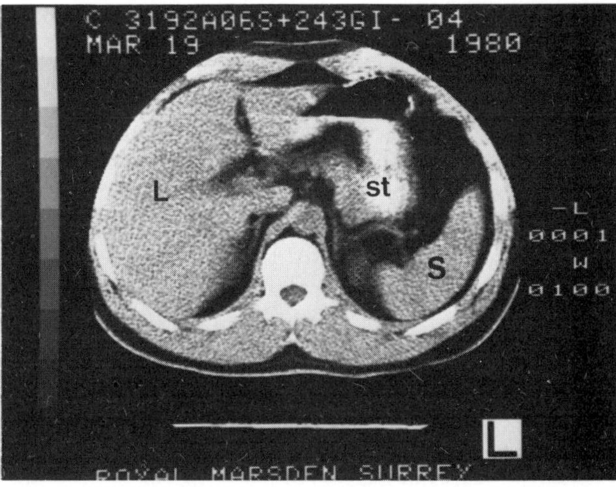

Fig. 7.10   Normal CT scan of upper abdomen, showing liver (L), spleen (S) and stomach (St). Intra-abdominal fat is seen as dark shadowing separating the soft tissues. With this amount of fat the soft tissue outlines are clearly seen. The stomach contains oral contrast medium. The aorta is enclosed by the crura of the diaphragm. The inferior vena cava (arrowed) is seen on the right of the aorta just as it emerges from the liver.

general, the fatter the patient the better the scan. In thin patients and especially in children absence of fat may produce a scan which is difficult or impossible to interpret.

When used for *primary diagnosis* CT can not only show the presence of an abnormality but may also determine its nature by distinguishing fat or fluid from soft tissue. Cysts (0 to +10 EMI units) and fatty masses (−40 to −20 EMI units) can thus be distinguished from solid tumours (+15 to +35 EMI units). The CT characteristics of a solid mass do not however usually permit precise diagnosis of the nature of the mass. Thus an inflammatory mass cannot usually be distinguished from a tumour. Benign and malignant tumours may have identical appearances.

Because of its ability to detect and define the shape, size and extent of masses, CT has rapidly found a place as a means of determining *the stage and extent of malignant disease* and for *monitoring response to treatment*. It has a unique role in *radiotherapy treatment planning* because of the way in which it shows not only the shape and size of the tumour but also the relation of the tumour to neighbouring structures.

Relationship to other techniques

CT of the body has three characteristics which increase its clinical effectiveness in relation to other imaging techniques:

1. It is only slightly operator-dependent. Although there are some minor technical problems associated with the preparation of the patient, positioning, etc., technically satisfactory images can be obtained after relatively little training.

2. It is not organ specific. All the tissues in a whole slice are examined. For example, an examination of the liver will include the lung bases, ribs and soft tissues, in addition to the spleen, adrenals, pancreas and other upper abdominal structures.

3. Most importantly, the images obtained in a great many patients can be understood by an untrained observer. The credibility of the examination is thus high so that reports are relatively easily accepted as a basis for decisions on management.

CT and ultrasound

The techniques are complementary. Where one or other is at its most effective there is no overlap. Thus the best use of CT is for brain scanning, while the best use for ultrasound is for the study of pregnancy. CT has, at present, no place in the investigation of heart disease, whereas echocardiography is a well established technique. CT is capable of examining any part of the body including the head and neck, lungs, mediastinum and bony structures, none of which can be examined satisfactorily with ultrasound. The only significant area of overlap is in the abdomen. Abdominal ultrasound examinations can fail because of interference from bony structures or excessive bowel gas or fat, none of which prevent CT.

The great advantages of ultrasound in relation to CT are that it is quicker, much more pleasant for the patient, less expensive and free of radiation hazard. The two disadvantages of ultrasound in the present stage of its development are that it is more dependent on the skill and expertise of the operator, and that the images are less readily understood by clinicians. In general, when both techniques are available and both are equally applicable, ultrasound will be used first, CT being reserved for those patients in whom ultrasound is unsuccessful or the result needs confirmation.

Technical considerations

A CT scanner should be used in the same way as any other diagnostic X-ray equipment, the technique being tailored to solve appropriate clinical problems. The number of scans and the intervals between scans will vary with the size of the area being examined and the size of the structure or lesion(s) being investigated. When the chest and abdomen are being scanned to exclude metastatic disease 35–40 scans may be required, while as few as 5 or 6 scans may be adequate to examine a known mass when monitoring response to treatment.

The examination is an outpatient procedure and the great majority of patients are not disturbed by it. A few find the machinery intimidating. Some find the taste of the oral contrast medium very unpleasant. Very occasionally a patient is too obese to enter the scanner.

A patient having a scan of the body can expect to be in the X-ray department for between $\frac{1}{2}$–$2\frac{1}{2}$ hours depending on the type of examination and the need for preparation. Using a scanner such as the EMI CT 5005 for body scans, throughput will vary between 7 and 10 patients in an 8-hour working day. Throughput may be higher using scanners with more rapid data processing.

Preparation of the patient

Patients having scans of the abdomen should have nothing to eat for four hours before the examination.

Before an examination of the abdomen patients are given oral contrast medium (usually 3 or 5 per cent Gastrografin) to opacify the bowel because an unopacified loop can easily be confused with a soft tissue mass. For the same reason, rectal Gastrografin is helpful when examining the pelvis. Gastrografin may persist mixed in the faeces in the large bowel for some days and unless cleared may hinder subsequent X-ray examinations.

Using scanners with a scan time of 18–20 seconds artefacts will degrade the image unless the patient can stop breathing for this period when the thorax or abdomen are being scanned. For abdominal scans patients are routinely given an anticholinergic agent, such as propantheline, buscopan or glucagon, to reduce peristalsis. Artefacts due to respiratory movement and peristalsis are very much reduced when faster scanners are used. Restless patients may need some sedation but must still be able to cooperate. Occasionally general anaesthesia is required even in adults. It is commonly needed if satisfactory scans are to be obtained in small children.

THE THORAX

Although conventional X-ray techniques effectively demonstrate most intrathoracic disease some problems are suitable for study with CT, especially those involving the mediastrinum.

The mediastinum

Evaluation of a mediastinal mass. This is one of the most effective uses of CT. Not only can the precise location of a mass be shown but also often its nature. For example, a prominent pericardial fat pad or a parapericardial cyst can be distinguished from a solid tumour mass by determining the CT number (Fig. 7.11). In the upper mediastinum vascular enhancement allows distinction between vascular lesions and soft tissue masses (Fig. 7.12). The same technique can be used to evaluate aortic aneurysms.

In patients where there is doubt as to whether the mediastinal outline is normal, CT can be decisive, proving or disproving the presence of an abnormal mass.

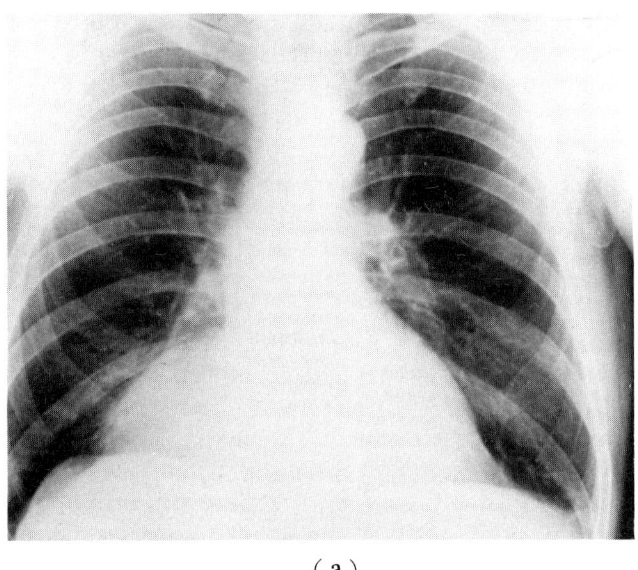

(a)

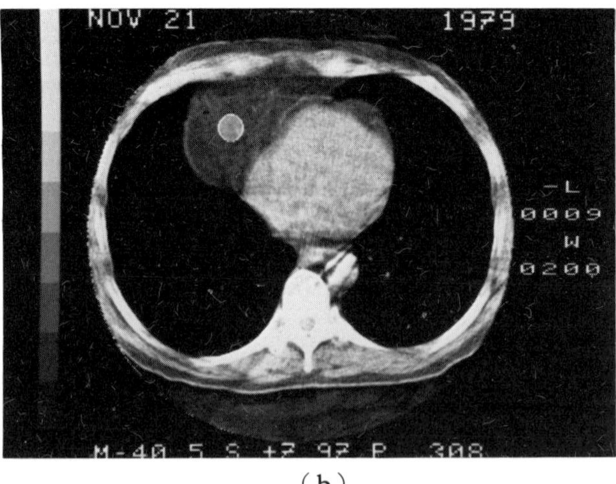

(b)

Fig. 7.11   (a) Mass in right cardiophrenic angle on routine chest X-ray, probably a fat pad.
(b) CT scan through the mass. Mass is much less dense than the heart. The mean CT number was −40
EMI units, confirming that the mass consisted of fat. The ringed shadow overlying the mass shows the area
within which the CT number was computed.

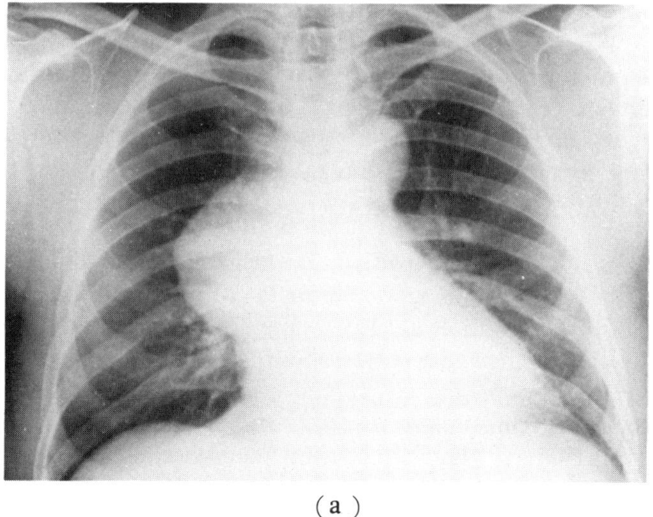

(a)

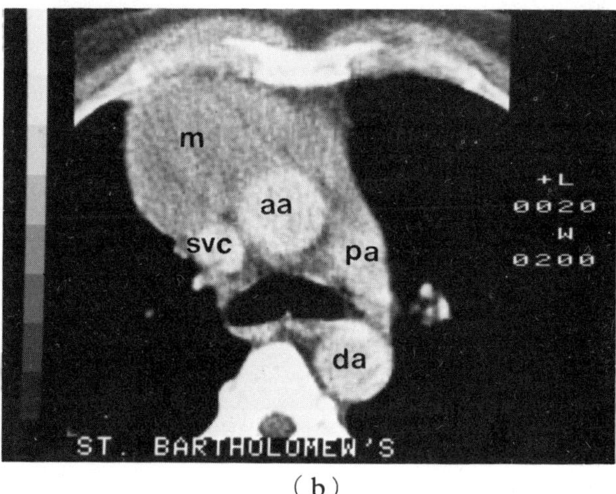

(b)

Fig. 7.12   (a) Right-sided anterior mediastinal mass on routine chest X-ray.
(b) CT scan at the level of the carina to exclude aneurysm. Intravenous contrast medium has been injected
to opacify the major vessels. A mass (m) of soft tissue density is seen lying in front of the superior vena cava
(svc) and ascending aorta (aa). Note pulmonary artery (pa) and descending aorta (da).

Occult mediastinal disease. CT can demonstrate masses not visible on conventional
tomography, especially those in the retrosternal space, such as thymomas (Mink et al,
1978) and enlarged lymph nodes (Crowe, Brown & Muhm, 1978; Husband et al,
1979). Enlarged nodes are also well shown elsewhere in the mediastinum, particularly
when they are silhouetted against the lung in sites such as the azygo-oesophageal
recess and the aortic pulmonary window (Heitzmann, Goldwin & Proto, 1977). CT is
the only technique that will demonstrate the retrocrural space and thus show lymph
node enlargement or tumour extension from one side of the diaphragm to the other.

The lungs
The lung fields are seen in cross-section without the superimposed shadows of the chest wall. The pulmonary vessels are clearly seen branching out from the hilum and vessels as small as 2 or 3 mm in diameter can be identified at the periphery. The costophrenic recesses are well shown. The depth of the posterior costophrenic recesses becomes obvious and emphasises the difficulty of examining this region with conventional radiography.

Pulmonary nodules. CT is more sensitive than whole lung tomography for detecting pulmonary nodules, nodules being visible in 15–20 per cent more patients with CT (Muhm et al, 1978; Husband et al, 1979) (Fig. 7.13). Nodules can be identified if their diameter is greater than that of neighbouring vessels so that nodules as small as 3 mm diameter can be diagnosed at the periphery of the lung. Whole lung tomography is a time-consuming investigation and often difficult to interpret, especially at the periphery where the earliest metastases tend to occur (Scholten & Kreel, 1977).

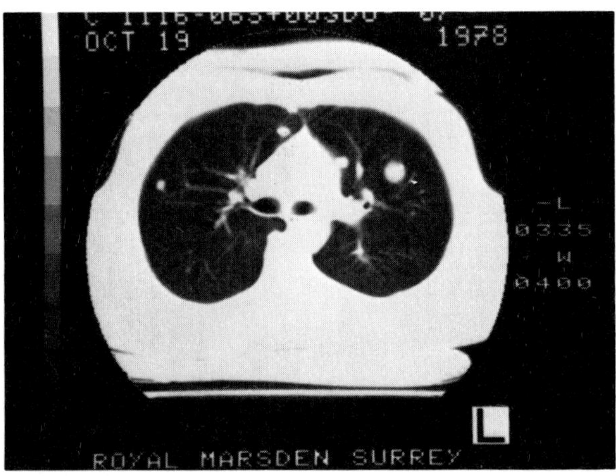

Fig. 7.13   Multiple pulmonary metastases. Only the larger lesion on the left was detected on whole lung tomography.

In the USA a considerable proportion of nodules prove to be a benign granulomata, such as histoplasmosis (Schaner et al, 1978). Under these circumstances small nodules cannot be confidently diagnosed as metastases. In the UK round nodules are rarely seen as incidental findings in patients without evidence of malignant disease. When multiple nodules occur in a patient with known malignancy the overwhelming likelihood is that they are metastases. It is, however, wise to be cautious when there are only one or two, especially if they are not uniformly round or are not lying at the periphery.

Computed tomography quite commonly reveals relatively large nodules (more than 1 cm diameter) which have not been detected on conventional radiographs. This occurs especially with masses lying in front of or behind the heart, or in the posterior costophrenic recesses.

At present CT does not appear to help in the diagnosis of the nature of a solitary pulmonary mass. It can however be useful in patients known to have bronchial carcinoma because the demonstration of unsuspected metastatic spread may prevent an unnecessary thoractomy.

Generalised disease. Standard radiography usually shows effusions, collapse and consolidation without difficulty but occasionally CT can be helpful in clarifying the underlying pathology, especially in patients with an opaque hemithorax. Airless lung can be distinguished from pleural fluid because it has the same density as other soft tissues. When consolidation is present with a patent bronchus the air bronchogram is clearly shown.

There is some evidence which suggests that CT may have a place in the diagnosis of diffuse interstitial pulmonary disease. Kreel (1976b) studying asbestosis and Putnam et al (1977) studying sarcoidosis report that interstitial changes are more readily visible on CT than on standard radiographs.

The pleura

Effusions appear as smooth elliptical shadows situated posteriorly if the patient is lying supine. Small effusions can be detected with CT when they are not evident on plain chest radiographs. Loculated effusions can be distinguished from solid masses by determination of the tissue density.

Pleural thickening may be difficult to distinguish from a small effusion unless scans are obtained in more than one position. CT is well suited to showing localised pleural lesions. Thus, Kreel (1976b) found that pleural plaques and calcification in asbestosis were more common on CT and appeared more extensive than on conventional radiographs.

THE ABDOMEN

The abdomen is relatively difficult to examine by conventional methods compared with the thorax and musculoskeletal system. For this reason, the majority of CT scans of the body are carried out to resolve abdominal problems. The value of the examination varies widely according to the type of problem the amount of intra-abdominal fat and the ability of the patient to cooperate. Large homogeneous structures like the liver, gallbladder, spleen and kidneys are well outlined. The technique is of particular value in the investigation of structures in the retroperitoneum.

The pancreas

CT is well suited to imaging the pancreas provided there is sufficient retroperitoneal fat. In practice, the technique has limitations. Even so, it seems to be the most effective technique currently available.

In some patients the gland lies almost horizontally and most of the body, tail and part of the head can be included on a single scan. In others, only part of the tail or body can be seen at any one time. When there is difficulty in identifying the gland the origin of the superior mesenteric artery is a useful landmark because it points to the body of the pancreas which lies in front of it (Fig. 7.14). The position of the head of the pancreas is confirmed by its relation to contrast medium lying in the second part of the duodenum.

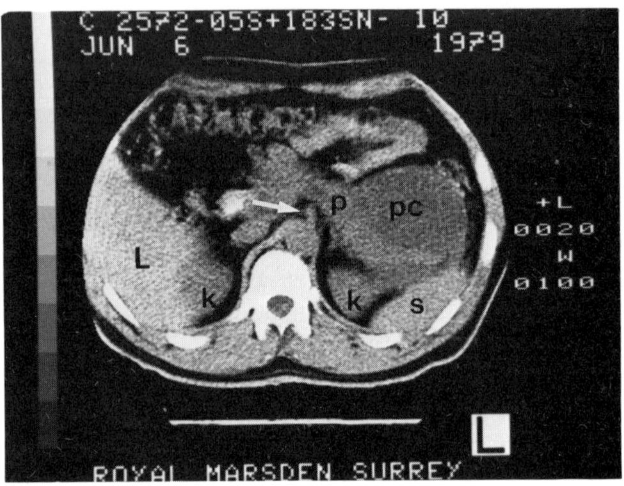

Fig. 7.14 Pancreatic pseudocyst (pc). Its low density distinguishes it from the tail and body of the pancreas (p). The origin of the superior mesenteric artery (arrowed) lies just behind the body of the pancreas.

Signs of pancreatic disease

The most important primary signs are:

1. *Enlargement* (Fig. 7.15). Generalised enlargement occurs in acute and chronic pancreatitis. Localised enlargement is associated with both pancreatitis and neoplasm, and occurs most commonly in the head of the pancreas. A mass in the head may be 3–4 cm in diameter before it distorts the outline and can be detected, but smaller masses can be detected in the body and tail.

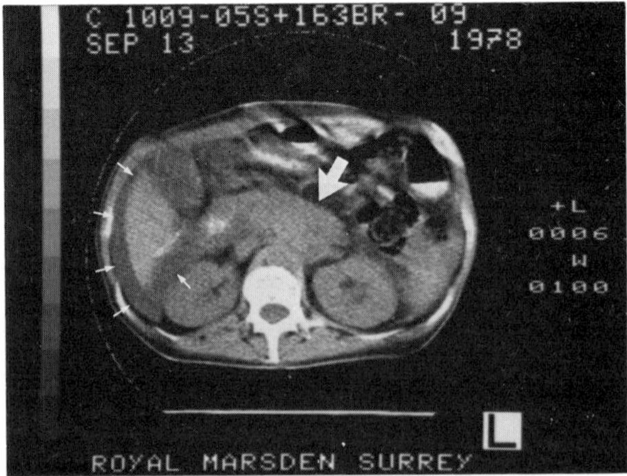

Fig. 7.15 Carcinoma of the body of the pancreas (large arrow). There is some ascites (small arrows) around the lower end of the liver.

2. *Alteration of density*. This occurs most obviously with pseudocysts which appear as well encapsulated lesions with well defined margins (Fig. 7.14). The contents have a density close to that of water. Abscesses and necrotic tumours can also have areas of low density but the density is rarely as low as that of a pseudocyst.

3. *Calcification*. This is evidence of chronic pancreatitis and is much more obvious on CT than on plain abdominal radiography. In one study calcification was observed on the CT scan when not visible on the plain abdominal radiography in 9 out of 50 patients with proven chronic pancreatitis (Ferrucci et al, 1979).

The secondary signs of pancreatic disease can also be important. Dilatation of the biliary tract may be the only evidence of a mass in the head of the pancreas which is too small to distort the outline of the gland. Lymph node enlargement or the presence of hepatic metastases may indicate that a pancreatic mass is a malignant tumour.

Differential diagnosis of pancreatic masses. As usual with CT it is easier to diagnose the presence of an abnormality than to determine its nature. A localised *solid mass* caused by a benign or malignant neoplasm may be indistinguishable from a mass due to pancreatitis. Calcification does not exclude carcinoma since pancreatitis and neoplasm may coexist. In the absence of tumour extension or metastatic spread the distinction between carcinoma and chronic pancreatitis cannot be made on the CT evidence alone. If a *low density mass* has the characteristic appearance of a pseudocyst and the clinical picture is appropriate, diagnosis usually presents no problem. If, however, the appearance is not absolutely characteristic it may not be possible to distinguish a pseudocyst from an abscess or a neoplasm with a large central area of necrosis.

Two other sources of confusion can lead to errors in the diagnosis of pancreatic masses. Firstly, masses arising in neighbouring structures, especially enlarged lymph nodes, can mimic pancreatic lesions. Secondly, neighbouring normal structures can be mistaken for lesions in the pancreas. The most common are loops of bowel not opacified with contrast medium. Overlying splenic vessels can also cause difficulty. Sometimes there is a fusiform bulge in the tail of a normal pancreas and this can be mistaken for a small tumour. Such errors were more common in the early days of body scanning but still occur.

The value of CT in pancreatic disease. In spite of the limitations of pancreatic imaging with CT the diagnostic accuracy is high. Accuracy rates for the diagnosis of carcinoma of the pancreas between 80 and 90 per cent were reported quite soon after the introduction of the technique (Haaga et al, 1977; Sheedy et al, 1977; Stanley, Sagel & Levitt, 1977).

Although CT can detect most carcinomas the scan is frequently normal in patients with chronic pancreatitis (Sheedy et al, 1977). Ferrucci et al (1979) confirmed the frequency of normal scans in chronic pancreatitis (16 per cent) and also emphasised the difficulty of distinguishing the nature of a pancreatic mass on CT. Twelve out of 50 patients with chronic pancreatitis showed only non-specific, diffuse or focal enlargement indistinguishable from a carcinoma.

Provided the limitations are borne in mind CT provides valuable information contributing to the diagnosis of almost all types of pancreatic disease. One exception is the diagnosis of functioning islet cell tumours. It was originally hoped that CT would solve this problem but the tumours are rarely detectable because they are usually too small to distort the outline of the gland.

CT and ultrasound of the pancreas. When a technically satisfactory examination can be obtained the overall accuracy of ultrasound in the diagnosis of pancreatic disease is comparable to that of CT (Husband, Meire & Kreel, 1977; Lee et al, 1979). The tail of the gland is, however, more readily shown by CT. The general advantages of ultrasound are such that it is likely to be used first, especially in thin patients. CT may be the investigation of first choice in obese patients and in those in whom a lesion is suspected in the tail of the gland.

The adrenal glands
The investigation of patients with possible adrenal disease is probably the most effective single use of CT in the abdomen. Other techniques for imaging the adrenals have considerable limitations so that CT, when available, is likely to be the investigation of choice in many patients.

The right gland lies immediately behind the inferior vena cava and just above the right kidney. The left gland lies behind the pancreas and in front of the top of the left kidney.

Adrenal masses
CT can be expected to demonstrate adrenal masses down to a size of 1.5–2.0 cm provided there is a reasonable amount of retroperitoneal fat (Fig. 7.16). Smaller masses can sometimes be identified.

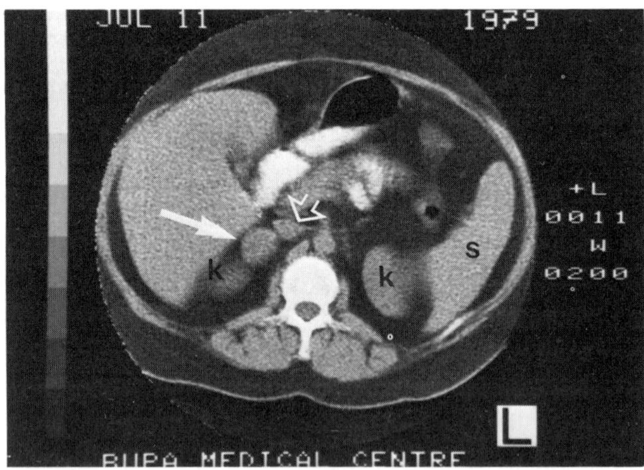

Fig. 7.16   3 cm tumour in right adrenal in patient with Cushing's syndrome (closed arrow). It lies behind the inferior vena cava (open arrow) and in front of the kidney (k).

The accuracy of diagnosis of the presence of an adrenal mass is high. Karstaedt et al (1978) were able to demonstrate all of 29 proven adrenal masses including 1 Conn's tumour 0.5 cm in diameter. Our own experience is closer to that of Dunnick et al (1979) who failed to show 3 out of 22 tumours. Two of these were small Conn's tumours, the other was a 3 cm phaeochromocytoma in a very thin patient. Occasionally adrenal tumours may be difficult to separate from masses arising from neighbouring structures, especially the kidney.

Use of CT in adrenal disease. In patients with Cushing's syndrome or with a possible phaeochromocytoma CT would seem to be the imaging method of choice. In both conditions tumours are likely to be large enough to be shown without difficulty. The glands are particularly clearly seen in Cushing's syndrome because of the excessive amount of retroperitoneal fat and tumours are readily distinguished from the normal or plump glands of bilateral hyperplasia. When looking for a phaeochromocytoma, scans through the adrenal area down to the aortic bifurcation will detect the great majority of tumours (Stewart et al, 1978). Venous sampling and arteriography would seem best reserved for patients in whom CT has failed to resolve the diagnostic problem.

In Conn's syndrome the tumours are often too small to demonstrate with any confidence using the slower scanners. Faster scanners capable of obtaining thinner slices are likely to be more accurate.

The ease with which adrenal tumours are demonstrated has emphasised the importance of the adrenals as a site of metastatic disease.

The kidney

Intravenous urography and ultrasound are very effective methods for imaging the kidney. CT is therefore rarely needed for the initial investigation of renal disease. It remains however an excellent way of demonstrating the renal and perirenal areas, and is a valuable tool for elucidating problems which have not been resolved by the simpler methods.

The kidneys are well displayed in cross-section by CT because they are surrounded by perinephric fat (Figs. 7.17 and 7.18). The hilum is seen as a central area of low density caused mainly by fat in the renal sinus. The calyces are not visualised without

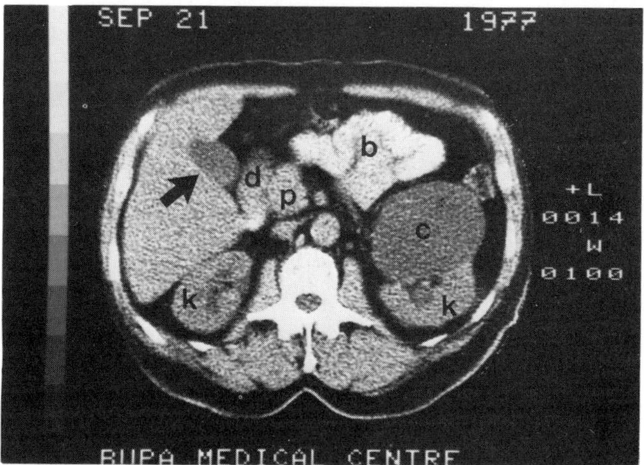

Fig. 7.17   8 cm cyst (c) on the anterior aspect of the left kidney. The mean CT number is +5 EMI units, close to that of water. The density of the cyst is similar to that of the gallbladder seen on the medial aspect of the liver (arrowed). Note the head of the pancreas (p) separated from the gallbladder by the second part of the duodenum (d). Part of the small bowel (b) is outlined with Gastrografin.

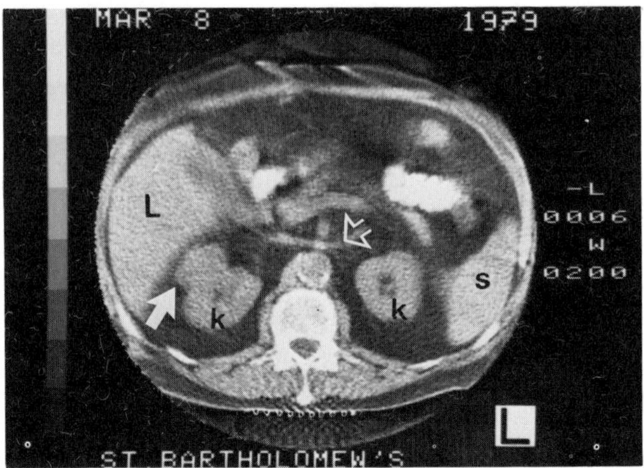

Fig. 7.18 A renal cell carcinoma (closed arrow) on the anterior surface of the right kidney. Its density is similar to that of other soft tissues. Note left renal vein crossing just in front of the aorta (open arrow). There is some aortic calcification.

the injection of intravenous contrast medium unless they are dilated. The contrast medium outlines the major parts of the pelvicalyceal system but little or no papillary/calyceal detail is shown.

Renal mass lesions

Simple cysts appear on CT as sharply defined mass lesions with a density close to that of water (Fig. 7.17). They are more readily detected on CT than on urography and one or more cysts are commonly found as incidental findings in examinations of the upper abdomen.

Tumours cannot usually be distinguished from the surrounding normal renal parenchyma unless they are large enough to distort the renal outline. Tumour calcification may be seen which is not seen on plain abdominal radiographs. Some tumours have a relatively less dense centre representing central necrosis. The majority of tumours take up contrast medium less well than the surrounding renal parenchyma and so appear more obvious after enhancement.

Occasionally tumours are shown by CT which have not been suspected on urography. Such masses usually originate from the surface of the kidney, growing outwards and causing very little calyceal distortion (Fig. 7.18).

Not all non-cystic masses are renal cell carcinomas. Abscesses, haematomas, hamartomas and other benign tumours, and granulomatous pyelonephritis can all have appearances which might be mistaken for carcinoma on CT. In addition, extrinsic masses such as retroperitoneal sarcomas or lymphoma adjacent to or invading the kidney can be confused with an intrinsic renal mass. Because of their fat content angiomyolipomas are one of the few tumours which permit a reasonably confident diagnosis on the CT appearance alone.

The differential diagnosis between cyst and tumour can almost always be made even on an unenhanced scan because of the difference in density and the presence or absence of a sharp margin; if in doubt, scans can be obtained after enhancement. Magilner and Ostrum (1978) reported that 145 consecutive renal masses with CT appearances characteristic of a cyst in which confirmation of the diagnosis was available all proved to be cysts.

Ultrasound is normally the first step in the evaluation of a mass lesion found at urography. CT can be used to resolve a diagnostic problem if ultrasound is inconclusive or if more information is needed about an echogenic mass.

The extent of a tumour. CT can show the extent of tumour spread into the perinephric tissues or the presence of metastases in lymph nodes or the liver. Renal vein and vena caval involvement can frequently be detected (see p. 128). CT thus provides a considerable amount of information about the extent and stage of a renal cell carcinoma, raising the possibility that in some patients it might replace renal arteriography as a preoperative investigation (Lowe et al, 1979).

CT is an excellent method of imaging the renal bed when investigating a patient for possible recurrence after nephrectomy. Other imaging techniques are of little value in this situation and CT would seem to be the investigation of choice (Bernadino et al, 1979).

Other renal lesions
Hydronephrosis is visible on CT even without the injection of contrast medium because the low density of the urine-filled dilated pelvis and calyces is distinct from the soft tissue density of the surrounding renal parenchyma. *Calculi* are obvious on CT even when very small. It is not uncommon to see calculi on CT which are 'non-opaque' on plain abdominal radiographs. When taken together with the plain abdominal films CT allows very precise definition of the position of stones and hence simplifies their location at surgery. CT has been recommended as a means of solving the problem of the *'non-functioning kidney'* (Forbes, Isherwood & Fawcett, 1978). *Major congenital abnormalities*, such as horseshoe kidneys and polycystic kidneys, are readily shown by CT but are usually equally well shown by other techniques.

Perirenal lesions
The fat-containing perinephric space is clearly seen in cross-section so that CT provides an excellent method for investigating a patient in whom there is suspicion of an abscess or other abnormality in the perinephric space. It is also an effective method for detecting fluid collections in relation to renal transplants (Kittredge, Brensilver & Pierce, 1978).

The aorta and inferior vena cava (Figs 7.10, 7.14 and 7.16)
The sharply defined outline of the aorta can be identified even in the thinnest patients. The inferior vena cava is sometimes more difficult to define. It varies widely in shape and size from a round structure which may be larger than the aorta to one that is flat and inconspicuous. The renal vein is frequently prominent as it crosses the front of the aorta to join the inferior vena cava behind the head of the pancreas (Fig. 7.18).

The aorta
Lack of clarity of the aortic outline is an important sign of retroperitoneal disease unless the patient is very thin. Conditions in which the contours are lost include lymphadenopathy, retroperitoneal fibrosis, tumours, haematomas and abscesses. Displacement, especially displacement forward from the spine, is also a useful sign usually of lymph node disease.

Aortic aneurysms are obvious on CT and their size can be accurately assessed (Gomes, Hakkal & Schellinger, 1978; Perrett & Sage, 1978). Haematoma from a leak is seen as a soft tissue mass spreading out retroperitoneally from the aortic margin. CT can provide information that is important when planning elective surgery by demonstrating the relation of the aneurysm to the renal arteries above and to the aortic bifurcation below (Dixon et al, 1980). Ultrasound for this purpose appears to be unreliable (Wheeler, Beachley & Ranniger, 1975; Perrett & Sage, 1978) and aortography is invasive.

The inferior vena cava
In patients with vena caval thrombosis due to tumour the vein is frequently seen to be enlarged (Marks et al, 1978). In the absence of enlargement a filling defect may be revealed after enhancement, especially if contrast medium is injected into the foot. CT cannot, however, detect microscopic tumour invasion and cannot be used to exclude involvement (Steel, Sones & Heffner, 1978).

The liver and biliary tract
Because of its generally uniform texture the liver would seem ideally suited to CT scanning. However, focal lesions frequently have a density very similar to that of the surrounding liver parenchyma and may be difficult to detect even on high quality scans. This together with the frequency of streak artefacts from the ribs and from gas in the stomach using slower scanners accounts for the fact that CT scanning of the liver has so far been less reliable than might have been hoped. Even so, other techniques for imaging the liver have serious limitations so that CT can frequently contribute to diagnosis and management.

The liver usually appears a little denser than other intra-abdominal organs. Portal venous radicles can frequently be identified as low density structures within it. The vessels tend to disappear after enhancement. The intrahepatic bile ducts are not visible unless they are dilated or contain air or are outlined with an appropriate contrast medium. The common bile duct may be diffcult to identify unless opacified. The gallbladder is seen as a low density structure on the inferomedial aspect of the right lobe of the liver.

Focal liver disease

Primary or secondary tumours are rarely large enough to distort the outline of the liver. They are diagnosed because they vary in density from the surrounding liver parenchyma (Fig. 7.19). They are usually seen as low density areas but are occasionally denser than the normal liver and some may calcify. The ease of diagnosis depends on the size of the lesion and the difference in density between it and the surrounding liver parenchyma. When the density difference is slight, even large lesions may be difficult to detect. Some lesions are isodense with normal liver tissue. This is particularly likely to occur with diffusely infiltrating hepatomas and in such cases the scan may appear normal unless the lesion is large enough to distort the outline of the liver.

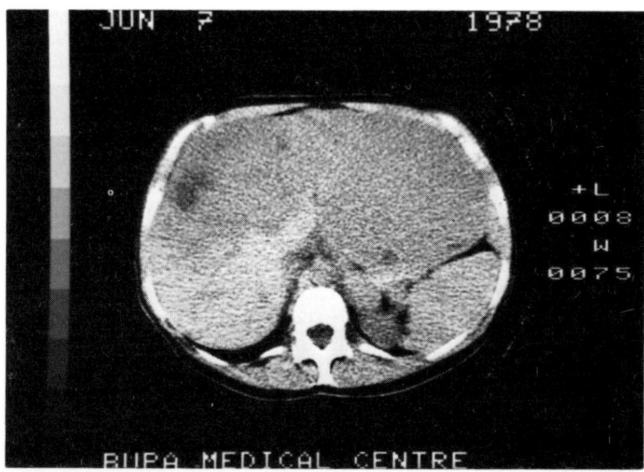

Fig. 7.19   A large hepatoma occupying the left lobe and much of the right lobe of the liver, with some areas of lower density representing areas of necrosis.

Tumours in the liver may be seen more distinctly after enhancement but sometimes they take up the contrast medium and may be obscured (Scherer et al, 1978; Moss et al, 1979). Occasionally enhancement shows a lesion not seen on the unenhanced scan (Moss et al, 1979).

Cysts can usually be distinguished from solid tumours but if less than 1.0–1.5 cm in diameter partial volume averaging may lead to the cyst appearing to be denser than expected and thus indistinguishable from a solid tumour.

Abscesses in the liver are usually less dense on CT than a tumour but denser than a cyst. There is, however, considerable overlap and a diagnosis of abscess cannot be made on the CT evidence alone.

Detection and differential diagnosis of focal liver disease. Cysts and abscesses can be detected without difficulty but even on good quality scans solid lesions may be difficult to demonstrate. In our experience, using a 20-second scanner, scans for the presence of metastatic disease in the liver are one of the most difficult types of scan to interpret. Accuracy rates of about 90 per cent for the detection of focal lesions have however been reported (Scherer et al, 1978; Snow, Goldstein & Wallace, 1979). Different types of solid lesion can rarely be distinguished one from another.

Diffuse liver disease
CT is at present of very little value in patients with diffuse liver disease. Only obvious enlargement or shrinkage or irregularity of outline can be identified with any confidence.

Fatty infiltration and *haemochromatosis* are associated with changes in the density of the liver. In fatty infiltration the density approaches that of fat but will vary according to the proportion of fat to normal liver tissue. The portal vessels stand out against the low density liver parenchyma, even on an unenhanced scan. In haemochromatosis and other conditions with iron overload the liver may appear denser than normal. Changes in density correlate well with iron content so that CT might have a place in monitoring progress (Houang et al, 1979; Chapman et al, 1980).

Gallbladder disease

Calcified gallstones may be seen when not visible on the plain radiograph. Many gallstones remain 'non-opaque' even with CT.

In the great majority of patients with *extrahepatic biliary obstruction* the intrahepatic ducts are dilated and the diagnosis is easily made by CT (Fig. 7.20). When only the

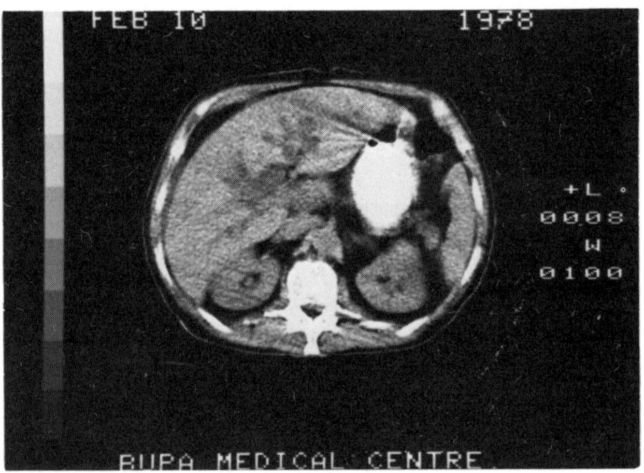

Fig. 7.20 Dilated bile ducts. The stomach is outlined with Gastrografin.

common duct is dilated the diagnosis may be more difficult to establish (Shanser et al, 1978). In many patients CT will not only show the appearance of obstruction but also its cause. Thus, Haaga & Reich (1978) were able to diagnose the cause of obstruction in 19 out of 25 patients with obstructive jaundice.

CT and other imaging techniques in disease of the liver and biliary tract. There is considerable overlap of the information provided by CT, ultrasound and isotope techniques. As might be expected the results of comparative studies of the three techniques in examination of focal liver lesions are conflicting (Grossman et al, 1977; Biello et al, 1978; Snow et al, 1979). It would seem appropriate at the present time to use isotope techniques and ultrasound as initial screening procedures when investigating the presence of focal liver lesions, reserving CT for patients in whom the diagnosis remains in doubt.

Cholecystography and ultrasound are effective methods of demonstrating the gallbladder and the presence of stones, and CT is rarely helpful. In the evaluation of jaundice, CT and ultrasound appear to be equally successful in demonstrating the presence or absence of obstruction (Goldberg et al, 1978).

The spleen

Cysts, calcification, infarcts, subscapsular haematomas, focal filling defects and rupture of the spleen can all be demonstrated. Diffuse involvement cannot however be detected so that CT is of very limited value in detecting splenic involvement in patients with lymphoma.

Computed tomography can frequently be the best imaging technique when investigating the left upper quadrant, which is a difficult area to elucidate by conventional methods. CT displays the tail of the pancreas, the spleen, the left kidney and adrenal and splenic hilar nodes, and also masses spreading from the stomach.

The alimentary tract

Of all the major organs, the bowel is the least well demonstrated by CT. Intraluminal lesions are not detectable unless the bowel is outlined with contrast medium, and even then only the largest lesions can be identified. On occasions, however, CT may be helpful in evaluating the extent of spread of a tumour beyond the bowel wall (Kressel et al, 1978).

In patients with *recurrent carcinoma of the rectum*, CT can produce unique information. The detection of recurrent carcinoma in such patients who have had abdominoperineal resection can be very difficult by other means. Interpretation of the scans is usually straightforward, although a recurrent mass sometimes has to be distinguished from bowel shadowing or from a localised mass of soft tissue remaining at the site of surgery (Husband, Hodson & Parsons, 1980).

Ascites, abscesses and haematomas

Ascites

Ascitic fluid has approximately the same density as water and is easily detected. It is first seen on upper abdominal scans as a crescentic shadow interposed between the liver and the diaphragm. When there are large amounts of ascites the fluid can act in rather the same way as fat, providing sufficient contrast to ouline the soft tissues.

Abscesses

The clinical diagnosis of intra-abdominal sepsis can be difficult and is one of the intra-abdominal problems to which CT can contribute most. Abscesses vary greatly in appearance from a collection of low density fluid to a mass of predominantly soft tissue density, possibly with only a small central area of low density. The specific feature which distinguishes an abscess from other masses or fluid collections is the presence of gas within the mass (Callen, 1979).

Computed tomography is applicable to the investigation of abscesses anywhere in the abdomen, but is particularly valuable for the demonstration of perinephric and psoas abscesses. Filly (1979) reviewed the place of CT, ultrasound and gallium-67 scanning for abscesses. Although CT appears to be the most accurate single method, a combination of the techniques is likely to be more effective.

CT can also be used as a guide for percutaneous catheter drainage (Haaga & Reich, 1978; Gerzof et al, 1979).

Haematomas
CT has a place in the evaluation of possible intra-abdominal haemorrhage including trauma. In the acute phase, a haematoma is seen as a mass of soft tissue density. As it becomes chronic it becomes less dense and may appear almost cystic.

Abdominal masses
The investigation of patients with palpable abdominal masses in whom no definite diagnosis has been made is one of the commonest indications for CT because CT can show the location of the mass and sometimes can determine its nature. It is particularly valuable in separating aneurysms from other causes of 'pulsatile' masses. The most striking feature of the use of CT in patients with abdominal masses is the confidence with which the presence or absence of a mass can be established when clinical examination is inconclusive.

Computed tomography can be used as a guide for percutaneous biopsy (Haaga & Reich, 1978; Ferrucci & Wittenberg, 1979). The display in the axial plane is ideal for guiding the needle. The technique is more precise than that using fluoroscopy or ultrasound. It is especially useful for small retroperitoneal lesions and for lesions in the pelvis (Fig. 7.21).

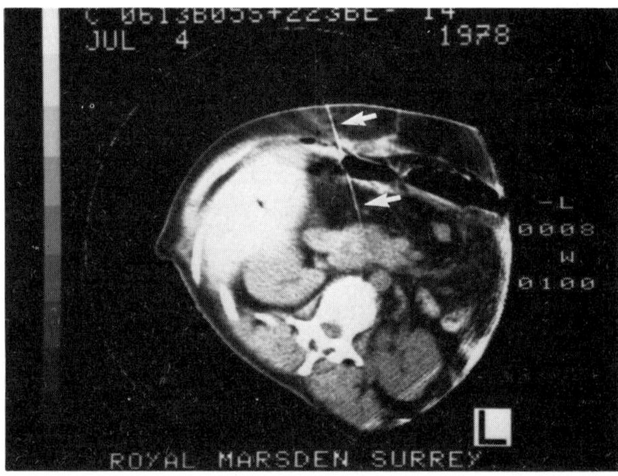

Fig. 7.21   Scan to confirm position of fine needle (arrows) during percutaneous aspiration biopsy of slightly enlarged head of pancreas. Biopsy established the diagnosis of carcinoma.

Lymph node disease of the abdomen and pelvis
The demonstration of lymph node enlargement is perhaps the commonest single indication for the use of CT, partly because the examination does not involve the discomfort and hazards of lymphography and partly because nodes are shown which are not accessible to lymphography.

The only feature which distinguishes abnormal from normal nodes is enlargement. They usually have a density similar to that of other soft tissues. CT provides no evidence about the internal architecture and so, unlike lymphography, cannot identify metastases in nodes of normal size.

The *para-aortic nodes* are the most easily examined because they are embedded in the retroperitoneal fat. Enlargement initially produces two distinct types of appearance. The commonest is observed as obliteration of the normal anatomical contours, the outlines of the aorta and inferior vena cava being lost early on. As enlargement increases the vessels are buried within the mass (Fig. 7.22). The psoas outline may

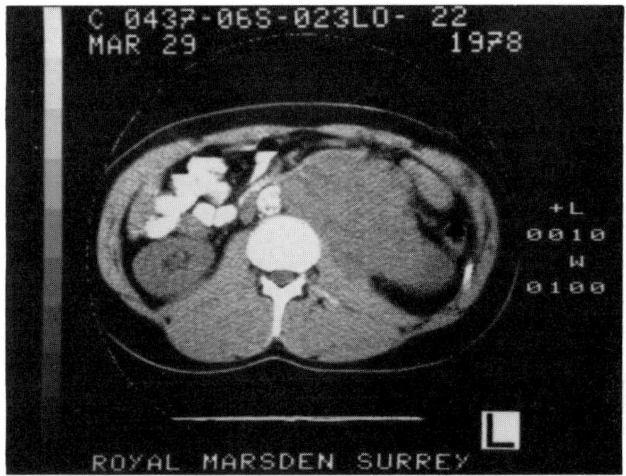

Fig. 7.22   Large mass of lymph nodes obscuring the aorta and left psoas muscle.

also be lost. Less commonly the nodes remain as discrete masses with margins clearly distinguished from neighbouring vessels. Early nodal involvement is most readily detected on the left of the aorta rather than on the right where the nodes tend to merge with the inferior vena cava and the head of the pancreas (Fig. 7.23).

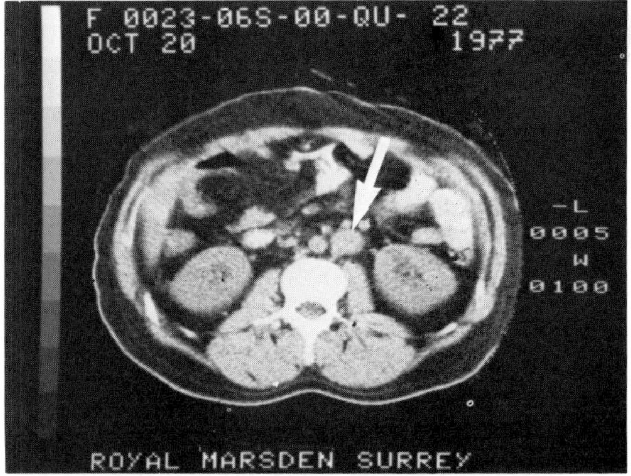

Fig. 7.23   Discrete lymph node mass (arrowed) to the left of the aorta.

Discrete nodal enlargement is seen in inflammatory disease and with benign hyperplasia in addition to lymphoma and metastatic disease. The more diffuse type of appearance seems only to occur in lymphoma and metastatic disease.

Nodes in other upper abdominal sites and in the pelvis. Lymphadenopathy can be demonstrated in any intra-abdominal site including nodes in the mesentery, porta hepatis, splenic and renal hila, and in the coeliac group of nodes. Enlargement of external iliac nodes is seen as a soft tissue bulge on the lateral pelvic wall just above the actabulum. Large internal iliac nodes are seen more posteriorly close to the obturator internus muscle.

In all these sites minor degrees of enlargement are more difficult to detect than in the para-aortic region.

Role of CT in lymph node disease

Computed tomography is more accurate in assessing lymph nodes involved with lymphoma than those involved with metastatic cancer because in the latter the nodes are frequently normal in size. Comparative sudies of CT and lymphography with the findings at staging laparotomy have shown that CT is as accurate as lymphography in detecting para-aortic node involvement in patients with lymphoma (Best et al, 1978; Lee et al, 1978; Earl et al, 1980). Both Best et al (1978) and Earl et al (1980) reported difficulty in excluding disease in nodes outside the para-aortic region because minor degrees of enlargement were difficult to distinguish from surrounding tissues.

Computed tomography is inferior to lymphography for detecting pelvic node metastases in patients with pelvic cancer. In a study of patients with carcinoma of the bladder CT missed metastases in 7 out of 11 patients with proven nodal involvement (Hodson, Husband & MacDonald, 1979). Lee et al (1978) studying patients with various types of pelvic cancer could find no evidence of node enlargement on CT in 6 out of 15 patients with proven nodal metastases.

Testicular tumours are an exception to the general rule that metastatic cancer is more difficult to identify on CT than on lymphography. Node involvement by such tumours is usually easily detected because they tend to cause gross enlargement and involve predominantly nodes in the upper para-aortic area. Husband et al (1979) report that CT findings correlate well with those at lymphography in this type of tumour but that CT will usually show disease beyond the reach of lymphography.

The pelvis

Computed tomography has not yet proved as fruitful a method of investigation for the pelvis as it has for the thorax and abdomen, partly because the pelvis is relatively accessible to physical examination and partly because much of the anatomy of the pelvis is not well suited to imaging by axial sections. As with ultrasound it is important that CT examinations of this region should be carried out when the bladder is distended. When the bladder is empty the small bowel occupies much of the pelvis and if unopacified is easily confused with a soft tissue mass. When the bladder is distended the low density urine acts as an effective contrast medium (Fig. 7.24). In some patients the bladder does not distend even after the injection of a diuretic and intravenous contrast medium may be needed. In males the seminal vesicles are outlined by fat separating them from the bladder and rectum (Fig. 7.24). In females the vaginal vault lies behind the bladder and can be identified more clearly when a tampon is inserted. This acts as a useful guide to the position of the uterus. The ovaries are situated on the side wall of the bony pelvis and cannot be identified unless enlarged.

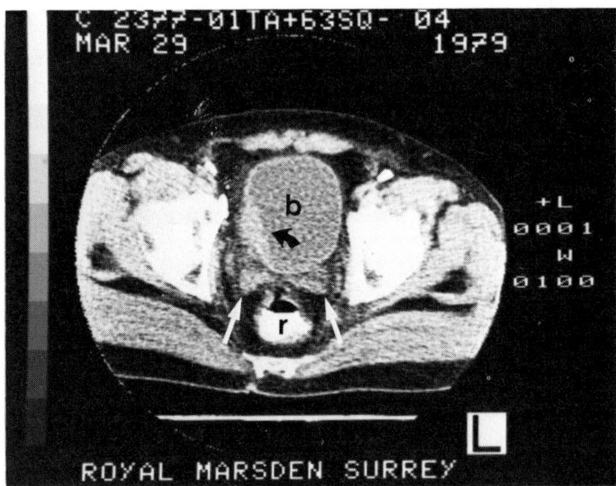

Fig. 7.24 Carcinoma of the bladder (black arrow) in a male. The bladder wall is thickened and the tumour is spreading into the perivesical tissues. The rectum (r) is filled with Gastrografin. Note the seminal vesicles (white arrows).

At present, CT of the pelvis is rarely useful for primary diagnosis. It can, however, be useful in the staging of tumours and in monitoring the response to treatment.

The bladder
Virtually the only indication for CT scans of the bladder is for the staging of known carcinoma. Studies correlating the CT findings with the pathological staging have shown that CT is more accurate than clinical staging, its main contribution being its capacity to detect extramural spread (Seidelmann, Cohen & Bryan, 1977; Hodson, Husband & MacDonald, 1979; Kellett et al, 1980). Kellett et al (1980) suggest that CT may be particularly helpful after radiotherapy in distinguishing a clinically frozen pelvis due to irradiation fibrosis from one due to tumour recurrence.

The uterus
Computed tomography has no place in the primary diagnosis of carcinoma of the cervix or uterus, nor is it of much value in the initial staging of early carcinoma of the cervix (Husband, J E unpublished data). As with bladder tumours, it appears to be useful in establishing the extent of disease after radiotherapy.

Other pelvic structures
Computed tomography is rarely required for the diagnosis of *ovarian cysts and tumours* but can be useful for monitoring the response of tumours to treatment. *Carcinoma of the prostate* cannot be distinguished from benign prostatic hypertrophy unless the tumour is advanced and has spread through the prostatic capsule into adjacent structures (Price & Davidson, 1979). *Pelvic lipomatosis* is strikingly displayed on CT because the grossly excessive fat fills most of the pelvis and the stretching of the sigmoid colon and compression and displacement of the bladder are very clearly shown.

The musculoskeletal system

Bones, muscles and other superficial soft tissues are well shown by CT and because of the large contrast differences interpretation tends to be relatively straightforward. In spite of this, the technique has been largely neglected as a means of investigating lesions of the musculoskeletal system. There is increasing evidence that it can often provide useful information not readily available using other methods, particularly when examining the spine and the bony pelvis, and when assessing the extent of tumours.

Tumours

Primary tumours. Computed tomography is of relatively little value in primary diagnosis. It is less effective than conventional radiography for defining the nature of a tumour in bone and it does not appear to help to distinguish between osteomyelitis and a malignant neoplasm (Berger & Kuhn, 1978). It can occasionally be useful by showing that a superficial mass consists of fat or by excluding a mass considered to be present on physical examination (Levine et al, 1979).

There are several reports suggesting that CT is the most effective method of determining the extent of a tumour, particularly when planning surgery. Its advantage over conventional radiography is due to its ability to show medullary spread as well as cortical involvement and to delineate the precise extent of soft tissue involvement (de Santos, Bernadino & Murray, 1979; Destouet, Gilula & Murphy, 1979; Levine et al, 1979).

Metastases are seen as lytic or sclerotic lesions and can be identified down to a size of about 1 cm. They are commonly observed in the vertebrae. They may be seen when conventional radiographs, including tomography, show no abnormality. This would suggest that CT might be useful when radiography is negative in the presence of a positive radiosotope scan. CT is not, however, a practical way of screening for metastases.

Trauma

In the assessment of fractures and dislocations of *the spine* CT can demonstrate involvement of the posterior elements which may be difficult to show with conventional radiography. Encroachment of bony fragments on the spinal canal and intervertebral foramina, and the presence of loose fragments can be accurately detected. CT avoids the manipulation normally needed to obtain satisfactory radiographs in this type of patient and is particularly valuable in patients with suspected fracture and possible instability of the cervical spine (McInerney & Sage, 1979).

Computed tomography is also useful in patients with pelvic fracture, particularly those in whom open reduction is considered for fractures involving the acetabulum (Lasda et al, 1978).

Other abnormalities

One of the commonest indications for CT of the spine is evaluation of possible spinal stenosis, especially when associated with degenerative changes or previous surgery (Lee, Kazam & Newman, 1978). Stenosis of the lateral recesses and exit foramina can be difficult to demonstrate by conventional techniques. There is increasing evidence to suggest that CT may have a part to play in assessing stenosis at these sites and in the investigation of low back pain (Sheldon, Sersland & Leborgne, 1977; Glenn et al, 1979; Burton et al, 1979).

In *congenital abnormalities* such as spinal dysraphism and diastematomyelia CT provides detailed information about the complex bone and soft tissue abnormalities which is not readily obtained by other means and which can be important when planning surgical management (James & Olliff, 1977). Studies of *bone densitometry* suggest that CT may provide a quantitative method of assessing metabolic bone disease (Bradley & Huang, 1978: Pullan & Roberts, 1978). It also seems possible that CT will come to have a place in the study of *muscle diseases* (Bulcke et al, 1979) and perhaps in disorders of fat metabolism.

Spinal canal
Poor contrast between the cord and the surrounding cerebrospinal fluid has up to now resulted in inadequate resolution of the canal contents without intrathecal contrast medium. The recent introduction of 'high resolution sector scanning' (Ethier et al, 1979) has resulted in more accurate demonstration of the cord and is of value in assessing cord lesions such as hydromyelia and tumour.

Computed tomography metrizamide myelography (CTMM) may be performed as a primary study or after conventional myelography. It gives localising information in the transverse plane and may be of help in showing the upper limit of an almost complete obstruction. In spinal dysraphism it provides accurate delineation of the relation of the complex abnormalities to the cord (Resjö et al, 1978). At present, replacement of conventional studies by CTMM is impractical and a sensible approach seems to be a combination of both types of investigation.

Computerised tomography in oncology
There are three ways in which CT contributes to the management of patients with known malignant disease, namely staging, monitoring response to treatment and radiotherapy treatment planning.

Staging
Computed tomography is an effective method for determining the extent of tumour in the paranasal sinuses (Forbes et al, 1978; Parsons & Hodson, 1979), nasopharynx (Thawley, Gado & Fuller, 1978) and larynx (Mancuso, Calcaterra & Hanafee, 1979), in the retroperitoneum (especially the kidney) and in the bladder. It is less effective for determining the extent of a tumour of the cervix and body of uterus, the ovaries, the lung and the gastrointestinal tract.

The role of CT in the assessment of lymph node involvement and of metastatic spread to lungs, liver and bone has already been discussed.

Monitoring response to treatment
Computed tomography is ideally suited to monitoring the change in size of a tumour in response to treatment. Tumours which are difficult to visualise by other methods can be scanned at the start of treatment to provide baseline information and the scans can be repeated during treatment so that shrinkage or growth of tumour can be assessed on sequential scans.

Radiotherapy treatment planning
The cross-sectional display of anatomy obtained by CT has obvious applications for radiotherapy planning (Hobday et al, 1979). The effect of CT varies with the site of the tumour and the size of the radiation field. Deep-seated intra-abdominal tumours are difficult to outline by conventional means and CT has clear cut advantages for planning. In other situations such as the lung where tumours are easy to localise by conventional films CT has much less impact. The more localised the proposed field the greater the value of CT.

REFERENCES

Berger P E, Kuhn J P 1978 Computed tomography of the musculoskeletal system in children. Radiology 127: 171–175

Bernadino M E, de Santos L A, Johnson D E, Bracken R B 1979 Computed tomography in the evaluation of post-nephrectomy patient. Radiology 130: 183–187

Best J J K, Blackledge G, Forbes W StC, Todd I D H, Eddleston B, Crowther D, Isherwood I 1978 Computed tomography of the abdomen in the staging and clinical management of lymphoma. British Medical Journal 2: 1675–1677

Biello D R, Levitt R G, Siegal B A, Sagel S S, Stanley R J 1978 Computed tomography and radionuclide imaging of the liver and colon: a comparative evaluation. Radiology 127: 159–163

Bradley J G, Huang H K 1978 Evaluation of calcium concentration in bones from CT scans. Radiology 128: 103–107

Bulcke J A, Termote J-L, Palmers Y, Croll A D 1979 Computed tomography of the human skeletal muscular system. Neuroradiology 17: 127–136

Burton C V, Heithoff K B, Kirkaldy-Wallace W, Range D 1979 Computed tomographic scanning and the lumbar spine. Spine 4: 356–368

Callen P W 1979 Computed tomographic evaluation of abdominal and pelvic abscesses. Radiology 131: 171–175

Chapman R W G, Williams G, Bydder G, Dick R, Sherlock S, Kreel L 1980 Computed tomography for determining liver iron content in primary haemochromatosis. British Medical Journal 1: 440–442

Crowe J K, Brown L R, Muhm J R 1978 Computed tomography of the mediastinum. Radiology 128: 75–87

de Santos L A, Bernadino M E, Murray J A 1979 Computed tomography in the evaluation of osteosarcoma: experience with 25 cases. American Journal of Roentgenology 132: 535–540

Destouet J M, Gilula L A, Murphy W A 1979 Computed tomography of long bone osteosarcoma. Radiology 131: 439–445

Dixon A K, Springall R G, Taylor G W, Fry I K 1980 Computed tomography of abdominal aortic aneurysms: determination of longitudinal extent. Clinical Radiology (in press)

Dunnick N R, Schaner E G, Doppman J L, Strott C A, Gill J R and Javadpour N 1979 Computed tomography of adrenal tumours. American Journal of Roentgenology 32: 43–46

Earl H M, Sutcliffe S B J, Fry I K, Tucker A K, Young J, Husband J E, Wrigley P F M, Malpas J S 1980 Computerised tomographic (CT) abdominal scanning in Hodgkin's disease. Clinical Radiology 31: 149–153

Ethier R, King D G, Belanger G, Taylor S, Thompson C 1979 Development of high resolution computed tomography of the spinal cord. Journal of Computer Assisted Tomography 3: 433–438

Ferrucci J T, Wittenberg J 1978 CT biopsy of abdominal tumours: aids to lesion localisation. Radiology 129: 739–744

Ferrucci J T, Wittenberg J, Black E B, Kirkpatrick R H, Hall D A 1979 Computed body tomography in chronic pancreatitis. Radiology 130: 175–182

Filly R A 1979 Detection of abdominal abscesses. Journal of the Canadian Association of Radiologists 30: 202–210

Forbes W StC, Fawcitt R A, Isherwood I, Webb R, Farrington T 1978 Computed tomography in the diagnosis of the paranasal sinuses. Clinical Radiology 29: 501–511

Forbes W StC, Isherwood I, Fawcitt R A 1978 Computed tomography in the evaluation of the solitary or unilateral non-functioning kidney. Journal of Computer Assisted Tomography 2: 389–394

Gerzof S G, Robbins A H, Birkett D H, Johnson W C, Pugatch R D, Vincent M E 1979 Percutaneous catheter drainage of abdominal abscesses guided by ultrasound and computed tomography. American Journal of Roentgenology 133: 1–8

Glenn W V, Rhodes M L, Altschuler E M, Wiltse L L, Kostanek C, Kno Y M 1979 Multiplanar display computerised body tomography applications in the lumbar spine Spine 4: 282–352

Goldberg H I, Filly R A, Korobkin M, Moss A A, Kressel H Y, Callen P W 1978 Capability of CT body scanning and ultrasonography to demonstrate the status of the biliary ductal system in patients with jaundice. Radiology 129: 731–737

Gomez M N, Hakkal H G, Schellinger D 1978 Ultrasonography and CT scanning: a comparative study of abdominal aortic aneurysm. Computerized Tomography 2: 99–109

Grossman Z, Wistow B, Bryan P, Dinn W, McAfee J, Kieffer S 1977 Radionuclide imaging, computed tomography and grey scale ultrasound of the liver: a comparative study. Journal of Nuclear Medicine 18: 327–333

Haaga J R, Alfidi R J, Havrilla T M, Tubbs R, Gonzales L, Meaney T, Corsi M 1977 Definitive role of CT scanning of the pancreas. Radiology 124: 723–730

Haaga J, Reich N E 1978 Computed tomography of abdominal abnormalities. CV Mosby, St Louis

Heitzmann E R, Goldwin R L, Proto A V 1977 Radiological analysis of the mediastinum utilising computed tomography. Radiologic Clinics of North America 15: 309–329

Hobday P, Hodson N J, Husband J E, Parker R P, MacDonald J S 1979 Computed tomography applied to radiotherapy treatment planning: techniques and results. Radiology 133: 477–482

Hodson N J, Husband J E, MacDonald J S 1979 The role of computed tomography in the staging of bladder cancer. Clinical Radiology 30: 389–395

Hodson N J, Husband J E 1980 The value of CT in the staging and management of pelvic tumours. In: Husband and Hobday (eds) European Seminars of Computerised Axial Tomography No. 2, CT in Oncology, Churchill Livingstone, Edinburgh

Houang M T W, Aruzena X, Skalicka A, Huehns E R, Shaw D G 1979 Correlation between computed tomographic values and liver iron content in thalassaemia major with iron overload. Lancet 1: 1322–1323

Husband J E, Hodson N J, Parsons C A 1980 The role of computed tomography in recurrent rectal tumours. Radiology 134: 677–682

Husband J E, Meire H B, Kreel L 1977 Comparison of ultrasound and computer assisted tomography in pancreatic diagnosis. British Journal of Radiology 50: 855, 862

Husband J E, Peckham M J, MacDonald J S, Hendry W F 1979 The role of computed tomography in the management of testicular teratoma. Clinical Radiology 30: 243–252

James H E, Olliff M 1977 Computed tomography in spinal dysraphism. Journal of Computer Assisted Tomography 1: 391–397

Karstaedt N, Sagel S S, Stanley R J, Melson G L, Levitt R G 1978 Computed tomography of the adrenal gland. Radiology 129: 723–730

Kellett M J, Oliver R T D, Husband J E, Fry I K 1980 Computed tomography as an adjunct to bimanual examination for staging bladder tumours. British Journal of Urology 52: 101–106

Kittredge R D, Brensilver J, Pierce J C 1978 Computed tomography in renal transplant problems. Radiology 127: 165–169

Kreel L 1976a The EMI whole body scanner: an interim clinical evaluation of the prototype. British Journal of Clinical Equipment 4: 220–227

Kreel L 1976b Computed tomography in the evaluation of pulmonary asbestosis. Acta Radiologica Diagnosis 17: 405–412

Kressel H Y, Callen P W, Montagne J-P, Korobkin M, Goldberg H I, Moss A A, Arger P H, Margulis A R 1978 Computed tomographic evaluation of disorders affecting the alimentary tract. Radiology 129: 451–455

Lasda N A, Levisohn E M, Yuan H A, Bunnell W P 1978 Computerised tomography in disorders of the hip. Journal of Bone and Joint Surgery 60-A: 1099–1102

Lee B C P, Kazam E, Newman A D 1978 Computed tomography of the spine and spinal cord. Radiology 128: 95–102

Lee J K T, Stanley R J, Sagel S S, Levitt R G 1978 Accuracy of computed tomography in detecting intra-abdominal and pelvic adenopathy. American Journal of Roentgenology 131: 311–315

Lee J K T, Stanley R J, Melson G L, Sagel S S 1979 Pancreatic imaging by ultrasound and computed tomography: a general review. Radiologic Clinics of North America 16: 105–118

Levine E, Lee K R, Neff J R, Maklad N F, Robinson R G, Preston D F 1979 Comparison of computed tomography and other imaging modalities in the evaluation of musculoskeletal tumours. American Journal of Roentgenology 131: 431–437

Love L, Churchill R, Reyne S C, Schuster G A, Moncada R, Kerkow A 1979 Computed tomography for the staging of renal carcinoma. Urologic Radiology 1: 3–10

Magilner A D, Ostrum B J 1978 Computed tomography in the diagnosis of renal masses. Radiology 126: 715–718

Mancuso A A, Calcaterra T C, Hanafee W N 1978 Computed tomography of the larynx Radiologic Clinics of North America 16: 195–208

Marks W M, Korobkin M, Callen P W, Kaiser J A 1978 CT diagnosis of tumour thrombosis of renal vein and inferior vena cava. American Journal of Roentgenology 131: 843–846

McInerney D P, Sage M R 1979 Computer-assisted tomography in the assessment of cervical spine trauma. Clinical Radiology 30: 203–206

Mink J H, Bein M E, Sukov R, Herrmann C, Winter J, Sample F, Mulder D 1978 Computed tomography of the anterior mediastinum in patients with myasthenia gravis and suspected thymoma. American Journal of Roentgenology 130: 239–246

Moss A A, Schrumpf J D, Schnyder P, Korobkin M, Shimshak R R 1979 Computed tomography of focal hepatic lesions: a blind evaluation of the effect of contrast enhancement. Radiology 131: 427–430

Muhm J R, Brown L R, Crowe J K, Sheedy P F, Hattery H R, Stephens D H 1978 Comparison of whole lung tomography and computed tomography for detecting pulmonary nodules. American Journal of Roentgenology 131: 981–984

Parsons C A, Hodson N 1979 Computed tomography in paranasal sinus tumours. Radiology 132: 641–645

Perrett L V, Sage M R 1978 Computed tomography of abdominal aortic aneurysms. Australia and New Zealand Journal of Surgery 48: 275–277

Price J M, Davidson A J 1979 Computed tomography in the evaluation of suspected carcinomatous prostate. Urologic Radiology 1: 39–42

Pullan B R, Roberts T E 1978 Bone mineral measurement using an EMI scanner and standard methods: a comparative study. British Journal of Radiology 51: 24–28

Putman C E, Rohman S L, Littner M R, Allen W E, Schachter E N, McLoud T C, Bein M E, Gee J B L 1977 Computerised tomography in pulmonary sarcoidosis. Computerized Tomography 1: 197–209

Resjö I M, Harwood Nash D C, Fitz C R, Chung S 1978 Computer tomographic metrizamide myelography in spinal dysraphism in infants and children. Journal of Computer Assisted Tomography 2: 549–558

Sagel S, Stanley R J, Evens R G 1976 Early clinical experience with motionless whole-body computed tomography. Radiology 119: 321–330

Schanger E G, Chang A E, Doppman J L, Conkle D M, Flye M W, Rosenberg S A 1978 Comparison of computed and conventional whole lung tomography in detecting pulmonary nodules: a prospective radiologic–pathologic study. American Journal of Roentgenology 131: 51–54

Scherer U, Rainier R, Eisenburg J, Schildberg F W, Meister P, Lissner J 1978 Diagnostic accuracy of CT in circumscript liver disease. American Journal of Roentgenology 130: 711–714

Scholten E T, Kreel L 1977 Distribution of metastases in the axial plane. A combined radiological–pathological study. Radiologica Clinica 46: 248–265

Seidelmann F E, Cohen W N, Bryan P J 1977 Computed tomographic staging of bladder cancers. Radiologic Clinics of North America 15: 419–440

Shanser J D, Korobkin M, Goldberg H I, Rohlfing B M 1978 Computed tomographic diagnosis of obstructive jaundice in the absence of intrahepatic ductal dilatation. American Journal of Roentgenology 131: 389–392

Sheedy P F, Stephens D H, Hattery R R, Muhm J R, Hartman G W 1976 Computed tomography of the body: initial clinical trial with EMI prototype. American Journal of Roentgenology 127: 23–51

Sheedy P F, Stephens D H, Hattery R R, MacCarty R 1977 Computed tomography in the evaluation of patients with suspected carcinoma of the pancreas. Radiology 124: 731–737

Sheldon J J, Sersland T, Leborgne J 1977 Computed tomography of the lower lumbar vertebral column. Radiology 124: 113–118

Snow J H, Goldstein H M, Wallace S 1979 Comparison of scientigraphy, sonography and computed tomography in the evaluation of hepatic neoplasms. American Journal of Roentgenology 132: 915–918

Stanley R J, Sagel S S, Levitt R G 1977 Computed tomographic evaluation of the pancreas. Radiology 124: 715–722

Steel J R, Sones P J, Heffner L T 1978 The detection of inferior vena caval thombosis with computed tomography. Radiology 128: 385–386

Stewart B H, Bravo E L, Haaga J, Meaney T F, Tarazi R 1978 Localisation of phaeochromocytomas by computed tomography. New England Journal of Medicine 299: 460–461

Thawley S W, Gado M, Fuller T R 1978 Computerised tomography in the evaluation of head and neck lesions. The Laryngoscope 88: 451–459

Wheeler W E, Breachley M C, Ranniger K 1975 Angiography and ultrasonography. A comparative study of abdominal aortic aneurysms. American Journal of Roentgenology 126: 95–100

7.3. Computed axial tomography of the brain
Jeffrey Gawler

In neurological practice, a plain radiograph of the head has limited diagnostic value for it displays the skull bones rather than the soft tissues which they protect. Human intracranial structures were first revealed on an X-ray by accident when Luckett (1913) reported a patient whose ventricular system was visible on a skull film because, as a sequel to trauma, it had filled with air. In 1918, Dandy exploited this chance finding and deliberately injected air directly into a patient's lateral ventricle to obtain a ventriculogram. The following year he showed that air introduced at lumbar puncture could be persuaded into the head to outline the ventricular system and subarachnoid space; a pneumo- or air encephalogram. Although both these techniques are still used to investigate certain neurological problems, their early clinical application carried sufficient risk to inspire Moniz (1927) to devise the technique of carotid arteriography. Isotope brain scanning, introduced in 1948 by Moore, provided a non-invasive method of investigating cerebral disease but it failed to produce the anticipated fall in demand for contrast procedures, and angiography or pneumoencephalography remained the diagnostic cornerstones for patients suspected of harbouring intracranial disease. Early in this decade Hounsfield (1973) introduced computerised X-ray scanning of the head, and the soft tissues within the skull became visible without recourse to contrast media. The technique involved no hazard or discomfort for the patient, and structural disease processes affecting the brain were identified with a clarity exceeding traditional methods. Neuroradiological practice was transformed overnight and Hounsfield was subsequently awarded the Nobel Prize for Medicine in recognition of his magnificent contribution to the investigation and management of patients with cerebral disease.

THE NORMAL EXAMINATION

A standard computerised scan (Fig. 7.25) provides a three dimensional display of the intracranial anatomy built up from a vertical series of transverse axial tomograms. Each tomogram (Fig. 7.26) represents a horizontal slice through the patient's head, reconstructed in terms of the X-ray density of the structures it contains. The technique is sufficiently sensitive to distinguish brain tissue from cerebrospinal fluid (c.s.f.) so that the ventricular system and many of the subarachnoid cisterns are visible. The lateral third and fourth ventricles are regularly seen but the aqueduct is normally too fine to resolve.

The posterior fossa cisterns (Fig. 7.27) provide important land marks which delineate the upper brainstem. The pontine cistern ventral to the pons continues postero-laterally on each side into the cerebellopontine angle cisterns. Rostrally the pontine cistern becomes continuous with the interpeduncular cistern lying between the cerebral peduncles and the crural cisterns which cap them. The quadrigeminal cistern overlies the posterior aspect of the midbrain and is prolonged around the brainstem as the ambient cisterns which open anteriorly into the crural cisterns. The quadrigeminal cistern is continuous superiorly with the cistern of the great vein of Galen which lies at the tentorial hiatus immediately behind the third ventricle. The lateral extremities of the Galenic cistern extend behind the pulvinar of the thalamus on each side as the lateral wings of the ambient cistern. The pineal projects backward into the cistern of the great vein and can be identified even when uncalcified. Posteriorly the Galenic cistern becomes continuous with the superior cerebellar cistern overlying the superior vermis immediately below the tentorium.

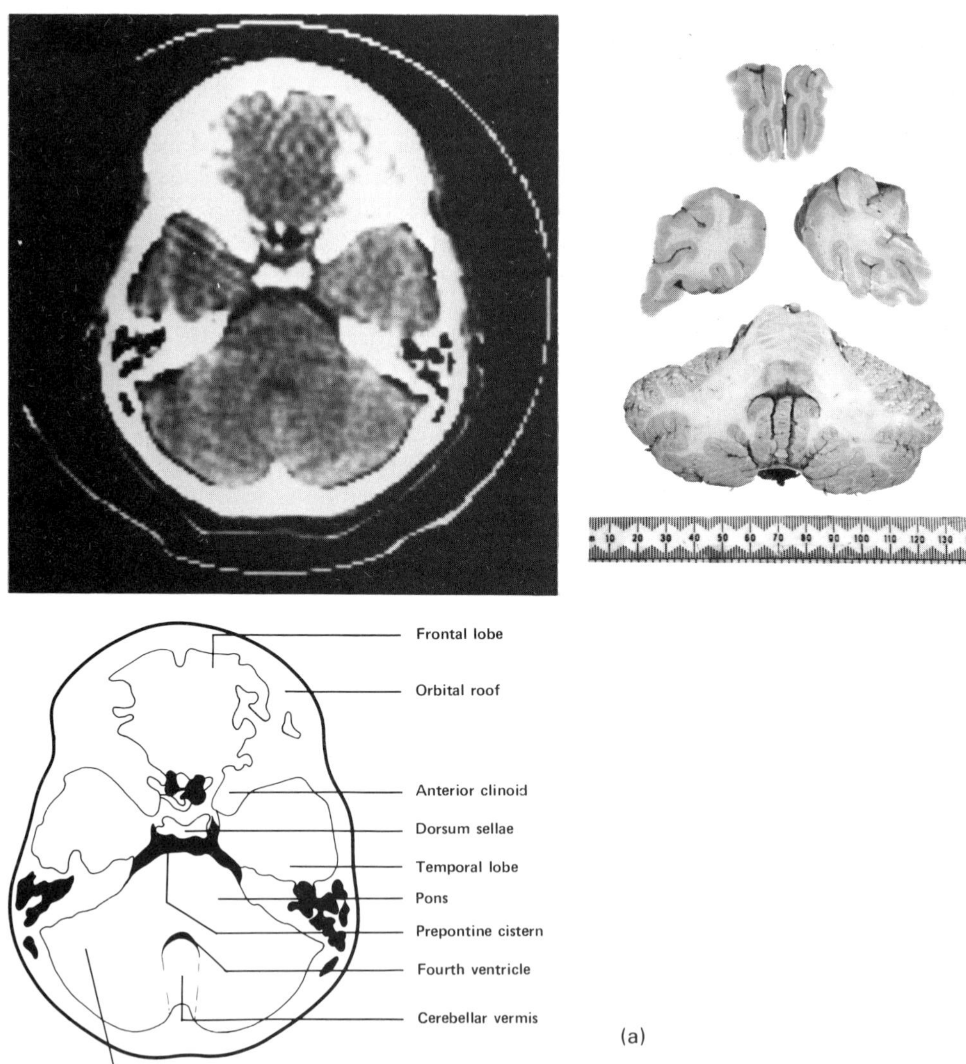

Fig. 7.25   (a) to (f) Vertical series of six normal transverse axial tomograms with equivalent brain slice and explanatory diagram.

In the supratentorial compartment the cisterns immediately above the sella are regularly identified, as are the insula cisterns which overlie the islands of Riel. Normal cortical sulci are made visible by the fluid that they contain and sometimes normal cerebellar suci can also be identified.

Computerised tomography detects the slight difference in X-ray absorption between grey and white matter and thus allows certain cerebral structures to be identified in their own right. The cortical grey matter mantle can be distinguished over the surface of the cerebral hemispheres not only subjacent to the skull but also as a midline band in relation to the interhemispheric fissure. The heads of the caudate nuclei are often seen as oval zones of grey matter density immediately lateral to the

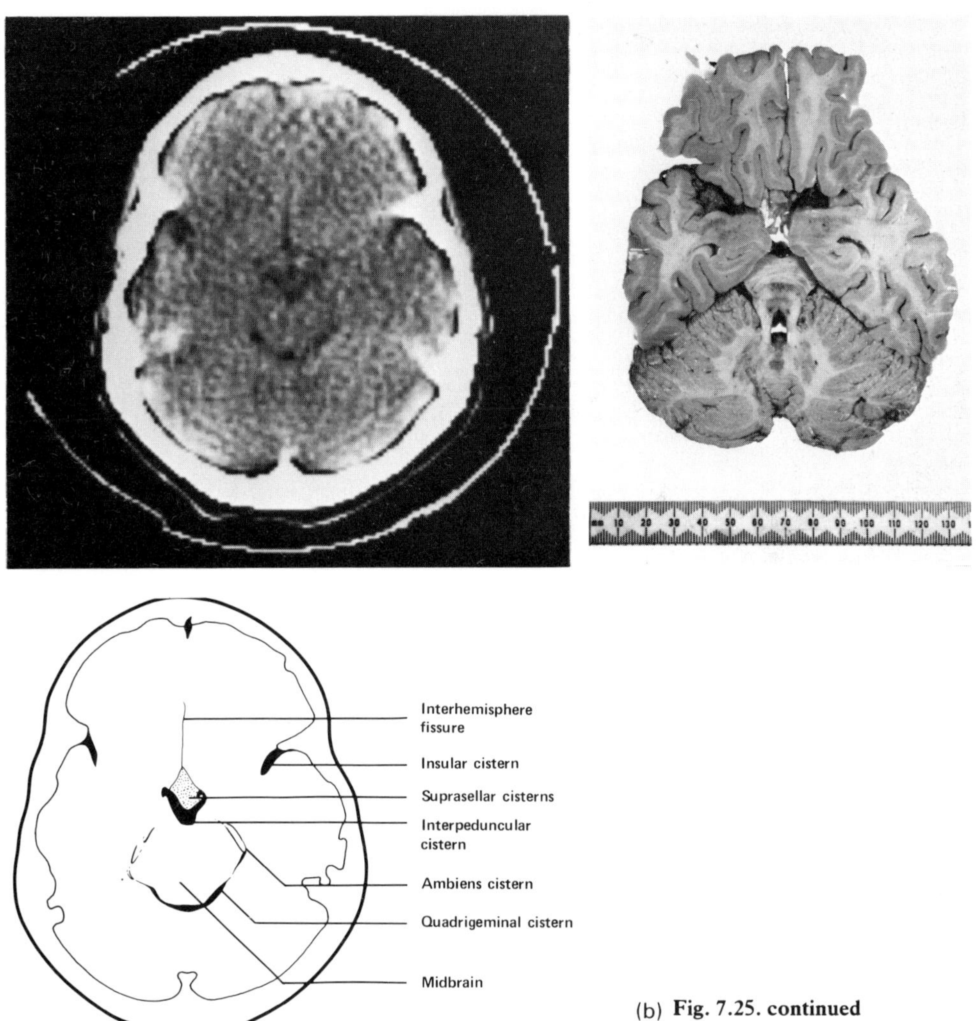

(b) **Fig. 7.25. continued**

ventricular frontal horns. Likewise, the thalami can usually be distinguished. Their medial margin is gauged from the third ventricle and the posterior aspect of the pulvinar is outlined by the trigone of the lateral ventricle and the wing of the ambient cistern. The lateral thalamic margin is defined by the posterior limb of the internal capsule. The putamen and globus pallidus (lentiform nuclei) are less well seen, and they merge laterally into the grey matter of the insula. The internal capsules are regularly seen as bands of white matter density. The anterior limb lies between the head of the caudate and the lentiform nucleus whilst the posterior limb intervenes between the thalamus and lentiform nucleus. It may be possible to identify the external capsule lateral to the lentiform nucleus. The septum pellucidum is visible between the anterior extremities of the lateral ventricles and at its posterior end the

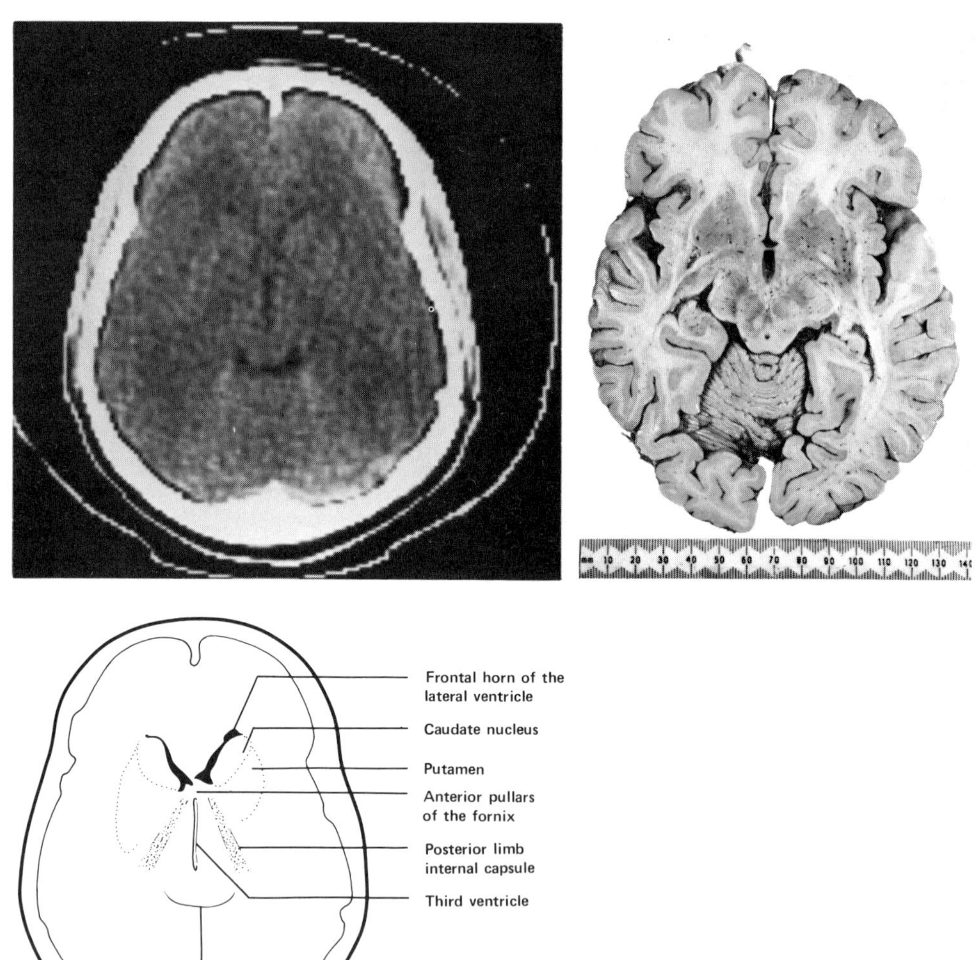

(c) **Fig. 7.25. continued**

anterior columns of the fornix are seen in the midline bulging into the posterior segments of the frontal horns. The foraminae of Munro open into the third ventricle at this site.

Scans taken after the intravenous injection of contrast outline some of the larger intracranial vessels. The anterior cerebral arteries are seen in the midline in the interhemispheric fissure immediately anterior to the septum pellucidum. The middle cerebral vessels can be seen in the lateral fissures and their branches in the insula cisterns. The basilar artery is usually apparent in the prepontine cistern and the posterior cerebral arteries are sometimes visible as they pass around the brainstem. The choroid plexuses in the third and lateral ventricles are highlighted and the great vein of Galen, inferior sagittal and straight sinuses are enhanced.

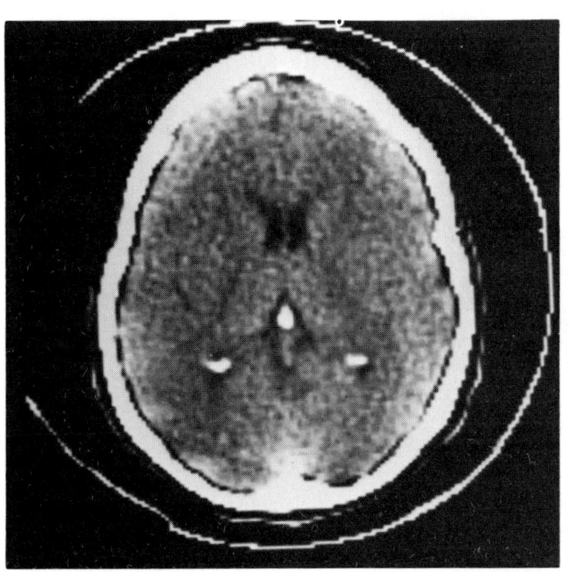

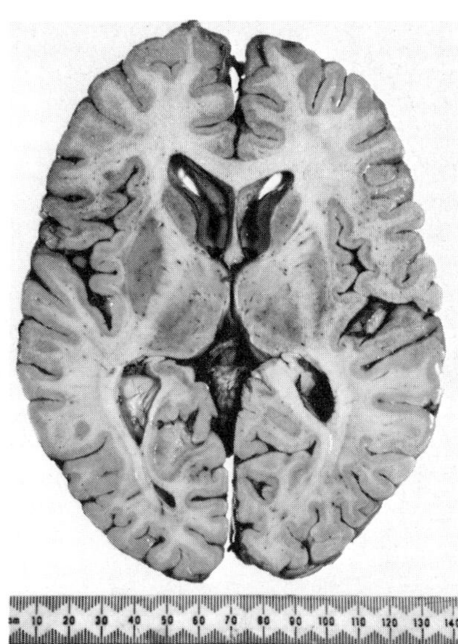

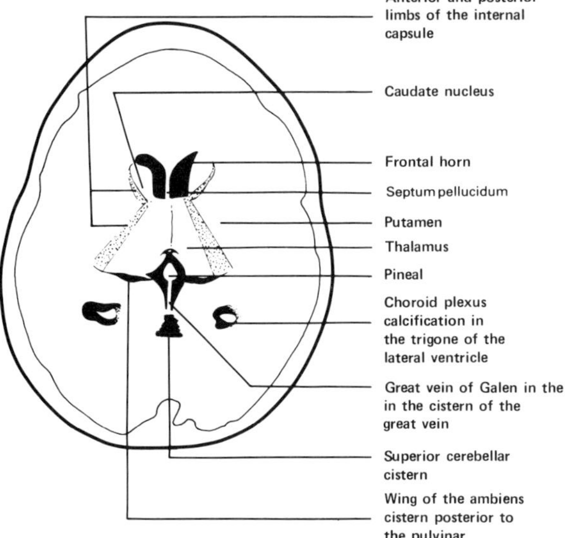

(d) **Fig. 7.25. continued**

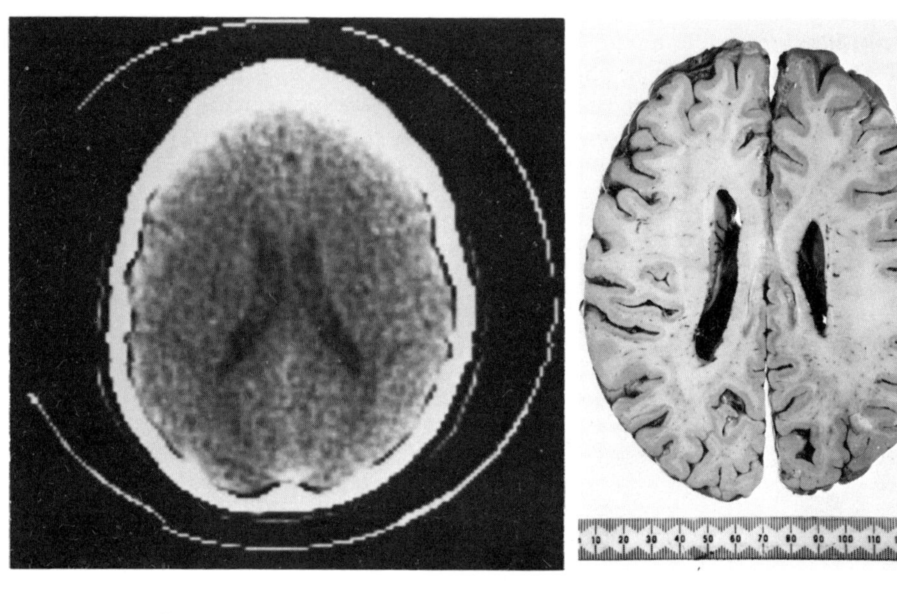

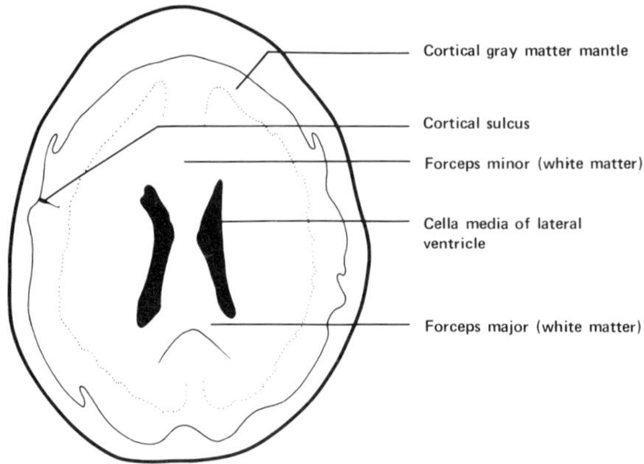

(e) **Fig. 7.25. continued**

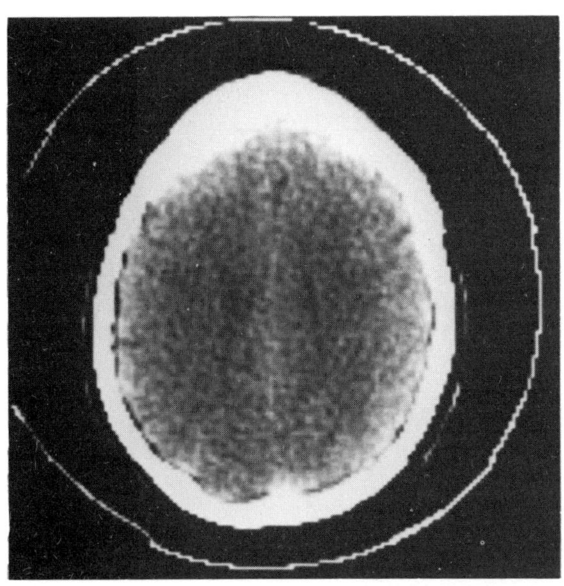

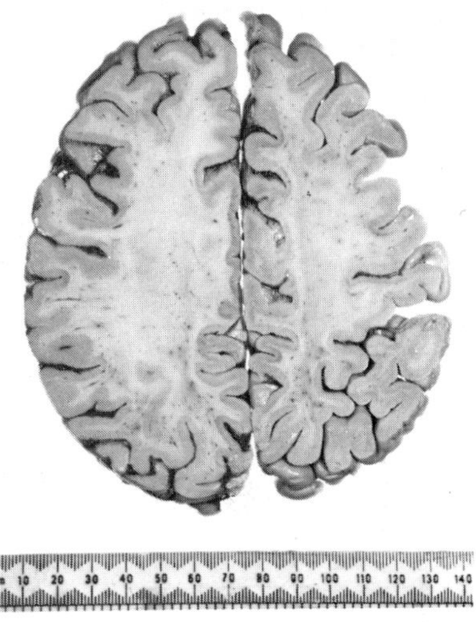

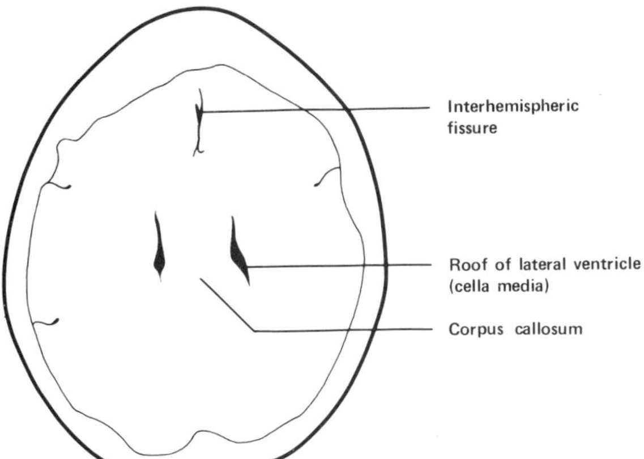

(f) **Fig. 7.25. continued**

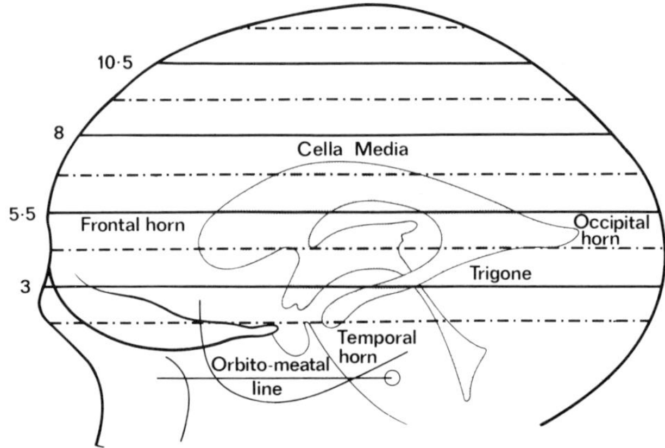

Fig. 7.26   Scan pairs are obtained at 3, 5.5, 8 and 10.5 cm above the orbitomeatal line thus providing a vertical series of eight tomograms.

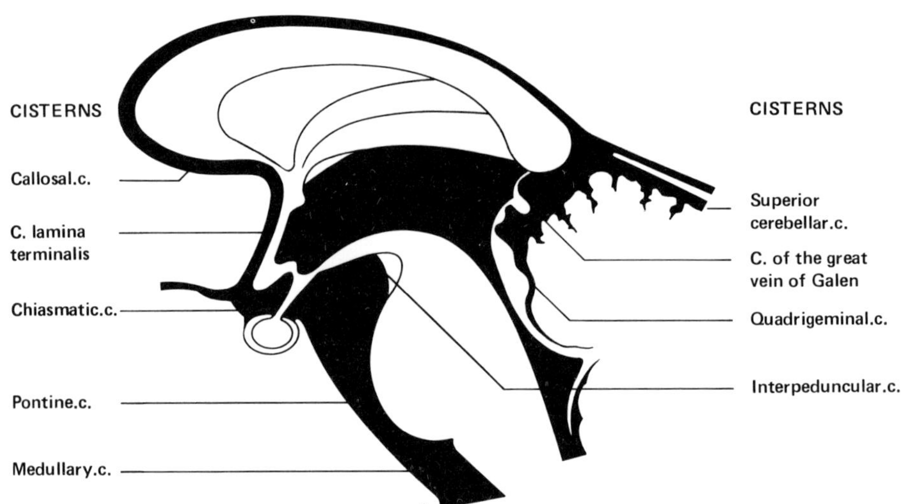

Fig. 7.27   Diagram of basal subarachnoid cisterns.

ABNORMAL SCANS

Cerebral atrophy

A diffuse loss of brain tissue leads to 'cerebral atrophy', an entity recognised by demonstrating enlargement of cortical sulci or dilatation of the ventricular system. These findings usually coexist but some patients have sulcal dilatation in isolation (cortical atrophy) while others show a non-obstructed dilated ventricular system with normal sulci (central atrophy or hydrocephalus ex vacuo). Cerebral atrophy is not a diagnosis, merely the visible end point of a spectrum of brain diseases and insults. Although a negative finding in the sense that no surgery is required, the recognition of cerebral atrophy is often helpful as it provides an explanation, albeit partial, for the patient's symptoms and signs.

Until the present decade pneumonecephalography was the only manner of demonstrating atrophic change in the brain during life. Because the procedure was unpleasant and there were attendant risks it was reserved for a minority of neurological patients who presented with rather specific problems. One category so investigated were those presenting with intellectual deterioration and unfortunately, for this reason, cerebral atrophy and dementia are now often equated.

As soon as computerised tomography was introduced it became clear that the method demonstrated cerebral atrophy. Comparative studies (Gawler et al, 1976) showed that computerised tomography and pneumoencephalography were equally reliable in this context. Moreover the computerised scan demonstrated the ventricular system, cortical sulci and subarachnoid space in an undisturbed condition so avoiding the distortions in ventricular size and sulcal appearances which were known to complicate pneumoencephalography. For this reason the computerised scan was particularly helpful in demonstrating either focal atrophy or generalised atrophy affecting various parts of the brain to a different degree.

For technical reasons it is not always possible to persuade air into the ventricular system at pneumoencephalography. When this occurs suspicions of pathological obstruction to the c.s.f. pathways are raised and formerly ventriculography would have been required to clarify this situation. Similarly cortical sulci are demonstrated at pneumoencephalography only when they fill with air and large sulci can be missed if filling is incomplete. Such diagnostic pitfalls are not relevant to orthodox computerised scanning for no contrast medium is needed to demonstrate these structures. By the same token however, the picture obtained is static and unlike pneumoencephalography there is no opportunity to observe the flow of contrast through the c.s.f. pathways.

The computerised scan appearances of cerebral atrophy include enlargement of the cortical sulci and it is important to obtain a vertex slice as the most prominent sulci may be apparent only at this level. Widening of the interhemispheric fissure and enlargement of the insula cisterns on each side are further indications of cerebral atrophy on computerised scans. The ventricular enlargement seen with cerebral atrophy usually has a rather different appearance than that which accompanies obstructive hydrocephalus, but further study is often required to make this distinction in patients who have ventricular dilatation alone.

Because there is no risk with computerised tomography it has allowed study of the cerebral anatomy in patients presenting with a wide range of neurological diseases including those such as migraine, where cerebral pathology is not anticipated. These studies have shown cerebral atrophy to be fairly commmon, particularly in older patients, and it is now clear that the finding does not necessarily indicate a dementing illness. Thus cerebral atrophy is a fairly common finding among those who present with epilepsy of late onset but psychometric evaluation in such patients is often normal. Claveria, Moseley & Stephenson (1977) have drawn attention to the poor correlation between mental function and the CAT scan appearances of cerebral atrophy. Thus intellectual function may be well preserved in patients who show fairly gross atrophy, while some patients with severe dementia have normal scans. Although it may be possible to show a broad correlation between the degree of ventricular dilatation and the level of intellectual impairment, it is important to underline that for an individual patient the demonstration of mild or moderate cerebral atrophy does not necessarily indicate a disease which will lead to progressive intellectual failure. When unexpected atrophic change is demonstrated by computerised scanning it is important that such patients have the benefit of metabolic screening tests to be sure that no potentially remediable underlying metabolic disease is reponsible for their problems. The demonstration of atrophy in patients with migraine supports the need to offer more enthusiastic control of individual attacks.

Hydrocephalus
Obstructive ventricular enlargement (Fig. 7.28) complicates a number of intracranial conditions and its recognition is often vital to their management. Before computerised tomography, ventriculography or pneumoencephalography was usually required to demonstrate a hydrocephalus although, rather less reliably, large ventricles could be shown on a carotid arteriogram. It was often difficult to plan the appropriate investigations in a patient who presented with symptoms and signs to suggest a posterior fossa tumour and commonly a number of separate procedures, each requiring an anaesthetic, were needed to define the tumour and assess the degree of hydrocephalus. In this context the computerised scan will not only demonstrate the tumour but also indicate the degree of hydrocephalus and whether an initial shunting procedure will be required before the tumour itself is dealt with. Similarly, patients with meningitis or subarachnoid haemorrhage can be screened without risk, so that a complicating hydrocephalus can be recognised and treated when necessary. Study of these patients has shown that hydrocephalus often develops shortly after a subarachnoid haemorrhage or during the acute phase of meningitis only to resolve later without treatment. Serial computerised scanning allows early recognition of the small minority of patients who do require a ventricular shunting procedure, either in the acute phase of a meningitic illness or after a subarachnoid haemorrhage when a chronic communicating hydrocephalus develops and produces clinical deterioration. Computerised tomography can be repeated without risk to the patient and it is therefore the ideal method of following patients whose hydrocephalus has been treated by a ventricular shunt. Such patients are at risk from a number of complications, for instance subdural haematoma, and the computerised scan will identify these as well as shunt failures with recurrent hydrocephalus. When lateral ventricular enlargement follows obstruction at the foramen of Munro it may be necessary to shunt both lateral ventricles independently. Previously it was difficult to assess the effects of this type of shunt but now the computerised scan can be used to give a clear picture of the ventricular anatomy so that failures of these complex shunts can be recognised promptly and corrected.

The orthodox computerised scan provides a static picture of the c.s.f. pathways and in some patients who show ventricular dilatation alone it is not possible to say whether this has an obstructive or an atrophic basis. Similarly when the drainage of the entire ventricular system is obstructed it may not be possible to identify the level of obstruction from the scan. Here ventriculography or pneumoencephalography can be of value in demonstrating obstruction, indicating its site and sometimes its nature; for example atresia of the exit foraminae of the fourth ventricle. Patients with normal pressure or communicating hydrocephalus present a particular problem in diagnosis and the pathophysiology of this entity remains obscure. Typical patients present with intellectual deterioration, gait disturbance and incontinence, and show a dilated

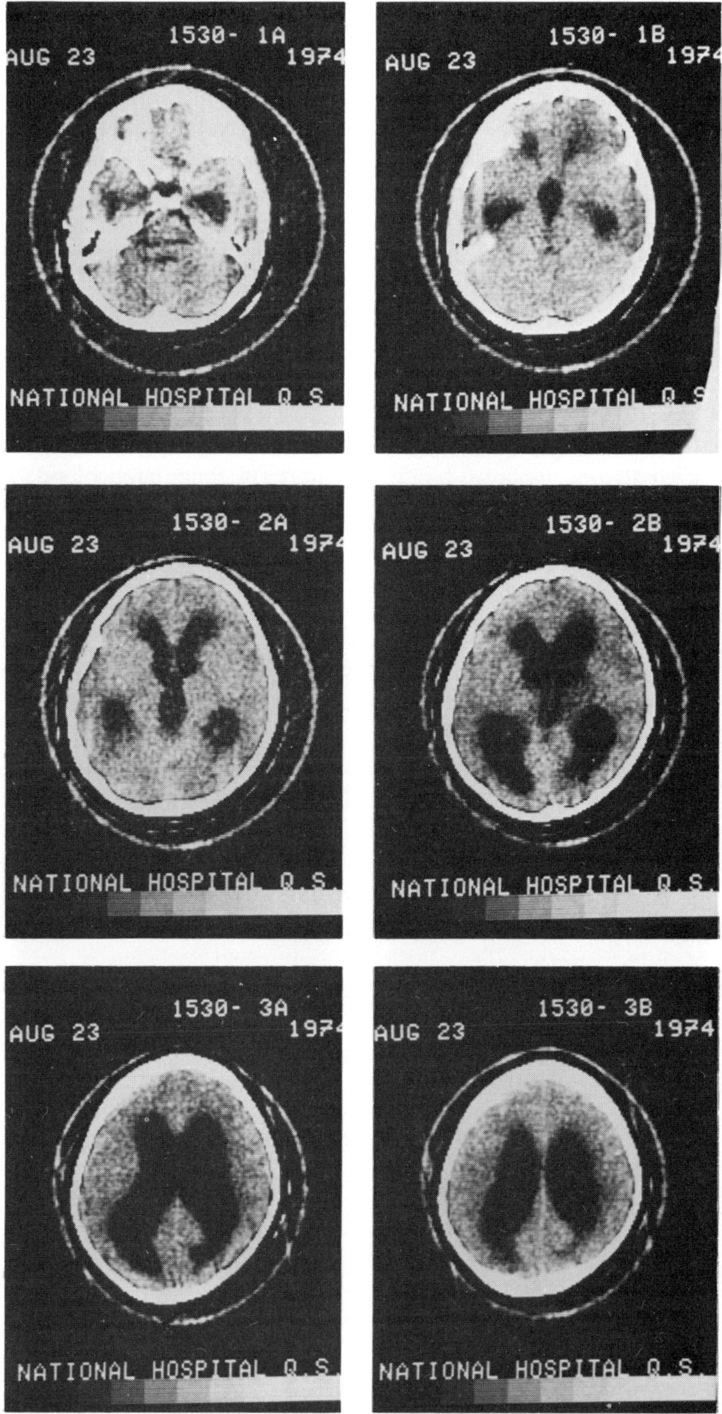

Fig. 7.28 Obstructive hydrocephalus involving the third and lateral ventricles caused by aqueduct stenosis.

ventricular system which communicates with the lumbar subarachnoid space at a
normal pressure. Some patients have obstruction to the flow of c.s.f. through the
tentorium while others are thought to have either convexity or absorption block.
Pneumoencephalography may demonstrate obstruction at the tentorium but in many
patients the study indicates only what has been apparent on the scan, namely a dilated
ventricular system. In these patients isotope cisternography has been used in an
attempt to demonstrate the obstruction of c.s.f. flow in the hope that patients who
would benefit from shunting could be identified. Along the same lines Greitz &
Hindmarsh (1974) developed a technique of using the computerised scan to follow the
flow of a water soluble contrast medium (Metrizamide) through the subarachnoid
pathways. They found this technique useful for investigating c.s.f. dynamics and in
the distinction between communicating hydrocephalus and cerebral atrophy.

Cerebrovascular disease

Computerised tomography provides invaluable diagnostic information among patients
who present with stroke. Because blood, particularly coagulated blood, is of greater
density than normal brain cerebral haemorrhage (Fig. 7.29) can be distinguished from
infarction or oedema which both reduce tissue density. The site distribution,

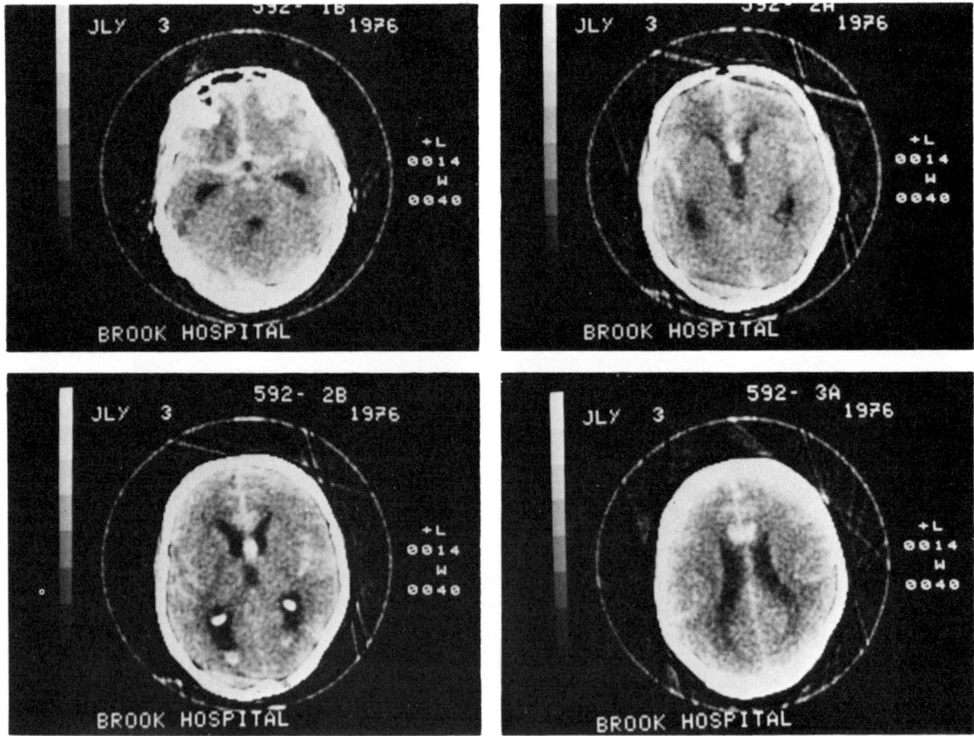

Fig. 7.29   Subarachnoid haemorrhage. Haematoma is present in the septum pellucidum and the anterior
aspect of the corpus callosum, which suggests bleeding from an anterior communicating artery aneurysm.
Blood is visible in the interhemispheric fissure anteriorly, the lateral fissures and insula cisterns. A little
blood has entered the ventricular system and has gravitated to occupy the occipital horns of the lateral
ventricles.

dimension and ventricular extension of cerebral haematomata can be defined with an accuracy not possible from other investigations. This information may prove life-saving, for it serves to identify those patients who might benefit from urgent surgical evacuation of their haematoma. Previously, the poor condition of many of these patients precluded contrast investigation and surgical management would not have been contemplated. For practical purposes, computerised tomography detects all macroscopic cerebral haematomata and because the increase in density that allows their recognition is apparent from the outset it is always possible to distinguish them from cerebral infarction in a patient who presents with stroke. The increase in density caused by a haematoma declines slowly and depending on the initial size of the lesion, disappears in one to four weeks. Large haematomata leave long term evidence of their presence; a cystic low density zone at the haematoma site, ipsilateral sulcal or ventricular enlargement and displacement of the ventricles to the side of the lesion. Small haematomata can resolve without trace.

Cerebral oedema and infarction both reduce tissue density. In those presenting with stroke the computerised scan may be normal during the first 24 to 48 hours and thereafter it may be possible to visualise the morphological changes of ischaemic necrosis (Fig. 7.30). It is estimated that the scan demonstrates 50–85 per cent of clinically suspected infarcts and the yield does depend on the timing of the scan. Because haemorrhages can always be recognised a diagnosis of infarction may be made by implication in those presenting with stroke, even though the computerised scan appears normal. The typical computerised scan appearances of infarction include progressive reduction in tissue density so that the lesion becomes more clearly defined and sharper at its periphery. Small low density lesions may disappear with time and it may not be possible to say whether this represents clearing of oedema or reabsorption of infarcted brain. In some patients it is possible to suggest the latter explanation since concomitant ventricular dilatation and sulcal enlargement develop. Mature infarcts usually remain as well defined areas of reduced density and sometimes a post-infarction cyst is apparent. These cysts may be distinct from or communicate with the ventricular system.

Infarcts in the brainstem are seldom demonstrated but at times there is associated cerebellar infarction which can be seen. Secondary haemorrhage into areas of infarction is easily detected and should serve as a contra-indication to anticoagulation when this is considered therapeutically.

A computerised scan is a helpful initial investigation among those who present with subarachnoid bleeding. The scan often shows localised intracerebral or subarachnoid haematomata whose position and distribution may indicate the source of bleeding (Fig. 7.29). Thus, rather characteristic haematoma patterns follow rupture of aneurysms at typical sites. Extensive intracerebral bleeding is simultaneously recognised and this may alter the management of an individual case either calling for urgent surgery to evacuate the haematoma or delaying angiography until there has been spontaneous improvement. After subarachnoid bleeding arterial spasm often leads to cerebral oedema and infarction; complications which can be recognised by scanning. Hydrocephalus often develops in the acute stage and although it seldom requires treatment in its own right follow-up scanning in the months after a subarachnoid haemorrhage will identify those patients who are likely to develop neurological damage as a consequence of chronic communicating hydrocephalus.

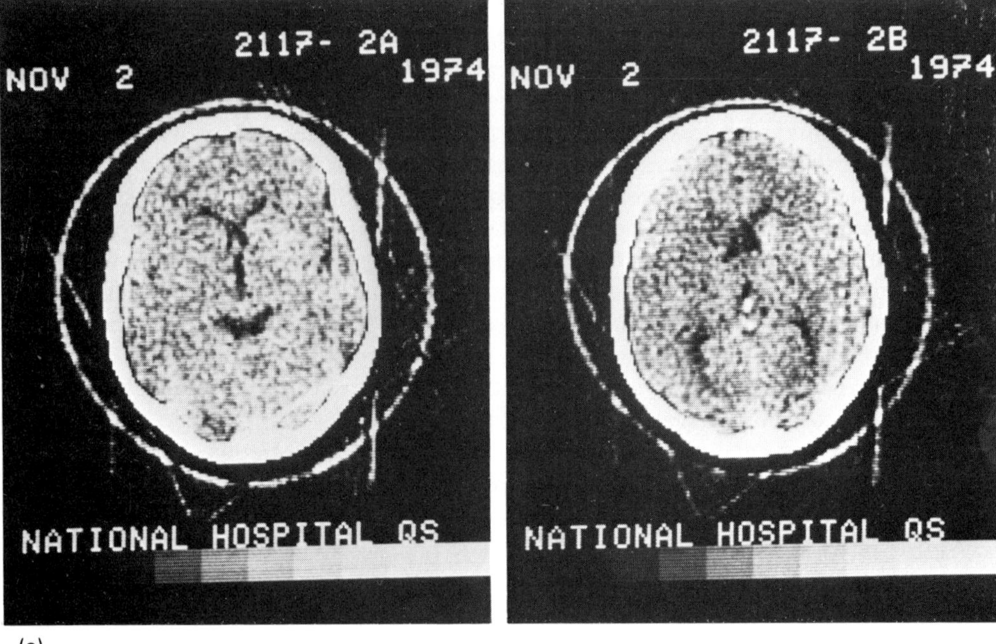

(a)

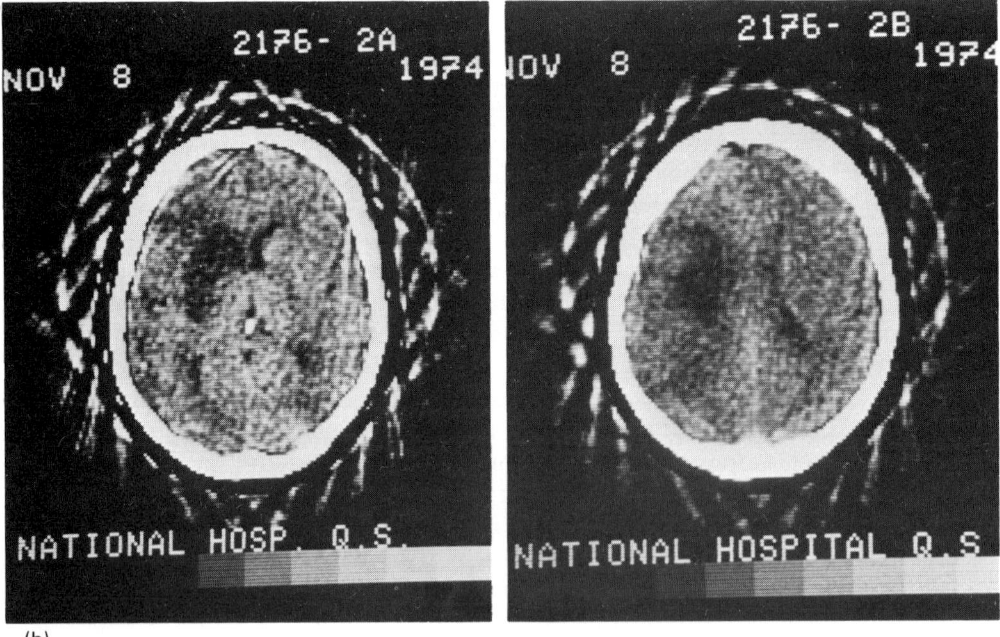

(b)

Fig. 7.30 (a) Scans obtained 24 hours after the onset of right hemiparesis with aphasia. No definite abnormality is visible although the frontal horn of the left lateral ventricle may be attenuated by local cerebral swelling.
(b) Scan of the same patient six days later showing an extensive left hemisphere infarct which involves the left caudate and lentiform nuclei together with the internal capsule and corona radiata.

After a subarachnoid haemorrhage, the patient may deteriorate suddenly either spontaneously, after angiography or after surgery. Under such circumstances a computerised scan provides a rapid, safe method of detecting rebleeding, operative haematoma, oedema or infarction and the appropriate treatment can be rapidly instituted; the patient is not exposed to further invasive investigations requiring anaesthetics.

The computerised scan may be helpful in those who present with transient ischaemic attacks for although the examination is usually negative it will detect the occasional patient who has an underlying tumour, for instance a meningioma. Some patients who present with transient neurological episodes do have multiple low density lesions and this obvious structural damage may increase the enthusiasm for invasive investigation seeking a surgically remediable cause for their recurrent attacks.

The computerised scan must be seen as the investigation of first choice in patients who present with strokes. Unfortunately strokes are common and access to computerised scanning facilities is limited so only a minority of patients benefit from this diagnostic advance. This is unfortunate because, contrary to popular misconception, our clinical diagnostic abilities in patients presenting with stroke are far from good. Thus ten to fifteen per cent of patients harbour intracranial tumours and our ability to distinguish cerebral haemorrhage from infarction is little better than chance. Although accurate diagnosis may not alter the management of the majority of stroke patients, the outlook of some can be improved by accurate diagnosis and appropriate surgical treatment. Angiography may be justified in others to detect lesions which may cause recurrent problems.

Among those with cerebrovascular disease angiography is still required to display the blood vessels themselves. This is true not only for those who present with subarachnoid haemorrhage where the investigation is undertaken to detect a source of bleeding, like an aneurysm or a vascular malformation, but also among certain patients who present with ischaemic episodes. In patients with aneurysmal subarachnoid haemorrhage ten per cent will have multiple aneurysms and the scan can be very helpful since the pattern of haematoma may indicate which aneurysm has bled and requires surgical treatment. In those with either recovered strokes or transient ischaemic episodes the computerised scan may indicate the arterial territory involved and so point to the vessel requiring angiographic study. Alternatively multiple lesions may implicate the heart or aorta as a source of embolic cerebral damage. Equally, multiple lesions may reflect small vessel disease and might serve as a contraindication to angiography among patients with hypertension or diabetes.

Craniocerebral trauma

The management of serious head injuries has been revolutionised by computerised scanning because the technique permits rapid diagnosis of conditions requiring surgical management. In the majority of patients it is possible to identify extracerebral or intracerebral haematomata and distinguish them from either cerebral oedema or contusion.

The density of subdural and extradural clots depends upon their physical characteristics; the degree of coagulation, clot lysis and the volume of fluid which they attract. The acute extradural haematoma, complicating a recent head injury is almost always visible as a high density lesion immediately subjacent to the skull. It presents a convex surface toward the underlying brain. Subdural haematomata may complicate a recent head injury but equally, particularly in older patients, they appear either spontaneously or some while after what may have been a fairly mild head injury. The acute subdural haematoma generally has a high density or one which is similar to the underlying brain; rarely it is less dense. The chronic subdural haematoma usually has a density similar to or less than the underlying brain. Subdural fluid collections have a flat or concave inner aspect overlying the hemisphere and cortical sulci are usually lost beneath the lesion (Fig. 7.31). The isodense subdural haematoma may lead to

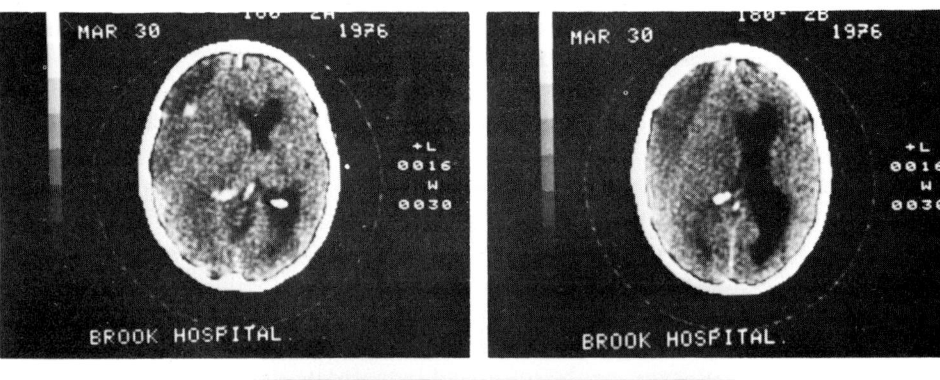

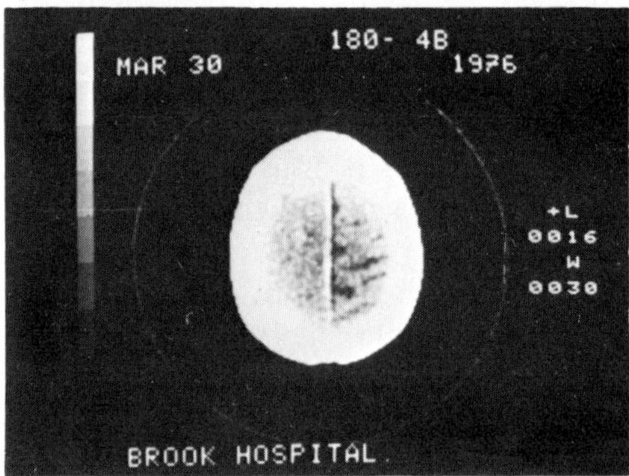

Fig. 7.31   Left sided chronic hypodense subdural haematoma. A tiny area of increased density over the surface of the hemisphere suggests recent fresh bleeding. The cortical sulci have been obliterated on the side of the lesion. Considerable hydrocephalus has developed and involves especially the right lateral ventricle.

difficulties in diagnosis since it cannot be seen in its own right, and this diagnosis should be suspected when the scan of a head injured, unconscious patient shows marked displacement of midline structures without an obvious lesion in the hemisphere on the appropriate side. When midline shift is associated with relatively unimpressive contusion it should be remembered that an isodense subdural haematoma may also be present, and under these circumstances it may be prudent to make exploratory burr holes on the affected side. Bilateral isodense subdural haematomas may lead to serious diagnostic errors since their balanced mass effect may lead to a midline ventricular system. When the ventricles are small but undisplaced it may not be possible to distinguish bilateral isodense subdural haematomata from bilateral cerebral swelling caused by oedema or heightened blood flow.

Cerebral contusion may produce single or multiple areas of reduced density and sometimes scattered small areas of high density imply additional patchy haemorrhage. These appearances are easy to distinguish from a well circumscribed intracerebral haematoma which might require surgical evacuation. In general, patients with contusions are best treated conservatively unless there is an associated extracerebral collection of blood.

Although widespread reduction in density suggesting cerebral oedema is seen in some cases after serious head injury others show obliteration of the ventricular system without other apparent change on the scan. Either cerebral oedema or an increase in cerebral blood volume have been suggested to explain these findings. With time, such patients may show increasing cerebral atrophy indicating widespread cerebral damage even though no focal abnormality has been visible. Serious cerebral damage may be present with a normal computerised scan, and it is thought that either brain stem injury or widespread axonal shearing is responsible for the fatal outcome in some of these cases.

In the majority of head injury patients a scan will identify those who require urgent evacuation of extracerebral or intracerebral haematomata, and only rarely is further investigation necessary before deciding on surgical management. When extensive contusion or widespread cerebral swelling is demonstrated by the scan further potentially harmful investigations can be avoided, and the patients can be treated medically with hyperventilation, Mannitol and dexamethasone. Communicating hydrocephalus may complicate serious head injury and this complication can be detected by serial scanning in appropriate patients.

Intracranial tumours
Most intracranial tumours are recognised by computerised scanning as areas of abnormal tissue density often with space-occupying effect, and for this reason their site, size and shape is generally shown with great accuracy (Fig. 7.32). The tissue density of many tumours can be increased by an intravenous injection of an iodine containing contrast medium and this may lead to better definition of a tumour, or infrequently, the appearance of a neoplasm which was not visible on the unenhanced scan. Enhancement can reflect iodine circulating in tumour blood vessels or concentration of iodine by the tumour consequent upon a breakdown in the blood-brain barrier. Enhancement often displays details of tumour morphology which would not be seen using the conventional neuro-radiological methods. Thus tumour capsules or nodules are particularly well shown and necrotic and cystic change can be defined. Calcification becomes visible long before it would be apparent on a conventional X-ray film. Cerebral oedema develops in the presence of many cerebral tumours and the reduction in tissue density which is causes is apparent on computerised scans. Oedema often appears to follow nerve fibre pathways so highlighting the tissue density differences between grey and white matter. Thus the internal and external capsules may become strikingly clear and undulating oedema may be seen extending into the cerebral convolutions. At times it can be difficult to distinguish low density tumour tissue from surrounding oedema particularly when contrast enhancement does not alter the density of the tumour itself. Under these

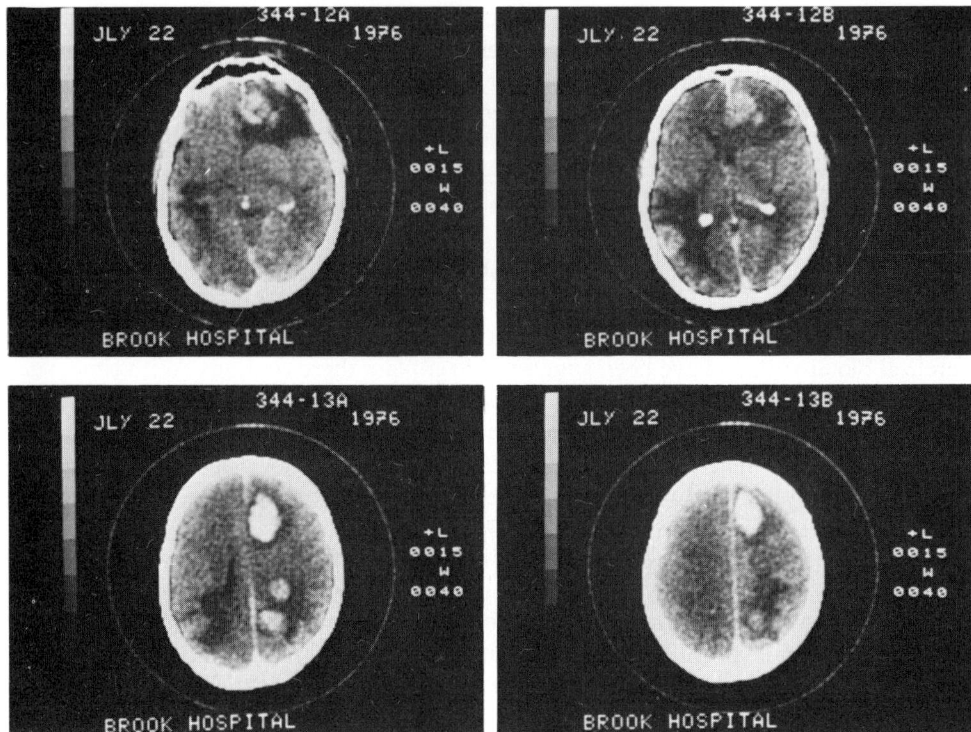

Fig. 7.32   Multiple cerebral metastases each producing considerable surrounding oedema.

circumstances further investigation for example, isotope scintigraphy or angiography, may be required in the hope of making this distinction.

Obstruction to the c.s.f. pathways caused by a tumour is easily seen. Hydrocephalus is often thought to complicate only tumours originating in the ventricular system or those developing in the posterior fossa where the aqueduct and the fourth ventricle become obstructed. In addition, however, hydrocephalus is often seen with large supratentorial tumours for they cause sufficient midline displacement to distort and obstruct the third ventricle. Under such circumstances the lateral ventricle on the side opposite the tumour may become strikingly dilated and contribute to the elevation of intracranial pressure.

The site, density and morphological characteristics of a tumour often allow its nature to be predicted. A meningioma, on the unenhanced scan, is usually of slightly higher density than surrounding brain. Calcification is occasionally apparent but cystic change is uncommon. Associated cerebral oedema may be inapparent or massive but the majority of tumours of this type show only a modest rim of reduced density. Following the intravenous injection of contrast there is generally marked homogenous enhancement to identify a clearly marginated mass which is often spherical. As meningiomata have a tendency to arise at certain sites tumour position may be important in diagnosis and occasionally they produce local changes in the bone, for example hyperostosis or erosion, which can be seen on the scan. These tumours are seldom missed on adequate enhanced computerised scans and the false negative results usually relate either to very small tumours, a centimetre or less in diameter, or those which are obscured by their close application to bone, for example in the supra and parasellar regions.

The appearance of a glioma depends upon its grade. Grade I tumours are most often of uniformly reduced density and they fail to enhance after contrast administration. More malignant tumours may show increased, decreased or mixed alterations in density and contrast enhancement is usual. Grade III and IV tumours are commonly necrotic or cystic centrally and show a ring-like capsule which enhances; tumour nodules may be visible centrally and odema is usually present at the periphery. Although a ring-like appearance is fairly typical of malignant gliomata it is also seen with metastases and cerebral abscesses. Irregular or multilocular cystic lesions are more often indicative of gliomata than metastases.

Metastases may be of greater, lesser or the same density as surrounding brain and even in a single patient lesions of different density may occur. Contrast enhancement is important here since it may define lesions not apparent on the unenhanced scan. Cystic lesions with ring-like enhancement are common and tumours may show considerable surrounding oedema.

Cerebral vascular malformations usually produce a mixture of high and low density and enhancement follows contrast administration. About one quarter of patients with angiomata have normal unenhanced scans and Terbrugge et al (1977) stress the need for contrast administration in patients where an angioma may be responsible for the clinical picture. Sometimes a curvilinear pattern is apparent after enhancement and this is highly suggestive of an angioma. Angiography is still required, however, to demonstrate the anatomy of lesions and identify the feeding vessels.

The larger acoustic nerve tumours, over two centimetres in diameter, should be visible on contrast enhanced scans of the posterior fossa. In the patients reported by Robins & Marshall (1978) only 15 per cent of acoustic tumours were visible on an unenhanced scan, while 60 per cent were seen after contrast administration, emphasising the need for iodine injection in these patients.

The larger, supra- and parasellar extensions of pituitary tumours are seen on computerised scans and here both contrast enhancement and very careful radiological technique are needed to obtain the best results. Because small tumours close to the skull floor are easily missed, a number of methods have been developed to improve diagnosis. Thin tomograms with variable angulation allow some tumours to be projected clear of the skull floor which obscures them and coronal scans can be of value. Further resolution may be obtained by positive contrast when computerised scans are obtained after the intrathecal administration of water soluble iodine (Metrizamide) (Drayer et al, 1977).

Computerised tomography is now the method of first choice for investigating all patients suspected of an intracranial mass lesion. The technique detects supra- and infratentorial tumours with a reliability which equals or exceeds the conventional neuro-radiological contrast procedures. Increasingly sensitive scans, careful technique and contrast enhancement have led to very low false positive and false negative rates. For many patients with intracranial tumours a computerised scan is the only preoperative investigation required. When the scan has clearly demonstrated a tumour the value of additional orthodox neuro-radiological contrast procedures is difficult to assess, and in practice depends upon the habits of the neurologist or neurosurgeon concerned. Although such tests may provide further information about a tumour, experience suggests they seldom alter the patient's management. On the other hand, many neurosurgeons prefer to obtain detailed information about the relationships of a tumour to blood vessels before craniotomy and they favour angiograms, particularly in patients with meningiomata when total excision is planned. Traditional contrast procedures are still required in some tumour suspects who have negative computerised scans. Thus either pneumoencephalography or positive contrast cisternography may be needed to demonstrate small acoustic or perisellar tumours, and medullary tumours may need these techniques or vertebral angiography to display them. Angiomata and vascular tumours, for example haemangioblastomata, may also require angiography for diagnosis.

Intracranial infection and cerebral inflammatory disease

Intracranial abscesses are visible on computerised scans as areas of abnormal density generally with space-occupying effect. The acute pyogenic abscess generally produces an extensive zone of reduced density on the unenhanced scan and following contrast injection ring-like enhancement generally delineates a vascular capsule. Abscesses are often multiloculate, and it is possible to distinguish their necrotic or pus-filled cores from surrounding cerebral oedema. In the acute situation a capsule is seldom clear before contrast is given but subacute and chronic abscess capsules may be apparent on the unenhanced scan. Homogenous as opposed to ring-like enhancement may be seen in chronic abscesses and tuberculomata. It must be stressed that abscess appearances may be indistinguishable from those of malignant gliomata and this remains an argument in favour of obtaining a tissue diagnosis in patients who are thought to have a glioma on the basis of the clinical picture and computerised scan. When the treatment of the cerebral abscess was monitored by conventional radiological methods it was traditional to instil Steripake into the evacuated capsule at the time of drainage so that abscess size could be measured on a skull X-ray. Steripake produces computerised scan artefacts and it is no longer desirable to use this material if computerised scanning is available to monitor progress. Serial scans in patients with multiple abscesses show that medical treatment alone can result in the resolution of quite sizeable lesions (Fig. 7.33). The same is true of tuberculomata.

Patients with encephalitis may have normal scans or show zones of low density. The appearances in herpes simplex encephalitis may be dramatic with a low density space occupying lesion occupying one temporal lobe. Patchy increases in density, probably due to bleeding, may be seen within such lesions. Contrast administration often produces no change although sometimes there is a little patchy enhancement visible. Rarely spherical, low density lesions occur in encephalitis and there is peripheral ring-like enhancement after contrast administration. Although such lesions may have little space occupying effect they are easily mistaken for metastases. Following encephalitis, particularly herpes encephalitis, there may be evidence of long-standing cerebral damage with the development of either cerebral atrophy or areas of permanently reduced density. Conversely, mild encephalitis may leave no clinical or radiological sequelae.

Acute pyogenic and viral meningitides are usually associated with a normal computerised scan. Hydrocephalus complicates some pyogenic infections, and although it

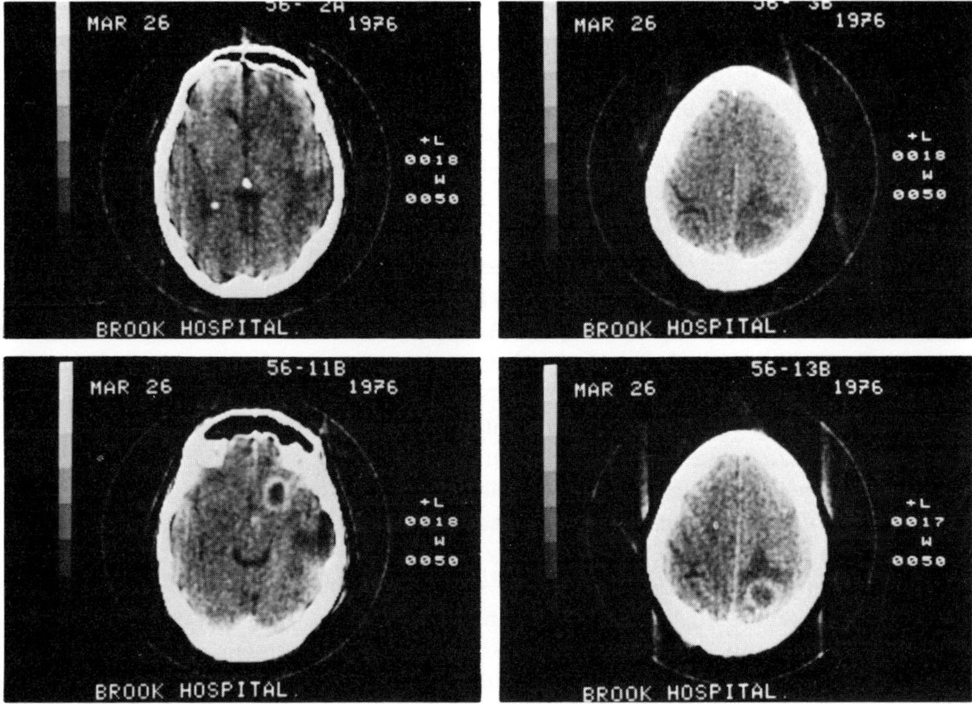

Fig. 7.33 Right frontal and parietal abscesses which developed during a septicaemic illness.
(a) The unenhanced scan shows areas of reduced density in the right hemisphere.
(b) Following intravenous injection of contrast the abscess capsules have been highlighted. The patient was treated conservatively with antibiotics and the scan returned to normal.

usually resolves with treatment serial scanning is sometimes required to detect those who develop communicating hydrocephalus. Meningeal enhancement in the basal regions has been described in patients with tuberculous meningitis, and a similar appearance may be seen in those with malignant meningeal infiltration.

The majority of patients with multiple sclerosis have normal computerised scans or examinations which reveal only cerebral atrophy. At times however areas of reduced attentuation are visible particularly in the periventricular white matter There is usually no change in these lesions after contrast administration. More impressive changes accompany white matter diseases of childhood, and the computerised scan in those with leucodystrophies show a striking diffuse reduction in white matter density, together with progressive cerebral atrophy. No enhancement occurs after contrast administration. Similar widespread changes have been described with disseminated necrotising leucoencephalopathy, postvaccinial encephalomeylitis, malignant hypertension and polycythaemia (Kendall, Clavarier & Quiroga, 1977).

CONCLUSION

A computerised tomogram should not be thought of in quite the same way as a conventional radiograph for it represents a mathematical reconstruction of anatomy in terms of X-ray absorption. Analysis of the pictures produced from phantoms and clinicopathological studies have shown that the reconstruction is highly reliable. It is, however, possible for areas to appear abnormal on the computed scan not because pathological tissue is present but because the reconstruction is in error. Aberrations of this type may arise if the patient moves during the examination, when certain faults develop in the apparatus and when a sequence of large density differences (as occurs with skull base tomograms) must be reconstructed. Fortunately most artefacts are easily recognised and with experience only a few give rise to serious diagnostic difficulties.

The computerised scan provices a brief, harmless and painfree means of studying the human brain under physiological conditions. A wide spectrum of intracranial diseases can be detected and the traditional neurological tests can often be avoided. This is an advantage not only for the patient, who avoids an anaesthetic and the risk of a conventional procedure, but there is also a measurable saving in medical time and hospital beds. The EMI scan often provides the most accurate information about the size and shape of a lesion, its local complications such as haemorrhage or oedema, and its more distant effects such as hydrocephalus or ventricular distortion. The findings often allow a specific histological diagnosis to be suggested. On the other hand, a normal EMI scan does not exclude intracranial pathology and when the clinical indications are present further studies using traditional techniques may be needed. In particular angiography remains the only means of identifying small aneurysms, defining the vascular anatomy in relation to aneurysms, angiomata or tumours. Pneumoencephalography may still be needed in the assessment of patients with hydrocephalus or those in whom small skull floor tumours are suspected.

Computerised scanning has revolutionised the diagnostic sequence traditionally used for neurological and neurosurgical patients: for the most part this sequence has been abbreviated and patients' management simplified. Further, it is to be hoped that computerised tomography will increase our understanding of neurological disease, and lead to therapeutic, as well as diagnostic advance.

REFERENCES

Claveria L E, Moseley I F, Stevenson J F 1977 The clinical significance of 'cerebral atrophy' as shown by CAT. In: Du Boulay G H, Moseley I F (eds) Computerised axial tomography in clinical practice. Springer Verlag, New York, p 213–216

Dandy W E 1918 Ventriculography following the injection of air into the cerebral ventricles. Annals of Surgery 68: 5

Drayer B P, Rosenbaum A E, Kennerdell J S, Robinson A G, Bank N O, Deeb Z L 1977 Computed tomographic diagnosis of supra-sellar masses by intrathecal enhancement. Radiology 123: 339

Gawler J, Du Boulay G H, Bull J W D, Marshall J 1976 Computerised tomography. A comparison with pneumoencephalography and ventriculography. Journal Neurology, Neurosurgery and Psychiatry 39: 203

Hounsfield G N 1973 Computerised transverse avial scanning (tomography). British Journal of Radiology 46: 1016

Kendall B E, Claveria L E, Quiroga W 1977 CAT in leukodystrophy and neuronal degeneration. In: Du Boulay G H, Moseley I F (eds.) Computerised axial tomography in clinical practice. Springer Verlag, New York, p 191–202

Luckett W H 1913 Air in the ventricles of the brain following fracture of the skull. Report of a case. Surgery Gynaecology Obstetrics 17: 237

Moniz E 1927 L'encephalographie arterelle, son importance dans la localisation des tumeurs cerebrales. Revue neurologie 2: 72

Moore G E (1948) Use of radioactive diiodofluorescein in the diagnosis and localisation of brain tumours. Science 107: 569

Robbins B, Marshall W H 1978 Computed tomography of acoustic neurinoma. Radiology 128: 367

Therbrugge K, Scoffi G, Ethler R, Melancon D, Tchang S, Milner C 1977 Computed tomography in arteriovenous malformations. Radiology 122: 703

8.1 Endoscopy: upper gastrointestinal endoscopy

Peter B. Cotton

The barium meal X-ray examination has dominated upper gastrointestinal tract diagnosis for more than 80 years. However the inherent fallibility of indirect radiographic information and the wish to have biopsy material for a histological diagnosis have together stimulated attempts to provide direct access to the oesophagus, stomach and duodenum. Rigid open tube oesophagoscopy, and the first attempts at gastroscopy, predated Roentgen. Semiflexible lens gastroscopes were introduced in the 1930s and 1940s and allowed a few experts to provide good diagnostic information, but these instruments never entered routine practice. The examinations were poorly tolerated, and even the experts had substantial blind areas. In the 1950s, the Japanese introduced the gastro-camera — a small camera which was swallowed by the patient but remained under mechanical control through a connecting shaft. About 20 photographs were taken blindly in different camera and patient positions, often providing a complete photographic survey of the stomach. The examinations were well tolerated and could be performed by relatively untrained staff, whose results could be monitored and reported by expert review of the photographs. The gastro-camera made an enormous impact in Japan, with its high incidence of gastric cancer, and is still used in mass screening programmes; it has not been popular elsewhere.

Gastrointestinal diagnosis has undergone a major revolution in the last 10 years as a result of the introduction of flexible fibreoptic instruments. While the principle of fibreoptic light transmission was first patented and developed in Britain (Baird, 1928; Hopkins & Kapany, 1954) the development of clinical instrumentation has resulted from the technical ingenuity of American and Japanese engineers.

Oesophagogastroduodenoscopy and colonoscopy are now routine procedures; (Cotton & Williams, 1980); instruments passed through the mouth can be guided directly into the biliary and pancreatic ducts. Macroscopic examination is routinely complemented by target biopsy and cytology, and fibrescopes are increasingly used as therapeutic tools — for the management of benign and malignant strictures, the removal of polyps, foreign bodies and gallstones, and for the application of haemostatic techniques in acute bleeding.

These rapid developments have produced their own problems. The precise indications for diagnostic and therapeutic procedures remains controversial. Standards vary widely, and training programmes are virtually non-existent.

PRINCIPLES OF FIBREOPTICS

Modern endoscopes are flexible because the image is carried by glass bundles, not by a series of lenses. Viewing bundles are 2–4 mm in diameter, and consist of many thousands of fine glass fibres. Light entering the face of each fibre is transmitted by multiple internal reflections (Fig. 8.1). An image is transmitted as a series of dots, rather like a newspaper photograph. Its quality depends upon the spatial orientation of the individual fibres being the same at both ends of the bundle. Each fibre is clad with glass of a lower optical density to prevent leakage of light; this cladding does not transmit light and is responsible for the fine mesh which is frequently apparent in a fibreoptic image. For these reasons, the quality of a fibreoptic image — although excellent — can never equal that obtained with a rigid lens system.

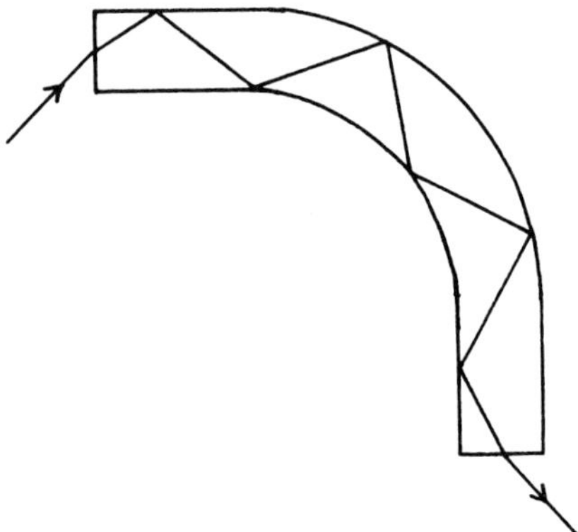

Fig. 8.1   Illustrating total internal reflection and light transmission through a glass fibre.

No view is obtained unless the organ is illuminated. Some early fibrescopes had bulbs in the tip; now light is transmitted from an external source through additional fibre bundles. Since they are not intended to transmit an image, the fibres of a light bundle are randomly arranged.

Instruments

Instruments for upper gastrointestinal endoscopy have a working length of about 1 metre, and an outside diameter of 9–13 mm. The distal tip can be deflected up to 200° by proximal manual controls (Fig. 8.2). As well as the image bundle, the shaft contains a second fibre bundle transmitting brilliant illumination from an outside source. There is also an operating (biopsy) channel (2–3 mm in diameter) for the passage of flexible forceps, cytology brushes and therapeutic devices. Air insufflation, water cleaning jets and suction are under direct finger tip control. All instruments are designed for photography with a proximal camera, and for use with teaching side arms.

Ranges of instruments are now available from many manufacturers. The only fundamental difference concerns the design of the distal tip — whether the lens faces forward or laterally. A forward viewing instrument is best for the oesophagus, and can be passed on through the stomach and into the duodenum. In the absence of a single term to describe the 'dyspeptic area' the examination of oesophagogastroduodenoscopy has been called panendoscopy, or OGD.

Until recently, the maximum deflection of the tip of the instrument was limited to 150°; it was then difficult to ensure a complete survey of the stomach and duodenum,

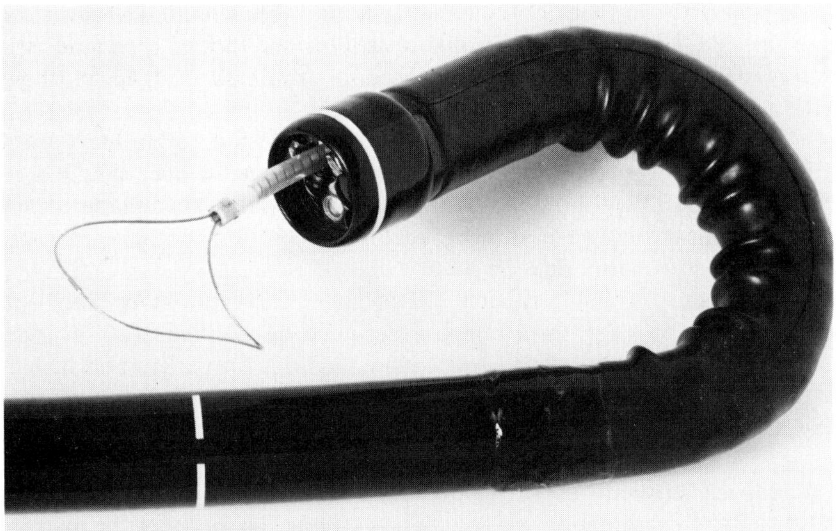

Fig. 8.2 Tip of a modern forward viewing oesophagogastroduodenoscope, showing 200° manoeuvrability, and a diathermy snare loop protruding from the biopsy channel.

and beginners had some relatively blind areas. Greater experience and newer instruments with 200° tip deflection have considerably reduced this potential problem; the experienced observer will expect to achieve a complete OGD in more than 95 per cent of patients. However there are still areas in which a side viewing endoscope may give more direct views (and more accurate biopsy sampling), particularly in patients with gastric or duodenal deformity due to scarring or previous surgery (Fig. 8.3). A side viewing instrument is also necessary for cannulation of the papilla of Vater. Compromise instruments have been designed to provide both

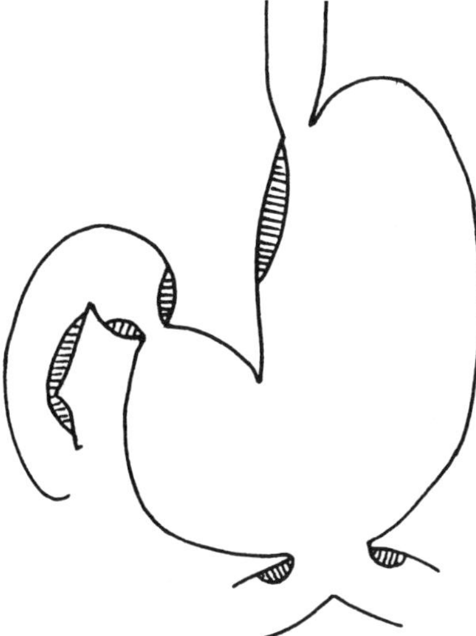

Fig. 8.3 Areas in which the beginner may find difficulty in obtaining a complete view with a forward viewing endoscope.

forward and lateral vision (with oblique facing or movable lenses). However a single all purpose upper GI instrument is probably an illusion. Indeed the trend is in the reverse direction, with a range of specialised instruments designed for specific purposes (e.g. children and therapeutic procedures).

Pending a major breakthrough in fibreoptic or television technology, the basic shape of instrumentation has now been established. There will be detailed refinements in the future, and we can hope for increasing durability and standardization of ancillary equipment—but we now have adequate tools for complete macroscopic examination and tissue sampling.

Instruments alone are not sufficient. Gastrointestinal endoscopy can only be performed reliably and safely in a purpose designed or adapted area, by properly trained medical and nursing staff, with adequate facilities for patient and instrument care (Cotton & Williams, 1980). Endoscopy under other circumstances is time-consuming, often inaccurate and sometimes dangerous.

Routine diagnostic procedures

Contraindications to examination are rare. The extreme flexibility of the instruments permits their use even in seriously ill and frail patients. Those with open infections are usually avoided, since problems of sterilisation have not yet been solved.

Most patients are examined on an outpatient basis. Mild sedation is usually given in Western countries, but is frequently unnecessary with the newer smaller instruments (Beavis, LaBrooy & Misiewicz, 1979). A relaxed friendly approach in a well designed and efficient department is acceptable to virtually all patients; general anaesthesia may be necessary in children, but should otherwise be used only in exceptional circumstances.

Complications are very rare, even in the frail and elderly. Perforation has been reported in 1 in every 1–5000 examinations (Schiller & Prout, 1976); it is usually due to inexperience or a therapeutic procedure such as oesophageal dilatation; many such accidents can be managed without surgical intervention. Fatility rates of 1 in 4–20 000 have been reported for diagnostic endoscopy—figures not dissimilar to those for intravenous cholangiography (Schiller & Prout, 1976; Ansell, 1970). These deaths have resulted from perforation, drug reactions, oversedation, and cardiovascular collapse. Emergency and complex therapeutic endoscopies carry additional risks.

Indications and results

Upper gastrointestinal endoscopy has become very popular throughout the world, but its precise indications and relationship to barium radiology remain controversial (Cotton, 1973; Knutson et al, 1978; Holdstock, Wiseman & Loehry, 1979; Killer-Walser et al, 1979). In general, endoscopy is still used selectively in Britain, for those patients in whom barium radiology does not answer the clinical question (Holdsworth et al, 1979; Moshakis & Hooper, 1978). Endoscopy is clearly appropriate when the barium meal shows a lesion of uncertain significance (antral or duodenal deformity) or something which may be incidental (hiatus hernia in a patient with pain but no heartburn). Endoscopy is also necessary when radiographs show a lesion (oesophageal stricture, gastric ulcer or tumour) which needs histological or cytological sampling. Some Japanese groups claim an accuracy of almost 100 per cent in the diagnosis and exclusion of malignant disease by endoscopic biopsy (Kasugai & Kobayashi, 1974).

The combination of the endoscopic, histological and cytological information should provide a correct diagnosis in more than 95 per cent of patients with oesophageal and gastric malignancy (Moshakis & Hooper, 1978; Winawer, Melamed & Sherlock 1976; Halter et al, 1977; Dekker & Tytgat, 1977). Precise techniques are important, and results improve with experience. This is particularly true in the recognition of small tumours; British gastroenterologists and surgeons have fallen behind their counterparts in many countries in the search for early gastric cancers (Miller & Kaufmann, 1975; Kawai, 1978).

The endoscopic yield in patients with 'barium negative dyspepsia' depends upon the relative expertise of the examiners involved, and on the selection of patients; many studies have reported finding lesions (mainly duodenal ulcers) in up to 30 per cent of such patients (Cotton, 1973; Stender et al, 1975). The selective use of endoscopy in the face of negative radiographs only for those patients with the most severe symptoms will increase the diagnostic yield of ulcers and tumours, but reduce the likelihood of diagnosing resectable cancer.

Barium radiographs are particularly difficult to interpret in patients who have previously undergone ulcer or tumour surgery. Endoscopy has become the prime diagnostic tool in this context, and in patients with occult and overt bleeding. Urgent endoscopy can define the source of bleeding in 80–90 per cent patients (Cotton, 1975), and the appearance of the lesion may also give important prognostic information (Foster, Miloszewski & Losowsky, 1978). The fact that the introduction of an accurate diagnostic technique has not apparently reduced the mortality in acute bleeding (Dronfield et al, 1977) is a reflection on current methods of treatment.

Gastrointestinal endoscopy is equally easy to perform in children, and is finding increasing application in the diagnosis of abdominal pain and bleeding. In babies we have used a fibreoptic bronchoscope, with little or no sedation; above about 2 years and into the mid-teens we usually employ general anaesthesia, although those with the greatest experience prefer standard sedation. Adult fibrescopes can be used below the age of 10, but specialised instruments are clearly preferable. The thinner paediatric endoscopes are also convenient in elderly and frail adults, and in patients with strictures.

Is the barium meal obsolete?
Oesophagogastroduodenoscopy is often indicated if the barium meal report is negative, positive or equivocal; why then do barium meals at all? Many gastroenterologists have already made a pragmatic decision to use endoscopy as the primary diagnostic tool, particularly in hospitals where there are substantial delays for contrast examinations. They know that they can clarify the situation rapidly, with biopsies as necessary, and see no purpose in doing a barium meal first. However, those same gastroenterologists would be quite unable to cope with the vast numbers of patients needing investigation were barium meals to cease overnight. The main advantage of the barium meal is its availability; it is easier for the patient in prospect, although in retrospect many patients prefer endoscopy because of the sedation. The costs of the two examinations are broadly similar. Barium radiology is theoretically safer than endoscopy since the direct complications are exceedingly rare. However, a wrong diagnosis carries its own hazards, and can be equally costly to the patient and community.

Against the availability and familiarity of the barium meal must be set the reasonable conviction that fibreoptic endoscopy performed by an expert should be more accurate, if only because he can take biopsy and cytology specimens. Studies comparing the relative diagnostic accuracy of endoscopy and radiology are difficult to perform, and even more difficult to interpret. Most series concern the use of endoscopy in selected cases, which inevitably exaggerate the inaccuracies of radiology. Endoscopy flourishes in hospitals where radiology is of poor standard — and vice versa. A difficult aspect of any comparative study is the diagnostic end-point; the accuracy of endoscopy is very high if the endoscopic diagnosis is assumed to be correct. Studies in which both procedures have been performed by the same individual carry more weight (Laufer, Mullens & Hamilton, 1975).

Endoscopy has stimulated many radiologists to improve their techniques, and to develop better methods such as the double contrast examination which does provide greater mucosal detail (Laufer, 1979). However, radiology can never provide the tissue samples which are important, not only in the diagnosis of malignancy, but also increasingly in the recognition and evaluation of mucosal dysplasia as a premalignant marker.

Barium radiology will maintain a small role in the investigation of patients with upper gastrointestinal obstruction (oesophageal and duodenal stenosis) and for the investigation of motility disturbances. However, in all other circumstances, endoscopy will gradually take over the prime diagnostic role as experience and facilities develop.

Is the rigid oesophagoscope obsolete?
Rigid tube oesophagoscopes have been used for generations, and are still popular with some British surgeons. Fibrescopes are certainly easier for the user and for the patient, and should be considerably safer; they can always be passed for the entire length of the oesophagus (at least up to any stricturing), and the examination can be extended into the stomach or duodenum where clinically indicated. Rigid instruments currently allow better suction and bigger biopsy samples; the importance of the latter has never been documented, and, in some elderly patients it may prove impossible or hazardous to even reach a lesion in the lower oesophagus. The rigid oesophagoscope will be obsolete within a few years, except for some examinations of the upper oesophagus, and for some therapeutic procedures.

Therapeutic upper gastrointestinal endoscopy
Colonoscopy polypectomy was the first, and remains the main therapeutic application of fibreoptic endoscopes, but many others are being developed and used in the upper gastrointestinal tract (Classen, Rosch & Farthmann, 1977). The simplest and safest method for dilating oesophageal strictures uses bougies passed over an endoscopically-sited guide wire; an extension of this technique allows insertion of a tube prosthesis through unresectable oesophageal and oesophagogastric tumours. This method provides good palliation, and is considerably safer than the surgical alternative (Atkinson, Ferguson & Parker, 1977; Hartog Jager, Bartelsman & Tytgat, 1977; Saunders, 1979). When necessary, foreign bodies can be removed from the oesophagus, stomach and duodenum using specially designed grasping forceps and a protective sleeve. Suture material at surgical anastomoses can be removed endoscopi-

cally by traction with or without diathermy. Treatment of peptic ulcers by superficial application or injection of drugs is at an experimental stage. Fibrescopes can be used to place tubes quickly into the stomach or duodenum for therapeutic purposes (enteral nutrition, or intestinal decompression) and to speed certain diagnostic procedures such as jejunal biopsy.

There has been increasing interest in the endoscopic treatment of patients presenting with haematemesis and melaena (Katon, 1976). Fibrescopes are now being used in many countries to inject sclerosing solutions into or around oesophageal varices. Many centres have used diathermy coagulation in bleeding ulcers, but animal work suggest that the depth of injury is difficult to control and there may be a risk of full thickness damage and perforation. Argon and Neodymium Yag lasers have been adapted for fibrescopes, and produce good haemostatis in experimental animals. Excellent clinical results are reported with the Nd-Yag laser (Kiefhaber, Moritz & Nath, 1979) but there is about 1 per cent risk of perforation. The Argon laser penetrates less deeply, and preliminary clinical results have been encouraging (Laurence et al, 1980; Table 8.1). However, many ulcers stop bleeding spontaneously, and randomised controlled trials are in progress to assess the real clinical impact of these new techniques.

Table 8.1   Results of Argon laser photocoagulation in patients actively bleeding from ulcers at the time of emergency endoscopy. Re-bled = clinical recurrence within same hospital admission. (from Laurence et al, 1980).

Ulcers	Total	Stopped	Re-bled
Spurting	36	25 (69 %)	3 (9 %)
Oozing	24	23 (96 %)	2 (8 %)
Total	60	48 (80 %)	5 (8 %)

Endoscopic retrograde cholangiopancreatography (ERCP)

Forward and lateral viewing endoscopes are easy to pass into the descending duodenum and provide excellent views; X-ray duodenography is now virtually obsolete. Peptic ulcers rarely occur beyond the bulb; the papilla of Vater and its associated ducts and diseases provide the main clinical interest (Cotton, 1977).

ERCP is a combined endoscopic and radiographic procedure, performed in the radiology department in close co-operation with an experienced radiologist. A lateral viewing duodenoscope is used to examine the duodenal loop and papilla of Vater in detail; biopsy and cytology specimens are taken as necessary. A small catheter is then passed through the instrument and into the orifice of the papilla under direct vision. Contrast materials are injected under fluoroscopic control and radiographs are taken of the biliary and/or pancreatic duct systems (Fig. 8.4). First popularised in Japan, the technique has now become routine in many countries, despite the fact that it is not easy to learn. With experience the success rate for cannulating the duct (or ducts) of interest rises from an average of 70 per cent to more than 90 per cent. Severe complications such as acute cholangitis and pancreatitis have been reported, but these are virtually confined to inexperienced examiners. During the last two years we have seen only one complication at diagnostic ERCP — a minor episode of pancreatitis — in more than 1000 examinations. Cholangitis can be prevented by keeping the procedure

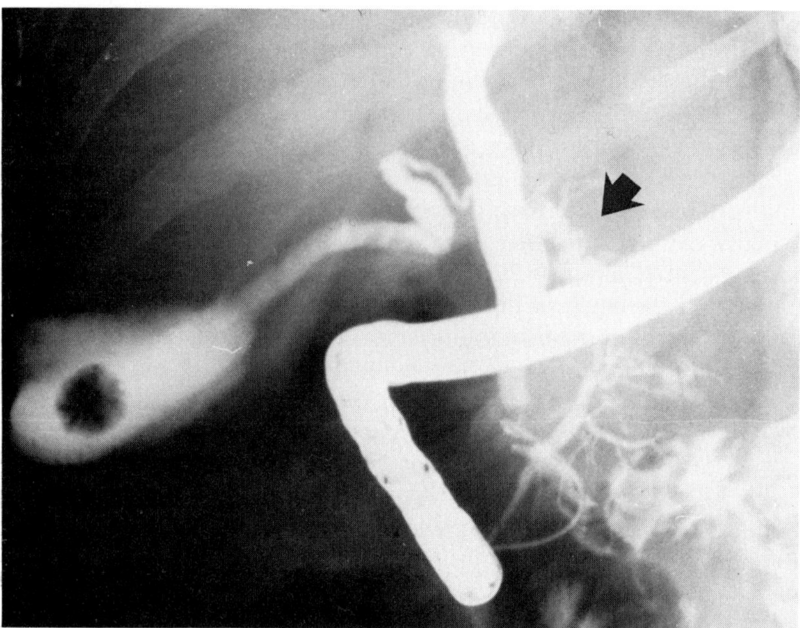

Fig. 8.4   Endoscopic retrograde cholangiopancreatography, showing the biliary system with a solitary stone in the gallbladder, and an obstructed pancreatic duct due to tumour (arrowed).

as sterile as possible, by the selective use of antibiotics, and by ensuring early drainage of any stagnant biliary system by endoscopic sphincterotomy or surgery. Pancreatography should not be performed in patients with pseudocysts (for fear of introducing infection) except as an immediately preoperative procedure.

ERCP has many potential diagnostic and therapeutic indications, but its actual use varies, depending on local interests and expertise (Cotton, 1977).

Pancreatography has an important role in defining and excluding major pancreatic and biliary duct abnormalities in patients with recurrent pancreatitis, and provides a logical basis for surgical management (Cotton & Beales, 1974). We have recently been impressed by the frequency of congenital pancreatic duct anomalies, such as pancreas divisum, which may itself be a cause of obstructive pancreatitis and pain (Cotton, 1980a) (Fig. 8.5). Pancreatograms show characteristic changes in advanced chronic pancreatitis; occasionally the differential diagnosis from cancer may prove difficult. Radiographs may be normal or only slightly abnormal in patients with recurrent pancreatitis at an early stage. Pancreatograms are virtually always markedly abnormal in patients with pancreatic cancer (Reuben & Cotton, 1979) and the diagnosis can be confirmed by juice or brush cytology (Fig. 8.6).

We have found ultrasonography and ERCP to be a particularly effective diagnostic combination in pancreatic disease (Cotton et al, 1980); we have abandoned pancreatic isotope scanning, and rarely use function tests and computed tomography, which has proved rather disappointing.

Many groups have found ERCP useful in the diagnosis of patients with jaundice; it provides information about the papilla and pancreas, as well as cholangiography and an opportunity to make a tissue diagnosis with biopsy and cytology. We have

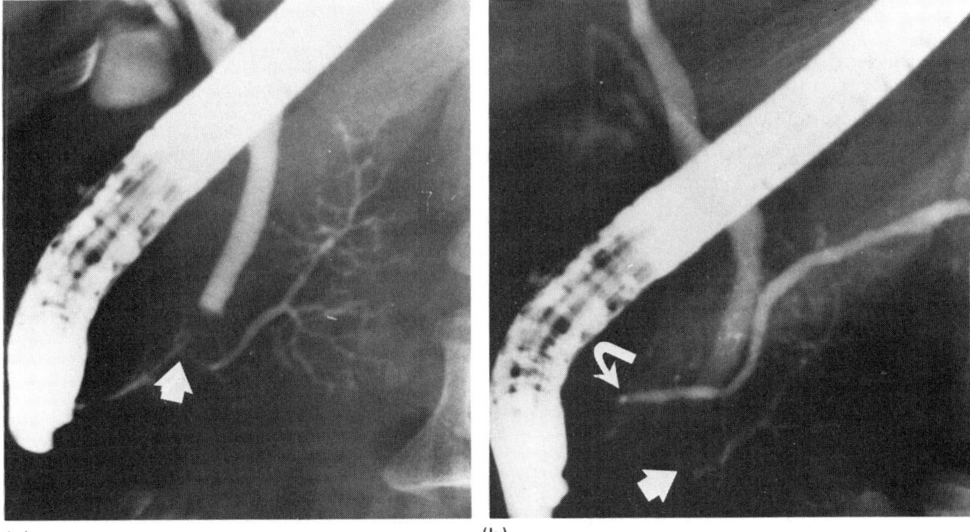

Fig 8.5 Patient with the congenital anomaly of pancreas divisum.
(a) Cannulation of the main papilla of Vater outlining the biliary system, and an isolated ventral pancreas.
(b) Cannulation of the accessary papilla (curved arrow) outlines the dorsal pancreatic duct system via
Santorini's duct. Contrast remains in the biliary system and ventral pancreas following previous
cannulation of the main papilla (arrowed).

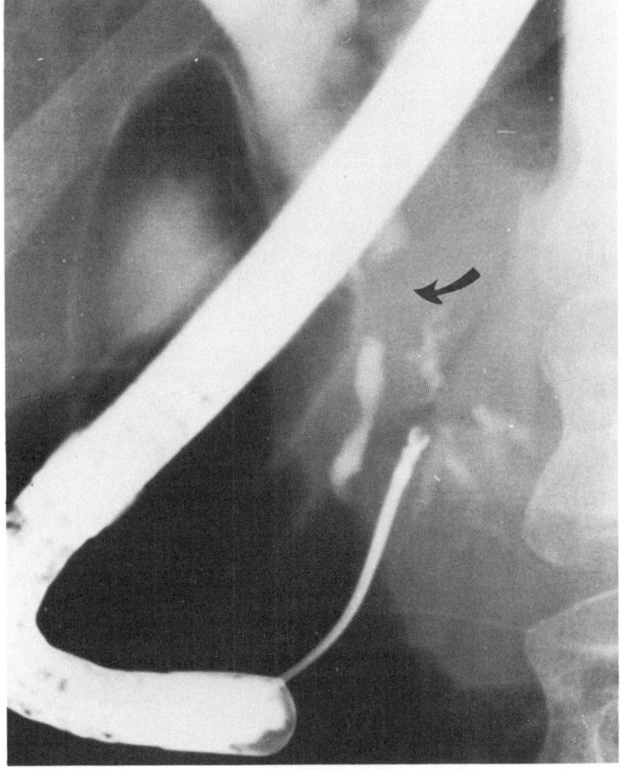

Fig 8.6 ERCP showing obstruction to the pancreatic duct due to a tumour, also causing stricturing of the
lower common bile duct (arrowed). Biopsy forceps have been passed up the pancreatic duct for histological
confirmation.

provided a definite diagnosis in 91 per cent of our last 150 jaundiced patients. ERCP is the best method for the diagnosis of cancer of the papilla of Vater; such tumours are clinically important since they may produce symptoms when very small and resectable. Fine needle percutaneous transhepatic cholangiography (PTC) is a simple technique, which should provide good cholangiograms in jaundiced patients with dilated ducts; it should be used as the first cholangiographic procedure when there is strong clinical or ultrasonographic evidence of obstruction, especially if the examiner can also perform transhepatic drainage (Dooley et al, 1979).

ERCP has the dominant role in jaundiced patients when there is no definite evidence of obstruction, and when gallstones are suspected, for then they can be removed directly by endoscopic sphincterotomy. Endoscopic cholangiography is particularly helpful in patients with symptoms after biliary surgery, whether or not they are jaundiced. Radiographs should be of higher quality than intravenous cholangiograms (Fig. 8.7) and the coincident gastroduodenoscopy and pancreatography may also be diagnostic. Duodenoscopic manometry provides another dimension to the investigation of postcholecystectomy pain.

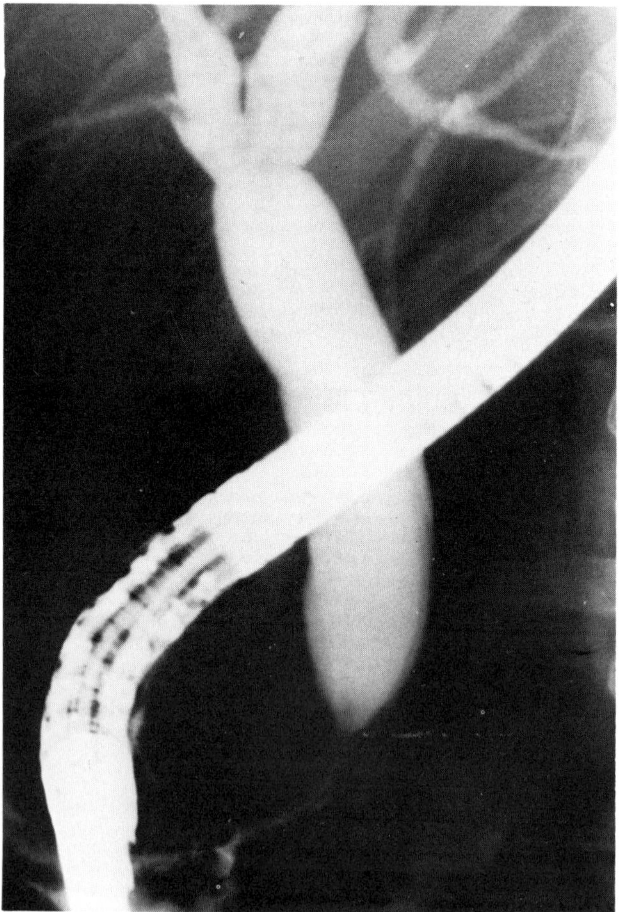

Fig. 8.7 Dilated biliary system shown on endoscopic retrograde cholangiography in a patient complaining of pain after cholecystectomy.

Endoscopic sphincterotomy for removal of gallstones

Endoscopic diathermy sphincterotomy has rapidly become popular in Europe since its description in 1974. When ERCP confirms the diagnosis of bile duct stones, the radiographic catheter is replaced by one incorporating a wire 'knife'; diathermy is applied to cut the roof of the papilla, to a length of about 15 mm, exposing the distal bile duct. Stones can be extracted directly with balloon catheters or baskets (Fig. 8.8) or allowed to pass spontaneously. Passage of stones can be monitored by repeat endoscopy, or via an indwelling transnasal biliary tube.

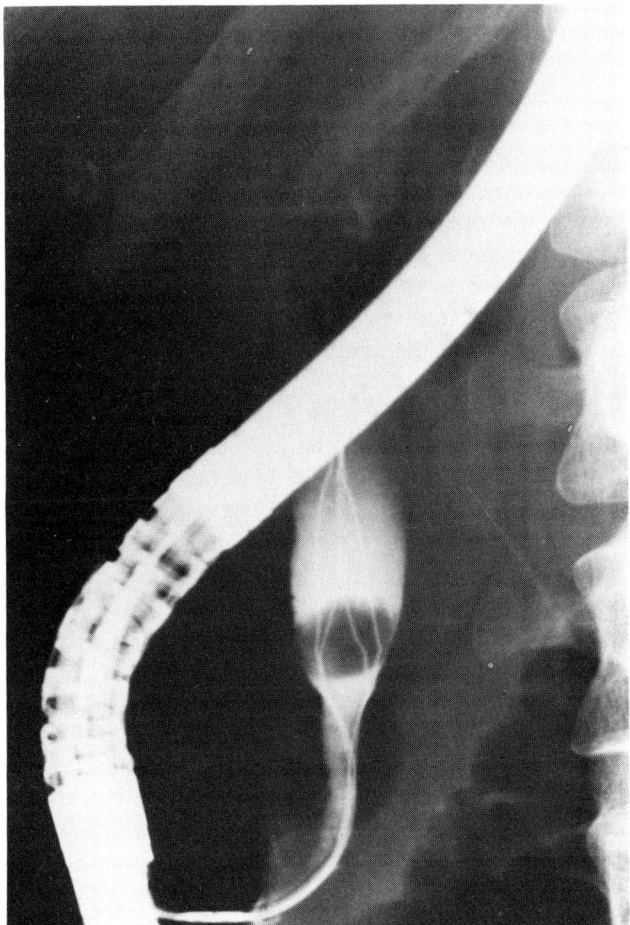

Fig. 8.8   Removal of a stone from the distal bile duct using a dormia-type wire basket after endoscopic sphincterotomy.

Many large series now report success rates for endoscopic sphincterotomy of around 95 per cent, and complete clearance of duct stones in over 90 per cent (Safrany, 1979; Cotton, 1980b). Complications of varying severity (including bleeding, pancreatitis and cholangitis) have been reported in 5–10 per cent of series; 2–3 per cent of patients have required emergency surgery, and the mortality rate varies from 0.6 to 2 per cent. Most of the patients treated have been elderly, or have had specific medical or surgical contraindication to further surgery; under these circumstances endoscopic sphincterotomy is certainly safer than operative duct exploration (Cotton, 1980b; Vellacott & Powell, 1979). Endoscopic sphincterotomy cannot claim to be safer than duct exploration in young and fit patients, and its use in this context must await follow-up studies of the long-term effects.

Sphincterotomy was initially used in patients with duct stones after cholecystectomy; it is being increasingly applied to those who still have gallbladders, to provide emergency drainage in patients with severe cholangitis or acute biliary pancreatitis. Cholecystectomy can be performed later with less risk, or postponed indefinitely in some very old patients. Sphincterotomy is also being used experimentally in the treatment of papillary and bile duct tumours, and in pancreatitis.

Choledochoscopy

Fibreoptic choledoschoscopes can be passed at operation into the bile duct to facilitate the diagnosis exclusion and removal of stones. Similar instruments can be passed down the T-tube track postoperatively to remove any residual stones.

The ever-ingenious Japanese engineers have now produced smaller fibrescopes which can be passed via the mouth, through the papilla and into the biliary (and pancreatic) ducts. The latest prototype provides excellent views and has an operating channel for tissue sampling and therapeutic applications.

Endoscopy of the small intestine

Endoscopy beyond the third part of the duodenum is difficult. Experimental instruments provide views of the proximal jejunum, and the prior passage of a transintestinal string can allow examination of the entire small bowel; indeed a few enthusiasts have made the complete trip from mouth to anus. Indications for small intestinal endoscopy are very rare. It is probably useful in a few patients with recurrent obscure bleeding; examination is then best performed at the time of laparotomy, when it is a simple matter to milk the intestine over the instrument.

Conclusion

Fibreoptic instruments have provided a major new dimension to the practice of gastroenterology. It is much easier now than 10 years ago to make a precise diagnosis in the oesophagus, stomach, duodenum, pancreas and biliary tree; it is also possible to demonstrate that some diseases are not present, which can be equally important. Fibrescopes provide new avenues for research, giving easy access to target mucosal specimens, and uncontaminated digestive secretions such as pancreatic juice (Denyer & Cotton, 1979).

Demands for diagnostic and therapeutic procedures continue to rise rapidly, putting considerable pressure on staff and facilities. In many countries this has led to the evolution of full time endoscopists, and of endoscopy as a subspeciality. In Britain, fibrescopes are still rightly regarded as tools for specialists with wider gastrointestinal training and interests. Preservation of this concept will require the appointment of more consultant physicians (and surgeons) with particular interest in gastroenterology.

REFERENCES

Ansell G 1970 Adverse reactions to contrast agents, scope of problem. Investigative Radiology 5: 374–384

Atkinson M, Ferguson R, Parker G C 1978 Tube intraducer and modified Celestin tube for use in palliative intubation of oesophago-gastric neoplasms at fibreoptic endoscopy. Gut 19: 669–671

Baird J L 1928 An improved method of and means for producing optical images. British Patent Specification 285: 738

Beavis A K, LaBrooy S, Misiewicz J J 1979 Evaluation of one visit endoscopic clinic for patients with dyspepsia. British Medical Journal 1: 1387–1389

Classen M, Rosch W, Farthmann E H 1979 Therapeutic endoscopy of the upper gastrointestinal tract. In: Jerzy Glass George B (ed) Progress in gastroenterology, vol 3. Grune and Stratton, New York, p 945–965

Cotton P B 1973 Fibreoptic endoscopy and the barium meal. Results and implications. British Medical Journal 2: 161–165.

Cotton P B 1975 Acute upper gastrointestinal haemorrhage. Endoscopy. In: Trulove S C, Goodman M J (eds) Topics in gastroenterology. Blackwells, London, p 9–23

Cotton P B 1977 Progress Report ERCP. Gut, 18: 316–341

Cotton P B 1980a Congenital anomaly of pancreas divisum can cause obstructive pain and pancreatitis. Gut 21: 105–114

Cotton P B 1980b Non-operative removal of bile duct stones by duodenoscopic sphincterotomy. British Journal of Surgery 67: 1–5

Cotton P B, Beales J S M 1974 Endoscopic pancreatography in the management of relapsing acute pancreatitis. British Medical Journal 1: 608–611

Cotton P B, Williams C B 1980 Practical gastrointestinal endoscopy. Blackwells, London

Cotton P B, Lees W R, Vallon A G, Cottone M, Croker J R, Chapman M 1980 Grey-scale ultrasonography and endoscopic pancreatography in pancreatic diagnosis. Radiology 134 (2): 453–459

Dekker W, Tytgat G N 1977 Diagnostic accuracy of fibre-endoscopy in the detection of upper intestinal malignancy. A follow-up analysis. Gastroenterology 73: 710–714

Denyer M E, Cotton P B 1979 Pure pancreatic juice studies in normal subjects and patients with chronic pancreatitis. Gut 20: 89–97

Dooley J S, Dick R, Olney J, Sherlock S 1979 Non-surgical treatment of biliary obstruction. Lancet i: 1040–1043

Dronfield M W, McIllmurray M B, Ferguson R, Atkinson M C, Langman M J S 1977 A prospective randomised study of endoscopy and radiology in acute upper gastrointestinal tract bleeding. Lancet i: 1167–1169

Foster D N, Miloszewski K J A, Losowsky M S 1978 Stigmata of recent haemorrhage in diagnosis and prognosis of upper gastrointestinal bleeding. British Medical Journal 1: 1173–1177

Halter W, Witzel K, Gretillat P A, Scheurer U, Keller M 1977 Diagnostic value of biopsy guided lavage and brush cytology in oesophagogastroscopy Digestive Diseases 22: 129–131

Hartog Jager, Den F C A, Bartelsman J F, Tytgat G N J 1979 Palliative treatment of obstructive oesophago-gastric malignancy by endoscopic positioning of a plastic prosthesis. Gastroenterology 77: 1008–1014

Hopkins H H, Kapany N S 1954 A flexible fibrescope using static scanning. Nature 173: 39

Holdstock G, Wiseman M, Loehry C A 1979 Open access endoscopy service for general practitioners. British Medical Journal 1: 457–459

Holdsworth C D, Bardhan K D, Balmforth G V, Dickson R A, Sladen G E 1979 Upper gastrointestinal endoscopy: its effects on patient management. British Medical Journal 1: 775–777

Kasugai T, Kobayashi S 1974 Evaluation of biopsy and cytology in the diagnosis of gastric cancer. American Journal of Gastroenterology 62: 199

Katon R M 1976 Experimental control of gastrointestinal haemorrhage via the Endoscope: A new era dawns. Gastroenterology 70: 272–277

Kawai K 1978 Screening for gastric cancer in Japan. Clinics in gastroenterology 7: 3 605–622

Killer-Walser R, Hess H, Wursch T G, Stuby K, Sonnenberg A, Bruhlmann W, Blum A L 1979 Fiberendoskopie und Radiologie bei Ulcus ventriculi, Magenkarzinom und Hiatuschernie: Fragestellung, Zeitpunkt und Assagekraft. Zchweizerische medizinische Wochenscrift 109: 3–6

Kiefhaber P, Moritz K, Nath G 1979 Endoscopic control of acute gastrointestinal haemorrhage by irradiation with a high power neodymium Yag laser (abs). International Medical Laser Symposium Detroit, March 1979

Knutson C O, Max M H, Ahmad W, Polk H C 1978 Should flexible fiberoptic endoscopy replace barium contrast study of the upper gastrointestinal tract? Surgery 84: 609–615

Laufer I 1979 Double contrast gastrointestinal radiology with endoscopic correlation. W B Saunders, England

Laufer I, Mullens J E, Hamilton J 1975 The diagnostic accuracy of barium studies of the stomach and duodenum — correlation with endoscopy. Radiology 115: 569–573

Laurence B H, Cotton P B, Armengol-Miro J R, Salord-Oses J C, LeBodic L, Sudry P, Fruhmorgen P, Bodem F 1980 Endoscopic laser photocoagulation for bleeding peptic ulcers. Lancet i: 124–125

Miller G, Kaufmann M 1975 Das Magenfruhkarzinom in Europa. 1170 Falle aus den Jahren 1968–1973. Deutsche medizinische Wochenschrift 100: 1946–1949

Moshakis V, Hooper A A 1978 The accuracy of endoscopic diagnosis of gastric carcinoma and the conventional barium meal. Clinical Oncology 4: 359–368

Rueben A, Cotton P B 1979 Endoscopic retrograde cholangiopancreatography in cancer of the pancreas. Surgery, Gynecology and Obstetrics 148: (2), 179–184

Safrany L 1979 Endoscopic treatment of biliary tract diseases. Lancet ii: 983–985

Saunders N S 1979 The Celestin tube in the palliation of carcinoma of the oesophagus and cardia. British Journal of Surgery 66: 419–421

Schiller K F R, Prout B J 1976 Schiller K F R, Salmon P R (eds). Hazards in modern topics in gastrointestinal endoscopy. William Heinemann, London

Stender V H St, Seifert E, Luska G, Otto P 1975 Vergleichende rontgenologische und endoskopische Diagnostik des ulcus ventriculi und duodeni. Fortschrift fur Roentgenstr 122: 381–385

Vellacott K D, Powell P H 1979 Exploration of the common bile duct: a comparative study British Journal of Surgery 66: 389–391

Winawer S J, Melamed M, Sherlock P 1976 Potential of endoscopy biopsy and cytology in the diagnosis and management of patients with cancer. Clinics in Gastroenterology 5: 3, 575–596

8.2 Fibreoptic colonoscopy and sigmoidoscopy

Christopher B. Williams

Fibre-endoscopy of the lower intestine has gradually emerged as a highly effective procedure which has transformed the clinical management of many patients with colorectal disorders. It has also given a much-needed stimulus to radiologists because the barium enema in general use is too often of low quality, with the emphasis on speed rather than accuracy. Colonoscopy presents a new option between initial screening procedures and surgery. The availability of this new option also makes it necessary for the clinician to reconsider which patients may benefit from earlier or more accurate diagnosis, and who may now avoid surgery. This chapter considers the interplay between the advantages and disadvantages of fibre-endoscopy and how it relates to radiology and well-tried techniques such as proctosigmoidoscopy and rectal biopsy.

Instrumentation

Because the colon is longer, more tortuous and elastic as compared with the upper gastrointestinal tract the majority of modern colonoscopes are more flexible than either gastroscopes or duodenoscopes. Advances in manufacturing technology allow them to retain full tip-angling capability whilst adapting to the flexures and loops of the colon. Finer glass fibres result in more flexible bundles with higher resolution, allowing a wider angle of view and longer life. The original colonoscopes were often difficult to manipulate round acute bends and often lasted only 100–200 examinations before major repairs were needed; modern instruments are easier for both patient and endoscopist and usually last 500 or more examinations without major overhaul. The limitations of colonoscopy are largely due to the mechanical difficulties of passing them and as the instruments have improved the usefulness of the procedure has rapidly increased.

Colonic fibre-endoscopes range in length from the 60–70 cm fibre-sigmoidoscope, through those of 110–140 cm medium or intermediate length, to the 165–185 cm 'long colonoscopes'. The shortest instruments deliberately restrict the extent of examination in the unsedated clinic patient, whereas only the variations in colonic anatomy from patient to patient and the skills of individual endoscopists determine how far the longer instruments can be inserted (Cotton & Williams, 1979). The long colonoscopes may be more easily looped inside the patient and are more awkward to handle during cleaning and use; they will usually reach to the caecum if required, which makes the long instrument the 'best-buy' for a hospital requiring a single instrument. Most centres performing colonoscopy acquire several different instruments so that a spare is always available, and they may then use a medium-length instrument as the 'work-horse' and a small diameter instrument for babies, for patients with strictures and 'ostomy' examinations. Two-channel instruments are available and occasionally useful because of the extra suction and instrumentation capacity in patients with massive bleeding or multiple polyps. Short fibre-sigmoidoscopes are mainly intended for diagnostic screening examinations, where comfort is of paramount importance and a relatively thin and 'floppy' instrument seems likely to prove the best.

Difficulties, limitations and complications of colonoscopy
The barium enema shows the differences in length of individual colons and, in particular, the variably tortuous sigmoid colon. What is not apparent, and not appreciated even by most endoscopists, is that it is the radiologically invisible *attachments* and mesenteries of the colon which determine how the bowel moves with the colonoscope inside it. At least 10 per cent of patients have a mobile descending colon with no retroperitoneal anchoring, which results in awkward looping of the instrument and pain for the patient; others have a colon acutely angulated by postoperative adhesions or fixed by inflammatory reactions complicating diverticular disease. Whereas barium will almost always flow to the caecum, passage of the colonoscope is unpredictably difficult or impossible in at least 5–10 per cent of patients with apparently 'normal' colons and the failure rate is greater in the presence of strictures or severe diverticular disease.

Since colonoscopy is a profound vagal stimulus it should be avoided in very sick patients, especially soon after myocardial infarction. The instrument stretches the colon wall and there is a significant danger of perforation if there is acute inflammation of the whole bowel wall, as will occur in any severe colitis (including Crohn's disease or acute diverticulitis) and the examination is therefore contraindicated in any such condition where there is abdominal tenderness to indicate full-thickness involvement. Even if limited inspection is possible, as in ischaemic or irradiation colitis, once the diagnosis is made the danger of damage will make it wiser to stop the procedure, examining the proximal bowel if necessary with X-ray.

Even if insertion is easy there are a number of circumstances in which accurate inspection is difficult or impossible (Fig. 8.9). In addition to the generally-known

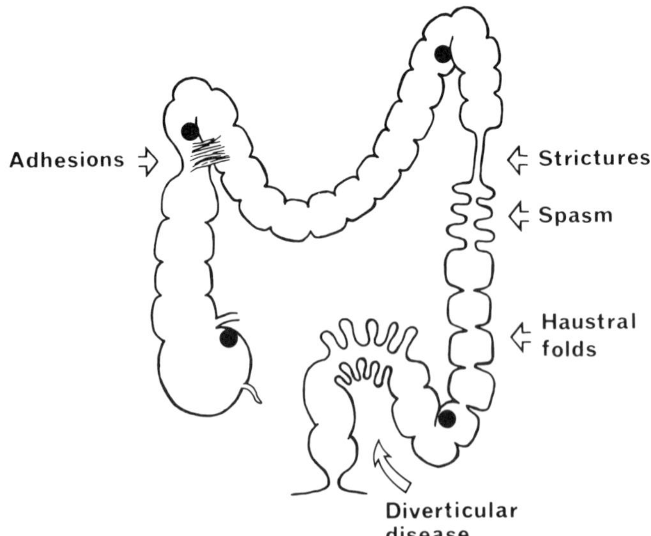

Fig. 8.9   The limitations of fibreoptic colonoscopy.

'blind-spots' for the endoscopist around acute flexures or in the capacious caecum, the presence of marked haustration, spasm or stricturing or fixed angulation due to adhesions or diverticular disease make it possible to miss lesions during colonoscopy. Thus, even though the endoscopist's view is certainly more accurate overall than the radiologist's (Thoeni & Menuck, 1977, Theuerkauf, 1978) it is highly desirable to have preliminary barium enema films available at the time of colonoscopy; if the endoscopy is in any way unsatisfactory it is equally possible for a check barium enema to follow immediately *after* the colonoscopy if CO_2 insufflation has been used.

The complications reported after colonoscopy are relatively few considering the technical difficulties of some examinations and the large numbers of polypectomies performed; they are, however, frequent enough to make it essential that patients are only referred for colonoscopy for sound clinical reasons. There is inevitably variation between different reported series, with mass surveys and those based on large endoscopy services showing fewer complications than some small personal series (Rogers et al, 1975; Frühmorgen & Demling, 1979). Diagnostic colonoscopy has been complicated by bowel perforation in approximately 1 per 500 examinations; although with modern, very flexible, instruments this rate should fall. The relatively large number of old and frail patients, often with adhesions and diverticula, makes occasional bowel damage almost inevitable. In some cases where the perforation is known to have been very small or due to a 'blow-out' of a diverticulum by air pressure, patients have been managed conservatively in view of the very clean colon after bowel preparation; however, in a few cases septic complications have been fatal (an approximate mortality of 1 per 5000 colonoscopies) suggesting that surgical repair is usually the best course. Since most colon polyps are stalked polypectomy is rarely complicated by perforation but at least 1 per 50 polypectomies is followed by haemorrhage, especially if the polyp is large.

Preparation of the patient
Some explanation of the procedure to the patient is highly desirable, with reassurance that it will not be allowed to be painful; many patients are otherwise highly apprehensive of an examination intended to go on longer and further than rigid proctosigmoidoscopy, of which they may have sour memories. Explanation and motivation also helps to ensure that the necessary bowel preparation regime is correctly followed; a half-hearted regime or a half-dose of purgative can only compromise the result of the examination. Limited preparation is possible for limited colonoscopy and two hypertonic phosphate enemas alone will normally clean all residue up to the splenic flexure, but for a completely clean colon tough measures are needed. Various centres have reported good results using isotonic saline (3–10 litres) which may be drunk or given by tube or a solution of 10 per cent mannitol (1 litre) which tastes better but may theoretically produce hydrogen gas with an explosion hazard (Bigard, 1979). The most common procedure is for one day of low residue diet and then clear fluids for the day before examination. A large dose of any purgative (castor oil, senna, bisacodyl, magnesium salts) is given the afternoon before and tap-water enemas administered just before the examination. Any preparation regime gives imperfect results in about 10 per cent of cases, but the endoscopist can usually interpret sufficiently well after aspiration and only 1–2 per cent of examinations fail because of poor preparation.

Medication

Sedation is often unnecessary for colonoscopy, but many patients seem to prefer a small dose of analgesic, as they would expect for a major dental procedure. With a short colon, or a confident patient, lack of sedation has obvious advantages in letting the patient leave unaccompanied afterwards, but this is unjustified if it results in a hurried or compromised examination. Most colonoscopists give a small intravenous dose of a sedative/analgesic combination at the start of the examination, which results in a comfortable and relaxed patient for the 10–15 minutes of instrumentation. The combination of intravenous administration of diazepam (5–10 mg) and pethidine (25–50 mg) provides satisfactory results which are short-lived, and gives a useful degree of amnesia for any trauma which may have occurred during the procedure; side-effects such as nausea are surprisingly rare and can occur even in the unsedated patient, due to the severity of the colonic stimulus. Any oversedation or respiratory depression can be quickly reversed with intravenous naloxone, and drowsy day-patients may be given an intramuscular dose which ensures they are fit to leave after a recovery period of only 10–20 minutes. Alternative regimes are used, such as neuroleptanalgesic combinations (droperidol and haloperidol) but appear to have no particular advantage and longer-lasting after effects.

The other important drugs hyoscine-n-butyl bromide (Buscopan) or glucagon are used to combat spasm. They are used during insertion in patients with severe diverticular disease with muscle spasm or more usually during examination or withdrawal if spasm may compromise an accurate view. Both are short-acting and therefore only given when required; at least the short action means that there are no after-effects.

Colonoscopic technique

Anyone with experience of fibre-endoscopy can rapidly learn the technique of insertion through the sigmoid colon. There may be surprise at the problems of steering the instrument tip in confined spaces with a sometimes imperfect view, and also in realising that the instrument shaft will loop if pushed in too fast. Colonoscopy is essentially little different from duodenoscopy, except that the distances involved are greater and the bends more numerous and unpredictable.

Passing out of the sigmoid colon, around the splenic and hepatic flexures and through the ileocaecal valve can be easy or very difficult; experience is only acquired by hours spent with the instrument in at least 50 patients and the necessary combination of patience, determination, delicacy, aggression and clinical common-sense. X-ray fluoroscopy will sometimes help to explain the endoscopist's difficulties or more precisely localise a lesion, but in general the endoscopist does better simply to use his eyes and hands intelligently, with occasional help from an assistant to compress any loop or change the patient's position. Modern instruments will follow loops and bends effortlessly that were unattainable with early colonoscopes or required particular tricks such as the 'alpha-loop' manoeuvre (which need now be rarely, if ever used).

Fluoroscopy does allow problem loops to be unravelled more quickly, the occasional use of the stiffening overtube to prevent them reforming, and is also very helpful while learning the technique. In 9 cases out of 10, however, the colonoscope will pass into the caecum (or as far as necessary) in 5–15 minutes without X-ray control and the current approach is to treat colonoscopy as a 'quick' examination like fibre-optic gastroscopy. The indications for colonoscopy are listed in Table 8.2.

Table 8.2   Indications for colonoscopy

Indications for colonoscopy as the primary procedure	
Rectal bleeding	— persistent
	acute (but of moderate degree)
Stomas	— ileostomies
	pouches
	colostomy patients
Polyp/cancer surveillance	— after sigmoid resection
	after polypectomy (selected patients)
	uretero-sigmoidostomies
	chronic extensive ulcerative colitis
Indications for colonoscopy after barium enema	
Abnormal barium enema	— for biopsy
Normal barium enema	— persistent bleeding
Inflammatory bowel disease	— selected cases
Polyps	— for attempted snare polypectomy

Colonoscopy as the primary procedure

There are relatively few indications, except as fibre-sigmoidoscopy in 'high-risk' patients, for first-line colonoscopy. This is mainly because of the limitations, complications and technical difficulties already discussed. The rewards of examination of patients with persistent rectal bleeding are detailed below, and allowing for careful clinical selection to exclude the great majority of patients bleeding from haemorrhoids or anal fissure (Williams & Thomson, 1977) colonoscopy might be justified in those who merit examination of the proximal colon. Barium enema would then be performed only in those where colonoscopy failed for technical reasons.

Relatively few reports have emerged of colonoscopy in acute rectal bleeding (Nuesch et al, 1976; Rossini & Ferrari, 1976) and in the presence of massive exsanguinating haemorrhage colonoscopy 'against the stream' is hopeless compared to the ease of angiography. In moderate haemorrhage however, especially if a two-channel colonoscope or one with a large diameter suction-channel is available, it is easy to attempt emergency colonoscopy since the bowel is self-cleansing. Not only may the bleeding site be localised but in a few cases where a polyp is the source, polypectomy has been possible.

Ileostomies and ileal pouches are easy to examine endoscopically, although it may be necessary to use a small diameter instrument and the examination may be of limited extent. Equally examination of the proximal colon through a colostomy is normally technically easy, which contrasts with the technical difficulties of obtaining high-quality barium examinations in the same patients; if the procedure is to check for polyps or synchronous cancer it seems logical to use colonoscopy for greater accuracy. This is especially so since the poor bowel preparation frequently found in these patients makes radiological interpretation very difficult but presents no problem in differential diagnosis to the endoscopist.

Other patients requiring surveillance for polyps and cancer should be considered for colonoscopic follow-up if the procedure is likely to be technically easy. After resection of the sigmoid colon colonoscopy becomes extremely quick and completely painless and the endoscopist is particularly accurate in inspecting (and if necessary biopsying) the anastomosis. Patients having once had polypectomy for an adenoma require long-term follow-up because of the significant risk of subsequently developing other lesions; those patients in whom total colonoscopy is easy are best served by repeated colonoscopy, which will identify smaller lesions than barium enema and allows simultaneous biopsy or removal of any polyp found.

Ureteric implantation into the sigmoid colon (ureterosigmoidostomy) carries a high long-term risk of development of carcinoma at the implantation site; with limited bowel preparation and no sedation it is easy to inspect, and if necessary biopsy, the ureteric orifices. The equivalent surveillance problem in patients with a chronic history of extensive ulcerative colitis is discussed below; since it depends mainly on the examination of mucosal biopsies colonoscopy is a more logical screening method than barium enema.

Screening for the presence of tiny polyps in members of a polyposis coli family is more accurate with the magnified close-up view of the colonoscope; left-sided examination should make or exclude the diagnosis. In all circumstances where biopsy confirmation or exclusion of minor abnormality is essential, colonoscopy could come first depending on the availability of the necessary expertise.

Colonoscopy after barium enema

X-ray abnormality
Colonoscopy is now usually indicated to inspect and biopsy equivocal abnormalities shown up on a screening barium enema and enlightened radiologists will suggest this instead of a repeat.

X-ray. In practice after the endoscopist's use of any necessary sedation or antispasmodics a 'stricture' or 'mucosal irregularity' may disappear and at least 5–10 per cent of 'polyps' shown on X-ray prove to be non-existent and probably due to misinterpretation of faecal residue or air bubbles. An important side-effect of the inter-relationship between X-ray and endoscopy should be to encourage radiologists to be freer with sedation or antispasmodics and more attentive to bowel preparation, thus avoiding such 'false-positive' errors.

Colonoscopic biopsies are very small due to the 2 mm diameter forceps imposed by the small channel of most colonoscopes, but large pieces can be taken from protuberant lesions by 'snare-biopsy', and brushing or washing cytology will help to sample a strictured area. Endoscopic photographs take a day or two in processing and therefore are usually of little clinical use; a few teaching centres with colour television facilities can make an immediate videotape of any endoscopically abnormal area for subsequent review. Otherwise it is one of the important limitations of the endoscopic assessment that the referring clinician receives only a written report of the procedure and (unlike X-ray) no other permanent record exists on which to make an independent judgement on the endoscopist's opinion.

Strictures, when confirmed, are usually passable and easily assessed, but may require the use of a thin instrument (such as a paediatric gastroscope or colonoscope). Failure to pass through and adequately inspect a stricture is recorded as a 'failed colonoscopy' since malignancy cannot be excluded. Brushing or washing cytology specimens may give a positive result in some impassable strictures. The majority of strictures referred for colonoscopy (including over three-quarters of those in chronic ulcerative colitis, hitherto regarded as highly likely to be malignant) prove to be benign to inspection, histological and cytological assessment (Hunt et al, 1978). This is an area of clinical management where colonoscopy and biopsy has wrought a revolution by removing the need for diagnostic laparotomy.

Diverticular disease, an all too common feature of elderly patients in Western society, presents considerable interpretative difficulty for the radiologist because of the associated muscle hypertrophy and deformity of the bowel. The endoscopist also experiences difficulty, but in insertion rather than interpretation, since once the bowel straightens out over the instrument on withdrawal an excellent view is obtained. The lumen is never strictured, although sometimes rigid and fixed. Such periocolic fixation causes failure of insertion in about 10 per cent of cases of diverticular disease and is also likely to weaken the instrument mechanically because of the difficulty in attempting to angle around fixed bends. Colonoscopy therefore is only indicated in patients with diverticular disease and pain/alteration of bowel habit if there is radiological suspicion of a coexistent carcinoma or the clinical possibility of inflammatory bowel disease. If there is persistent bleeding in a patient with diverticular disease, however, this will prove in about 40 per cent of cases referred for colonoscopy to be due to hidden pathology such as polyps, cancer or inflammatory disease. Persistent minor bleeding is very rarely due to the diverticula bleeding, true diverticular bleeding being usually massive and self-limiting.

In a few patients with severe diverticular disease there is seen at colonoscopy to be superficial reddening and friability of the mucosal folds between orifices, apparently due to mucosal trauma secondary to the muscular disorder. Biopsies of these areas may show minor inflammatory or traumatic features; minor bleeding may continue intermittently without sinister significance and no treatment is called for.

Unexplained rectal bleeding
Thirty-five to fifty per cent of patients referred because of persistent red rectal bleeding unexplained on rigid proctosigmoidoscopy or barium enema are found on colonoscopy to have an abnormality, usually in the sigmoid colon, (Hunt, 1978; Tedesco et al, 1978). Such bleeding will usually be mixed in with the stool or visible during proctosigmoidoscopy. Black melaena without red bleeding is invariably upper gastrointestinal in origin.

Ten per cent of patients who bleed persistently are found on colonoscopy to have a missed colon cancer, 15–20 per cent a polyp, and 15 per cent have other missed abnormalities such as inflammatory bowel disease (including irradiation colitis) or angiodysplasia. The radiological failure is most frequently due to an error in interpretation, often compounded by poor technique or bowel preparation; any lesion present is frequently visible on review of the original films, partly hidden by overlapping folds of sigmoid colon or by overlying barium-filled terminal ileum (Fig. 8.10).

The rectum is included in the endoscopic examination because 'solitary' traumatic ulcers and even cancers can be missed on proctosigmoidoscopy. Modern colonoscopes can be retroverted in the rectum to give an unusual view of haemorrhoids which are, even in this group, the commonest cause of haemorrhage. Occasionally the cause of iron-deficiency anaemia is found, usually in the right colon, including minor inflammatory disease and caecal carcinoma or angiodysplasia.

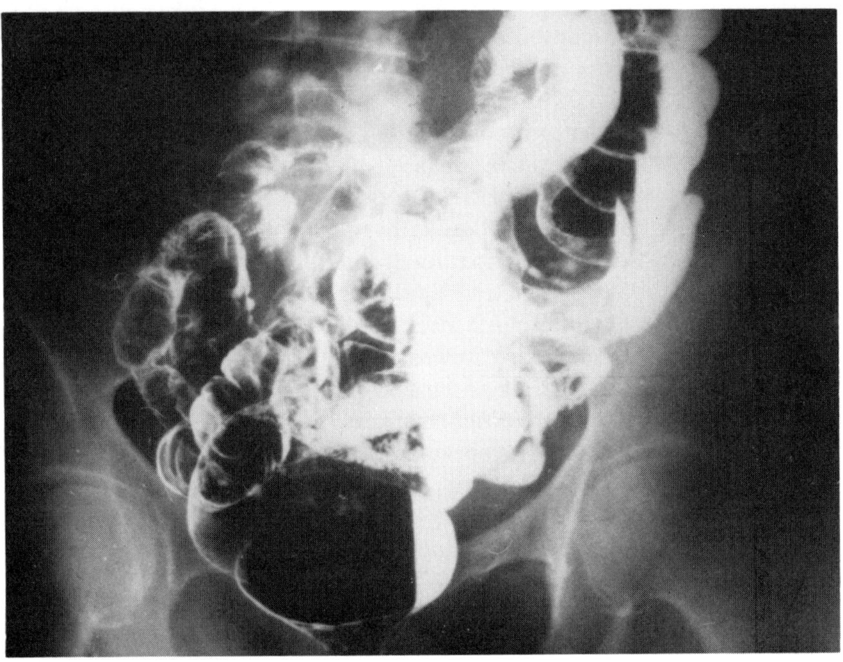

Fig. 8.10   A limitation of barium enema — overlapping of terminal ileum and redundant sigmoid colon.

Haemangiomas and angiodysplasia are by their nature flat on the mucosal surface, therefore invisible on barium enema and often poorly seen even on angiography. Most haemangiomas are visible in the rectum, colonoscopy only being helpful to define extent before surgery. Some vascular lesions may however be isolated and very small, either a red circular patch 5–7 mm in diameter or a characteristic 'spider' telangiectasis spreading from a central vessel. They are easily seen and unless these are very numerous may be lifted up and electrocoagulated using the 'hot-biopsy forceps' (Rogers, 1976).

Inflammatory bowel disease
Inflammatory bowel disease of any type is usually adequately assessed by conventional means of proctosigmoidoscopy, rectal biopsy and barium enema (Laufer, Mullens & Hamilton, 1976). In certain cases, such as those with absolute or relative rectal sparing or mild extensive disease, assessment can be very wrong and it is possible to have mild total colitis with a normal barium enema. Invariably however, there will be clinical features which will suggest this possibility, such as anaemia, raised sedimentation rate or mild abnormality of the rectal biopsy; it is unnecessary to colonoscope all patients with symptoms suggesting only a spastic colon.

Chronic extensive ulcerative colitis patients, with a somewhat increased risk of developing colon carcinoma, are suitable for surveillance by periodic colonoscopy with multiple mucosal biopsies in an attempt to demonstrate any evidence of dysplasia or early precancerous change (Lennard-Jones et al, 1977). An increasing number of centres report success in isolating seriously at-risk patients who are then submitted for prophylactic surgery, whereas about 90 per cent of patients appear to be at no obvious risk. Such studies are, however, still in the phase of academic assessment and not all pathologists have the requisite interest and skills. The endoscopist's role is primarily in taking biopsies; he will rarely see endoscopic evidence of any cancer or precancerous lesion since these are frequently intramucosal.

Crohn's disease, by its nature, is a patchy disorder which frequently spares the rectum and if the characteristic ulcers are superficial they are easily missed by the radiologist. In colour the red margin and white centre of a typical 'aphthoid' ulcer may be only 1–2 mm in diameter but have a characteristic appearance, being flat and set in an otherwise normal mucosa, which differentiates it from all other ulcerating conditions (such as infective colitis) which have more generalised inflammation with different ulcer appearance or distribution (Williams & Waye, 1978). Although the endoscopic appearance may be characteristic the biopsies rarely contain diagnostic granulomas, these being found in only 10 per cent in our overall experience, although in 25 per cent or more of patients in the early acute stage of the disease (Geboes & Vantrappen, 1975). It is therefore best to ensure that marginal biopsies are taken of the smallest ulcers seen and to anticipate difficulties in interpretation. It is also essential that the pathologist receives representative biopsies in *any* patient who may have inflammatory bowel disease, since diagnostic granulomas can be found unexpectedly even in an apparently typical example of 'ulcerative colitis'.

As with ulcerative colitis only selected patients with known or suspected Crohn's disease require colonoscopy, in those with deep ulcers or fissuring colonoscopy may even be hazardous. By contrast minor disease, doubtful abnormality in the terminal ileum or possible recurrent disease at a previous anastomosis may be more accurately assessed by colonoscopy than X-ray, although usually the radiologist will make the initial examination.

Polypectomy
The most important single justification for the role of colonoscopy lies in the non-operative management of colonic polyps for purposes of cancer prevention (Wolff & Shinya, 1978). Of polyps seen at colonoscopy, 80 per cent prove to be adenomas of which 4 per cent already contain invasive carcinoma (Gillespie et al, 1979) and 1 per cent are 'polypoid carcinomas', where malignant tissue completely displaces any previous adenoma (Muto, Bussey & Morson, 1975). Only polyps with a base or stalk over 2 cm diameter present any difficulty for snare removal, this may have to be in multiple portions in the largest lesions to avoid risks of bleeding or perforation. Only about 2 per cent of individual polyps prove to be endoscopically unremovable. The small numbers of patients found to have five or more adenomas should be treated with suspicion and every care taken to ensure that there are not many 1–3 mm tiny adenomas present which might suggest the need for surgical management. The endoscopic 'dye-spray' technique is useful for this purpose, layering a thin layer of

dilute blue dye or ink on the mucosa surface and showing up any tiny lesions for biopsy.

The technicalities of polypectomy rarely present a problem in the average 1–2 cm pedunculated polyp, and the procedure usually takes about 30 minutes on an outpatient basis. Electrocoagulation is visible after a short application of low-power (and inherently safe) diathermy current, which is not felt at all by the patient. The severed polyp head is conveniently retrieved using the snare loop or suction onto the instrument tip and pulled out for histological examination, multiple large polyps requiring multiple reinsertions, although smaller ones can be diathermied and sampled with 'hot-biopsy' (Williams, 1973) or sucked out into a trap in the suction line. Only when polyps of 2 cm or greater diameter are seen on the prior X-ray is the stalk likely to be large, with the possibility of bleeding; such patients are admitted overnight with blood available. If bleeding occurs this is usually immediately visible after transecting the stalk, which can be restrangulated with the snare. Secondary haemorrhage is very rare but may surprise the patient 5–14 days after removal of a large polyp; he should be warned of the possibility and the potential need for an emergency visit to hospital. During personal experience of over 1500 snare polypectomies only 12 patients required blood transfusion for haemorrhage, 3 of them eventually being submitted to operation; a single patient sustained bowel perforation during insertion of the instrument and there was no mortality. Compared to the inconvenience and the expected morbidity and mortality of operation on all patients with significant-sized polyps these results speak for themselves.

Many polyp patients are elderly and a poor operative risk. For this reason even when invasive carcinoma is found in the head of a polyp the pathologist may be able to prove that it has been adequately removed and that the risks of surgery are greater than the unlikely possibility of resectable metastases. Colonoscopy thus can sometimes resect 'early' colon cancer as well as help to prevent it or diagnose it earlier.

Paediatric colonoscopy

Rather surprisingly, total colonoscopy with a single-channel colonoscope is relatively easy for anyone with experience of adult colonoscopy, in children from the age of 2 years upwards (Burdelski, 1978); in babies it is usually desirable to have a small diameter instrument. General anaesthesia is unnecessary and after an oral or intramuscular premedication the usual valium/pethidine intravenous combination is given in a slightly reduced dose; the child will have total amnesia for the procedure.

Colonoscopy seems particualry justified in children with possible or probable inflammatory bowel disease, an increasingly common occurrence even in the 3- to 6-year-old range. Otherwise a general anaesthetic is given for sigmoidoscopy and rectal biopsy and a separate barium enema performed, usually of relatively poor quality since children are said not to tolerate the formal air-contrast technique well. During the colonoscopy biopsies and photographs are taken for documentation, including examination of the rectum with representative biopsies. Therapeutic polypectomy or electrocoagulation procedures are as easy in children as in adults.

Research applications

The colonoscope offers a new means of introducing tubes, balloons or electrodes into any part of the colon and the distal few centimetres of the terminal ileum. Biopsy specimens can be taken from any point for studies, such as immunofluorescence histochemistry, immunoassay or bacteriological culture. In addition, clinical, pharmaceutical, genetic and epidemiological studies can only benefit from the ability to visualise and sample small mucosal abnormalities at an early stage. Just as endoscopy is now the accepted way of monitoring ulcer-healing in the upper gastrointestinal tract limited colonoscopy with photography and biopsy may be the most logical way of assessing the response of conditions such as inflammatory bowel disease during drug future trials.

Fibre-sigmoidoscopy

The existence of fibre-sigmoidoscopes and the principles of limited bowel preparation and fibre-sigmoidoscopy have already been covered. The rigid proctosigmoidoscope, safe, cheap, quick and easy to use, will doubtless remain the method of choice for screening proctoscopy examinations of the anorectum and the taking of rectal biopsies. In 'high-risk' patients, however (including those with rectal bleeding, polyps, previous cancer surgery or a family history of colon cancer or polyposis) the slight extra trouble of fibre-sigmoidoscopy will be richly rewarded by a doubled or trebled yield of pathology in a relatively 'blind' area for the radiologist (Marks, 1978).

Fibre-sigmoidoscopy, reaching in a number of patients to the descending colon or splenic flexure without sedation and with a 60 cm instrument, takes only 5–6 minutes. As increasing numbers of physicians and surgeons are familiar with fibreoptic instruments the present technical difficulties will be overcome so that most gastrointestinal medical or surgical clinics will have an instrument available and keep back a few patients for examination at a suitable moment in the outpatient session. Already in some parts of the world there are enthusiasts (not always in private practice) who claim to be using the short fibreoptic instrument as a routine; before this is realistic in ordinary circumstances, the instruments will need to be easier to handle and clean, more robust, but also smaller and so more comfortable for the patient.

The future

Trials are in progress to evolve a self-propelled colonoscope, but this seems an unlikely prospect for the foreseeable future. Further modifications in instrument design will certainly occur, which will improve the insertion characteristics and accuracy of view, but some patients will remain difficult or impossible to examine.

As more clinicians become familiar with the possibilities and limitations of the colonoscope and the rewards for combining with high-quality barium enema, the two procedures will be increasingly linked; the combination of fibre-sigmoidoscopy to view the distal colon followed by immediate air-contrast films to show the overall appearance and proximal colon is humane and practical.

Patients requiring colonic investigation now have a number of possible preparation, medication and examination regimes available to them and for future investigations individual case records could be marked to indicate the most suitable combination on the basis of prior experience. The clinician needs to adopt a more flexible view of what can now be done in the colon, and to select colonoscopy and fibre-sigmoidoscopy for the many patients in whom it is indicated.

REFERENCES

Bigard M A, Gaucher P, Lassalle C 1979 Fatal colonic explosion during colonoscopic polypectomy. Gastroenterology 77: 1307–1310

Cotton P B, Williams C B 1980 Practical gastrointestinal endoscopy. Blackwell Scientific Publications, London

Fruhmorgen P, Demling L 1979 Complications of diagnostic and therapeutic colonoscopy in the Federal Republic of Germany. Results of an enquiry. Endoscopy II: 146

Geboes K, Vantrappen G 1975 The value of colonoscopy in the diagnosis of Crohn's disease. Gastrointestinal Endoscopy 22: (1) 18–23

Gillespie P E, Chambers T I, Chan K W, Doronzo F, Morson B C, Williams C B 1979 Colonic adenomas — a colonoscopic survey. Gut 20: 240–245

Hunt R H 1978 Colonoscopy in unexplained rectal bleeding. Clinics in Gastroentrology 7: 685

Hunt R H, Teague R H, Swarbrick E T, Williams C B 1975 Colonoscopy in the management of colonic strictures. British Medical Journal 2: 360–361

Laufer I, Mullens J E, Hamilton J 1976 Correlation of endoscopy and double contrast radiography in the early stages of ulcerative and granulomatous colitis. Radiology 118: 1–5

Lennard-Jones J E, Morson B C, Ritchie J K, Shove D C, Williams C B 1977 Cancer in colitis — assessment of the individual risk by clinical and histological criteria. Gastroenterology 7: 1280–1289

Marks G, Boggs W, Castro A F, Gathright J B, Ray J E, Salvati E 1979 Sigmoidoscopic examinations with rigid and flexible fibreoptic sigmoidoscopes in the surgeons' office. Diseases of the colon and rectum 22: (3) 162

Muto T, Bussey H J R, Morson B C (1975) The evolution of cancer in colon and rectum. Cancer 36: 2251–2270

Nuesch H J, Kobler E, Jenny S, Sauberli H, Deyhle P 1976 Emergency coloscopy. Acta Endoscopica 6: 161–163

Rogers B H G, Adler F 1976 Haemangiomas of the caecum. Gastroenterology 71: (6) 1079–82

Rogers B H G, Silvis S E, Nebel O T, Sugawa C, Mandelstam P 1975. Complications of flexible fibreoptic colonoscopy and polypectomy. Gastrointestinal Endoscopy 22: 73–77

Rossini F P, Ferrari A 1976 Emergency coloscopy Acta Endoscopica 6: 165–168

Tedesco F J, Waye J D, Raskin J B, Morris S J, Greenwald R A, 1978 Colonoscopic evaluation of rectal bleeding: a study of 304 patients. Annals of Internal Medicine 89: 907–909

Theuerkauf F J 1978 Rectal and colonic polyps relationships via colonoscopy and fibre-sigmoidoscopy. Diseases of the colon and rectum, 21: 2–7

Thoeni R F, Menuck L 1977 Comparison of barium enema and colonoscopy in the detection of small colonic polyps. Radiology 124: 631–635

Williams C B, Waye J D 1978 Colonoscopy in inflammatory bowel disease, Clinics in Gastroenterology 7: 701–717

Williams J T, Thomson J P S 1977 Ano-rectal bleeding: study of causes and investigative yields. The Practitioner 329: 327

Wolff W I, Shinya H 1975) Definitive treatment of malignant polyps of the colon. Annals of Surgery 182: 516–525

8.3 Bronchoscopy

Stewart W. Clarke

Hippocrates first suggested intubation for asphyxia and Killian implemented this suggestion by removing a foreign body through a rigid open tube bronchoscope 25 centuries later, in 1897. Latterly the rigid bronchoscope has been used chiefly for the diagnosis of lung cancer.

The flexible fibreoptic bronchoscope was developed in Japan after the gastroscope and was introduced to Western practice in the early 1970s, first in the USA, then in Europe. This has stimulated much renewed interest in bronchoscopy which has recently been widely reviewed in a supplement of Chest (1978).

RIGID BRONCHOSCOPY

The standard rigid bronchoscope (Fig. 8.11) is about 40 cm in length and 7 to 11 mm in diameter for adults with smaller models for children. The basic open tube has changed little since its inception. However, the various attachments have been

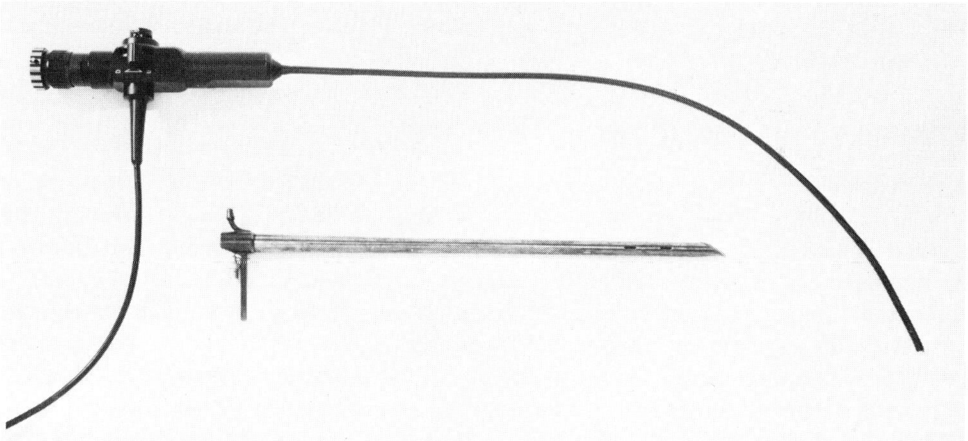

Fig. 8.11 Rigid and fibreoptic bronchoscopes.

improved with distal illumination often with a fibreoptic light-carrier bundle, built-in instrument channels through which suction tubes can be inserted, and ventilation connections. Additionally telescopes have been greatly improved giving forward oblique (30 degree) and lateral (90 degree) views. In particular the Hopkins (Storz) telescopes utilising a new rod lens optical system give an outstanding view.

Most bronchoscopists using this instrument now do so with the patient fully anaesthetised, local anaesthesia being too uncomfortable for the patient. It is often said that few if any patients ever had more than one rigid bronchoscopy under local anaesthesia. Ventilation is carried out using the Sanders intermittent positive-pressure venturi system (Carden, 1978) which has revolutionised the technique permitting controlled ventilation and avoiding the previous 'smash and grab' apnoeic manoeuvre. Insertion is usually accomplished with the patient lying supine and the neck hyperextended. The operator stands or sits at the head end of the patient and introduces the bronchoscope into the right side of the mouth lifting the cricoid cartilage forward, indentifying the larynx and thence passing the tube down the trachea. Passage may be difficult in patients with a short thick neck, small mouth or prominent teeth or in those with diseases of the spine such as cervical spondylosis or ankylosing spondylitis. Other relative contraindications are severe heart disease, aortic aneurysm, metastases of the cervical spine, neck deformities and general poor condition (Sackner, 1975).

Complications of rigid bronchoscopy include haemorrhage, bronchial or tracheal perforation, subglottic oedema, bronchospasm and loss or breakage of instruments (e.g. swabs, forceps). Several of these complications are the results of introducing a straight rigid tube down a canal which has a right angled bend (the oropharynx) at its origin and for this reason rigid bronchoscopy requires a high degree of technical skill.

The rigid bronchoscope allows satisfactory visualisation and biopsy of the bronchial tree to the level of the origins of the segmental lower lobe bronchi. However, only the orifice and 0.5–1 cm of the inferior aspect of the right and left upper lobe bronchi may be seen and their segmental orifices inspected through the right angled telescope. A biopsy can be done simply in the lower lobe and now also in the upper lobe with the Storz deflecting device and flexible biopsy forceps which can be angled at 90° with the telescope in place.

FLEXIBLE FIBREOPTIC BRONCHOSCOPY

The flexible fibreoptic bronchoscope has been developed into a refined instrument (Fig. 8.11) with a mobile tip remotely controlled from the body of the instrument and a centre channel for injection of saline or lignocaine, or for instance aspiration of secretions or the passage of the biopsy forceps. Tip deflection ranges from 130°–180°, the higher figure being usually in one direction only (Berci, 1978). The instrument has a viewing eyepiece with adjustable focus and a collar for attachment of a parallel teaching 'scope or camera. A lever at the hub controls bidirectional tip flexion which combined with rotation allows precise angulation and location in the bronchial tree. Illumination is provided by a remote cold light source transmitted along non-coherent (non-aligned) fibre bundles to the tip. The object thus illuminated can be seen by the observer through coherent (aligned) fibre bundles transmitting the image to the eye without distortion. The view is better than that seen directly through the rigid bronchoscope though not as good as that through the telescope since the interface between the multiple glass fibres gives a coarse-grain appearance which is emphasised on photographs taken through the fibreoptic instrument. However, the depth of insertion is much greater than with the rigid bronchoscope and includes the upper lobes, an area hitherto difficult to explore.

Technique
At first the fibreoptic bronchoscope was introduced through the rigid bronchoscope as a flexible telescope. This technique has proved too cumbersome for routine use and it now has few advocates.

Transnasal insertion
The majority of fibreoptic bronchoscopists (60 per cent) favour the transnasal route (Clarke, 1977) possibly the simplest and most satisfactory method. The patient is carefully evaluated beforehand, with appropriate chest X-rays and simple pulmonary function tests (Forced Expired Volume in one second, FEV_1, Peak Expiratory Flow Rate, PEFR). After a four-hour fast, premedication with Onmopon (papaveretum) 10–20 mg and Scopolamine (hyoscine) 0.2–0.4 mg is given intramuscularly one hour before bronchoscopy. Onmopon produces analgesia, sedation and useful suppression of the cough reflex while Scopolamine (or atropine) blocks vagal activity, dries secretions and diminishes the chance of vagally induced cardiac dysrrhythmia. Pethidine and atropine may be used in the hypoxic or elderly patient in whom respiratory depression should be avoided. Intravenous diazepam may be required occasionally.

The procedure is described fully to the patients since they are conscious and must co-operate throughout. The preferred position is with the patient supine at 45° on a couch, the bronchoscopist standing in front and to the right hand of the patient. Some prefer the patient flat and to stand behind while others prefer a dental chair. The nose, pharynx and larynx are anaesthetised with lignocaine aerosol, which is unpalatable but effective.

The bronchoscope is checked, the shaft lubricated with lignocaine gel 2 per cent, and then passed under direct vision through the inferior meatus of the nose the nasopharynx behind the epiglottis and onto the larynx. Thereafter 4 per cent lignocaine (2 ml) is injected through the centre channel to anaesthetise the vocal cords. The bronchoscope is gently inserted through the open cords during deep breathing with a no-touch technique to avoid coughing. The trachea and bronchi are anaesthetised with 2 per cent lignocaine to minimize cough and discomfort. Local anaesthetic applied to the pharynx, larynx and tracheobronchial mucosa is absorbed rapidly, giving peak blood levels 10 to 15 minutes later comparable with those achieved by intravenous injection (Perry, 1978). These levels are rarely toxic, however, if the dose is less than 200–400 mg.

The vocal cords are inspected carefully during quiet breathing and phonation, whereupon cord paralysis can be seen clearly. After passing through the cords the trachea is inspected, then the carina for sharpness and mobility during deep breathing and coughing; fixity can be seen without the need to probe the carina, a point often doubted by rigid bronchoscopists. Thereafter the right main, upper lobe, middle lobe and lower lobe bronchi are inspected distally to segmental level followed by a similar routine on the left side. The site of any suspected lesion is scrutinized particularly keenly and appropriate biopsies taken (usually 3–6 of either forceps, brush or both) together with a routine sputum trap specimen from the suction line. Secretions and blood can be aspirated often helped by lavage with sterile saline (5–10 ml). Despite the small size of the centre channel (2–2.6 mm) with high pressures, fluid can be aspirated at more than 1 l/min^{-1} and oxygen delivered at more than 8 l/min^{-1} if required. The procedure takes an average of 30 minutes depending on the nature of the problem. The patient can drink about one hour later after the local anaesthetic has worn off and leave the hospital escorted two to four hours later, if a day case.

The side effects include adverse reaction to the premedication or lignocaine, haemoptysis, laryngospasm, bronchospasm and postbronchoscopy fever. These are uncommon and often due to poor technique. In a series of 25 000 cases, Credle, Smiddy & Elliot (1974) noted an incidence of complications of 0.2 per cent minor, 0.08 per cent major and 0.01 per cent mortality.

To check patient acceptability, Johnson, Hodson & Clarke (1978) asked 60 patients to complete a questionnaire; 27 per cent found it not unpleasant, 55 per cent mildly so and 18 per cent very, nasal pain being the major complaint (37 per cent). However, 77 per cent of patients thought a repeat acceptable if indicated.

Transoral insertion
Some bronchoscopists prefer the transoral route either passing the bronchoscope directly or through an endotracheal tube. For instance, this is the commonest method in Japan, though only accounting for 20 per cent in the USA (Credle et al, 1974). The 'transoral' exponents argue that while it is no less acceptable it is appreciably safer, enabling the bronchoscope to be withdrawn and reinserted easily in the event of fogging or blockage and ensuring a patent airway should haemorrhage be severe. These views are not born out in practice. Moreover, direct transoral is less easy than transnasal insertion since the tip of the bronchoscope slides around the oropharynx causing discomfort and gagging.

Other methods
With general anaesthesia the bronchoscope may be inserted through the endotracheal tube ($>8.5\,mm$ diameter) via a T-piece and examination easily done, though flexibility is somewhat impaired by the endotracheal tube. Similarly in the intensive care unit with a ventilated patient bronchoscopy can be done easily for bronchial toilet.

Comparison of rigid and fibreoptic bronchoscopy
There are few valid direct comparisons between rigid and fibreoptic bronchoscopy since the former is used mainly by surgeons and the latter by physicians. At the Brompton Hospital the number of rigid and fibreoptic bronchoscopies were comparable from 1st July, 1974 till 30th June, 1975. Subsequently the number of fibreoptic bronchoscopies has increased by five to sixfold over rigid bronchoscopies (Fig. 8.12). Taking the criteria of a positive bronchial biopsy in patients with lung cancer, Webb & Clarke (1980) found positive histology in 72 per cent of fibreoptic and 51 per cent rigid. The improved yield was chiefly for upper lobe lesions, reflecting the flexibility of the fibreoptic bronchoscope, while the size of the biopsy forceps seemed to have no effect. These figures confirm the superiority of the fibreoptic bronchoscope. Removal of foreign bodies and severe haemorrhage may require rigid bronchoscopy still.

INDICATIONS FOR BRONCHOSCOPY

The introduction of the fibreoptic bronchoscope with a simplified technique and better vision has led to a widening of the indications for bronchoscopy. Hitherto the

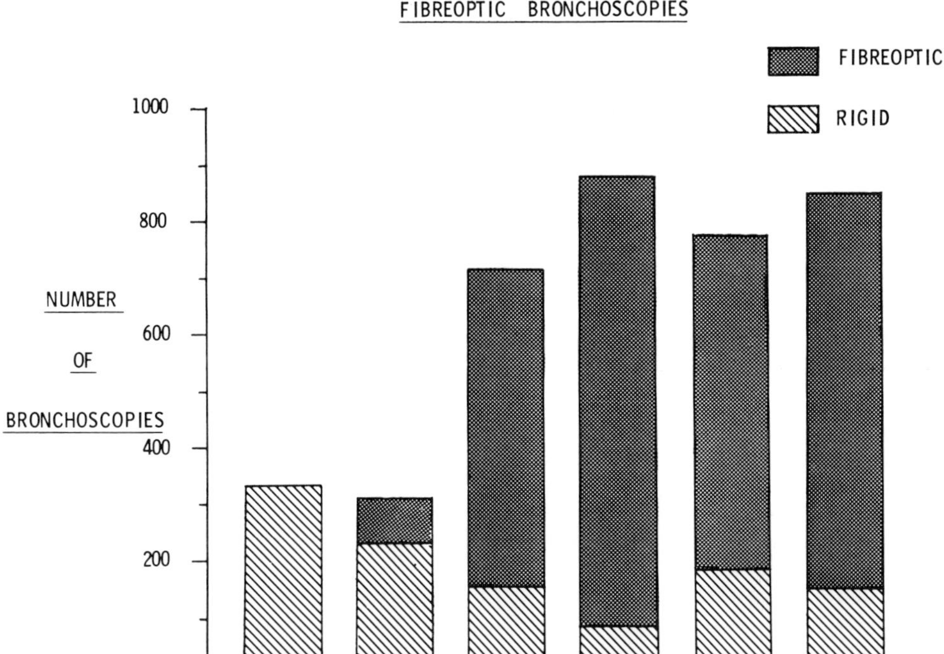

Fig. 8.12   Number of rigid and fibreoptic bronchoscopies in a six-year period at the Brompton Hospital.

investigation was used chiefly for the diagnosis of bronchial carcinoma and occasionally for foreign body removal and aspiration — surgical bronchoscopy. Now many other lung conditions for which surgery has no role can be investigated easily — medical bronchoscopy.

Symptomatic presentation

In a representative series of patients (Knight & Clarke, 1979) the major presenting symptoms were cough 38 per cent with sputum in 25 per cent, haemoptysis 36 per cent, chest pain 27 per cent, dyspnoea 27 per cent wheezing 7 per cent malaise 7 per cent and no symptoms in 3 per cent.

Cough is a reserve protective mechanism augmenting mucociliary clearance from the central regions of the bronchial tree. Common causes of cough include upper and lower respiratory infection, chronic bronchitis and bronchial asthma. However, cough may be a feature of bronchial carcinoma, adenoma, lung collapse or inhaled foreign body. Therefore, in any patient in whom cough is persistent and unexplained, bronchoscopy should be considered in the light of the clinical examination and chest X-ray findings.

Sputum production if unexplained is an indication for smear, culture and cytology and possible bronchoscopy.

Haemoptysis is commonly caused by respiratory infection and chronic bronchitis. Nevertheless, in high-risk smokers (> 20 cigarettes daily and > 45 years of age) this symptom may be the hallmark of bronchial carcinoma. Examination at the time of haemoptysis may be useful since blood may be tracked to the site of origin at least to segmental level. This is particularly valuable if the chest X-ray is clear. With more profuse haemoptysis it may be difficult to keep the field clear to determine the site of origin, particularly so if the patient is coughing. In these cases elective bronchoscopy should be done later. Other causes of haemoptysis include bronchiectasis, pulmonary infarction, pulmonary hypertension and mycetoma.

Chest pain in lung disease is usually pleuritic in type or dull and poorly defined when involving lung parenchyma, hilar regions or mediastinal structures. Of itself it does not constitute a definite indication for bronchoscopy.

Dyspnoea is commonly present with heart failure, severe airways obstruction or significant lung collapse and as such it is usually associated with other clinical and radiographic features necessitating bronchoscopy.

Wheeze is not always due to asthma and a high degree of suspicion should be retained particularly if features are atypical or if in fact the noise is stridor indicating upper airways obstruction. Spirometry may also help in defining this symptom though bronchoscopy is the definitive investigation.

In the same series other presenting symptoms include weight loss, voice change (laryngeal paralysis), superior vena caval obstruction, arthralgia, night sweats, neurological symptoms and unexplained finger clubbing.

Radiographic presentation

The findings on chest X-ray often constitute the main indication for bronchoscopy. Thus Knight & Clarke (1979) found a 'shadow' in 45 per cent, a mass-lesion in 22 per cent, an area of collapse in 17 per cent, old pulmonary tuberculosis in 12 per cent, a normal chest X-ray in 11 per cent and pleural effusion in 6 per cent of their patients.

Of particular interest are the 11 per cent of patients in whom chest X-ray was normal and it should be remembered that by no means is this investigation infallible since central bronchial or early more peripheral tumours may fail to show. In these cases a high index of suspicion is required. Old pulmonary tuberculosis is often a source of disquiet since haemoptysis may occur with minor intercurrent infection or occasionally reactivation; the lesion may shed squamous cells also and lead to scar cancer.

A visual diagnosis of inflammatory change was made in 28 per cent, tumour 26 per cent, normal bronchial tree 22 per cent, bronchial stenosis 9 per cent, mucus plugging or hypersecretion 5 per cent, crowding or distortion of bronchi 3 per cent, and localised bleeding 3 per cent. Endobronchial tuberculosis and sarcoidosis, bronchial adenoma, tracheobronchomegaly, tracheopathea-osteoplastica, mycetoma and extrinsic compression were also seen.

Biopsy results yielded normal tissue in 25 per cent, tumour in 23 per cent, inflammatory tissue in 7 per cent, squamous metaplasia in 5 per cent, tuberculosis in 2 per cent and sarcoidosis in 1 per cent. The results of brush biopsy were less impressive since on the vast majority of occasions forceps biopsy alone was undertaken. In some centres brushings may give the highest single yield (Kvale, Bode & Kini, 1976) while in others the majority of diagnoses depend on forceps biopsies (Zavala, 1975). With the combination of multiple prebronchoscopic sputum examinations followed by bronchoscopy with biopsy, brush and sputum trap the diagnosis should be made in almost 100 per cent of patients with lung cancer, (Kvale, 1978).

With respect to bacteriology, whichever way the bronchoscope is passed the tip will be contaminated by commensals from the upper airways. Further the local anaesthetic appears to inhibit bacterial growth (including tuberculosis). This may explain the low yield of pathogens in most studies. Careful technique with a special shielded brush yields better results (Wimberley, Faling & Bartlett, 1979). Nevertheless this is a good method for diagnosing opportunistic infection with Pneumocystis carinii for instance (Kvale, 1978).

Transbronchial lung biopsy (Fig. 8.13)
This technique has been facilitated by the introduction of the fibreoptic broncho-scope. The method of insertion is the same with the exception that the patient lies flat under a fluoroscope which is used to guide the biopsy forceps. In diffuse lung disease the forceps are advanced fully, then withdrawn 2 cm and opened, being advanced during deep inspiration and closed at end-expiration, before being withdrawn (Stableforth & Clarke, 1977). Several specimens may be taken from different sites on the same side. For localised lesions larger than 2 cm in diameter the forceps may be positioned accurately by rotating the fluoroscope or patient though lesions of this size lie at the limits of the technique. Lung tissue can be recognised by its tendency to fluff on suspension whereas bronchial tissue is denser and sinks.

Transbronchial biopsy should be attempted with caution in uncooperative patients, uraemic patients and in those with uncorrected bleeding disorders or in whom increased hypoxaemia would be a major risk despite supplemental nasal O_2.

Stableforth et al (1978) reported 55 patients who underwent transbronchial biopsy. Lung or tumour tissue was obtained in all with diagnostic histology in 35 (64 per cent) and either normal lung tissue or tissue showing non-specific changes in 20 (36 per cent). The usual complications of haemorrhage (50 ml) were seen in 1 patient (2 per cent) and pneumothorax in none. Dividing the patients into those with diffuse or local disease, a histological diagnosis was obtained in 78 per cent of the former but only 50 per cent of the latter. With diffuse shadowing sarcoidosis was predominant followed by carcinoma either primary or secondary, fibrosing alveolitis, eosinophilic pneumo-nia, extrinsic allergic alveolitis, eosinophilic granuloma, asbestosis, pneumoconiosis, and Pneumocystis pneumonia. With localised shadowing carcinoma was first followed by irradiation fibrosis, pulmonary tuberculosis and organising pneumonia. These figures are broadly in agreement with those quoted by Zavala (1978).

This is a very useful technique and is probably the safest and best means of undertaking lung biopsy. The drawbacks are the small amount of tissue obtained and the degree of crush artefact which may make distinction between the different types of fibrosing alveolitis for instance rather difficult. For this reason open or drill lung biopsy may be preferred if indications are sufficiently strong. Stableforth et al (1978) give a useful comparative list of current lung biopsy methods.

Herf, Suratt & Arora (1977) reviewing the deaths and complications associated with

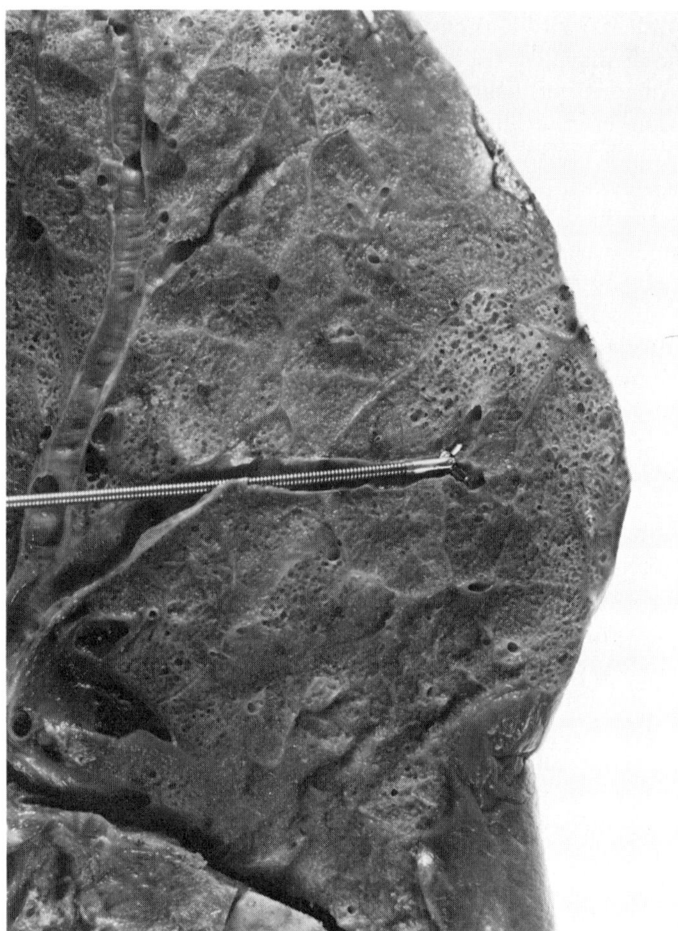

Fig. 8.13 Transbronchial lung biopsy — showing forceps positioned in a post-mortem lung. (Reproduced by permission of the Editor of the British Journal of Hospital Medicine.)

transbronchial biopsy in multiple centres in North America noted pneumothorax in 5.5 per cent and haemorrhage (> 50 ml) in 1.3 per cent of patients, accounting for nine deaths (0.2 per cent) of whom eight had coagulation disorders. Full coagulation studies and the platelet count should be obtained and the deficiencies corrected in all patients before the procedure.

SPECIFIC INDICATIONS FOR FIBREOPTIC BRONCHOSCOPY

Early diagnosis of lung cancer with normal chest X-ray
In this group rigid bronchoscopy may fail to visualise the lesion unless it is central and fibreoptic bronchoscopy require a time consuming search with a series of careful brushings and microbiopsies from the segmental and lobar spurs (subcarinae) (Marsh et al, 1978). Sanderson et al (1974) described 13 patients in all of whom fibreoptic bronchoscopy demonstrated the lesion, 6 requiring repeat bronchoscopy and 3

showing multiple tumours. Marsh et al (1978) studied 33 patients. In 4 the source was the upper respiratory tract (1 nasopharynx and 3 larynx), in 21 a segmental bronchus, and in 5 the lobar or main bronchus. In the remaining 3 patients the origin remained obscure. The segmental bronchus may be an important site of a small early carcinoma or lesion in situ appearing as an area of slight roughening only, often almost undistinguishable from bronchoscopic trauma. Localised friability, loss of mucosal sheen, thickening and irregularity of the bronchial spurs, or interruption distortion or obliteration of the normal longitudinal folds, may all indicate an early carcinoma. Furthermore the extent in situ may be more widespread than actually visible. These lesions appear to hold a good prognosis though proof positive of this is awaited. Nevertheless, early localisation with the fibreoptic bronchoscope is being emphasised.

Lung cancer may be staged by repeat bronchoscopy during the therapeutic regime and knowledge of the individual response may produce more precise effective treatment.

Diagnosis of sarcoidosis

Sarcoidosis is a relatively common disease presenting most often with bilateral hilar lymphadenopathy (BHL) with or without radiographic lung shadowing. The differential diagnosis includes tuberculous lymphadenopathy or lymphoma and in either case the distinction is important though obtaining histological proof may be difficult. Recent reports have suggested a high histological yield (> 90 per cent) with fibreoptic bronchoscopy and transbronchial lung biopsy in cases with BHL and lung shadowing (Koerner et al, 1975); however, this figure falls to 44–55 per cent with BHL and clear lung fields (Poe et al, 1979). Endobronchial plaques of sarcoid tissue may be seen in the absence of parenchymal chest X-ray changes often leading to cough and occasional wheeze. Relatively normal looking bronchial mucosa may yield granulomata and random biopsy is useful. This has now become the method of choice for the histological confirmation of most cases of sarcoidosis.

Bronchopulmonary lavage in treatment and diagnosis

Bronchopulmonary lavage was first used for treating pneumonia, then bronchiectasis, chronic bronchitis, cystic fibrosis, lung abscess and bronchial asthma. With earlier techniques lavage was performed through an endotracheal tube, a Carlens bronchospirometry catheter or a rigid bronchoscope with the patient anaesthetized and ventilated, using varying volumes of saline (50 ml to 10 l) and additives such as acetylcysteine, heparin and sodium iodide (Ramirez, 1966). The benefits of this treatment in pulmonary alveolar proteinosis for instance are considerable (Editorial, 1979). With the other conditions improvement is debatable and the technique not without hazard.

Segmental lavage through the fibreoptic bronchoscope, as suggested by Sackner (1975), has the merit of direct vision and the safety of local anaesthesia. It can be done routinely at diagnostic bronchoscopy using aliquots of 5–10 ml saline to wash out secretions including mucus plugs, often asthmatic or aspergillotic in origin. Additionally, lavage can be safely done in acute severe asthmatics refractory to other intensive treatment or in more chronic severe asthmatics, though the documented results are sparse and inconclusive. Nevertheless, at times the removal of mucus plugs may be life saving.

More recently there has been a surge of interest in the diagnostic value of bronchopulmonary lavage, whereby living lung cells can be obtained with a relatively non-invasive technique. Using five 60 ml aliquots of saline Davis et al (1976) found an average cell yield of 12×10^6 in non-smokers (consisting of 93 per cent macrophages, 60 per cent lymphocytes and 1 per cent polymorphs) and 25×10^6 in smokers. The scavenging and secretory activities of alveolar macrophages, their interaction with lymphocytes and the effects of drugs (e.g. halothane and lignocaine) and noxious agents (e.g. bacterial endotoxins and tobacco smoke) can be investigated. Serial samples can be obtained to assess the state of cellular and humoral lung defences against inhaled allergens, bacteria, inorganic particles, drugs and smoking. Finally lavage may give useful information additional to lung biopsy (transbronchial or other type) or even provide an alternative method of diagnosis in diffuse pulmonary diseases such as sarcoidosis, fibrosing alveolitis and pneumoconiosis. For instance an increase in lavage lymphocytes appears to predict a favourable corticosteroid response, while an increase in eosinophils and/or neutrophils alone predicts failure, in cryptogenic fibrosing alveolitis (Haslam et al, 1980). Lavage cell profiles may be valuable therefore in selecting therapy.

Diagnosis of opportunistic infections
Bronchoscopy may be used to make a firm diagnosis in lung infections when conventional tests including sputum examination, transtracheal aspiration and serological tests have failed and the patient is deteriorating despite intensive treatment. However, the technique is particularly useful with opportunistic infection in the compromised host such as the patient immunosuppressed after renal or bone marrow transplantation or undergoing cytotoxic chemotherapy for cancer or lymphoma. Often the presentation is insidious with fever, minimal chest symptoms such as cough and scant sputum and diffuse lung shadowing. The differential diagnosis includes Pneumocystis carinii pneumonia, candidiasis, aspergillosis, tuberculosis and other infiltrative lung conditions and pulmonary oedema.

The standard bronchoscopy technique is used with brush and transbronchial lung biopsy. There is an overall positive diagnostic rate of about 74 per cent (Cunningham et al, 1977) though in individual conditions this varies widely with up to 100 per cent for Pneumocystis pneumonia. It is now the method of choice in confirming the diagnosis in these patients and is preferable to percutaneous aspiration which has a much higher risk of pneumothorax. Particularly care must be taken in handling the specimens (Kvale, 1978) and close liaison with the laboratories is necessary.

Training (Sackner, 1975)
Fibreoptic bronchoscopy is relatively easy to learn. The average doctor needs about three months training, starting with practice in a model bronchial tree to familiarize himself with the instrument. He should then attend a series of bronchoscopies (including transbronchial biopsy) viewing through a parallel teaching attachment before undertaking one himself. After doing 50 bronchoscopies under supervision he should be reasonably competent. Often passage through the nose or mouth is the hardest part to master. In practice junior staff coming afresh to the technique learn quickly. Those experienced in rigid bronchoscopy learn slowly, often trying to graft the fibreoptic technique onto the rigid technique. In fact, the two techniques are quite

dissimilar though the bronchial tree is common to both. Spacial orientation within the bronchial tree is particularly important with the fibreoptic bronchoscope and an effort must be made to relate the position of the tip to the fixed landmarks particularly the carina, the right and left main bronchi and the posterior longitudinal muscle and anterior cartilaginous rings. The tip of the bronchoscope can then be located precisely whatever the position of the patient and bronchoscopist.

Cost

The fibreoptic bronchoscope is more expensive and less durable than the rigid instrument. Nevertheless, when assessing its cost-effectiveness the simplicity of the technique and the ability to do it as an outpatient procedure must be born in mind. Rigid bronchoscopy involves theatre facilities, anaesthetists and usually bed occupancy all of which involve expensive resources. A previous comparison (Clarke, 1977) yielded a relatively low figure for the cost of this investigation comparable with chest tomography for instance.

Research

Fibreoptic bronchoscopy has stimulated lung research. Tracheal mucus velocity can be measured either with teflon discs inserted and observed through the bronchoscope (Sackner, 1975) or with radioactive particles inserted alone and monitored by external counters (Chopra et al, 1979). Regional gas exchange can be measured by precise placement of the bronchoscope tip and may have clinical application where lung surgery is contemplated (Williams et al, 1979). Alveolar cell physiopathology may be studied after lavage as discussed above. The fibreoptic bronchoscope has provided a simple means of entrée into the lung which should continue to stimulate a wide variety of further research.

REFERENCES

Berci G 1978 Flexible fiber and rigid (pediatric) bronchoscopic instrumentation and documentation. Chest 73: supplement, 768–775

Carden E 1978 Recent improvements in techniques for general anaesthesia for bronchoscopy. Chest 73: supplement, 697–700

Chest 1978 Diagnostic and therapeutic applications of the bronchoscope. 73: supplement, 685–778

Chopra S K, Taplin G V, Elam D, Carson S A, Golde D 1979 Measurement of tracheal mucociliary transport velocity in humans — smokers versus non-smokers (preliminary findings). American Review of Respiratory Disease 119: 205

Clarke S W 1977 Medical bronchoscopy — using the fibreoptic bronchoscope. In: Besser G M (ed) Advanced medicine, 13th edn. Pitman Medical, Tunbridge Wells, p 230–248

Credle W F, Smiddy J F, Elliott, R C 1974 Complications of fibreoptic bronchoscopy. American Review of Respiratory Disease, 109: 67–72

Cunningham J H, Zavala D C, Corry R J, Keim L W 1977 Trephine air drill, bronchial brush, fiberoptic transbronchial lung biopsies in immunosuppressed patients. American Review of Respiratory Disease 115: 213–220

Davis G S, Brody A R, Landis J N, Graham W G B, Craighead J E, Green G M 1976 Quantitation of inflammatory activity in interstitial pneumonitis by bronchofiberscopic pulmonary lavage. Chest 69: supplement 265–266

Editorial 1979 Bronchopulmonary lavage. British Medical Journal 2: 690

Haslam P L, Turton C W G, Heard B, Lukoszek A, Collins J V, Salsbury A J, Turner-Warwick M 1980 Bronchoalveolar lavage in pulmonary fibrosis: comparison of cells obtained with lung biopsy and clinical features. Thorax 35: 9–18

Herf S M, Suratt P M, Arora N S 1977 Deaths and complications associated with transbronchial lung biopsy. American Review of Respiratory Diseases 115: 708–711

Johnson N McI, Hodson M E, Clarke S W 1978 Acceptability of fibreoptic bronchoscopy under local anaesthesia. The Practitioner 221: 113–114

Knight R K, Clarke S W 1979 An analysis of the first 300 fibreoptic bronchoscopies at the Brompton Hospital. British Journal of Diseases of the Chest 73: 113–120

Koerner S K, Sakowitz A J, Appelman R I, Becker N H, Shoenbaum S W 1975 Transbronchial lung biopsy for the diagnosis of sarcoidosis. New England Journal of Medicine 293: 268–270

Kvale P A, Bode F R, Kini S 1976 Diagnostic accuracy in lung cancer: Comparison of techniques used in association with flexible fiberoptic bronchoscopy. Chest 69: 752–757

Kvale P A 1978 Collection and preparation of bronchoscopic specimens. Chest 73: supplement 707–712

Marsh B R, Frost J K, Erozan Y S, Carter D 1978 Diagnosis of early bronchogenic carcinoma. Chest 73: supplement 716–717

Perry L B 1978 Topical anaesthesia for bronchoscopy. Chest 73: supplement 691–693

Poe R H, Israel R H, Utell M J, Hall W J 1979 Probability of a positive transbronchial lung biopsy result in sarcoidosis. Archives of Internal Medicine 139: 761–763

Ramirez R J 1966 Bronchopulmonary lavage — new techniques and observations. Diseases of the Chest 50: 581–588

Sackner M A 1975 Bronchofiberscopy. American Review of Respiratory Disease 111: 62–88

Sanderson D R, Fontana R S, Woolner L B, Bernatz P E, Payne W S 1974 Bronchoscopic localization of radiographically occult lung cancer. Chest 65: 608–612

Stableforth D E, Clarke S W 1977 Transbronchial biopsy through the flexible fibreoptic bronchoscope. British Journal of Hospital Medicine 18: 460–466

Stableforth D E, Knight R K, Collins J V, Heard B E, Clarke S W 1978 Transbronchial lung biopsy through the fibreoptic bronchoscope. British Journal of Diseases of the Chest 72: 108–114

Webb J, Clarke S W 1980 A comparison of biopsy results using rigid and fibreoptic bronchoscopes. British Journal of Diseases of the Chest 74: 81–83

Williams S J, Pierce R J, Davies N J H, Denison D M 1979 Methods of studying lobar and segmental function of the lung in man. British Journal of Diseases of the Chest 73: 97–112

Wimberley N, Faling L J, Bartlett J G 1979 A fiberoptic bronchoscopy technique to obtain uncontaminated lower airways secretions for bacterial culture. American Review of Respiratory Disease 119: 337–343

Zavala D C 1975 Diagnostic fiberoptic bronchoscopy: Techniques and results of biopsy in 600 patients. Chest 68: 12–19

Zavala D C 1978 Transbronchial biopsy in diffuse lung disease. Chest 73: supplement 727–733

9.1 Immune complexes in disease

B. A. Pussell

Immune complexes are antigen–antibody aggregates that are formed as part of an immune response and in this respect they represent a humoral mechanism for the elimination of circulating antigen and are therefore physiological. Immune complex disease results from the deposition of immune complexes in tissues not normally responsible for their clearance. The ensuing inflammation and altered function occurs as a result of a common pathological mechanism which is mostly independent of the type of antigen initiating such responses. The first part of this chapter considers the reasons for the diversity of clinical manifestations of immune complex disease. Although exact mechanisms are unknown the complexity of clinical manifestations is reflected by the complexity of the antigen–antibody interaction at the immuno-chemical level.

The second part of this chapter will deal with tests for immune complexes used in diagnosis and management. Recent advances in technology have led to the development of a large number of tests which measure immune complexes in the sera of patients in a variety of diseases.

ROLE OF IMMUNE COMPLEXES IN DISEASE

The concept of circulating immune complexes causing disease arose from the classical experiments on acute and chronic serum sickness in rabbits (Dixon, Feldman & Vazques, 1961). However, today, many diseases with varied clinical manifestations are labelled immune complex disorders and it is necessary to review some of the immune complex diseases in experimental animals and in man to determine the serological and pathological findings that justify a variety of disorders being included in this category. The heterogeneity of these disease manifestations may be explained by a multitude of factors including the nature of the immune complex, the biological properties of the complex, the host response and the fate of the complex. By a consideration of all these factors it may be possible to gain insight into the origin of such heterogeneity.

Pathogenicity of immune complexes

Acute serum sickness
Although von Pirquet in 1911 attributed serum sickness to a serum factor it was not until the classical experiments of Dixon and colleagues (reviewed by Wilson & Dixon, 1971) 50 years later that the pathological mechanisms were defined. In these experiments rabbits were given an intravenous injection of a large amount of radiolabelled bovine serum albumin (BSA). Figure 9.1 illustrates such an experiment.

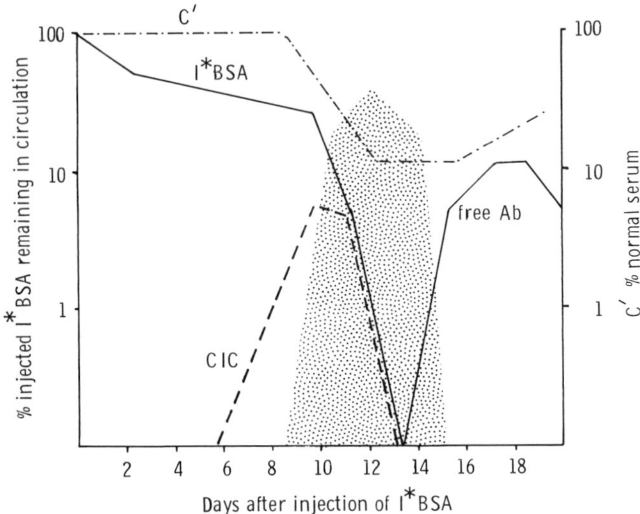

Fig. 9.1   Acute serum sickness in rabbit. C' — haemolytic complement. I* BSA — radio-labelled bovine serum albumin. CIC — circulating immune complexes. Free Ab. — free antibody to BSA. The hatched area indicates the duration of vasculitis and nephritis that occurred when BSA antigen was circulating complexed with antibody.

The labelled antigen disappeared from the circulation in three phases: the first early phase reflects intravascular–extravascular equilibration, the second normal catabolism followed by a rapid third phase due to antibody production and consequent immune elimination. It was during this third phase that immune complexes were detected in the circulation, that complement consumption occurred and that shortly afterwards, vasculitis and glomerulonephritis could be found. The causative role of immune complexes in this experimental model was suggested by the demonstration of antigen, antibody and complement in the lesions. Such changes were not seen in animals whose antibody response was deficient or absent. Following the elimination of the antigen the tissues healed and the animals survived, indicating a self-limiting process that subsided following the elimination of antigen.

Chronic serum sickness
This disease was produced in rabbits by the daily injection of BSA antigen (Wilson & Dixon, 1971). The amount of antigen injected was calculated so that it exceeded the amount of antibody produced. Chronic glomerulonephritis was seen in all animals in which an antibody response occurred. The amount of antigen deposited in the kidneys increased 10- to 15-fold immediately before the onset of the proteinuria again suggesting that the immune complexes formed were responsible for the tissue damage. This increased rate of deposition in the kidney also implied a failure of normal reticulo-endothelial system (RES) clearance. When a constant amount of antigen was injected daily the development of disease depended upon the immune response of the animal (reviewed by Germuth & Rodriguez, 1973). In animals that had either a very good antibody response or no response at all there was no disease, but animals that mounted a relatively weak antibody response developed immune complex glomerulonephritis and an analysis of their sera following the injection of

antigen demonstrated immune complexes of between 500 000 and 900 000 daltons which persisted for up to 24 hours. In animals that developed an intermediate antibody response mesangial deposition and proliferation occurred. Analysis of their sera showed immune complexes of about one million daltons persisting for up to six hours. Such experiments therefore emphasise the differences in size of complex, ratio of antigen to antibody, circulation time and host response that all play a role in the development of disease.

These experiments illustrate the capacity of experimental immune complexes to produce a variety of disease whose histological appearances are similar to that found in human glomerulonephritis and they provide a theoretical basis for the current view that many forms of glomerulonephritis in man are mediated by immune complexes. Such disease requires continued antigen exposure. In man the antigen may be endogenous, e.g. autoantigens as in systemic lupus erythematosus or exogenous, e.g. chronic infection such as an infective endocarditis or hepatitis B virus infection.

Infective endocarditis
Infective endocarditis is a good human model of an immune complex disease and is comparable to chronic serum sickness in experimental animals. Lesions that at one time were thought to have been due to microemboli are now clearly shown to result from immune complex deposition (Reed & Williams, 1977) and antigen, antibody and complement have been identified in glomerular deposits. Tests for circulating immune complexes are nearly always positive and generally parallel the course of the disease (Bayer et al, 1979; Cabane et al, 1979). As yet there has been no report of the identification of an antigen in circulating immune complexes in infective endocarditis, however, it is interesting that Harkiss, Brown & Evans (1979) have reported circulating immune complexes containing staphlococcus albus antigen in the clinically similar disease, shunt nephritis. Abatement of the immune complex disease in infective endocarditis usually follows appropriate therapy and tests for immune complexes become negative following successful therapy. As in chronic serum sickness chronic antigenaemia is essential for the induction of the clinical manifestations of immune complex disease in infective endocarditis.

Nature of an immune complex
The nature of immune complexes depends upon the nature of the constituent antigen and antibody, their relative concentrations and their binding properties.

The antigen
Antigens are defined as substances that will bind to specific antibodies or sensitised lymphocytes. They may be mono or polyvalent depending on the number and position of the antigenic determinants. Monovalent antigens will only bind one antibody molecule and therefore are unable to form large complexes. Since about six amino acids are sufficient to constitute an antigen site, large molecules may have many different antigenic determinants or many repeating single determinants. The antigenic site is usually formed as a result of the secondary and tertiary structures of polypeptide chains and need not necessarily be confined to a single polypeptide chain. Alteration of such secondary and tertiary structures, e.g. unfolding, may lead to a loss of antigenicity.

The antibody
Antibody molecules are immunoglobulins of IgG, IgM, IgA, IgE and IgD classes. The antigen binding site is located in the variable, F'ab region of the molecule. There are two such regions on IgG and 10 on IgM molecules. This is quite separate from the portion of the molecule (the Fc region) capable of interacting with complement and cell receptors. The strength of the bond between antigen and the F'ab portion of the molecule is termed the affinity and this varies during an immune response. Early in antibody production the affinity tends to be low but with time and repeated exposure to antigen this increases. Antigen–antibody avidity refers to the number of binding sites on the antibody molecule. Antibody affinity and avidity are important parameters of immune complex formation, responsible for many of their biological properties (see below).

Antigen–antibody lattice
The physical size of an antigen–antibody complex depends upon the degree of lattice formation. With divalent IgG antibodies lattice formation is related to the concentration and valency of antigen, the concentration of antibody and the affinity of the interaction. In states of gross antigen excess the complexes formed are small and soluble and consist of two antigens to one antibody. At concentrations of antigen and antibody at or near equivalence (with polyvalent antigens and antibodies of high affinity) very large complexes are formed which readily precipitate. Varying degrees of antigen excess therefore produce complexes of varying size and solubility. Lattice formation is important in determining the biological properties of complexes.

Biological properties of immune complexes
The biological properties of antigen–antibody complexes are largely independent of the type of antigen. Their effects are mediated via the antibody part of the complex being presented to the various receptors in the complexed form.

Complement fixation
The complement system is a series of plasma proteins which interact in a similar fashion to the blood clotting system and is the best understood mediator of humoral allergic injury. Activation occurs by two pathways:

1. The *classical* pathway (the first to be described) is activated by immune complexes binding to the first component, C1q, which triggers a sequence of enzymatic interactions leading to the cleavage of the third component, C3.

2. A second pathway, the *alternative* pathway, has now been delineated in which C3 can be cleaved independently of C1 by the action of substances such as polysaccharides (e.g. endotoxin) as well as complexes of IgA.

Both pathways normally 'tick-over' at a slow rate under the control of inhibitor proteins and are activated either by increasing the rate of formation or by stabilisation of the activated products (Properdin and C3 nephritic factor are stabilisers of the alternative pathway). Activation of complement on the surface of a cell or bacterial wall will lead to the binding of the late components (C5 to C9) which cause cytolysis. However, other active products are generated during activation which are potent mediators of inflammation. C3a is anaphylotoxic and C5a is chemotactic whilst C3b is responsible for immune adherance.

The fixation of complement by immune complexes requires a lattice containing two or more antibody molecules (Haakenstad & Mannik, 1977). IgM and IgG-1 and IgG-3 subclasses are very efficient at binding the first component of the classical pathway of complement (C1q). Aggregates of IgG and IgA have been shown to activate the alternative pathway of complement (Muller-Eberhard, 1975). Activation of complement is a potent mediator of tissue damage as a result of the generation of anaphylotoxins and chemotactic factors. The vasculitis of acute serum sickness can be completely abrogated by prior complement depletion. Such treatment does not prevent immune complex deposition in tissues but prevents the polymorphonuclear cell-dependent damage.

In experimental animals, the clearance of complexes from the circulation is independent of complement (Mannik, Haakensted & Arend, 1974) although it may be an important secondary mechanism for clearance in the diseased state.

Complement is capable of dissolving or solubilising immune complex precipitates. This function of complement was first described by Miller & Nussenzweigh (1975). Complement dissolution is absolutely dependent on an intact alternative pathway but is enhanced by classical pathway activation. The process of dissolution probably occurs by the interposition of C3 molecules causing disruption of the lattice structure and this mechanism may be important in the inactivation of tissue bound complexes. The phlogistic role of such dissolved complexes are as yet unknown. Bartolotti et al (1979) have recently tested this property in the sera of patients with immune complex disease. They were able to show that solubilisation was defective in the sera of such patients and, in serial studies, these abnormalities were associated with disease activity.

Other humoral receptors

The formation of antiglobulins or rheumatoid factors is a common feature of immune complex disease although their role in disease is less well understood. It is possible that by interacting with complexes, antiglobulins may increase the lattice and therefore either enhance their clearance by the reticulo-endothelial system (see below) or enhance their interaction with complement. Such effects may be beneficial and in this respect Hill et al (1978) in a study of morphological correlations in systemic lupus erythematosus found only mild lesions in patients with rheumatoid factor suggesting that the rheumatoid factor was protective.

The formation of immunoconglutinins — antibodies to activated complement components — may similarly lead to further aggregation of complement-containing immune complexes and alter their biological properties.

Reticulo–endothelial system interactions

The properties necessary for efficient RES clearance of immune complexes have been extensively reviewed by Haarkenstad & Mannik (1977) and will be summarised here.

The removal of immune complexes from the circulation by the RES depends upon the lattice of the complex, the nature of the antibody and antigen and on the status of the RES. A large lattice greater than two antibody molecules was shown (Mannik et al, 1974) to be removed quickly from the circulation by the liver. In healthy animals this removal was not influenced by prior complement depletion. Immune complexes formed with IgG[1] and IgG[3] subclasses were shown to bind to monocyte Fc receptors whereas IgG^2, IgG^4, and other immunoglobulins were not. This binding depended upon an intact Fc region. By reducing and alkylating the antibody molecule the immune complexes, although unaltered in antigen binding properties and lattice formation, were no longer removed from the circulation. Clearance of antigen from the circulation may occur independently of antibody formation, e.g. native or denatured DNA injected into unimmunised animals was removed very quickly (Mannik et al, 1974).

The status of the RES is important in the removal of immune complexes. The concept of a saturable RES requires that there be a finite number of receptors. That saturation could occur in vivo was suggested by Wilson & Dixon (1971) in the studies of chronic serum sickness referred to previously. Mannik et al (1974) by injecting preformed complexes into experimental animals were able to show that the rate of removal followed first order kinetics and that the removal mechanism was saturable. Recently Frank et al (1979) and Lockwood et al (1979) have demonstrated defective splenic function in patients with immune complex disease. Lockwood et al (1979) have also shown that this defective splenic function could be reversed by plasma-exchange and that it correlated with immune complex levels and clinical disease activity. It is also possible that RES function may be under genetic control, thus a primary defect in RES function may lead to the persistence of immune complexes in the circulation (see discussion of host response).

Other cellular interactions
Immune complexes are capable of interacting with a variety of cells other than those of the RES described above via surface receptors for IgG or complement.

Human platelets interact with immune complexes via their surface IgG receptor. This results in platelet aggregation and release of platelet factors capable of activating the clotting system. Immune complexes are not capable of interaction with the clotting system except via their action on platelets. This property of platelets has been used to develop a test for circulating immune complexes (see p. 212).

Polymorphonuclear neutrophils also have receptors for the Fc region of IgG. Binding of immune complexes leads to their phagocytosis, or if they are part of a large surface, to release of proteolytic enzymes into the surrounding medium. This latter process is believed to be important in mediating tissue damage in immune complex disease (WHO Scientific Group, 1977). Neutrophil involvement also occurs indirectly by the activation of complement by immune complexes leading to the release of the complement chemotactic factor C5a.

Eosinophils and basophils also have receptors for immunoglobulin and degranulate on stimulation. Henson & Cochrane (1971) were able to show that one of the requirements for injury in experimental acute serum sickness was an interaction of the antigen with an IgE antibody on the surface of basophils that led to the release of vasoactive amines from platelets. This illustrates the complex relationships that exist between humoral and cellular mediators following immune complex formation.

Lymphocytes also bear receptors for the Fc region of IgG whilst receptors for C3 are found on the B lymphocyte subpopulation. Sjögren et al (1971) suggested that immune complexes could modify cell mediated immune responses against autologous tumours. They postulated that immune complexes could block or suppress lymphocyte transformation and the generation of tumour specific cytotoxicity and were able to show that there was a relationship between the levels of immune complexes and residual tumour. Immune complexes may also influence the afferent side of the immune response. Pepys (1976) has shown that the C3 component of complement is necessary in the induction of thymus dependent antibody production and by activating complement immune complex uptake by germinal centres in the spleen may be enhanced leading to continued antibody production.

Localisation of immune complexes
Immune complexes occur in tissues because of their formation in situ or because of deposition from the circulation. In situ formation results from local antigen release or local antigen deposition. The Arthus reaction is an example of local immune complex formation. Following the subcutaneous injection of antigen into an individual with a high titre of circulating antibody to that antigen an immune complex forms locally and leads to an area of inflammation termed an Arthus reaction.

The effect of lattice and immune complex size has been studied by Haakensted & Mannik (1977). Large lattice complexes persisting in the circulation were necessary for glomerular deposition. Large complexes led to deposition in the mesangial region whilst smaller complexes were deposited in the capillary loop.

Immune complexes may lodge more readily at sights of previous injury. In experimental immune complex nephritis in rats Couser et al (1978) have shown an increase in immune complex deposition following a previous glomerular injury induced by an aminonucleoside — a substance which produces a minimal change nephrotic syndrome in experimental animals. An immune complex may localise because of antigen specific affinity for a particular tissue. Izui, Lambert & Miescher (1976) demonstrated an affinity for glomerular basement membrane and collagen of DNA and suggested that this might be a basis for local formation of DNA-anti-DNA complexes in systemic lupus erythematosus.

Host response
Soothill (1975) and Peters & Lachmann (1974) proposed that the development of nephritis was a consequence of a defect of the immune response which led to the persistence of antigen–antibody complexes in the circulation. However, the recent development of tests for circulating immune complexes have proved disappointing in regard to idiopathic nephritis. This of course may be related to the specificity of the tests and will be discussed in the second part of this chapter. The host response to an antigen may be defective because of a deficiency of complement, a defect in antibody response, a deficiency in cell mediated immunity or a defective reticulo–endothelial system.

Hypocomplementaemia
Peters et al (1973) proposed that complement deficiency was the common factor that led to nephritis in patients with the syndrome of secondary deficiency of C3 (associated with the presence of C3 nephritic factor), partial lipodystrophy and membranoproliferative nephritis. There is a susceptibility to infection in hereditary

C3 deficiency and therefore a propensity to develop persistence of immune complexes in the circulation. In this respect Pussell et al (1980) have recently observed a family with hereditary C3 deficiency, increased susceptibility to infection and nephritis. In the generation of such disease the infection need not be overt but must provide a persistent source of antigen to induce chronic immune complex formation. In this same family circulating immune complexes were detected by the C1q binding assay. Susceptibility to immune complex disease is also seen in other complement deficiency states: SLE-like illness is associated with C2 deficiency, C1r and C1s deficiency and C4 deficiency; a patient with C1r deficiency also had chronic glomerulonephritis (Lachmann & Hobart, 1978). An increased susceptibility to immune complex disease has been reported in C1 inhibitor deficiency where uncontrolled complement activation led to a secondary deficiency of complement. Although the inheritance of some complement components (e.g. C2) is linked to the immune response genes such studies suggest that it is the absence of complement, due either to hereditary deficiency or secondary activation, that predisposes to the development of immune complex disease.

Deficient antibody response
Soothill & Steward (1971) have shown that mice prone to chronic immune complex disease caused by chronic viral infection tend to produce antibody of low affinity. As already discussed low affinity antibody is poor at lattice formation and hence poorly eliminated by the reticulo–endothelial system.

In the experimental model of chronic serum sickness where the animals were given a constant dose of antigen (Germuth & Rodriguez, 1973) there was considerable variation in disease. In those animals that failed to produce or produced a high affinity antibody there was no renal disease, in those animals that produced a low affinity antibody response an immune complex type of glomerulonephritis occurred. The development of disease was therefore related to the immune response of the animal.

Cell-mediated deficiency
The idea that immune complexes might induce a secondary deficiency in cell mediated immunity was suggested by Taylor & Basten (1976). It was known that antigen–antibody complexes persisted on the surface of T cells in sensitised animals and thereby suppressed antibody formation. They proposed that immune complexes activated suppressor T cells which then induced the release of substances (perhaps from macrophages) that caused suppression of both T and B cell function. The existance of deficient cell-mediated immunity in the presence of circulating immune complexes may contribute to the production and persistance of the antigen–antibody complexes.

Defective reticulo–endothelial function
RES blockade is a feature of both experimental and human immune complex disease and the presence of immune complexes in the circulation is thought to reflect a failure of their clearance by the RES. Although other factors such as the type and affinity of antibody may explain this failure there remains the possibility that in some individuals there is a diminished clearance capacity of the RES. Thus a failure of RES clearance may lead to the persistence of immune complexes in the circulation formed in

response to a number of environmental antigens for example, food antigens. Recently Levinsky (personal communication) has demonstrated post prandial circulating immune complexes in patients with Henoch–Schonlein disease. Although he also demonstrated increased amounts of immune complexes in normal controls the patients were unable to effectively clear their postprandial complexes.

TESTS FOR CIRCULATING IMMUNE COMPLEXES

Human immune complex disease should be classified as such only when the specific antibodies and antigens causing the inflammation have been identified. In a small number of instances this has been carried out by elution studies on specimens obtained at biopsy or autopsy or by immunofluorescent techniques using specific antisera to the suspected antigen. However, these procedures are rarely possible in the diagnosis of immune complex diseases and hence evidence for an immune complex aetiology has relied on more indirect methods such as the demonstration of immunoglobulin and complement by immunofluorescent techniques in sites known to be associated with immune complex deposition, e.g. glomerular capillary loop, blood vessels, skin and synovium. Even these methods depend upon the availability of tissue for study. Hence secondary phenomena, such as the measurement of complement components have been employed in the diagnosis and management of immune complex disease.

With the recent techniques which enable circulating immune complexes to be measured, it had been hoped to simplify the diagnosis and management of immune complex disease. That this is not yet entirely the case illustrates again the complexity of the problem. As a result of the widespread application of these tests many more diseases have now been added to those identified as due to immune complexes. Although excellent correlations have been reported between immune complexes and disease activity (Pussell et al, 1978; Woodroffe et al, 1979; Haslam et al, 1979; Gamble et al, 1979; Harkiss et al, 1979; Cabane et al, 1979 and Bayer et al, 1979), there is also a frequent lack of correlation especially with respect to glomerulonephritis (reviewed by Border, 1979). There are several explanations for such lack of correlation: (a) the circulating complexes may not be the damaging ones but merely reflect the presence of tissue bound damaging complexes; (b) the currently available methods may fail to detect the damaging complexes either because of insensitivity or non-reactivity; (c) the appearance of tissue damage may depend upon another independent factor such as vasodilatation, before the complexes are deposited and the development of disease is therefore associated with this other factor; (d) the immune complexes may appear infrequently in the circulation and hence be missed during sampling. Conversely the demonstration of immune complexes in the circulation does not necessarily implicate them in the pathogenesis of the disease under study. The aim of the second part of this chapter is to consider some of the available tests, their sensitivity, specificity and clinical correlation.

Methods for detection of immune complexes
Methods for the detection of immune complexes may, generally, be classified into antigen-specific and antigen-non-specific (see Table 9.1). Antigen-specific methods require that the antigen be known or suspected before applying the particular tests, e.g. hepatitis B antigen. The antigen-non-specific methods are based on various

Table 9.1   Antigen-non-specific methods for detection of immune complexes in body fluids

Physical properties:	(usually combined with immunochemical analysis)	
	Ultracentrifugation ⎱	depends on physical size
	Gel filtration ⎰	
	Cryoprecipitation	
	Polyethylene glycol precipitation	
Interaction with humoral receptors:		
	Complement	C1q binding assay (C1q BA)
		C1q solid phase assay (C1q SP)
		C1q deviation test (C1q DV)
		C1q latex inhibition assay (C1q LI)
		conglutinin solid phase assay (Kg SP)
		conglutinin fluid phase assay (Kg FP)
	Antiglobulin	RF latex inhibition
		MRF binding assay
Interaction with cellular receptors:		
	Complement dependent	Raji cell assay
	Fc dependent	Platelet aggregation test

distinct properties of the complexed molecules that are not shared by the free antigen or antibody. It is proposed therefore to discuss those antigen-non-specific tests most commonly reported in the literature. A more complete description of immune complex assays has been given by Zubler & Lambert (1978).

Physical properties
These methods rely on separation from normal serum constituents by the characteristics of size or increased precipitability in certain conditions. Following separation the complexes may then be subjected to further immunochemical analysis.

Separation on the basis of size by ultracentrifugation or gel filtration with subsequent demonstration of immunoglobulin or complement in heavily sedimenting positions has been applied to the study of immune complexes (Amlot, Slaney & Williams, 1976). The sensitivity of such methods is high although the technique is cumbersome allowing only a few samples to be analysed at any one time.

Alterations of solubility by cryoprecipitation or polyethylene glycol (PEG) precipitation are simple techniques that do not require highly sophisticated equipment. Cryoglobulins are often found in immune complex disease when large volumes of blood are tested. The demonstration of complement components and occasionally antigens (Levo et al, 1977) in the cryoprecipitates has provided evidence for their immune complex nature. PEG causes precipitation of proteins according to their size. Immunochemical analysis of the precipitates or an increase in the amount of the precipitate (Creighton, Lambert & Miescher, 1973) has been shown to correlate with clinical immune complex disease. Further manipulation of the PEG precipitate such as its ability to cause complement consumption (PEG complement consumption test) has also been applied to the study of disease (Harkiss et al, 1979). The major problem of such methods is their lack of specificity although Harkiss et al (1979) have overcome this problem by combining this test with the identification of specific antibody and antigen in the precipitate.

Interaction with humoral receptors

Interaction with C1q, the first component of the classical complement pathway forms the basis of one of the most widely used immune complex assays. This test which uses purified human C1q may be performed in the fluid phase ([125]I C1q binding assay of Zubler et al, 1976) or the solid phase (C1q solid phase assay of Hay, Nineham & Roitt, 1976). Although other substances (e.g. DNA, heparin, endotoxin) may also bind C1q, in practice these occur at concentrations below the range of sensitivity of the test or do not react under the conditions of the assay. C1q also forms the basis for two inhibition assays. The first tests the ability of immune complex sera to inhibit the uptake of C1q into sensitised sheep red cells (Sobel, Bokisch & Muller–Eberhard, 1975), and the second tests the inhibition by complexes of C1q dependent agglutination of IgG-coated latex particles (Cambiaso, Ricconi & Masson, 1977).

Interaction with conglutinin. Conglutinin is a protein found in bovine serum which has the exclusive property of binding to fragments of activated C3. As with C1q both solid phase (Kg–SP, Casali et al, 1977) and fluid phase analyses (Kg–FP, Lachmann et al, 1979) have been described. Non-immune complex associated fragments of C3 will bind to conglutinin but under the conditions of the test these do not interfere (personal observation).

Interaction with antiglobulins, such as rheumatoid factors is the basis of a number of assays. Cambiaso et al (1977) have combined a rheumatoid factor with C1q in an automated inhibition assay. The use of monoclonal rheumatoid factors prepared from the sera of patients with lymphoproliferative diseases has been shown to have a higher specificity for complexed IgG (Winchester, Kunkel & Angello, 1971). Again both solid phase (Gabriel & Angello, 1977) and fluid phase assays (Barrett & Naish, 1979) have been described.

Interaction with cellular receptors
The use of such techniques requires the preparation and/or maintenance in tissue culture of various cell lines. Standardisation of the cells must be made regularly because of changes in function caused by alterations in metabolism. Interaction of immune complexes with cells occurs via receptors for the Fc region of IgG or complement fragments. The cells used for these assays have surface antigens which may react with antibodies in the test sera and thus give false positive reactions, e.g. antiplatelet and anti-lymphocyte antibody in SLE may react with platelets and Raji cells giving false positive tests for immune complexes.

The Raji cell assay (Theofilopoulos, Wilson & Dixon, 1976) was developed from cells from a patient with a lympho-proliferative disorder. These lymphoid cells have receptors for the Fc region of IgG as well as complement (C3b, C4 and C1q). The binding of immune complexes in the assay is mostly by the complement receptors. Labelled anti-human immunoglobulin is then used to identify the bound immune complexes. The presence of antilymphocyte antibodies interacting with the Raji cell may lead to false positive results. This test is theoretically the cellular counterpart of the conglutinin binding assay and would therefore be expected to give a good correlation. In diseases such as SLE and vasculitis this is indeed the case (WHO Collaborative Study, 1978) but in rheumatoid arthritis there is no correlation — the Raji cell assay being more frequently positive. One possible explanation is the requirement of the conglutinin assay for immune complex bound C3b which has been inactivated by C3b inactivator.

The platelet aggregation test described by Penttinen (1977) utilises the Fc receptor on human platelets. Immune complex containing serum will cause aggregation of platelets. The degree of aggregation is determined by serial dilutions of patients serum. Many factors other than immune complexes have been shown to interfere with this test (Zubler & Lambert, 1978). Native C1q and rheumatoid factors, as well as high levels of immunoglobulin can cause platelet aggregation.

Evaluation of immune complex assays
The WHO Collaborative Study (1978) attempted to assess 18 separate immune complex assays by dispatching test and control sera to the laboratories where the individual tests were first described. The sera included normal human sera, aggregated human globulin of various sizes and concentrations, pathological sera from patients with SLE, RA, vasculitis, glomerulonephritis, thrombocytopenic purpura, Crohn's disease, various tropical infectious diseases, various forms of cancer and sera containing interfering substances such as free DNA and lipopolysaccaride. Of the 18 assays analysed only 6 methods distinguished aggregated human globulin from normal sera, were unaffected by the interfering substances and were generally best at discriminating between normal and pathological sera. The methods were 5 complement-based assays (C1q BA, C1q SP, C1q DV, Kg–SP and Raji cell assays) and 1 antiglobulin-based assay (monoclonal RF inhibition assay). Although other assays gave very good results in some instances, e.g. C1q latex inhibition in schistosomiasis and neutrophil inhibition test in filariasis, the 6 methods detected abnormalities most frequently in all pathological sera and generally correlated well with each other in individual diseases. For these reasons the ensuing comments will be confined to these 6 tests.

Sensitivity
Many tests for immune complexes are expressed in terms of their ability to bind to a simulated complex and the most commonly used is heat-aggregated human IgG in normal human serum. Such a procedure leads to a wide variety of aggregate sizes and includes unaggregated monomeric IgG in the preparation. For these reasons the use of heat aggregated IgG as an index of sensitivity may lead to variations among assays and affect the reproducibility. However, the WHO Collaborative Study (1978) were able to show that a range of relative concentrations from $1-100\,\mu g$ gave a clear-cut dose-response curve in most assays. Although there was some variation the overall sensitivity was satisfactory.

The quantitation of complexes in sera in terms of an equivalent amount of heat aggregated IgG should not be taken to reflect the total quantity of complexes present in the sera but the amount reactive in the assay. Differences between assays in their ability to detect aggregated IgG does not necessarily reflect differences in their ability to detect complexes in sera. The C1q binding and conglutinin binding assays have a

10-fold difference in sensitivity with respect to heat aggregated IgG but when both tests were used to examine sera from a number of patients with SLE there was a significant correlation between the two assays (Pussell et al, 1978).

Specificity
The use of antigen-non-specific methods for detecting immune complexes may lead to false positive results because of interaction with interfering substances. Aggregated immunoglobulins, which may be generated as a result of poor handling of serum samples, are capable of interacting with all assays. Also highly polyanionic substances such as DNA, lipopolysaccharide and heparin will bind C1q. The WHO Collaborative Study attempted to assess the effects of these potential interfering substances. They were able to show that of the C1q based assays only the C1q deviation test was significantly affected by the addition of DNA and none were affected by lipopolysaccharide. Woodroffe et al (1977) also assessed the effect of heparin and endotoxin on the C1q binding assay. Although both of these substances caused a false positive effect they did so only at high concentrations.

Methods based on interactions with cell surface receptors (Raji cell assay) may be influenced by the presence of antibodies directed at the cell surface. The very high incidence of positivity of the Raji cell assay in SLE may be caused by the presence of antilymphocyte antibodies (the Raji cell is a lymphoid cell) and Woodroffe et al (1977) were able to show a correlation between lymphocytoxicity and Raji cell assay positivity. Although the findings were not conclusive they suggested that lymphocytotoxic antibodies contributed to the high positivity in SLE of the Raji cell assay.

Clinical correlations
Serial studies using more than one assay, correlated with clinical and other laboratory findings have provided the strongest evidence for the value of these assays in the diagnosis and management of patients with immune complex disease. It must be stressed again, however, that the finding of immune complexes in the circulation does not necessarily implicate them in the pathogenesis of the disease.

Systemic lupus erythematosus. A number of groups have reported the association of immune complexes and clinical disease activity (Levinsky, Cameron & Soothill, 1977; Pussell et al, 1978; Zubler & Lambert, 1978; Woodroffe et al, 1979). In the majority of patients the level of immune complexes correlated with disease activity and a good response to therapy was associated with a reduction in their levels. As yet the presence of immune complexes demonstrated by one particular assay has not been shown to be associated with particular organ involvement. However, Levinsky & Soothill (1979) by assaying sera fractionated by gel filtration have shown that patients with lupus nephritis had complexes of intermediate (1×10^6 daltons) and large size (4×10^6 daltons) whereas those without renal involvement had only the large complexes. Further applications of immune complex assays may provide clues as to the origin of the heterogeneity of disease in SLE.

Rheumatoid arthritis is associated with similar findings (Zubler et al 1976, Nineham et al, 1979). Immune complexes correlate with active joint inflammation and with extra-articular manifestations. Nineham et al (1979) also showed that improvement in clinical disease and reduction in immune complexes occurred following the introduction of gold therapy. Immune complex assays have also been used as a diagnostic aid in RA. The incidence of positivity in seropositive and seronegative rheumatoid arthritis far exceeds that of ankylosing spondylitis, osteoarthritis and other patients with inflammatory arthritis caused by gout, chondrocalcinosis and infection (Zubler & Lambert, 1978). Williams et al (1979) using the clearance of heat-damaged red cells as a marker of RES function studied 26 patients with rheumatoid arthritis. In 11 of 13 patients with active disease the clearance of the damaged red cells was prolonged and there was an inverse correlation with immune complexes detected by C1qB assay. In the patients with inactive disease the red cell clearance was normal and only 4 of 13 had detectable immune complexes. A serial study of one patient illustrated the clear association between disease activity, red cell clearance and immune complexes.

Infective endocarditis was discussed earlier in this chapter. The measurement of immune complexes in this protoype immune complex disease has shown the expected high incidence of positivity and correlation with therapy (Cabane et al, 1979). Indeed immune complex assays also have diagnostic value as well as a place in monitoring therapy in this disease.

Glomerulonephritis. Recently Border (1979) reviewed the published reports of immune complexes in various forms of glomerulonephritis. The highest incidences of positivity were found in glomerulonephritis associated with systemic disease, e.g. acute poststreptococcal glomerulonephritis, SLE and vasculitis. Patients with idiopathic glomerulonephritis had a low incidence of positivity, the notable surprising exception being minimal change nephrotic syndrome — a disease in which immune deposits in the glomeruli are usually absent. Predictably low incidences of positivity were found in antibody mediated Goodpasture's syndrome and IgA nephropathy where most assays are incapable of detecting IgA complexes. However, low incidences were also found in membranous glomerulonephritis, focal glomerulonephritis, membranoproliferative glomerulonephritis and other forms of chronic glomerulonephritis where immune deposits in the renal biopsy are frequently found by immunofluorescent techniques, and there was poor correlation between the assays used. Possible explanations for such disorders have been considered earlier. One further possibility is that the concept of circulating immune complexes depositing in the glomerulus may be wrong and that immune deposits may result from local formation by antibody reacting with glomerular bound or trapped antigens. Such a mechanism has been demonstrated experimentally (Golbus & Wilson, 1979). The place of assays for immune complexes in idiopathic glomerulonephritis await the results of serial studies. Initial reports in adult idiopathic nephrotic syndrome (Border, 1979) have failed to show correlation with disease activity and response to therapy. The finding of immune complexes in a patient with glomerulonephritis may therefore indicate the presence of an associated systemic disease.

Miscellaneous. There are many other diseases in which immune complexes have been shown to be of prognostic or diagnostic value, e.g. infectious disease and cancer. These topics have been recently reviewed (Reed & Williams, 1977; Rossen & Barnes, 1978; Zubler & Lambert, 1978).

Conclusion

Although there are many unanswered questions regarding the part played by immune complexes in immune complex disease the application of tests for such complexes has added to our understanding and management of patients with a variety of diseases. As yet the tests are not diagnostic but are adjuncts to diagnosis. A single estimate is of less value than serial studies and the application of more than one assay is necessary to compensate for the heterogeneity of the immune complexes. In certain diseases serial testing for immune complexes helps in management.

However, several problems remain unsolved and these are fundamental to the nature of immune complex disease rather than the usefulness of the tests. Does the heterogeneity of immune complexes explain the heterogeneity of disease? Are the circulating complexes pathogenic or merely markers of other pathogenic tissue bound complexes? Why are immune complexes deposited in a particular organ? What is the role of the host in the clearance of immune complexes?

ACKNOWLEDGEMENTS

I am grateful to Professor D. K. Peters and Dr B. D. Williams for helpful discussion and criticism in the preparation of this article. I also wish to acknowledge the advice given by Dr S. R. Bartolotti, Dr C. M. Lockwood, Dr A. J. Pinching, Dr A. J. Rees and Mr N. Amos. Mrs C. Bateson kindly typed the manuscript.

REFERENCES

Amlot P L, Slaney J M, Williams B D 1976 Circulating immune complexes and symptoms in Hodgkin's disease. Lancet i: 449–451

Barratt J, Naish P 1979 A simple radiolabelled rheumatoid factor binding assay for the measurement of circulating immune complexes. Journal of Immunological Methods 25: 137–146

Bartolotti S R, Pussell B, Dash A, Peters D K 1979 Complex dissolution: An assay for complement function and immune complex load. Kidney International 16: 92 (abs)

Bayer A S, Theofilopoulos A N, Eisenberg R, Dixon F J, Guze L B 1976 Circulating immune complexes in infective endocarditis. New England Journal of Medicine 295: 1500–1505

Bayer A S, Theofilopoulos A N, Tillman D, Dixon F J, Guze L B 1979 Use of circulating immune complex levels in the serodifferentiation of endocarditic and nonendocarditic septicaemiais. American Journal of Medicine 66: 58–62

Border W A 1979 Immune complex detection in glomerular disease. Nephron 24: 105–113

Cabane J, Godeau P, Herreman G, Acar J, Digeon M, Bach J F 1979 Fate of circulating immune complexes in infective endocarditis. American Journal of Medicine 66: 277–282

Cambiaso C L, Riccomi H, Masson P L 1977 Automated determination of immune complexes by their inhibitory effect on the agglutination of IgG-coated particles of rheumatoid factor or C1q. Annals of the Rheumatic Diseases 36 (Suppl): 40–44

Casali P, Bossus A, Carpentier A N 1977 Solid-phase enzyme immunoassay or radioimmunoassay for the detection of immune complexes based on their recognition by conglutinin: Conglutinin binding test. Clinical and Experimental Immunology 29: 342–354

Couser W G, Jermanovich N B, Belok S, Stilmant M M, Hoyer J R 1978 Effect of aminonucleoside nephrosis on immune complex localisation in autologous immune complex nephropathy in rats. Journal of Clinical Investigation 61: 561–572

Creighton W D, Lambert P H, Miescher P A 1973 Detection of antibodies and soluble antigen–antibody complexes by precipitation with polyethylene glycol. Journal of Immunology 111: 1219–1227

Dixon F J, Feldman J D, Vazquez J J 1961 Experimental glomerulonephritis. The pathogenesis of a laboratory model resembling the spectrum of human glomerulonephritis. Journal of Experimental Medicine 113: 899–920

Frank M M, Hamburger M I, Lawley T J, Kimberley R P, Plotz P H 1979 Defective reticuloendothelial system Fc-receptor function in systemic lupus erythematosus. New England Journal of Medicine 300: 518–523

Gabriel A, Agnello V 1977 Detection of immune complexes. The use of radioimmunoassay with C1q and monclonal rheumatoid factor. Journal of Clinical Investigation 59: 990–1001

Gamble C N, Wiesner K B, Shapiro R F, Boyer W J 1979 Immune complex pathogenesis of glomerulonephritis and pulmonary vasculitis in Becket's disease. American Journal of Medicine 66: 1031–1039

Germuth F G J, Rodriguez E 1973 Immunopathology of the renal glomerulus. Little Brown & Co, Boston

Golbus S, Wilson C B 1979 Experimental glomerulonephritis induced by in situ formation of immune complexes in glomerular capillary wall. Kidney International 16: 148–157

Haakenstad A D, Mannik M 1977 The biology of immune complexes. In: Talal N (ed) Autoimmunity, 1st edn. Academic Press, New York, p 277–360

Harkiss G D, Brown D L, Evans D B 1979 Longitudinal study of circulating immune complexes in a patient with staphylococcus albus induced shunt nephritis. Clinical and Experimental Immunology 37: 228–238

Haslam P L, Thompson B, Mohammed I, Townsend P J, Hodson M E, Holborow E J, Turner-Warwick M 1979 Circulating immune complexes in patients with cryptogenic fibrosing alveolitis. Clinical and Experimental Immunology 37: 381–390

Hay F C, Nineham L J, Roitt I M 1976 Routine assay for the detection of immune complexes of known immunoglobulin class using solid phase C1q. Clinical and Experimental Immunology 24: 396–400

Henson P M, Cochrane C G 1971 Immune complex disease in rabbits: the role of complement and of a leukocyte dependent release of vasoactive amines from platelets. Journal of Experimental Medicine 133: 554–571

Hill G S, Hinglais N, Tron F, Bach J F 1978 SLE — Morphologic correlations with immunologic and clinical data at the time of biopsy. American Journal of Medicine 64: 61–79

Izui S, Lambert P H, Miescher P A 1976 In vitro demonstration of a particular affinity of glomerular basement membrane and collagen for DNA. A possible basis for a local formation of DNA anti-DNA complexes in systemic lupus erythematosus. Journal of Experimental Medicine 144: 428–443

Lachmann P J, Hobart M J 1978 Complement genetics in relation to HLA. British Medical Bulletin 34: 247–252

Lachmann P J, Macanovic M, Harkiss G, Brown D L 1979 The use of bovine conglutinin as a reagent for detecting immune complexes. In: Peeters H (ed) Protides of biological fluids vol 26. Pergamon Press, Oxford, p 37–41

Levinsky R J, Cameron J S, Soothill J F 1977 Serum immune complexes and disease activity in lupus nephritis. Lancet i: 564

Levinsky R J, Soothill J F 1979 The heterogeneity of immune complexes in disease. In: Peters H (ed) Protides of the biological fluids vol 28. Pergamon Press, Oxford, p 243–246

Levo Y, Gorevic P D Kassab H J, Zucker-Franklin D, Franklin E C 1977 Association between hepatitis B virus and essential mixed cryoglobulinaemia. New England Journal of Medicine 296: 1501

Lockwood C M, Worrledge S, Nicholas A, Cotton C, Peters D K 1979 Reversal of impaired splenic function in patients with nephritis or vasculitis (or both) by plasma exchange. New England Journal of Medicine 300: 524–530

Mannik M, Haakenstad A O, Arend W P 1974 The fate and detection of circulating immune complexes. In: Brent L, Holborow J (ed) Progress in immunology II, vol 5. North Holland Publishing Company, Amsterdam, p 91–101

Miller G N, Nussenzweig V 1975 A new complement function: solubilization of antigen–antibody aggregates. Proceedings of the National Academy of Sciences (Wash) 72: 418

Muller–Eberhard H J 1975 Complement Annual Review of Biochemistry 44: 697–724

Nineham L J, Hay F C, Male D K, Roitt I M, Young A, Perumal R 1979 Immune complexes in rheumatoid arthritis: correlations with clinical features and effects of gold. In: Peeters H (ed) Protides of biological fluids, vol 28, Pergamon Press, Oxford, p 179–182

Penttinen K 1977 The platelet aggregation test. Annals of the Rheumatic Diseases 36 (Suppl): 55–58

Pepys M B 1976 Role of complement in the induction of immunological responses. Transplant Review 32: 93–120

Peters D K, Lachmann 1974 Immunity deficiency in the pathogenesis of glomerulonephritis. Lancet i: 58–60

Peters D K, Williams D G, Charlesworth J A, Boulton-Jones J M, Sissons J G P, Evans D J, Kourdsky O, Morel-Maroger L 1973 Mesangiocapillary nephritis, partial lipodystrophy and hypocomplementaemia. Lancet ii: 535

von Pirquet C E 1911 Allergy. Archives of Internal Medicine 7: 259–288

Pussell B A, Bourke E, Marwan Nayef, Morris Susan, Peters D K 1980 Complement deficiency and nephritis. Report of a family. Lancet i: 675–677

Pussell B A, Lockwood C M, Scot D M, Pinching A J, Peters D K 1978 The value of immune complex assays in diagnosis and management. Lancet ii: 359–365

Reed W P, Williams R C 1977 Immune complexes in infectious disease. Advances in Internal Medicine 22: 49–72

Rossen R D, Barnes B C 1978 Measuring serum immune complexes in cancer. Annals of Internal Medicine 88: 570–571

Sjögren H O, Hellstram I, Bansal S C, Hellstrom K E 1971 Suggestive evidence that 'blocking antibodies' of tumour-bearing individuals may be antigen–antibody complexes. Proceedings of the National Academy of Sciences of the United States of America 68: 1372–1375

Sobel A T, Bokisch V A, Muller-Eberhard H J 1975 C1q deviation test for the detection of immune complexes, aggregates of IgG and bacterial products in human sera. Journal of Experimental Medicine 142: 139–150

Soothill J F 1975 Immunity deficiency syndromes. In: Gell P G H, Coombs R A, Lachmann P J (eds) Clinical aspects of immunology, 3rd edn. Blackwell scientific publications, Oxford, England

Soothill J F, Steward M N 1971 The immunological significance of the heterogeneity of antibody affinity. Clinical and Experimental Immunology 9: 193–199

Taylor R B, Basten A 1976 Suppressor cells in humoral immunity and tolerance. British Medical Bulletin 32: 152–157

Terman D S, Buffaloe G, Mattioli C, Cook G, Tillquist R, Sullivan M, Ayus J C 1979 Extracorporeal immunoadsorption: initial experience in human systemic lupus erythematosus. Lancet ii: 824–826

Theofilpoulos A N, Wilson C B, Dixon F J 1976 The Faji cell radioimmune assay for detecting immune complexes in human sera. Journal of Clinical Investigation 57: 169–182

WHO Immunology Unit. A WHO collaborative study for the valuation of eighteen methods for detecting immune complexes in serum. Journal of Clinical Laboratory Immunology 1: 1–15

WHO Scientific Report 1977 The role of immune complexes in disease. No 606 World Health Organisation, Geneva

Wilson C B, Dixon F J 1971 Quantitation of acute and chronic serum sickness in the rabbit. Journal of Experimental Medicine 134: 7s–18s.

Williams B D, Pussell B A, Lockwood C M, Cotton C 1979 Defective reticuloendothelial system function in rheumatoid arthritis. Lancet i: 1311–1314

Winchester R J, Kunkel H G, Agnello V 1971 Occurrence of gamma-globulin complexes in serum and joint fluid of rheumatoid arthritis patients: use of monoclonal rheumatoid factors as reagents for their demonstration. Journal of Experimental Medicine 134: 286s–295s

Woodroffe A J, Border W A, Theofilopolous A N, Gotze O, Glassock R J, Dixon F J, Wilson C B 1977 Detection of circulating immune complexes in patients with glomerulonephritis. Kid Int 12: 268–278

Woodroffe A J, Foldes M, McKenzie P K, Thompson A J, Seymour A E, Clarkeson A R 1979 Serum immune complexes and disease. Australian and New Zealand Journal of Medicine 9: 129–135

Zubler R H, Lambert P-H 1978 Detection of immune complexes in human diseases. Progress in Allergy 24: 1–48

Zubler R H, Nydegger U, Perrin L H, Fehr K, McCormick J, Lambert P-H, Miescher P A 1976 Circulating and intra-articular immune complexes in patients with rheumatoid arthritis. Correlation of ^{125}I-C1q binding activity with clinical and biological features of disease. Journal of Clinical Investigation 57: 1308–1319

9.2 Plasma exchange in immunologically mediated disease

A. J. Pinching

In recent years, plasma exchange has become an important means of treating and of investigating a variety of diseases. This procedure, which has been greatly facilitated by the development of cell separators, is unique in being able to produce an acute and substantial alteration in the internal macromolecular environment. Its principal application in immunological disease has been in the removal of autoantibodies and immune complexes (Table 9.2). However, the depletion pari passu of other plasma proteins, many of which are mediators of inflammatory injury, has proved valuable, especially in fulminating disease. This chapter presents a current appraisal of the technique, its rationale and hazards and a more detailed analysis of its contribution to certain specific immunological disorders.

Table 9.2 Disorders successfully treated by plasma exchange

A. Antibody-mediated diseases
  (i) Autoantibody
        Anti-glomerular basement membrane disease
        Myasthenia gravis
        Herpes gestationis
        Pemphigus vulgaris (?)
        Idiopathic thrombocytopenic purpura (?)
        Autoimmune haemolytic anaemia (fulminant) (?)
        B-cell antibody mediated hypogammoglobulinaemia
        Graves's disease
        Insulin-resistant diabetes (type B)
  (ii) Alloantibody
        Factor VIII antibodies
        Rhesus isoimmunisation

B. Immune complex mediated diseases
        Rapidly progressive nephritis
          Microscopic polyarteritis
          Wegener's granulomatosis
          Henoch-Schönlein purpura (?)
          Idiopathic
        Systemic lupus erythematosus
        Mixed essential cryoglobulinaemia
        Cutaneous vasculitis
        Rheumatoid arthritis (?)

C. Other diseases
        Raynaud's phenomenon
        Scleroderma (vascular) (?)
        Guillain-Barré syndrome (?)
        Asthma (?)
        Renal transplant rejection (?)

GENERAL CONSIDERATIONS

The technique

Plasma exchange is effected by separating whole blood into plasma and cellular components by centrifugation and returning the cellular elements to the patient with plasma or plasma fractions from healthy donors. Plasmapheresis, strictly speaking, involves the removal of plasma without plasma substitution, volume being replaced if necessary by crystalloid. It is possible to perform plasma exchange using handpacks, but this is laborious and cell separators have greatly simplified the procedure. Two methods of exchange exist, one continuous (e.g. IBM, Aminco) and other semicontinuous (Haemonetics). In the former, the centrifugation chamber is thin, providing a small extracorporeal compartment, thus allowing blood to be separated continuously; for plasma exchange, cells are returned directly to the patient together with donor plasma, while the patients plasma is removed. In the semicontinuous system, a larger centrifugation bowl is used, the patient's blood volume being maintained by infusion of replacement plasma. The bowl is first filled with blood and then plasma is constantly removed from the central upper part of the bowl, while more whole blood flows into the bowl from the patient. This continues until the bowl contains packed cells and a small layer of plasma; the contents of the bowl are then returned to the patient and the cycle is restarted. This system, while maintaining stable circulating volume, causes fluctuations in haematocrit and therefore the haemoglobin must be adequate before starting the procedure. Blood entering the separator is heparinised, but little heparin returns to the patient as it is largely removed with the plasma.

Arteriovenous access

The technique is dependent upon adequate blood flow from the patient, and there are a variety of methods for achieving this, all of which may present problems. Peripheral vein-to-vein exchange may be used in patients with large forearm veins if only a small number of exchanges is planned, for most veins will not tolerate daily puncture with large gauge needles for more than one to two weeks. In patients with renal disease particular care has to be taken as preservation of veins for possible use in long-term haemodialysis is essential. Femoral vein catheters may give poor flows and are a source of infection in immunosuppressed patients. While the risk of infection with subclavian catheters is smaller, it is still present.

The alternative to vein-dependent methods is the creation of an arteriovenous shunt or fistula. Shunts provide excellent flow and are convenient but are likewise a source of infection in immunosuppressed patients. If time is available for the maturing of an arteriovenous fistula before immunosuppression and plasma exchange are started, and if a long series of exchange is planned (i.e. non-fulminating disorders), then this is the method of choice.

Plasma solutions

The most commonly used replacement solution in plasma exchange is plasma protein fraction (PPF); this is Cohn fraction 5, being, in effect, a pasteurized albumin solution. Its bland protein composition renders it virtually free of allergic effects and its mode of preparation makes the risk of infection such as Hepatitis B negligible. Fresh-frozen plasma (FFP) may also be used, either throughout to replete normal globulins, or, more usually, 2–3 units at the end of exchange to restore adequate levels of clotting factors in selected patients (see Hazards of Plasma Exchange).

The use of PPF and FFP in exchange have quite different effects (Moran et al, 1977). With FFP only abnormal plasma constituents or proteins present in excess are depleted and deficient plasma factors may be replaced. PPF, however, whilst removing abnormal proteins, leaves most globulins at subnormal levels (Keller & Urbaniak, 1978; Lockwood et al, 1979a). Plasmapheresis, with crystalloid replacement, may be performed in patients with normal renal function when infrequent exchanges are performed, but is inadvisable in the presence of renal failure or when intensive daily exchanges are being carried out. It should be recognised that the effects of plasmapheresis, as opposed to plasma exchange, on protein metabolism may differ.

Frequency and duration of exchange

In principle the frequency and duration of exchange should be based on the distribution of the substance to be removed in body fluid compartments, its rates of equilibration between the plasma and other compartments and its rate of regeneration. For instance, immune complexes are predominantly intravascular, so equilibration with other fluid compartments is not an important factor (Rossen et al, 1977). On the other hand, autoantibodies have a significant extravascular distribution, both free and bound, and re-equilibration following each plasma exchange leads to an early rise in plasma levels (Lockwood et al, 1979a) and will determine the frequency of exchanges necessary (usually daily). The rate of antibody synthesis or immune complex generation will tend to determine the length of a course of exchange.

In practice the frequency and duration of exchange are of necessity determined by evidence of active tissue damage rather than the levels of initiators of injury; it seems that immune complex mediated disease (Lockwood et al, 1977a; 1977b; 1979a) requires less plasma exchange than comparable autoantibody mediated disease (Lockwood et al, 1976; 1977a; 1977b; Rees, Lockwood & Peters, 1979). In both immune complex and antibody mediated disease, the rate of generation of the immunopathogenetic factor is clearly influenced by concurrent immunosuppressive therapy.

Concurrent therapy

There are two basic objectives of concurrent therapy; one is to minimise the tissue injury resulting from autoantibodies or immune complexes and the other is to reduce or abolish their generation. Both steroids and immunosuppressive agents (cyclophosphamide and azathioprine) probably reduce tissue injury by their anti-inflammatory action. Immunosuppressive agents are principally used, however, to reduce the rate of synthesis of autoantibody or the antibody component of immune complexes.

As an experiment to evaluate the role of humoral factors in a particular disease or to assess its short-term therapeutic role, plasma exchange alone may be appropriate. However, in most clinical situations the main reason for using plasma exchange is the rapidity of its effects and the provision of time for drug therapy to become effective. The acute effects of plasma exchange may also enhance the activity of other agents. There is a theoretical basis for considering that plasma exchange and immunosuppression may be synergistic and this arises from two quite separate experiments. It is known that plasma removal following active immunisation leads to feedback stimulation of antibody production (Bystryn, Schenken & Uhr, 1971), so that if this were to apply to autoantibody synthesis plasma exchange would, by promoting cell division by the responsible clone, render it sensitive to the effects of cytotoxic agents (suicidal proliferation). On the other hand, experiments in guinea pigs have shown that if one antibody subclass is administered to an animal it stimulates the formation of another antibody subclass (Hall et al, 1977), suggesting that antibody synthesis is itself dependent upon the presence of antibody. Strangely these different theories both lend support to the use of plasma exchange regimens but their applicability to the treatment of disease in man remains to be established.

Hazards of plasma exchange
Plasma exchange is very well tolerated by patients and symptoms during the procedure are rare. With the routine addition of calcium (0.45 mmol/unit) and potassium (1.4 mmol/unit) to PPF, paraesthesiae and cramps are unusual. With PPF the incidence of anaphylactic or allergic reactions is negligible but with FFP they are a significant hazard. Other hazards of plasma exchange arise largely from the extracorporeal circuit — air embolism, clotting of the centrifugation bowl, etc. — and from infection related to arteriovenous access. Arteriovenous shunts in immunosuppressed patients have considerable practical advantages but despite extreme vigilance in detecting and treating local infections early their use is associated with a high incidence of significant infections sometimes complicated by septicaemia. A significant number of septicaemic episodes are seen in patients with long-line (femoral or subclavian) venous exchanges. Patients at Hammersmith Hospital are currently being evaluated to determine the relative role of corticosteroids, immunosuppressive agents, renal failure and plasma exchange in the genesis of infection in general (Cohen, Pinching, Rees & Peters, in preparation); it appears that plasma exchange per se does not compound the risks of infection due to drugs.

Bleeding is rarely a problem in plasma exchange with PPF despite the considerable reduction in clotting factors (Keller & Urbaniak, 1978; Lockwood et al, 1979a). There is a high risk with extreme thrombocytopenia or when there is a fresh bleeding point such as a visceral biopsy or peptic ulcer. In such cases the use of 2–3 units of FFP at the end of exchange appears to avert haemorrhagic complications. Patients with haemoglobin levels of, or less than, 8 gm/100 ml who are on the semicontinuous separator, should be transfused before exchange. Drug dosage does not usually need to be adjusted in patients on plasma exchange, even for protein bound drugs, as their distribution throughout their body and their continued administration maintain adequate drug levels; for example in myasthenia gravis, anticholinesterase drugs are not sufficiently depleted by exchange as to lead to deterioration even in cases of the congenital form who do not benefit from exchange (Pinching, Peters & Newsom-Davis, 1976).

General objectives
Plasma exchange plays two, but not mutually exclusive, roles: it may be to establish the role of a humoral substance in the pathogenesis of a disease or it may be therapeutic. The sudden exchange of the plasma milieu will produce acute changes in circulating proteins, etc., and evidence for pathogenicity may emerge from longitu-

dinal correlation between the clinical response and the presence or otherwise of putative initiators (autoantibody or immune complex) or mediators of injury (acute phase proteins, complement components, clotting factors, kinins etc.). While the possible benefit of removal of abnormal substances such as autoantibody or immune complex is self-evident, plasma exchange in conditions of unknown pathogenesis may identify involvement of humoral factors and lead to the development of assays for their estimation. Furthermore, the transient and extensive depletion of other plasma proteins (Keller & Urbaniak, 1978; Lockwood et al, 1979a) by plasma exchange with PPF may be beneficial whether they are initially present at normal or elevated levels. For instance, acute phase proteins, many of them involved in the inflammatory response and essential for the mediation of tissue injury, are simultaneously depleted. The resulting anti-inflammatory effect may be of particular value in fulminating disease such as in rapidly progressive nephritis in which there is little time before the acute changes become irreversible.

The extent to which autoantibody titre needs to be reduced depends upon the severity and reversibility of injury and also the threshold above which the antibody is pathogenic in any individual. This threshold may not be static, as has been indicated by the observations of infection-provoked relapse in quiescent antiglomerular basement membrane (anti-GBM) disease (Rees, Lockwood & Peters, 1977), in which intercurrent infection reduces the threshold for tissue damage. In immune complex disease, intrinsic mechanisms for the removal of circulating immune complexes may be defective; plasma exchange may lead to restoration of normal clearance (Lockwood et al, 1977a, b). Infection is also an important precipitant of relapse in immune complex disease, and may be associated with the reappearance of circulating immune complexes and probably with alterations in clearance mechanisms (Pinching et al, 1980).

The rate of autoantibody synthesis varies considerably so that the need for exchange and immunosuppression have to be tailored to the individual judged by clinical evidence of organ damage. The titres of autoantibody or immune complex do, however, indicate the alterations in putative initiators of disease and high levels may help to explain unusually long periods of activity, while active disease and low levels may indicate the possibility of superimposed infection. In non-fulminating diseases the duration of plasma exchange may, in part, be determined by theoretical considerations of synergism between plasma exchange and immunosuppression because the amount of plasma exchange required to produce immediate clinical remissions may differ from that needed for long-term benefit.

Monitoring

There are two aspects of disease that need to be monitored in patients undergoing plasma exchange. Firstly, detailed, frequent, serial assessment of target organ function and damage, as for example serum creatinine and urine deposit in renal disease, or pulmonary function tests and chest radiology in pulmonary diseases, and secondly, the frequent serial assay of putative initiators and mediators. When possible this will include not only specific autoantibodies and immune complexes but also the assessment of intrinsic regulatory functions such as antibody synthesis and clearance mechanisms for immune complexes. Assays for antiglomerular basement membrane antibodies and acetylcholine receptor antibodies have been used extensively in monitoring patients with anti-GBM disease (Rees et al, 1979) and myasthenia gravis (Dau et al, 1977; Newsom-Davis et al, 1978) respectively. Similarly assays for circulating immune complexes (C.I.C.s) including Clq binding, conglutinin and rheumatoid factor binding assays have been used to monitor therapy (Lockwood et al, 1977a; Pussell et al, 1978). A new method for investigating splenic clearance of labelled heat-damaged or antibody-coated red cells, which probably require the same clearance mechanism as that for immune complexes, has been developed (Frank et al, 1979; Lockwood et al, 1979b). The correction of defective clearance, seen in patients with autoallergic disease following plasma exchange, is one of the most intriguing observations yet made; it may reflect either a specific effect on splenic macrophages or be due to the removal of I.C.s which are blocking splenic clearance.

DISEASES INVOLVING AUTOANTIBODY

Antiglomerular basement membrane disease

The most familiar form of this disease is Goodpasture's syndrome, characterised by rapidly progressive glomerulonephritis and lung haemorrhage (Rees et al, 1979), which is often but not always associated with the presence of circulating anti-GBM antibodies and linear immunofluorescent staining for IgG on renal glomerular and pulmonary alveolar basement membranes. While the disease may present in several ways, both the lung haemorrhage and the nephritis are often fulminant: severe hypoxia and/or renal failure may develop within a few days of onset. In the great majority of cases that have been untreated or treated with corticosteroids or immunosuppressive agents alone, death resulted rapidly from lung haemorrhage or renal failure, unless dialysis was available. This dismal outcome reflects the rapidity with which widespread and, in the case of the kidney, irreversible changes result from the tissue fixation of anti-GBM antibody.

It is in such an adverse setting that plasma exchange was first shown to be of value in fulminating autoallergic disease (Lockwood et al, 1976); the speed with which plasma exchange could reduce the level of circulating anti-GBM antibody and the humoral mediators of inflammation made this a most logical application of the procedure. The concurrent use of steroids and immunosuppressive agents was also rational in that it might not only reduce further tissue damage but also decrease antibody synthesis. The introduction of this regimen led to a substantial improvement in the outcome. Twenty-six consecutive patients have been treated at Hammersmith Hospital (Lockwood et al, 1976; 1977b; 1979a; Rees et al, 1979) with intensive daily plasma exchange (for periods of 10–50 days), combined with a standard regimen of prednisolone (60 mg daily) and immunosuppressive agents (cyclophosphamide 3 mg/ kg and azathioprine 1 mg/kg). Pulmonary haemorrhage was controlled in 18 out of 19 patients. Of 11 patients with deteriorating renal function but who were not anuric at the time of starting plasma exchange, the downward trend in renal function was reversed and function improved in 10. The two failures were in patients with serious systemic infection and inadequate plasma exchange, in one case directly related to the problem of vascular access. Six patients had stable but impaired renal function with evidence of active nephritis and in these renal function was maintained and examination of the urine deposit showed resolution of nephritic changes. The remaining patients were anuric at presentation and showed no evidence of renal recovery. The fulminating nature of the disease untreated was indicated on several occasions by complete loss of renal function within a few days of preliminary investigations; if the disease is suspected, diagnosis and treatment are a matter of the utmost urgency if organ function is to be preserved.

Similar experiences had been reported in two other centres (Walker et al, 1977; Kincaid Smith & D'Apice, 1978; Johnson et al, 1978), and it is clear that the natural history of this disease precludes any attempt to identify the particular roles of plasma exchange and other agents, especially as there are strong theoretical grounds for not doing so. However, in a few patients in whom plasma exchange has to be temporarily discontinued before the disease is fully under control due to difficulties of vascular access the ensuing relapse, and the remission after the reintroduction of exchange, demonstrate the importance of the exchange itself in the early stage of therapy. The roles of the various agents used in plasma exchange regimens have also been brought out by observations on small numbers of patients from centres where unsatisfactory results have been reported. Less than intensive plasma exchange in the early stage did not prevent the onset of irreversible renal failure in one instance, when, in the face of deterioration following cessation of exchange, the procedure was not reintroduced (McLeish, Maxwell & Luft, 1978). In another study, plasma exchange was used in one patient without concurrent drug therapy until renal function had been lost (Swainson et al, 1978), and this suggests that combination therapy is indeed necessary to control simultaneously the several aspects of the immunopathological derangement.

Autoantibody is produced over quite a short period but is very destructive and if the patients can be tided over this period without loss of organ function, the long-term prognosis is very satisfactory. If patients lose all renal function, transplantation may be considered once the autoantibody has definitely disappeared from the circulation, as recurrence of the disease in transplanted kidneys occurs only in patients with circulating autoantibody. Recurrence of disease in transplanted kidneys has however been successfully treated with a plasma exchange regimen (Swainson et al, 1978) and possibly even prevented (Cove-Smith et al, 1978).

Patients with anti-GBM disease who have active lung haemorrhage and/or nephritis (if not anuric) should always be treated with intensive daily plasma exchange, corticosteroids and immunosuppression. The rarity of the disease and the different problems of the management of these severely ill patients, make it essential that therapy is conducted in specialised centres.

Myasthenia gravis
In myasthenia gravis, in which the characteristic weakness and fatiguability of the disease is chronic, alterations in the patient's clinical state occur more gradually than in anti-GBM disease; this has enabled more detailed evaluation of the role of different treatment schedules as well as an investigation of the immunopathogenesis of the disease. Recent studies have indicated that the disorder results from interference with acetylcholine receptors at the motor endplate (reviewed by Drachman, 1978 and Pinching, 1978). The presence of acetylcholine receptor antibodies in a large proportion of myasthenic patients and the development of an experimental model of myasthenia in animals immunised with acetylcholine receptor preparations suggested

that these antibodies play a pathogenetic role. Although other clinical studies had indicated that antibodies are pathogenic, it was not until the use of plasma exchange to produce abrupt falls in the antibody titre was associated with marked clinical improvement that the importance of these antibodies was confirmed (Pinching et al, 1976). Plasma exchange as a method of investigation is ideally suited to this problem. The striking clinical improvement following plasma exchange alone, and the natural history of the disease after exchange indicate a close correlation in individual patients between the level of antibody and the clinical state (Newsom-Davis et al, 1978). It now appears that the antibodies have two effects, causing, firstly, some destruction of the motor-endplate and also blockade of the remaining acetylcholine receptors, probably by an allosteric effect from the antibody-binding site to the acetylcholine binding site (Lindstrom & Lambert, 1978).

Large numbers of patients have now been treated in several centres (Pinching et al, 1976; Dau et al, 1977; Newsom-Davis et al, 1978; 1979a and 1979b; Behan et al, 1979; Newsom-Davis & Vincent, 1979) — largely those suffering from the severe generalised form of the disease. Recent studies have concentrated on the most appropriate timing, frequency and duration of plasma exchange and the best combination therapy. As in anti-GBM disease, the use of immunosuppressive agents seemed logical to reduce antibody production and to avoid any rebound phenomenon following antibody removal (which has been seen in some myasthenic patients following exchange alone). Immunosuppressive agents (usually azathioprine) do indeed, when used alone, cause a gradual reduction in antibody titre over periods of several months (Newsom-Davis et al, 1979b; Newsom-Davis & Vincent, 1979). Corticosteroids have also been shown to be beneficial in many patients with myasthenia gravis (Moran, Johns & Campa, 1976; Drachman, 1978), and although the mechanism of this is uncertain their effect is probably peripheral rather than specifically immunosuppressive. Many patients show pronounced benefit from corticosteroids in the short-term and remain well in the long-term on small maintenance doses, even though antibody levels are unaffected.

For this reason, studies in which the steroid dosage remains the same when plasma exchange and immunosuppressive drugs are introduced, can be used to evaluate the role of antibody. If plasma exchange and immunosuppression are combined with the introduction of/or simultaneous increment in steroid therapy as in a recent study (Behan et al, 1979), the effect of several mechanisms affecting pathogenesis is being observed. The differences in results seen with regimens including an increase in steroids and those in which steroids are not altered may indicate that, as in anti-GBM disease, the combination therapy produces optimal benefit, but comparative studies are required. Some investigators have suggested that prolonged initial exchange may lead to better longer-term remissions, but other studies (Newsom-Davis & Vincent, 1979) have not confirmed this; apart from the possible avoidance of rebound, no evidence of synergism between plasma exchange and immunosuppressive therapy as currently used as been demonstrated in most patients (Newsom-Davis et al, 1979b).

Although the role of plasma exchange in myasthenia is still unclear, patients with severe disease, poorly controlled on conventional therapy, merit consideration of plasma exchange and immunosuppression. The rapid improvement with plasma exchange in patients, even with severe myasthenia, suggests it may be particularly helpful in respiratory myasthenic crises. Its rapid action can also be used to increase ventilatory function in patients with acute fulminating disease who are proceeding to thymectomy. Patients with no detectable circulating antibody, such as those with congential myasthenia (Vincent & Newsom-Davis, 1979) or 'burnt-out' myasthenia, are unlikely to benefit from plasma exchange or immunosuppression. Clinical trials of plasma exchange in a few larger centres will finally determine its place in therapy.

Miscellaneous antibody-mediated diseases
The applications of plasma exchange to other antibody-mediated diseases have, with the notable exception of rhesus disease, been less important than the foregoing and have tended to be more of scientific than therapeutic interest. Two auto-antibody-mediated skin diseases, Herpes gestationis (Carruthers & Ewins, 1978) and pemphigus vulgaris (Ruocco et al, 1978; Cotterill et al, 1978), have been studied using plasma exchange. Patients appeared to benefit from the procedure but there is as yet no indication of a therapeutic role emerging for plasma exchange. Plasma exchange has also been applied with benefit to autoimmune thyroid disease in which an autoantibody appears to be implicated in the development of ophthalmic Graves's disease and pretibial myxoedema (Dandona et al, 1979a and 1979b). Patients who benefitted were those with rapidly progressive ophthalmopathy whereas those with long-standing changes did not. Patients with the rare insulin resistant form of diabetes and acanthosis nigricans (type II) which is associated with autoantibodies to insulin receptors (Flier, Kahn & Roth, 1979) have been treated with plasma exchange and the removal of antibody has been elegantly monitored by studies of the effect on receptor function in vitro (Muggeo et al, 1979).

The use of plasma exchange in haematological disorders associated with the presence of autoantibody such as idiopathic thrombocytopenic purpura and autoimmune haemolytic anaemia has been limited, largely because the response to other therapeutic measures such as steroids or splenectomy is so often satisfactory. Nevertheless, it does seem that in some severely affected patients plasma exchange may offer valuable short-term control (Branda et al, 1978; Gordon-Smith and the late Dr Sheila Worlledge, personal communication).

Plasma exchange as an attempt to reduce the fetal mortality from rhesus isoimmunisation was probably the first truely immunological application of the technique (Clarke et al, 1970; Fraser et al, 1976; Graham-Pole, Barr & Willoughby, 1977). Mothers with grossly elevated antibody levels whose fetuses are at extremely high risk from intrauterine death or severe hydrops may be given plasma exchange to reduce maternal antibody titre. This reduces fetal mortality and may enable intrauterine exchange transfusion of the fetus to be postponed until it is sufficiently mature to tolerate the procedure more safely. It may even obviate the necessity for fetal exchange transfusion and reduce the severity of disease in the neonate. As the antibody wanes following delivery, there is no rationale for concurrent immunosuppression.

Plasma exchange has also been used in the removal of alloantibodies arising in haemophiliacs who have received multiple factor VIII transfusions (Pintado, Jaswell & Walter-Bowie, 1975; Cobcroft, Tamagnini & Dormandy, 1977). These antibodies act as factor VIII inhibitors and become clinically significant in the treatment of bleeding episodes with factor VIII. If the inhibition prevents control of bleeding, plasma exchange offers a useful means for reducing the titre of alloantibody. As the titre of antibody wanes rapidly when factor VIII is not being given, there is generally no justification for concurrent immunosuppression. This particular application of plasma exchange has emphasised the fact that the control of antibody synthesis differs in the case of allo- and autoantibodies and cautions the extrapolation from studies of one to the other, and from experimental immunisation to autoallergic disease.

IMMUNE COMPLEX DISEASE

Rapidly progressive glomerulonephritis

This form of nephritis, when not associated with GBM antibodies, is generally seen in systemic vasculitic diseases such as Wegener's granulomatosis, polyarteritis (microscopic) or Henoch-Schönlein purpura, although it may occur in isolation. The progression of the nephritis with only an abnormal urine deposit to renal failure may be more insidious than with anti-GBM disease and be marked by periods of reduced activity, but a fulminating course also occurs. The finding of complement and immunoglobulins in the glomeruli and/or vessels on renal biopsy and the frequency detection of C.I.Cs (e.g. by Clq binding assay) strongly suggests that immune complexes are involved in immunopathogenesis and probably initiate injury; a marked increase in acute phase proteins is also characteristic.

Patients with these disorders have sometimes been successfully treated in the past using steroids and/or immunosuppressive agents, occasionally in combination with anticoagulants or antiplatelet agents. However the results have not always been satisfactory and some patients with fulminant disease responded poorly to drugs alone. Following the successful application of plasma exchange to the histologically similar anti-GBM disease, and in view of the C.I.Cs and pronounced acute phase response, it seemed appropriate to investigate the use of plasma exchange in such patients. Pilot studies (Lockwood et al, 1977a; 1977b; 1979a) showed encouraging results which suggested that patients responded to plasma exchange and drug therapy more rapidly and to a greater degree than with drugs alone. This applied not only to the renal involvement but also to other aspects of systemic disease. Several patients with severe disease who would not have been expected to respond to drugs alone made a favourable response. However, the fact that patients may respond to drugs alone has led to the setting up at Hammersmith Hospital of a randomised controlled trial of plasma exchange and drugs, and drugs alone, stratified according to the severity of renal failure. Meanwhile other groups have recorded similarly encouraging results from uncontrolled series (Becker et al, 1977; Rossen et al, 1977; Kincaid-Smith & d'Apice, 1978; Harmer et al, 1979).

In a preliminary analysis of 33 patients treated by combined plasma exchange and immunosuppression at Hammersmith Hospital, including many patients not entered into the trial (Pinching et al unpublished observations), 18 of whom needed dialysis, 24 showed improved renal function; of those not responding, 4 died of hypoxia before the renal response could be assessed and 4 had needed dialysis for more than 10 days before therapy had been introduced. Extrarenal manifestations (pulmonary haemorrhage, granulomata, ocular, aural disease, myopathy and nervous system involvement) were seen to improve in 27 of the 31 patients in whom they occurred, the remainder dying early of hypoxia. This improvement was associated with the rapid disappearance of C.I.Cs and decrease in the acute phase response; splenic clearance of abnormal red cells also improved (Lockwood et al, 1979a and 1979b). Despite initial improvement, mortality was high, often due to multiple causes, including hypoxia (6), lack of renal support for patients without renal recovery (2), infection (9), myocardial failure (1) and late relapse (2). Of the remainder, most have remained well, although several have had minor relapses, often provoked by infection and usually responding to prompt increments in therapy.

Relatively short-term plasma exchange (usually 3–14 days) may be needed to control disease, in contrast to anti-GBM disease. The improvement in renal function is also more rapid and more substantial than that seen in anti-GBM disease. Anuria or the need for dialysis in immune complex rapidly progressive glomerulonephritis do not necessarily imply irreversibility, although if present for more than 10 days before therapy, recovery of function is rare. Patients with a critical degree of hypoxia from pulmonary involvement before treatment have fared poorly despite initial improvement in some.

It is clear that specific therapy should be introduced where possible before organ function is critically compromised not only because the response is less good, but also because the incidence of infective complications rises with the need for organ support such as dialysis or ventilation. The contribution of infection to morbidity and mortality and in provoking relapses make this the single most important problem in the management of these heavily immunosuppressed patients. It is doubtful whether plasma exchange increases the risk of infection due to drugs alone but this aspect of the problem is currently being evaluated (Cohen, Pinching, Rees & Peters, in preparation). The results both of this further study and of the controlled trial to determine the effect of plasma exchange must be awaited before firm recommendations can be made.

Systemic lupus erythematosus

Immune complexes are implicated in the pathogenesis of system lupus erythematosus (SLE) although autoantibody formation is also a feature. Many of the manifestations of this protean disease (e.g. rash, arthropathy) are readily controlled with conventional agents including anti-inflammatory drugs, antimalarials and low dose steroids. Similarly, many patients with renal or other systemic manifestations may be managed satisfactorily with high dose steroids. The role of immunosuppressive agents is more arguable as the risk of infection is particularly high and their benefit has not been established. There are however a few patients who respond poorly to or relapse despite corticosteroids; these patients generally have severe and often fulminating disease — particularly diffuse glomerulonephritis causing renal failure, cerebral lupus or rare pulmonary involvement. Plasma exchange can be readily justified in such cases. Unfortunately, special problems apply to SLE in the evaluation of new therapies — in particular the tendency for spontaneous remission, the response to early treatment which is often delayed and the fact that intercurrent infections, to which these patients are especially prone, may enhance disease activity. These features in severely ill patients have made controlled evaluation of plasma exchange extremely difficult, while patients in whom such features of the disease are minimal tend not to require this therapy.

Verrier-Jones et al (1976) have used small volume infrequent plasma exchange in eight patients with SLE and observed clinical improvement in four in whom C.I.Cs were detectable; an extension of this study, with additional patients, has recently been published and emphasizes the heterogeneity of the patient population (Verrier-Jones et al, 1979). Nine patients with severe active disease have been treated at Hammersmith Hospital with a more intensive regimen of 4-litre daily plasma exchanges as used in rapidly progressive nephritis, but generally omitting immunosuppressive agents (some already reported by Lockwood et al, 1977b, 1979a and 1979b). In four cases plasma exchange and steroid therapy were introduced simultaneously but in five plasma exchange was only introduced after failure to respond to, or relapse following, adequate periods of high-dose steroid therapy. Eight patients had diffuse lupus nephritis with renal failure, three had severe cerebral lupus and two had significant pulmonary involvement; eight had C.I.Cs and all had evidence of complement consumption. In three of the four treated concurrently, very rapid resolution was seen, at a rate and to a degree unexpected with steroids alone. Four of the five treated with exchange after failure of steroids, showed resolution of active disease in all sites and renal function improved substantially. This response was associated with the disappearance of C.I.Cs, reversal of splenic blockade (Lockwood et al, 1979b) and the correction of complement abnormalities and the time course strongly suggested that the introduction of plasma exchange was responsible. Moran et al (1977) have suggested on the basis of studies on two patients with haematological complications of SLE that the use of FFP rather than PPF for exchange may be beneficial, possibly by repleting complement components.

While these results are encouraging, the great majority of patients with SLE are readily and satisfactorily treated with corticosteroids alone. The use of plasma exchange, other than for clinical research purposes, should be restricted to those patients in whom a tolerable dose of corticosteroids is inadequate.

Miscellaneous conditions

Patients with other putative immune complex diseases have also been treated with plasma exchange. Two cases of cutaneous vasculitis, one with evidence of circulating immune complexes and complement consumption and the other with systemic manifestations, have been controlled using plasma exchange intermittently, once every four to six weeks without immunosuppressive therapy. Improvement of complement abnormalities and disappearance of immune complexes followed in one and in both correction of defective splenic function following plasma exchange occurred (Lockwood et al, 1970a and 1977b). Patients with cryoglobulinaemia may benefit from plasma exchange, although the level of cryoglobulins often rises rapidly after exchange. One patient (Lockwood, 1979) showed a reduction in the temperature of precipitation of the cryoglobulin despite little overall change in its quantity, so that precipitation in vivo, even in the extremities, was unlikely; this effect was associated with clinical improvement (healing of large leg ulcers). Immunosuppression is certainly an important adjunct to plasma exchange in such patients.

A recent study of 12 patients with active rheumatoid arthritis using a combination of plasma exchange and gold or penicillamine showed induction of remission in all 10 cases on this combination, and improvement was maintained for several months (Wallace et al, 1979); 2 patients not receiving these drugs did not have sustained benefit. The 10 who responded had not been helped by drugs alone before plasma exchange. A regimen of thrice weekly exchanges for 3 weeks, twice weekly exchanges for 3 weeks and weekly exchanges for a further 5 weeks was used. The removal of lymphoid cells during exchange in some of the patients appeared not to confer additional benefit. An interesting observation was that while the early more frequent exchanges reduced levels of C.I.Cs and inflammatory mediators, these returned to pre-exchange levels in the later phase of treatment but without relapse. The problems of assessing disease activity in rheumatoid arthritis are considerable and plasma exchange may have a substantial placebo effect, so further controlled studies are awaited with interest.

DISEASES OF UNCERTAIN PATHOGENESIS

Long-term relief of Raynaud's phenomenon has been shown to occur after relatively little plasma exchange, used alone (Talpos et al, 1978; O'Reilly et al, 1979), and the duration of benefit (three to four days) makes it unlikely to be due to the reduction of plasma viscosity — which is short-lived (Kilpatrick et al, 1978). Some of these patients had scleroderma and several other patients with vascular complications of scleroderma have shown similar improvement in an uncontrolled pilot study. The only other aspect of this condition which may benefit is the rapidly progressive arthropathy and the hand changes; it seems inherently unlikely that plasma exchange will reverse established sclerotic changes. Further experience of rapidly progressive scleroderma, especially in those patients with vascular complications, is now needed. The pathogenesis of Raynaud's phenomenon is unknown but the results of plasma exchange indicate that humoral factors are involved; the long-lasting improvement following exchange appears to result from correction of reduced deformability of red cells although the mechanism whereby plasma exchange produces it is uncertain (Dodds et al, 1979).

Reports of benefit from plasma exchange in Guillain-Barré syndrome are encouraging (Brettle et al, 1978; Levy, Newkirk & Ochoa, 1979). In view of the poor response to steroids reported in a recent controlled trial (Hughes et al, 1978), they merit further study although the natural history of the disease poses great problems in evaluation. Cases of relapsing Guillain-Barré syndrome in particular have benefitted rapidly from plasma exchange (Levy et al, 1979; Legg, N. J., personal communication).

It is hoped that the identification of humoral mediators may follow these observations. Although there is a single case report of the effect of plasma exchange in a patient with asthma (Gartmann, Grob & Frey, 1978), it is not sufficiently detailed to allow proper evaluation and further results on this are awaited.

Despite initial encouraging results (Cardella et al, 1977), renal transplant rejection, whose pathogenesis is not fully understood, shows no lasting benefit from plasma exchange (Cardella et al, 1978). The transient effect observed, probably results from depletion of mediators alone rather than any basic effect on the initiation of rejection. If this were the case it would indicate that the longer-lasting benefit from plasma exchange in other conditions cannot be attributed to depletion of mediators alone.

Conclusions

Plasma exchange provides a means of investigating and treating a wide variety of immunologically mediated diseases. Its usual therapeutic role is likely to be in the acute management of these diseases, due to its rapid and marked effects on plasma constitution, but it should always be considered as only one part of a treatment regimen. Careful selection and monitoring of patients under such treatment and the restriction of this experience to a limited number of centres with the facilities to monitor such patients will enable experience to be gained rapidly. In this way clinical and experimental indications for the procedure and its optimal mode of use can most quickly and economically be achieved.

ACKNOWLEDGMENTS

I am grateful to Dr C. M. Lockwood, Dr A. J. Rees, Dr B. Pussell, Dr J. Newsom-Davis and Dr A. Vincent for generous advice and discussions concerning plasma exchange and to Professor D. K. Peters for his unstinting guidance throughout.

REFERENCES

Becker G J, d'Apice A J F, Walker R G, Kincaid-Smith P 1977 Plasmapheresis in the treatment of glomerulonephritis. Medical Journal of Australia 2: 693–696

Behan P O, Shakir R A, Simpson J A, Burnett A K, Allan T L, Haase G 1979 Plasma exchange combined with immunosuppressive therapy in Myasthenia gravis. Lancet ii: 438–440

Branda R F, Tate D Y, McCullough J J, Jacob H S 1978 Plasma exchange in the treatment of fulminant (autoimmune) thrombocytopenic purpura. Lancet i: 688–690

Brettle R P, Gross M, Legg N J, Lockwood C M, Pallis C 1978 Treatment of acute polyneuropathy by plasma exchange. Lancet ii: 1100

Bystryn J C, Schenken I, Uhr J H W 1971 A model for regulation of antibody synthesis by serum antibody. In: Amos B (ed) Progress in immunology. New York, Academic Press, p 630–636

Cardella C J, Sutton D, Uldall P R, deVeber G A 1977 Intensive plasma exchange and renal transplant rejection. Lancet i: 264

Cardella C J, Sutton D, Falk J A, Katz A, Uldall P R, deVeber G A 1978 Effect of intensive plasma exchange on renal transplant rejection and serum cytotoxic antibodies. Transplant Proceedings 10: 617–619

Carruthers J A, Ewins A R 1978 Herpes gestationis: studies on the binding characteristics activity and pathogenetic significance of the complement fixing factor. Clinical and Experimental Immunology 31: 38–44

Clarke C A, Elson C J, Bradley J, Donohoe W T A, Lehane D, Hughes-Jones N C 1970 Intensive plasmapheresis as a therapeutic measure in rhesus immunised women. Lancet i: 793–798

Cobcroft R, Tamagnini G, Dormandy K M 1977 Serial plasmapheresis in a haemophiliac with antibodies to factor VIII. Journal of Clinical Pathology 30: 763–765

Cohen J, Pinching A J, Rees A J, Peters D K In preparation. Infection and immunosuppression: a study of the infective complications of 75 patients with immunologically mediated disease.

Cotterill J A, Barker D J, Millard L G, Robinson E A 1978 Plasma exchange in the treatment of pemphigus vulgaris. British Journal of Dermatology 98: 243

Cove-Smith J R, McLeod A A, Blamey R W, Knapp M S, Reeves W G, Wilson C B 1978 Transplantation, Immunosuppression and Plasmapheresis in Goodpasture's syndrome. Clinical Nephrology 9: 126–128

Dau P C, Lindstrom J M, Cassel C K, Denys H H, Shev E E, Spitler L E 1977 Plasmapheresis and immunosuppressive therapy in Myasthenia gravis. New England Journal of Medicine 297: 1134–1140

Dandona P, Marshall N J, Bidy S P, Nathan A, Havard C W H 1979a Successful treatment of exophthalmos and pretibial myxoedema with plasmapheresis. British Medical Journal i: 374–376

Dandona P, Marshall N J, Bidy S P, Nathan A W, Harvard C W H 1979b Exophthalmos and pretibial myxoedema not responding to plasmapheresis. British Medical Journal ii: 667–668

Dodds A J, O'Reilly M J G, Yates C J P, Cotton L T, Flute P T, Dormandy J A 1979 Haemorrheological response to plasma exchange in Raynaud's syndrome. British Medical Journal ii: 1186–1187

Drachman D B 1978 Myasthenia gravis. New England Journal of Medicine 298: 136–142, 186–193

Flier J S, Kahn C R, Roth J 1979 Receptors, antireceptor antibodies and mechanisms of insulin resistance. New England Journal of Medicine 300: 413–419

Frank M M, Hamburger M I, Lawley T J, Kimberly R D, Plotz P H 1979 Defective reticulo-endothelial system Fc-receptor function in systemic lupus erythematosus. New England Journal of Medicine 300: 518–523

Fraser I D, Bothamley J E, Bennett M O, Airth G R, Lehane D, McCarthey M, Roberts F M 1976 Intensive antenatal plasmapheresis in severe rhesus isoimmunisation. Lancet i: 6–8

Gartmann J, Grob P, Frey M 1978 Plasmapheresis in severe asthma. Lancet ii: 40
Graham-Pole J, Barr W, Willoughby M L N 1977 Continuous flow plasmapheresis in management of severe rhesus disease. British Medical Journal i: 1185–1188
Hall C L, Colvin R B, Carey K, McCluskey R T 1977 Passive transfer of autoimmune disease with isologous IgG$_1$ and IgG$_2$ antibodies to tubular basement membrane in strain XIII guinea pigs. Journal of Experimental Medicine 146: 1246–1260
Harmer D, Finn R, Goldsmith H J, Bone J M, Forbes A W 1979 Plasmapheresis in fulminating crescentic nephritis. Lancet i: 679
Hughes R A C, Newsom-Davis J M, Perkin G D, Pierce J M 1978 Controlled trial of Prednisolone in acute polyneuropathy. Lancet ii: 750–753
Johnson J P, Whitman W, Briggs W A, Wilson C B 1978 Plasmapheresis and Immunosuppressive agents in antibasement membrane antibody-induced Goodpasture's syndrome. American Journal of Medicine 64: 354–359
Keller A J, Urbaniak S J 1978 Intensive plasma exchange on the cell separator: effects on serum immunoglobulins and complement components. British Journal of Haematology 38: 531–540
Kilpatrick D, Fleming J, Clyne C, Thompson G R 1978 Reduction of blood viscosity following plasma exchange. Atherosclerosis 32: 301–306
Kincaid-Smith P, d'Apice A J F 1978 Plasmapheresis in rapidly progressive nephritis. American Journal of Medicine 65: 564–566
Levy R L, Newkirk R, Ochoa J 1979 Treatment of chronic relapsing Guillain-Barré syndrome by plasma exchange. Lancet ii: 741
Lindstrom J, Lambert C H 1978 Content of acetylcholine receptor and antibodies bound to receptor in Myasthenia gravis, experimental auto-immune Myasthenia gravis and the Eaton-Lambert syndrome. Neurology (Minneapolis) 28: 130–138
Lockwood C M, Rees A J, Pearson T A, Evans D J, Peters D K, Wilson C B 1976 Immunosuppression and plasma-exchange in the treatment of Goodpasture's syndrome. Lancet i: 711–715
Lockwood C M, Rees A J, Pinching A J, Pussell B, Sweny P, Uff J, Peters D K 1977a Plasma exchange and immunosuppression in the treatment of fulminating immune-complex crescentic nephritis. Lancet i: 63–67
Lockwood C M, Rees A J, Pussell B, Peters D K 1977b Experience of the use of plasma-exhange in the management of potentially fulminating glomerulonephritis and SLE. Experimental Haematology, 5 Supplement, 117–136
Lockwood C M 1979 Plasma exchange in cryoglobulinaemia. Kidney International 16: 522–530
Lockwood C M, Pussell B, Wilson C B, Peters D K 1979a Plasma exchange in nephritis. Advances in Nephrology 8: 383–418
Lockwood C M, Worlledge S, Nicholas A, Cotton C, Peters D K 1979b Reversal of impaired splenic function in patients with nephritis or vasculitis (or both) by plasma exchange. New England Journal of Medicine 300: 524–530
McLeish K R, Maxwell D R, Luft F C 1978 Failure of plasma exchange and immunosuppression to improve renal function in Goodpasture's syndrome. Clinical Nephrology 10, 71–73
Mann J D, Johns T R, Campa J F 1976 Longterm administration of corticosteroids in Myasthenia gravis. Neurology (Minneapolis) 26: 729–740
Moran C J, Parry H F, Mowbray J, Richards J D M, Goldstone A H 1977 Plasmapheresis in systemic lupus eythematosus. British Medical Journal i: 1573–1574
Muggeo M, Flier J S, Abrams R A, Harrison L C, Deisserroth A B, Kahn C R 1979 Treatment by plasma exchange of a patient with autoantibodies to the insulin receptor. New England Journal of Medicine 300: 477–480
Newsom-Davis J, Pinching A J, Vincent A, Wilson S G 1978 Function of circulating antibody to acetyl-choline receptor in myasthenia gravis: investigation by plasma exchange. Neurology (Minneapolis) 28: 266–272
Newsom-Davis J, Vincent A 1979 Combined plasma exchange and immunosuppression in Myasthenia gravis. Lancet ii: 688
Newsom-Davis J, Ward C D, Wilson S G, Pinching A J, Vincent A 1979a Plasma exchange: short and long-term benefits? In: Dau P C, Clark E C (eds) 1st International Conference on Plasmapheresis and the Immunobiology of Myasthenia gravis. Boston, Houghton-Mifflin, p 198–211
Newsom-Davis J, Wilson S G, Vincent A. Ward C D 1979b Long-term effects of repeated plasma exchange on Myasthenia gravis. Lancet i: 464–468
O'Reilly M J G, Talpos G, Roberts V C, White J M, Cotton L T 1979 Controlled trial of plasma exchange in treatment of Raynaud's syndrome. British Medical Journal 1: 1113–1115
Pinching A J 1978 Diseases of the neuromuscular junction: pathophysiological mechanisms in Myasthenia gravis and the Eaton–Lambert syndrome. In: Legg N J (ed) Neurotransmitter systems and their clinical disorders. Academic Press, New York, London.

Pinching A J, Peters D K, Newsom-Davis J 1976 Remission of myasthenia gravis following plasma exchange. Lancet ii: 1373–1376

Pinching A J, Rees A J, Pussell B A, Lockwood C M, Mitchison R S, Peters D K 1980 Relapses in Wegener's granulomatosis — the role of infection

Pintado J, Jaswell H G, Walter-Bowie E J 1975 Treatment of life-threatening haemorrhage due to acquired factor VIII inhibitor. Blood 46: 535–541

Pussell B A, Lockwood C M, Scott D M, Pinching A J, Peters D K 1978 Value of immune complex assays in diagnosis and management. Lancet ii: 359–363

Rees A J, Lockwood C M, Peters D K 1977 Enhanced allergic tissue injury in Goodpasture's syndrome by intercurrent bacterial infection. British Medical Journal ii: 723–726

Rees A J, Lockwood C M, Peters D K 1979 Nephritis due to antibodies to GBM. In: Kincaid-Smith P, d'Apice A J F, Atkins R C (eds) Progress in glomerulonephritis. J. Wiley and Son, New York

Rossen R D, Hersh E M, Sharp J T, McCredie K B, Gyorkey F, Suki W N, Eknoyan G, Reisberg M A 1977 Effect of plasma exchange on circulating immune complexes and antibody formation in patients treated with cyclophosphamide and prednisone. American Journal of Medicine 63: 674–682

Ruocco V, Rossi A, Argeniziano G, Astarita C, Alviggi L, Farzati B, Papaleo G 1978 Pathogenicity of the intercellular antibodies of pemphigus and their periodic removal from the circulation by plasmapheresis. British Journal of Dermatology 98: 237–241

Swainson C P, Robson J S, Urbaniak S J, Keller A J, Kay A B 1978 Treatment of Goodpasture's syndrome by plasma exchange and immunosuppression. Clinical and Experimental Immunology 32: 233–242

Talpos G, Horrocks M, White J M, Cotton L T 1978 Plasmapheresis in Raynaud's Disease. Lancet i: 416–417

Verrier-Jones J, Cumming R H, Bucknall R C, Asplin C M, Fraser I D, Bothamley J, Davis P, Hamblin T J 1976 Plasmapheresis in the management of systemic lupus erythematosus. Lancet i: 709–711

Verrier-Jones J, Cumming R H, Bacon P A, Evers J, Fraser I D, Bothamley J, Tribe C R, Davis P, Hughes G R V 1979 Evidence for a therapeutic effect of plasmapheresis in patients with systemic lupus erythematosus. Quarterly Journal of Medicine 48: 555–576

Vincent A, Newsom-Davis J 1979 Absence of anti-acetylcholine receptor antibodies in congenital myasthenia gravis. Lancet i: 441–442

Walker R G, d'Apice A J F, Becker G J, Kincaid-Smith P, Crasswell D W T 1977 Plasmapheresis in Goodpasture's syndrome with renal failure. Medical Journal of Australia i: 875–879

Wallace D J, Goldfinger D, Gatti R, Lowe C, Fan P, Bluestone R, Klinenberg J R 1979 Plasmapheresis and lymphoplasmapheresis in the management of rheumatoid arthritis. Arthritis and Rheumatism 22: 703–710

10. Bone marrow transplantation

H. Grant Prentice

The haemopoietic system in man is thought to be dependent upon a population of pluripotential stem cells (PSC) which, through their committed counterparts, give rise to myelopoiesis (formation of red blood cells, granulocytes, monocyte and platelets) and to stem cells of the lymphoid system. The PSC is an infrequent cell ($< 1:10\,000$) in post embryonal human bone marrow and has the defined capabilities of both self replication and differentiation. Density gradient separation studies in the dog show a cell, resembling a small lymphocyte but with a distinct electron microscopic appearance (Körbling et al, 1979) within a fraction capable of marrow reconstitution, which may be the PSC. Bone marrow transplantation concerns the transfer of this pluripotential cell to correct congenital or acquired defects of bone marrow including rescue from otherwise lethal chemotherapy and radiotherapy.

History
In the late 1940s Jacobsen et al (1950) demonstrated, in the mouse, that shielding of the spleen provided protection from supralethal irradiation. This was at first misinterpreted as demonstrating a splenic protective 'factor'. Subsequent work by Lorenz et al (1951) showed similar protection by transfer of viable bone marrow cells. These studies stimulated in the 1950s and early 60s heroic clinical therapeutic attempts for patients with bone marrow failure, including radiation accident victims (Mathé et al, 1959) and patients with leukaemia. These early attempts (reviewed by Bortin, 1970) were largely disastrous, since transplant immunology was still in its infancy, and the unmatched grafts either failed to 'take' or were followed by fatal graft versus host disease (GvHD).

The investigators returned to the laboratory while the histocompatibility complex in animals and man was elucidated. By the late 1960s it was again possible to return to human bone marrow transplantation and at last a therapeutic potential was identified (Fefer et al, 1974). This chapter deals with the advances in bone marrow transplantation made in the last decade.

METHODS AND SOME OBSTACLES TO SUCCESSFUL BONE MARROW TRANSPLANTATION

Bone marrow donors and HLA typing
Work in animals (Epstein et al, 1968) clearly indicated that matching for the major histocompatibility complex (MHC) was a prerequisite for successful bone marrow transplantation.

Human leukocyte A (HLA)

The MHC in man is represented by serologically defined cell surface antigens A + B (+ C) and the D antigen defined in the mixed lymphocyte culture (MLC). The genetic code for this complex is carried on the no. 6 chromosome where the loci are closely linked. The function of these structures is thought to be concerned with antigenic recognition and presentation in immune reactivity. The genetic loci are inherited in a simple mendelian dominant fashion with one A + B ($\pm$ C) and one D (making one haplotype) inherited from each parent (see Fig. 10.1 which illustrates the inheritance of the serologically defined structures in a model family).

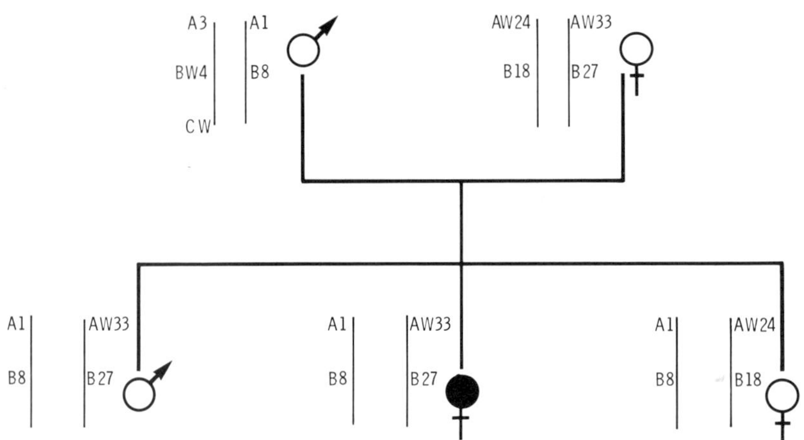

Fig. 10.1   Serological HLA (A + B + C) typing. The patient and her brother have inherited the same haplotypes.

Because of occasional crossovers the chance of compatibility between any two siblings is slightly less than 25 per cent. D locus compatibility is currently determined in a two-way mixed lymphocyte reaction (MLR) in which, in turn, potential donor and recipient lymphocytes act as stimulator or responder. The stimulator cells are inactivated by mitomycin C or irradiation and a response is identified by the incorporation of tritiated thymidine.

Since, with rare exceptions in the last decade (Dupont et al, 1979) successful transplantation has only been undertaken between genotypically compatible siblings, and the mean family size in the United Kingdom is now only 1.8, the chance of a compatible sibling donor is roughly 20 per cent. HLA antigens are not unlimited and some combinations are more common than others. D antigens are relatively few (Van Rood & Van Leeuwen, 1976) and may be more relevant. Unfortunately a D typed panel must await the production of suitable antisera for testing on a large scale. Red cell incompatibility is not a bar to marrow transplantation.

Patient and donor requirements*

Few transplants have been successful if the patient is older than 40. He or she must be

---

* A donor panel has been established by the Anthony Nolan Fund Laboratories under the direction of Dr D. C. O. James (Telephone: 01–937–1433) where 25 000 people are typed for A + B + C antigens and the results stored on a computer facility.

in good general health, in particular myocardial insufficiency, irreversible renal or hepatic disease are contraindications to the procedure.

The legal position for donors, especially children, is not yet clearly defined, but it is vital to obtain fully informed consent. Examination by an independent paediatrician if the potential donor is below the age of consent is mandatory.

Bone marrow harvest procedure

The technique employed most extensively is that described by Thomas & Storb (1970). Some minor modifications to simplify the procedure are:

1. The anaesthetised donor is anticoagulated with heparin, eliminating clotting in the aspirate and the requirement for extensive filtration. The theoretical risks are outweighed by prevention of deep vein thrombosis.

2. Conventional Salah or Jamshidi needles may be used.

3. No more than 5 ml is aspirated at each site to reduce blood dilution of stem cells. A total of 500 to 600 ml of marrow is required to achieve the minimum nucleated marrow cell count of 2×10^8/kg recipient weight and is obtained mainly from the pelvis.

4. Simple filtration is through an inverted adapted platelet giving set (Fenwal FKX 2134) which is attached direct to the collection bag containing tissue culture medium. The procedure takes 45–60 minutes. The donor has some discomfort for 12–24 hours, but the loss of this bone marrow carries no haematological consequences.

Following completion of the appropriate immunosuppressive or antileukaemic therapy the marrow is infused intravenously through a standard blood giving set.

Supportive care

Considerable advances have been made recently in the support of patients with bone marrow failure. After bone marrow transplantation supportive care is needed for more than three weeks.

For intravenous access a right atrial catheter is inserted via the internal jugular vein and fed out through a skin tunnel on the anterior chest wall. The catheter is used for blood product transfusion, antibiotic administration and parenteral nutrition, as well as for all venous blood sampling. A luer-type cap is applied after heparinisation when not in use, and the patient remains mobile. Septicaemic complications are rare even when the catheter is left in situ for up to six months.

Decontamination and protective isolation have been shown to protect granulocytopenic patients from exogenous pathogens (Rodrigquez et al, 1978). Single rooms with toilet and washing facilities in which the filtered air is under positive pressure are used by most groups. Prior to entry patients undergo bacterial decontamination as follows; daily baths with addition of an iodine-containing solution. Groins and axillae are sprayed with chlorhexidine, and chlorhexidine cream is applied to the vaginal area and to the nose. Gastrointestinal decontamination includes mouth washes with chlorhexidine 0.2 per cent solution, and the FRACON (Framycetin, Colistin, Nystatin) regimen (Storring et al, 1977) which is one effective method of gastrointestinal tract sterilization. Only sterile food and drinks are allowed. Strict reverse barrier isolation procedures are followed.

From the 30th day after marrow transfusion patients may be given prophylactic cotrimoxazole therapy to prevent pneumocystis carinii infection (Hughes et al, 1977).

With blood product support accidental engraftment by foreign lymphocytes and subsequent graft versus host disease is prevented by X-irradiation (1500 rads) to all blood products until donor engraftment is confirmed.

Platelet concentrates are used to maintain a count $> 20 \times 10^9/l$. Most units use random platelet donations, and there is good reason to think that this may have certain advantages over HLA matched single donor platelets (Ness & Perkins, 1979).

Prophylactic granulocytes reduce infection in the granulocytopenic host (Clift et al, 1978), but their use is not always practical. In any event granulocyte concentrates are given to patients with fever who fail to respond to the antibiotic/antifungal treatment, the ideal source being the marrow donor.

Nutritional support is required for optimum marrow engraftment (Stuart & Sensenbrenner, 1979). More rapid engraftment is likely to reduce the incidence of infection. Parenteral nutrition should be given if more than 10 per cent of the original body weight is lost. Patients routinely receive multiple vitamin preparations including vitamin K_1 weekly.

Infection is the immediate cause of death in the majority of patients undergoing bone marrow transplantation (Winston et al, 1979). A pathogen is isolated in less than 50 per cent of febrile episodes and most groups therefore use an empirical antimicrobial regime as soon as appropriate blood culture, mouth, stool, skin and urine samples are taken.

Gentamicin and carbenicillin or ticarcillin are given initially; if pseudomonas is not isolated the penicillin is discontinued. Continued fever at 48 hours requires the addition of antifungal drugs (miconazole and flucytosine) if candida has ever been isolated from any site. At 72 hours metronidazole may be added as an antianaerobic bacterial agent and therapeutic granulocytes are also indicated. Gas liquid chromatography of serum for candida products, is now proving an invaluable rapid guide to treatment.

Interstitial pneumonitis is a major cause of death in bone marrow transplant recipients. It is almost certainly multifactorial in origin but the single most frequent association is with cytomegalovirus infection (Neiman et al, 1973) for which no proven therapy is yet available. Other pathogens which may be isolated from lung biopsies are herpes simplex and herpes zoster which respond readily to acycloguanosine, a new, effective, antiviral agent (Selby et al, 1979). Pneumocystis carinii is best treated with high dose cotrimoxazole.

Graft versus host disease (GvHD)

Despite matching for the major histocompatibility complex and post engraftment immunosuppressive therapy, GvHD occurs in up to 80 per cent of recipients and is the main cause of death in more than 25 per cent (Thomas et al, 1977a). Yunis et al (1976) using various tissues depleted of T-lymphocytes, in a murine system, demonstrated their requirement in this reaction. Activation of these lymphocytes must involve minor histocompatibility antigens, some of which are now recognised, such as those coded for by the sex chromosomes (Storb, Prentice & Thomas, 1976). The reaction has been likened to the two stage lymphocytolysis test in vitro (Beschorner et al, 1978) in which the responding lymphocytes undergo activation and proliferation followed by target cell necrosis. Some clues to the 'natural' control of this phenomenon are apparent from the identification of deficiency of suppressor T-cells in the acute disease, with restoration of numbers prior to cessation of disease activity (Reinherz et al, 1979).

Acute graft versus host disease (aGvHD)

HISTOLOGICAL FEATURES

Excellent reviews of GvHD are presented by Thomas et al (1975b) and Lerner et al (1974) in which the Seattle group grade both the clinical phenomena and the histology on a scale 0–IV, according to severity. The main target organs are skin, gastrointestinal tract and the liver. A rash is usually the first manifestation and may occur as early as one week after marrow infusion. A peculiar initial distribution of the rash on the palms of the hands and soles of the feet, helps differentiate it from the many other causes of pruritic rashes (especially antibiotic allergy) in these patients. The Seattle group stage the skin lesion as (+) maculopapular rash over < 25 per cent of body surface, (+ +) 20–50 per cent, (+ + +) generalised erythroderma and (+ + + +), erythroderma with bullous formation and desquamation. Clinical assessment of liver involvement ranges from stage (+) bilirubin 34–51 μmol/l to (+ + + +) bilirubin > 255 μmol/l and the gut stage (+) > 500 ml diarrhoea per day (+ +) > 1000 ml (+ + +) > 1500 ml to stage (+ + + +) with severe abdominal pain, with or without ileus. The histological staging ranges in the skin from (+) with basal vacuolar degeneration to (+ + + +) with frank epidermal loss and the liver (+) < 25 per cent degenerate interlobular bile ducts to (+ + + +) > 75 per cent. The gut in stage (+) shows dilation of glands and single cell necrosis of epithelial cells to (+ + + +) with diffuse microscopic mucosal denudation. The overall clinical grade 0–IV is assessed as a composite of the individual organ clinical and histological staging.

Lymphocytic bronchitis described by Beschorner et al (1978) is often complicated by secondary bacterial pneumonia.

Haematological manifestations include, in most patients, a premonitary eosinophilia and occasionally peripheral T-lymphocytosis. Thrombocytopenia is uniform and recurrence of marrow hypoplasia frequent.

Although the pattern is variable, early onset GvHD is usually severe. Grade II or greater GvHD is often fatal with a survival of only 15 per cent. Although there is no clear temporal division between the acute and chronic diseases, acute GvHD is uncommon beyond six weeks.

Chronic graft versus host disease (cGvHD)
This syndrome is probably due to donor, stem cell derived, immunecompetent T-lymphocytes, which have been processed by the recipient thymus. The main target organs include the skin, which initially shows a lichen planus-like lesion which may go

on to scleroderma affecting the limbs and face predominantly. The skin shows a triad of telangiectasia, atrophy and hyperpigmentation. Liver function tests shows an obstructive picture which can go on to cirrhosis. Xerostomia and xerophthalmia are frequent. Malabsorption is not usually severe. Autoimmune haemolysis and thrombocytopenia occur frequently. Failure of immune reconstitution with increased susceptibility to infection is common. Circulating immune complexes are found in many patients and were associated with fatal mesangiocapillary glomerulonephritis in one case (Prentice, unpublished).

The prevention of GvHD

SUPPRESSION OF RESPONDING CELLS

Methotrexate was shown in a murine model (Uphoff, 1958) to reduce the incidence and severity of GvHD when given after marrow infusion. This work was expanded by the Seattle group (Thomas & Storb, 1971), and this drug, in intermittent doses for three months, is now widely used as standard GvHD prophylaxis (often combined with folinic acid rescue). Despite this a 70–80 per cent incidence of GvHD is still seen.

Antilymphocyte globulin was shown to have some effect on established GvHD by the Seattle group (Storb, Weiden & Thomas, 1974). It was not successful prophylactically (Weiden et al, 1979b) but, as newer specific monoclonal antisera becomes available, this approach may prove valuable.

Cyclosporin A is a fungal polypeptide with powerful in vitro and in vivo immunosuppressive properties (Borel et al, 1977). It is currently being studied in the prevention of GvHD and there are very encouraging preliminary results (Powles et al, 1980). Specific tolerance is not induced in a canine skin graft model (Deeg et al, 1979), but this aspect of its use in bone marrow transplantation awaits evaluation.

SELECTIVE ELIMINATION OF IMMUNE COMPETENT LYMPHOCYTES

One of the earliest methods was to exploit the different densities of stem cells and lymphocytes. This approach was pioneered by Dicke, Hooft & Van Bekkum (1968) in murine and primate models.

With highly purified anti-T sera Thierfelder's group in Munich have used this to treat donor bone marrow in vitro to remove T lymphocytes, firstly in dogs, and now in man with promising preliminary results (Rodt et al, 1979).

The Royal Free team are now using monoclonal antibodies derived from mouse or rat hydbridoma clones (Köhler & Milstein, 1975) which react with human T-lymphocytes. Following incubation with the donor marrow in vitro and subsequent reinfusion into recipient it has been hoped that removal of coated T-cells could be achieved. Initial attempts with an IgM antibody were unsuccessful probably because of failure of in vivo opsonization. Subsequent work with an IgG_2 mouse antibody (OKT_3, Ortho Pharmaceuticals) appears more promising; this antibody binds complement and can be used to lyse T-lymphocytes in vitro under optimal conditions.

All of these methods are designed to eliminate immune competent T-lymphocytes from the marrow and prevent acute GvHD. It is assumed that subsequent recovery of

T-lymphocytes from the donor PSC will involve recipient thymus maturation, with some hope that this will modify host recognition and GvHD.

Treatment of established GvHD
Acute graft versus host disease, if mild (I) may resolve with continued methotrexate 'prophylaxis'. Grades II–IV GvHD are usually progressive. Initially encouraging results with antithymocyte globulin treatment (Storb, Weiden & Thomas, 1974) have not been confirmed (Weiden et al, 1979b). Cyclosporin A has been used in five patients with established GvHD (Powles et al, 1978). Although clearing of the skin lesions was dramatic, only one of the five patients survived.

Nine patients with established grade II–IV GvHD have been treated with very high doses of methyl prednisolone by i.v. bolus injections (20 mg/kg i.v. 12 hourly) (Prentice et al, 1980) Seven patients showed complete resolution, one responded partially (but developed chronic GvHD of skin and liver) and in one there was no response. With improvement in the lesions, the dose was halved every 48 hours. One patient had a fatal recurrence of acute GvHD on steroid withdrawal.

Interestingly the most recent controlled trial between antithymocyte globulin and corticosteroids in Seattle showed a superior effect for modest doses of steroids (Weiden et al, 1979b).

Chronic GvHD sometimes responds to conventional doses of corticosteroids which are best given in combination with azathiaprine.

THE INDICATIONS FOR BONE MARROW TRANSPLANTATION

Aplastic anaemia
Considerable debate still surrounds the pathophysiology of idiopathic aplasia; the subject is well reviewed by Geary (1979). The theory of a microenvironmental structural defect must be disputed in view of the beneficial effect of bone marrow transplantation. On the other hand evidence for an immune environmental cause is compelling:

1. Recovery of autologous marrow, following rejection of allogeneic marrow, in some patients with aplasia given immunosuppressive conditioning regimes (Thomas et al, 1975a), a phenomenon now confirmed by many other groups.

2. Response to antithymocyte globulin and to intensive immunosuppressive therapy with high dose steroids, or cyclophosphamide (see other therapies).

3. Evidence for the presence of both humoral and cell mediated inhibition. Incubation of normal bone marrow with patient sera (Barrett et al, 1978) and marrow coculture experiments (Ascensao et al, 1976) demonstrate profound inhibition of the normal marrow in some cases.

4. Occasional failure of syngeneic (identical twin) marrow engraftment, such as that illustrated by a patient with post-hepatitis aplasia reported by the Royal Marsden Hospital Transplant Team (1977), in which initial attempts with bone marrow infusion alone or following azathioprine therapy failed, with successful engraftment only following intensive cyclophosphamide treatment.

Morley et al (1978) show, on the other hand, impressive data in their sophisticated assay system employing bleomycin sensitivity, for residual DNA damage in lymphocytes of patients with aplastic anaemia. Presumably these are the progeny of defective pluripotential stem cells. In theory DNA damage could lead to altered surface antigen structures and evoke an immune response, thus the two main hypotheses are not necessarily mutually exclusive.

Aplasia following drug and radiation damage or that associated with chromosomal defects (Fanconi's anaemia) and idiopathic aplasia are all amenable to marrow transplantation.

The single most important factor in selecting a patient for bone marrow transplantation is the presence of a bad prognosis. Various criteria have been proposed to identify severe aplasia, the most commonly employed are those of Camitta et al (1975) who include

1. Neutrophil count of less than $0.5 \times 10^9/l$
2. Platelet count of less than $20 \times 10^9/l$
3. Reticulocyte count less than 1 per cent (corrected for PCV).

If two of three parameters are present, in a patient with a hypoplastic bone marrow in which more than 65 per cent residual cells are 'non-haemopoietic', then without bone marrow transplantation there is an 80 per cent risk of death in the first year.

Severe post-hepatitic aplasia carries a 90 per cent mortality and is an absolute indication for bone marrow transplant (Camitta et al, 1974).

Syngeneic (identical twin) transplantation

If, without prior immunosuppressive drugs the donor marrow is rejected, an immune reaction directed against the bone marrow pluripotential stem cell is probable and immunosuppressive therapy as for allogeneic grafting should be undertaken and the transplant procedure repeated. Five successful transplants from identical twins are reviewed by Storb (1978). At the time of his report these patients were well 1–16 years later.

Allogeneic (MHC identical) transplantation

Marrow transfusions between 'matched' non-identical siblings will be rejected unless immunosuppressive therapy is given prior to the transfusion. The most commonly used regimen is that originally developed by Santos (Santos et al, 1970) in which cyclophosphamide in high dosage (50 mg/kg body weight is given on 4 consecutive days). This is preceded (24 hours) by infusion of donor buffy coats cells, since cyclophosphamide is known to be most immunosuppressive when given one day after exposure to donor tissue antigens. Thirty-six hours after completion of the chemotherapy donor marrow can be infused.

The outcome of 110 transplants in Seattle for aplasia were detailed by Storb et al (1978). The preparative treatment included cyclophosphamide or in a few patients total body irradiation (TBI). A high initial mortality in the first three months was associated with either graft rejection or GvHD. Sixty patients died, including 27 following graft rejection and 22 with GvHD. Fifty patients (45 per cent) had survived from 2 to 73 months. Nine had evidence of chronic GvHD, the rest had returned to normal health.

Similar results have been obtained by many other teams. Thus, the main residual problems preventing total success in aplastic anaemia are bone marrow graft rejection and GvHD.

Bone marrow graft rejection does not occur in patients with severe combined immune deficiency (SCID). Despite the immunosuppressive therapy referred to earlier, graft rejection is the single most important problem in aplastic anaemia both in North America and Europe. Storb, Prentice & Thomas (1977) identified patients with a high risk of graft rejection. Important factors were a positive relative response index (RRI) in the MLC, indicating sensitization against the donor antigens and low numbers of bone marrow cells infused (less than 3×10^8/kg recipient weight). A positive RRI is likely in patients who have been transfused with blood products from relatives or those who have been multitransfused. Thus, avoidance of transfusions and early referral are prerequisites for transplantation. Subsequent to October 1975 the Seattle group have used standard cyclophosphamide immunosuppressive therapy for those with a low risk of rejection; these patients have a 14 per cent rejection rate with 77 per cent survival (Storb, 1979). High-risk sensitised patients were initially treated with procarbazine, antithymocyte globulin and total body irradiation, or with cyclophosphamide and total body irradiation. This drastically reduced the rejection rate (10 per cent), but survival was not improved because of the complications of GvHD and interstitial pneumonitis. Subsequently the high risk patients have been treated with cyclophosphamide, as for the non-sensitised patients, but following bone marrow infusion this has been boosted by transfusion of 2×10^8 viable peripheral blood mononuclear leucocytes/kg daily for three to five days. With this treatment the Seattle team have been able to reduce the rejection rate in sensitised patients to 14 per cent with an increased survival of 67 per cent. The overall survival rate after bone marrow transplantation in aplastic anaemia since 1975 in Seattle has now reached 73 per cent helped by a concurrent reduction in the mortality from GvHD.

Kersey et al (1979) using total lymphoid irradiation (TLI) in addition to cyclophosphamide have encouraging preliminary results in the prevention of rejection in a group of patients at high risk.

Other treatments
Many groups have now demonstrated that androgenic hormones are of little value in severe aplastic anaemia (Lynch et al, 1975). Following the observation of marrow recovery after cyclophosphamide in spite of donor graft rejection, cyclophosphamide has been used alone, with success, in two of four patients (Santos, Elfenbein & Tutschka, 1979), supporting the hypothesis of an immune basis for the aplasia.

Encouraging results from the use of antilymphocyte globulin (ALG) (Speck et al, 1977) are the subject of a current European Bone Marrow Transplantation Group (EBMT) trial. Alternative non-myelotoxic immunosuppression with very high dose methyl prednisolone has been followed by rapid marrow recovery in 6 of 11 patients with severe aplastic anaemia (Bacigalupo et al, 1979).

Leukaemia
Bone marrow transplantation for leukaemia was not originally conceived as a therapeutic manoeuvre in its own right, but as a means of rescuing patients from otherwise lethal therapy, due to permanent marrow aplasia. A subsequent anti-leukaemic effect (see Graft v Leukaemia) of allogeneic marrow derived lymphoid cells has now been identified.

Antileukaemia treatment (conditioning regime)
The first 10 patients transplanted in end-stage leukaemia by the Seattle group (Thomas et al, 1977b) were treated first with 1000 rads total body gamma-irradiation (TBI). There was only one long term survivor suggesting that the antileukaemic effect of radiotherapy alone was inadequate, despite the fact that it reaches 'sanctuary' sites such as the central nervous systems (c.n.s.). Cyclophosphamide (60 mg/kg on two consecutive days) was added with an apparent increase in the antileukaemic effect. Most groups now use this regimen. The intensive SCARI (Cytosine Arabinoside, 6-Thioguanine, Daunorubicin, Cyclophosphamide and total body irradiation) programme (UCLA Transplant Team 1977) has a greater antileukaemic effect, which is offset by increased toxicity. 36 to 48 hours after the last cyclophosphamide treatment patients have total body irradiation (TBI).

TOTAL BODY IRRADIATION (TBI)
Following animal work, the Seattle group used 1000 rads (midpoint dose) total body irradiation, administered by horizontally opposed ^{60}Cobalt sources at 5.5 and later 8.0 rads/minute (Thomas, Storb & Buckner, 1976). Most centres have only a single source and the patient must therefore be turned to achieve a homogenous dose. The only major diversion from this technique has been made by Kersey's group in Minnesota (Kim et al, 1977) and the Royal Free team who use a Linear accelerator delivering X-rays at a much higher dose rate (25 rads/minute), when a total dose of 750 rads midpoint dose is given. The shortened procedure (30–40 minutes) improves patient comfort, and does not interfere with the day to day running of the radiotherapy department. A theoretical disadvantage is that of an increased incidence of pneumonitis. Kersey (personal communication) has found the incidence of pneumonitis to be related to the pretransplant condition of the patient and the extent of previous therapy. In a recent series of 13 patients early in the course of treatment, with minimal disease, they have seen only 2 patients with pneumonitis; they were both obese and infected.

The immediate toxicity includes transient nausea and vomiting, skin erythema and salivary gland swelling. The long-term side effects include sterility and cataract formation and, of more concern, a theoretical likelihood of second malignancies.

In addition to prophylactic (anti-GvHD) intravenous methotrexate, intrathecal methotrexate is now given because of some late c.n.s. relapses.

Results

ACUTE LEUKAEMIA
The original large series of patients treated in Seattle (Thomas et al, 1977c), with relapsed and refractory acute leukaemia, identified a therapeutic phenomenon previously not described, which was indicated by a change in the shape of the survival curve. The curve now showed three components. There were initial early deaths attributable to the complications of the procedure, i.e. bone marrow failure or GvHD with some deaths due to resistant leukaemia or the poor general condition of the patient. In the second phase from 130 days to 2 years death was mainly attributable to recurrent leukaemia. From two years onwards there was a true plateau (at 16 per cent, which 'constitutes an operational definition of cure' in this group of patients who have

had no maintenance thereapy from the time of the procedure. Currently (Thomas et al, 1979a) 14 of 100 recipients of allogeneic marrow and 6 of 16 recipients of syngeneic marrow (Fefer et al, 1977) are in continuous remission from 3 to more than 8 years.

The ability to cure acute leukaemia by this method encouraged both the Seattle group (Thomas et al, 1979a and 1979b) and others to extrapolate the manoeuvre to patients in remission who could be identified as having a bad prognosis. In acute myeloblastic leukaemia it is currently possible to achieve up to 85 per cent complete remission regardless of age (Rees et al, 1977). However only one-third of patients are aged under 40, of whom only 20–30 per cent will have an MHC identical sibling, and are thereafter candidates for marrow transplant. In acute lymphoblastic leukaemia the overall prognosis at presentation for those who achieve complete remission is greater than 50 per cent at five years using conventional chemotherapy and CNS radiotherapy (Pinkel, 1979). Certain groups of patients can be identified as having a worse prognosis; these include those over the age of 10 (Pinkel, 1979), patients with a high tumour load at presentation or T and B cell subtypes as opposed to the better prognostic type common ALL (cALL) (Chessells, Hardisty & Rapson, 1977), males (Baumer & Mott, 1978) and those who have undergone at least one relapse (Cornbleet & Chessells, 1978).

It was surmised, correctly, that transplantation of patients with a bad prognosis during the remission phase would be beneficial because of reduced leukaemia cell load and their better general condition. The major residual problems remain those of GvHD and interstitial pneumonitis. The published and unpublished results for the Seattle group, the Royal Marsden Hospital, the Royal Free Hospital and others are pooled in Figure 10.2 which shows the approximate range of the survival curves within each group of patients compared with the outcome for patients achieving remission with AML seen by most groups (but see other therapies). The Seattle group

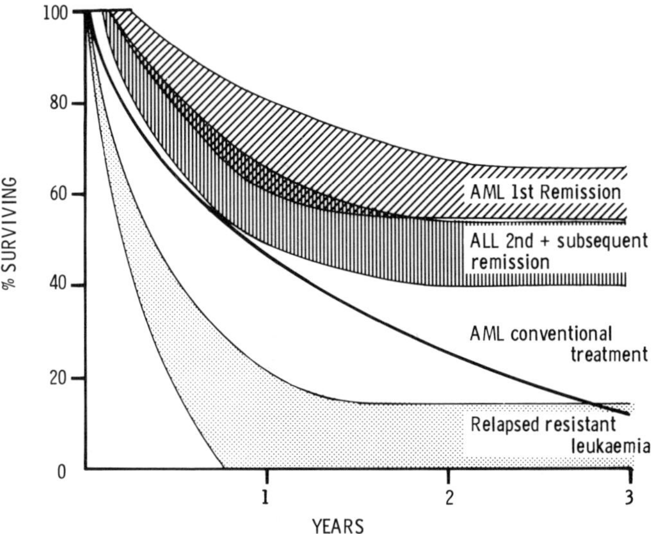

Fig. 10.2 'Plateau effect' of bone marrow transplantation for leukaemia. Compilation of published and unpublished results from several centres.

(Thomas et al, 1979a) have found that, with transplantation in remission, relapses occur in the first 12 months only and thereafter they have a plateau at 63 per cent for patients with acute myeloblastic leukaemia, that is 12 of 19 patients. There has been only 1 leukaemic relapse and 5 deaths due to interstitial pneumonitis (complicating severe GvHD in 4). In acute lymphoblastic leukaemia (Thomas et al, 1979b) 22 patients were transplanted in their second or subsequent remission, 10 relapsed from 68 to 281 days following the procedure. There is a projected survival at two years of 50 per cent for this group of patients with the prospect that most will be cured of their disease. Identification of patients with lymphoblastic leukaemia with bad prognosis, for whom bone marrow transplantation in first remission would be the treatment of choice, may improve these results.

CHRONIC GRANULOCYTIC LEUKAEMIA (C.G.L.)

This disease affects a younger population and although busulphan has improved the quality of life, survival has not been extended beyond a median of three years. Four patients have been successfully grafted during the chronic phase from identical twins by the Seattle group following antileukaemic treatment with dimethyl busulphan, cyclophosphamide and total body irradiation (920 rads). Elimination of the CGL cells is demonstrated by the fact that no Ph^1 positive cells have been detected subsequently. These patients have remained in remission (Fefer et al, 1979) from 22–31 months.

Graft versus Leukaemia (GVL)

Barnes & Loutit (1957) demonstrated an antileukaemic effect of allogeneic but not syngeneic marrow in CBA leukaemia bearing mice. The initial data in man Sanders & Thomas, 1978) was obscured by deaths mainly due to GvHD. Subsequently sophisticated analytic methods (Weiden et al, 1979) in 242 syngeneic and allogeneic transplants reported from Seattle demonstrate a relapse rate $2\frac{1}{2}$ times less in patients with significant GvHD compared with those with none or only mild disease, but unfortunately there was no difference in survival. With a reduction in the incidence of GvHD from 1977 onwards this group see as yet no apparent loss of antileukaemic effect. Odom et al (1978) have reported the disappearance of lymphoblastic leukaemia which had relapsed following allogeneic female into male transplants in two patients. This was associated in both patients with GvHD. It is to be hoped that in the future the introduction of more effective methods of preventing GvHD will not abolish the antileukaemic effect.

Other therapies

Unless the complications of allogeneic bone marrow transplantation such as GvHD can be overcome and widespread use of non-related donors is feasible, the future of allogeneic bone marrow transplantation for acute leukaemia will be limited. Freireich's group in Houston (Freireich et al, 1976) devised, in 1970, a strategy which involved the reintroduction of intensive chemotherapy for adults with acute leukaemia who had been in complete remission for more than 60 weeks. This 'late intensification' therapy proved to be well tolerated and allowed patients to discontinue chemotherapy. Of 44 patients thus treated more than 70 per cent remained in remission for one to five years. Freireich clearly demonstrates the improving propsects of patients treated in ideal conditions with modern chemotherapy and has recently presented data (Keating et al, 1979) to show that 24 per cent of patients achieving complete remission between 1971 and 1973 are five-year survivors, with the implication that many of these have been cured of their disease.

AUTOLOGOUS BONE MARROW TRANSPLANTATION

The possibility of increasing the therapeutic effect, by harvesting and storing autologous (own) bone marrow at low temperature, prior to chemotherapy and radiotherapy, has been long recognised (Kurnick et al, 1958). Interest lapsed however because of a lack of effective treatment until more recently (reviewed by Graze & Gale, 1978). Storage of autologous marrow in liquid nitrogen ($-196°C$) using cryoprotective agents now allows for sophisticated programmes to be devised. Haematological recovery can be accelerated with reinfusion of marrow after high dose (sublethal) chemotherapy when compared with a control group receiving the same drugs without marrow reinfusion (McElwain et al, 1979).

Several groups are exploring the use of autologous bone marrow transplantation in leukaemia. The first proven application has been in the re-establishment of chronic phase disease, in chronic granulocytic leukaemia, following the successful therapy of acute transformation (Buckner et al, 1978), by reinfusion of stored chronic phase marrow.

The use of stored remission marrow from patients with acute leukaemia in relapse would carry distinct advantages of avoiding GvHD and would overcome the problem of finding a suitable donor. So far, however, there is no evidence of long term cures, despite attempts to remove any residual leukaemic cells by physical separation techniques (Dicke et al, 1979).

Immunological removal of residual leukaemic cells is under investigation. Antisera directed against surface membrane antigens are used either to produce target cell lysis (Thierfelder et al, 1979) or effect physical removal. Most attention is at present

Table 10.1 Miscellaneous indications for allogeneic bone marrow transplantations

Disease	Defect	Reference
Severe combined immune deficiency (SCID) syndrome	Heterogenous group with congenital lymphoid T ± B cell deficiencies. Some have deficiency of enzyme ADA	O'Reilly et al, 1978
Wiskott-Aldrich disease	Eczema, thrombocytopenia and failure of humoral immunity	Bach et al, 1978
Chediak-Higashi anomaly	Albinism, defect in membrane bound intracellular organelles. Progressive pancytopenia	Theoretical
Sickle-cell disease	Amino-acid substitution in β-globin chain	
Thalassaemia major	β-globin chain synthesis defect	
Pure red-cell aplasia	—	
Paroxysmal nocturnal haemoglobinuria including aplasia	Acquired red cell membrane sensitivity to complement haemolysis	See Aplasia
Osteopetrosis	Congenital deficiency of osteoclasts	Ballet et al, 1977

Or any other life threatening disease in which the defect is attributable to the marrow PSC or its progeny directed to the T (thymic) lymphoblastic leukaemias which express surface antigens different from those on myeloid precursors. Since some of those leukaemic cells fail to express thymocyte/T cell antigens, of theoretical interest is the characterisation of antigenic structures of the surface of the pluripotential stem cell. If unique antigens are present on this rare cell, it will be possible to raise antisera against them, which would then be used to effect a physical separation and allow a transplant of autologous 'pure' stem cells.

REFERENCES

Ascensao J, Kagan W, Moore M, Pahwa R, Hansen J, Good R 1976 Aplastic anaemia: evidence for an immunological mechanism. Lancet i: 669–671

Bach F H, Albertini R J, Joo P, Anderson J L, Bortin M M 1968 Bone marrow transplantation in a patient with Wiskott-Aldrich syndrome. Lancet ii: 1364

Bacigalupo A, Giordano D, Van Lint M T, Vimercati R, Marmont A M 1979 Bolus methyl prednisolone in severe aplastic anaemia. New England Journal of Medicine 300: 501–502

Ballet J J, Griscelli C, Courtris C, Milhaud G, Maroteaux P 1977 Bone-marrow transplantation in osteopetrosis. Lancet ii: 1137

Barnes D W H, Loutit J F 1957 Treatment of murine leukaemia with X-rays and homologous bone marrow. British Journal of Haematology 3: 241–252

Barrett A J, Faille A, Saal F, Balitrand N, Gluckman E 1978 Marrow graft rejection and inhibition of growth in culture by serum in aplastic anaemia. Journal of Clinical Pathology 31: 1244–1248

Baumer J H, Mott M G 1978 Sex and prognosis in childhood acute lymphoblastic leukaemia. Lancet ii: 128–129

Beschorner W E, Saral R, Hutchings G H, Tutschka P J, Santos G W 1978 Lymphocytic bronchitis associated with graft-versus-host disease in recipients of bone-marrow transplants. New England Journal of Medicine 299: 1030–1036

Borel J F, Feurer C, Magnee C, Stähelin H 1977 Effects of the new anti-lymphocytic peptide cyclosporin A in animals. Immunology 32: 1017–1025

Bortin M M 1970 A compendium of reported human bone marrow transplants. Transplantation 9: 571–587

Buckner C D, Stewart P, Clift R A, Fefer A, Neiman P E, Singer J, Storb R, Thomas E D 1978 Treatment of blastic transformation of chronic granulocytic leukaemia by chemotherapy, total body irradiation and infusion of cryopreserved autologous marrow. Experimental Haematology 6: 96–109

Camitta B M, Nathan D G, Forman E N, Parkman R, Rappeport J M, Orellana T D 1974 Post-hepatitic severe aplastic anemia — an indication for early bone marrow transplantation. Blood 43: 473–483

Camitta B M, Rappeport J M, Parkman R, Nathan D G 1975 Selection of patients for bone marrow transplantation in severe aplastic anaemia. Blood 45: 355–363

Chessells J M, Hardisty R M, Rapson N T, Greaves M F 1977 Acute lymphoblastic leukaemia in children: classification and prognosis Lancet ii: 1307–1309

Clift R A, Sanders J E, Thomas E D, Williams B, Buckener C D 1978 Granulocyte transfusions for the prevention of infection in patients receiving bone-marrow transplants. New England Journal of Medicine 298: 1052–1057

Cornbleet M A, Chessells J M 1978 Bone-marrow relapse in acute lymphoblastic leukaemia in childhood. British Medical Journal 2: 104–106

Deeg H J, Storb R, Gerhard-Miller L, Shulman H M, Weiden P L, Thomas E D 1979 Cyclosporin A, A powerful immunosuppressant in vivo and in vitro in the dog, fails to induce tolerance. Transplantation, in press

Dicke K A, Van Hooft J I M, Van Bekkum D W 1968 The selective elimination of immunologically competent cells from bone marrow and lymphatic cell mixtures. Transplantation 6: 562–570

Dicke K A, Spitzer G, Peters L, McCredie K B, Zander A, Verma D S, Vellekoop L, Hester J 1979 Autologous bone-marrow transplantation in relapsed adult acute luekaemia. Lancet i: 514–517

Dupont B, O'Reilly R J, Pollack M S, Good R A 1979 Use of HLA genotypically different donors in bone marrow transplantation. Transplantation Proceedings XI: 219–224

Enno A, Darrell J, Hows J, Catovsky D, Goldman J M, Galton D A 1978 Co-trimoxazole for prevention of infection in acute leukaemia. Lancet ii: 395–397

Epstein R B, Storb R, Ragde H, Thomas E D 1968 Cytotoxic typing antisera for marrow grafting in littermate dogs. Transplantation 6: 45–58

Fefer A, Thomas E D, Buckner C D, Storb R, Neiman P, Glucksberg H, Clift R A, Lerner K G 1974 Marrow transplants in aplastic anemia and leukemia. Seminars in Haematology II: 353–371

Fefer A, Buckner C D, Thomas E D, Cheever M A, Clift R A, Glucksberg H, Neiman P E, Storb R 1977 Cure of hematologic neoplasia with transplantation of marrow from identical twins. New England Journal of Medicine 297: 146–148

Fefer A, Cheever M A, Thomas E D, Boyd C, Ramberg R, Glucksberg H, Buckner C D, Storb R 1979 Disappearance of Ph^1-positive cells in four patients with chronic granulocytic leukemia after chemotherapy, irradiation and marrow transplantation from an identical twin. New England Journal of Medicine 300: 333–337

Freirech E J, Bodey G P, McCredie K B, Hersh E M, Gehan E A, Hart J, Gutterman J U, Rodriguez V, Smith T, Hester J P 1976 Developmental therapy in adult acute leukemia. Archives of Internal Medicine 136: 1417–1421

Geary C G, Testa N G 1979 Pathophysiology of marrow hypoplasia. In: Geary C G (ed) Aplastic anaemia. Baillière Tindal, London

Graze P R, Gale R P 1978 Autotransplantation for leukemia and solid tumours. Transplantation Proceedings, X, 177–184

Hughes W T, Kuhn S, Chaudhary S, Feldman S, Verzosa M, Aur R J A, Pratt C, George S L 1977 Successful chemoprophylaxis for pneumocystis carinii pneumonitis. New England Journal of Medicine 297: 1419–1426

Jacobson L O, Simmons E L, Marks E K, Robson M J, Bethard W F, Gaston E O 1950 The role of the spleen in radiation injury and recovery. Journal of Laboratory and Clinical Medicine 35: 746–770

Keating M J, Bodey G P, McCredie K B, Freireich E K 1979 Five year survival and remission duration in adult acute myelogenous leukemia (AML). Proceedings of the American Society for Clinical Oncology 20: 416, Abstract C-517

Kersey J H, Krivit W, Nesbit M E, Ramsay N K C, Coccia P F, Levitt S H, Kim T H 1979 Combined cyclophosphamide-total lymphoid irradiation compared to other forms of immunosuppression for human marrow transplantation. In: Baum S J, Ledney G D (eds) Experimental hematology today 1979, ch 23. Springer-Verlag, Berlin, New York

Kim T H, Kersey J, Sewchand W, Nesbit M E, Krivit W, Levitt S H 1977 Total-body irradiation with a high-dose-rate linear accelerator for bone-marrow transplantation in aplastic anemia and neoplastic disease. Radiology 122: 523–525

Köhler G, Milstein C 1975 Continuous cultures of fused cells secreting antibody of predefined specificity. Nature 256: 495–497

Körbling M, Fliedner T M, Calvo W, Ross W M, Northdurft W, Steinbach I 1979 Albumin density gradient purification of canine hemopoietic blood stem cells (HBSC): Long-term allogeneic engraftment without GvH-Reaction. Experimental Hematology, 7: 277–288

Kurnick N B, Montano A, Gerdes J C, Feder B H 1958 Preliminary observations on the treatment of postirradiation hematopoietic depression in man by the infusion of stored autogenous bone marrow. Annals of Internal Medicine 49: 973–986

Lerner K G, Kao G F, Storb R, Buckner C D, Clift R A, Thomas E D 1974 Histopathology of graft-vs.-host reaction (GvHR) in human recipients of marrow from HL-A-matched sibling donors. Transplantation proceedings VI: 367–370

Lorenz E, Uphoff D, Reid T R, Shelton E 1951 Modification of irradiation injury in mice and guinea pigs by bone marrow injections. Journal of the National Cancer Institute 12: 197–201

Lynch R E, Williams D M, Reading J C, Cartwright G E 1975 The Prognosis in Aplastic Anemia. Blood 45: 517–528

Mathe G, Jammet H, Pendic, B, Schwarzenberg L, Duplan J-F, Maupin B, Latarjet R, Larrieu M-J, Kalic D, Djukic Z 1959 Transfuions et greffes de moelle osseuse homologue chez des humains irradies a haute dose accidentellement. Revue Francaise Etudes Cliniques et Biologiques IV: 226–238

McElwain T J, Hedley D W, Burton G, Clink H M, Gordon M Y, Jarman M, Juttner C A, Millar J L, Milsted R A V, Prentice G, Smith I E, Spence D, Woods M 1979 Marrow autotransplantation accelerates haematological recovery in patients with malignant melanoma treated with high-dose Melphalan. British Journal of Cancer 40: 72–80

Morley A, Trainor K, Seshadri R, Sorrell J 1978 Is aplastic anaemia due to abnormality of DNA? Lancet ii: 9–12

Neiman P, Wasserman P B, Wentworth B B, Kao G F, Lerner K G, Storb R, Buckner C D, Clift R A, Fefer A, Fass L, Glucksberg H, Thomas E D 1973 Interstitial pneumonia and cytomegalovirus infection as complications of human marrow transplantation. Transplantation 15: 478–485

Ness P M, Perkins H A 1979 Therapeutic complications in acute myelogenous leukemia. New England Journal of Medicine 301: 557

Odom L F, Githens J H, Morse H, Sharma B, August C S, Humbert J R, Peakman D, Rusnak S L, Johnson F B 1978 Remission of relapsed leukaemia during graft-verus-host reaction. A 'graft-versus-leukaemia reaction' in man? Lancet ii: 537–540

O'Reilly R J, Pahwa R, Dupont B, Good R A 1978 Severe combined immunodeficiency: Transplantation approaches for patients lacking an HLA genotypically identical sibling. In: Gale R P, Opelz G (eds) Immunobiology of bone marrow transplantation, vol 2. Grune & Stratton, New York

Pinkel D 1979 The Ninth Annual David Karnofsky Lecture. Treatment of acute lymphocytic leukemia. Cancer 43: 1128–1137

Powles R L, Clink H, Sloane J, Barrett A J, Kay H E M, McElwain T J 1978 Cyclosporin A for the treatment of graft-verus-host disease in man. Lancet ii: 1327–1331

Powles R L, Clink H M, Spence D, Morgenstern G, Watson J G, Selby P J, Woods M, Barrett A, Jameson B, Sloane J, Lawlor S D, Kay H E M, Lawson D, McElwain T J, Alexander P 1980 Cyclosporin A to prevent graft-versus-host disease in man after allogeneic bone marrow transplantation. Lancet i: 327–329

Prentice H G, Bateman S, Bradstock K F, Kendra J, Hoffbrand A V 1980 High dose methyl prednisolone therapy in established acute graft versus host disease. BLUT. In press

Rees J K H, Sandler R M, Challener J, Hayhoe F G J 1977 Treatment of acute myeloid leukaemia with a triple cytotoxic regime: DAT. British Journal of Cancer 36, 770–776

Reinherz E L, Parkman R, Rappeport J Rosen F S, Schlossman F 1979 Aberrations of suppressor T cells in human graft-versus-host disease. New England Journal of Medicine 300: 1061–1068

Rodriguez V, Bodey G P, Freireich E J, McCredie K B, Gutterman J U, Keating M J, Smith T L, Gehan E A 1978 Randomized trial of protected environment — prophylactic antibiotics in 145 adults with acute leukemia. Medicine 57: 253–266

Rodt H, Netzel B, Kolb H J, Janka G, Haas R J, Rieder I, Belohradsky B, Thierfelder S 1979 Suppression of graft-versus-host disease (GvHD) by incubation of bone marrow grafts with anti-T-cell globulin. In: International Society of Haematology European and African Dvision Fifth Meeting, Abstracts III: 86

Royal Marsden Hospital Bone-Marrow Transplantation Team 1977 Failure of syngeneic bone-marrow graft without preconditioning in post-hepatitis marrow aplasia. Lancet ii: 742–744

Sanders J E, Thomas E D 1978 Bone marrow transplantation for acute leukaemia. In: Clinics in Haematology 7: 295–311

Santos G W, Burke P J, Sensenbrenner L L, Owens A H, Jr 1970 Rationale for the use of cyclophosphamide as an immunosuppressant for marrow transplants in man. In: Bertelli A, Monaco A P (eds) Pharmacological treatment in organ and tissue transplantation. Amsterdam, Exerpta Medica Foundation 24–31

Santos G W, Elfenbein G J, Tutschka P J 1979 Bone marrow transplantation — present status. Transplantation Proceedings XI: 182–188

Selby P J, Powles R L, Jameson B, Kay H E M, Watson J G, Thorton R, Morgenstern G, Clink H M, McElwain T J, Prentice H G, Corringham R, Ross M G, Bridgden D 1979 Parenteral acyclovir therapy for herpesvirus infections in man. Lancet ii: 1267–1270

Slavin S, Gottlieb M, Strober S, Bieber C, Hoppe R, Kaplan H S, Grumet F C 1979 Transplantation of bone marrow in outbred dogs without graft-versus-host disease using total lymphoid irradiation. Transplantation 27: 139–142

Speck B, Gluckman E, Haak H L, Van Rood J J 1977 Treament of aplastic anaemia by antilymphocyte globulin with and without allogeneic bone-marrow infusions. Lancet ii: 1145–1148

Storb R, Gluckman E, Thomas E D, Buckner C D, Clift, R A, Fefer A, Glucksberg H, Graham T C, Johnson F L, Lerner K G, Neiman P E, Ochs H 1974 Treatment of established human graft-versus-host disease by antithymocyte globulin. Blood 44: 57–75

Storb R, Prentice R L, Thomas E D 1977 Marrow transplantation for treatment of aplastic anemia. An analysis of factors associated with graft rejection. New England Journal of Medicine 296: 61–66

Storb R, Prentice R L, Thomas E D 1977 Treatment of aplastic anemia by marrow transplantation from HLA identical siblings. Journal of Clinical Investigation 59: 625–632

Storb R, Thomas E D, Weiden P L, Buckner C D, Clift R A, Fefer A, Goodell B W, Johnson F L, Neiman P E, Sanders J E, Singer J 1978 One-hundred-ten patients with aplastic anemia (AA) treated by marrow transplantation in Seattle. Transplantation Proceedings, X: 135–140

Storb R (for Seattle Marrow Transplant Team) 1979 Decrease in the graft rejection rate and improvement in survival after marrow transplantation for severe aplastic anemia. Transplantation Proceedings XI: 196–198

Storring R A, McElwain T J, Jameson B, Wiltshaw E, Spiers A S D, Gaya H 1977 Oral non-absorbed antibiotics prevent infection in acute non-lymphoblastic leukaemia Lancet ii: 837–840

Strober S, Slavin S, Gottlieb M, Zan-Bar I, King D P, Hoppe R T, Fuks Z, Grumet F C, Kaplan H S 1979 Allograft tolerance after total lymphoid irradiation (TLI). Immunological Review 46: 87–112

Stuart R K, Sensenbrenner L L 1979 Adverse effects of nutritional deprivation on transplanted hematopoietic cells. Experimental Hematology 7: 435–442

Thierfelder S, Rodt H, Thiel E, Hoffmann-Fezer G, Netzel B, Haas R J, Wündisch G F, Bender-Götze, Ch 1979 Immunologic markers for classification of leukemias and non-Hodgkin lymphomas. In Gross R, Hellriegel K-P (eds) Recent results in cancer research. Springer-Verlag, Berlin, New York

Thomas E D, Storb R 1970 Technique for human marrow grafting. Blood 36: 507–515

Thomas E D, Storb R 1971 The effect of amethopterin on the immune response. Annals New York Academy of Science 186: 467–474

Thomas E D, Storb R, Buckner C D 1976 Total-body irradiation in preparation for marrow engraftment. Transplantation Proceedings VIII: 591–593

Thomas E D, Storb R, Clift R A, Fefer A, Johnson L, Neiman P E, Lerner K G, Glucksberg H, Buckner C D 1975a Bone-marrow transplantation. New England Journal of Medicine, 292: 832–843

Thomas E D, Storb R, Clift R A, Fefer A, Johnson L, Neiman P E, Lerner K G, Glucksberg H, Buckner C D 1975b Bone-marrow transplantation New England Journal of Medicine 292: 895–902

Thomas E D, Buckner C D, Banaji M, Clift R A, Fefer A, Flournoy N, Goodell B W, Hickman R O, Lerner K G, Neiman P E, Sale G E, Sanders J E, Singer J, Stevens M, Storb R, Weiden P L 1977la One hundred patients with acute leukemia treated by chemotherapy, total body irradiation, and allogenic marrow transplantation. Blood 49: 511–533

Thomas E D, Fefer A, Buckner C D, Storb R 1977b Current status of bone marrow transplantation for aplastic anemia and acute leukemia. Blood 49: 671–681

Thomas E D, Flournoy N, Buckner C D, Clift R A, Fefer A, Neiman P E, Storb R 1977c Cure of leukemia by marrow transplantation. Leukemia Research 1: 67–70

Thomas E D, Sanders J E, Flournoy N, Johnson F L, Buckner C D, Clift R A, Fefer A, Goodell B W, Storb R, Weiden P L 1979a Marrow transplantation for patients with acute lymphoblastic leukemia in remission. Blood 54: 468–476

Thomas E D, Buckner C D, Clift R A, Fefer A, Johnson F L, Neiman P E, Sale G E, Sanders J E, Singer J W, Shulman H, Storb R, Weiden P L 1979b Marrow transplantation for acute non-lymphoblastic leukemia in first remission. New England Journal of Medicine 301: 597–599

UCLA Bone Marrow Transplantation Group 1977 Bone marrow transplantation with intensive combination chemotherapy/radiation therapy (SCARI) in acute leukemia. Annals of Internal Medicine 86: 155–161

Uphoff D E 1958 Alteration of homograft reaction by A-methopterin in lethally irradiated mice treated with homologous marrow. Proceedings of the Society of Experimental and Biological Medicine 99: 651–653

Van Rood J J, Van Leeuwen A 1976 Major and minor histocompatibility systems in man and their importance in bone marrow transplantation. In: Dupont D, Good R A (eds) Immunobiology of bone marrow transplantation vol 1. Grune & Stratton, New York, p 103–110

Weiden P L, Flournoy N, Thomas E D, Prentice R, Fefer A, Buckner C D, Storb R 1979a Antileukemic effect of graft-versus-host disease in human recipients of allogeneic-marrow grafts. New England Journal of Medicine 300: 1068–1073

Weiden P L, Doney K, Storb R, Thomas E D 1979b Antithymocyte globulin (ATG) in human marrow transplantation. Experimental Hematology 7: 102

Winston D J, Gale R P, Meyer D V, Young L S 1979 Infectious complications of human bone marrow transplantation. Medicine 58: 1–31

Yunis E J, Fernandes G, Smith J, Good R A 1976 Long survival and immunologic reconstitution following transplantation with syngeneic or allogeneic fetal liver and neonatal spleen cells. In: Dupont B, Good R A (eds) Immunobiology of bone marrow transplantation vol 1. Grune & Stratton, New York p 173–177

11. Organ transplantation

R. Y. Calne

RENAL TRANSPLANTATION

In September 1979 an important anniversary was celebrated at the Peter Bent Brigham Hospital in Boston, namely the 25th year after the first kidney graft was performed in man. In the 1950s the technique of kidney grafting was well established in animals and the inevitable rejection that grafts between individuals of the same species who were not twins was also recognised. Autografted kidneys transplanted from and to the same individual and skin grafts transplanted between identical twins were not rejected and if surgery was satisfactory were accepted permanently. This was the background which led Doctors Murray, Merrill & Harrison (1956) to perform the first kidney graft between identical twins at Peter Bent Brigham Hospital. One of the twins suffered from terminal renal failure and the other twin gave one of his normal kidneys. As anticipated, the results of such transplants were excellent, the only complication in surgically successful cases was the development of the patient's own disease which occasionally occurred in the transplant.

Transplants between individuals who were not identical twins tended to do very badly with the immunosuppression then in vogue, namely total body irradiation. There were only isolated good results reported with grafts between non-identical twins using X-ray immunosupression. The use of azathioprine combined with steroids changed the whole picture. It now became possible to get excellent results in a proportion of patients with transplanted kidneys coming even from unrelated donors. This new immunosuppressive regimen, together with the introduction of recurrent dialysis, enabled kidney transplantation to be established as a therpaeutic endeavour. A proliferation of research in basic immunology and in particular the development of tissue typing for the HL-A system permitted clinicians to select donors where there were theoretical expectations of better results than organs taken at random.

Donor compatability
The predicted value of tissue typing was, however, disappointing in selecting kidneys from unrelated donors but was of great importance in intrafamilial grafting particularly between siblings. Serological methods provide definition of antigens at two subloci of the sixth human chromosome, the A and B series. When these are matched between siblings the result of kidneys grafting is nearly as good as between identical twins. Some 80 per cent would be functioning at five years. There is a one in four chance of a pair of siblings having identical HL-A antigens.

Recently, new techniques have become available to test for the so-called D sublocus of the same chromosome complex. This previously had been determined with somewhat less precision by cell culture methods which took several days to perform.

Now, results with D related or DR serological tissue typing, are exciting a great deal of interest and already there are suggestions that this system is of more importance in predicting kidney grafting results than the A and B systems. Moreover, the number of antigens defined at the DR locus are much less than the A and B, so the chances of obtaining a good match are correspondingly better. The effects of prior blood transfusion are also of interest. It is known that following transfusions of blood, which are commonly necessary in patients with chronic renal failure, antibodies quickly appear in the serum which react against transplantation antigens. Similar antibodies may appear following sensitization by kidney graft or multiple pregnancies. In general, patients with high titres of antibodies do not do as well following grafting as those who have not developed antibodies and if there is a specific cross-match, namely that the patient's serum destroys the white cells of the donor, then the outlook for a graft is very poor and virtually instantaneous rejection may occur.

Patients who have received blood transfusions and have not produced antibodies do exceptionally well following kidney grafting and argument has taken place as to whether this is due to a specific inhibition of immune capacity or whether the blood transfusions have merely acted as an antigenic stimulus, selecting good and bad responders. Certainly as a group, patients who have received blood transfusion do better than patients who have not, but since methods of selecting a negative cross match preclude grafting a kidney in the face of antibodies directed against that kidney, the debate continues, but most centres now give blood transfusions to their patients on dialysis.

One of the depressing features of organ grafting has been the lack of progress in overall results in the past decade, although the percentage of patients surviving now has improved. The principle has been accepted that if a kidney is undergoing severe rejection, immunosuppression should not be pushed too hard but rather the kidney should be sacrificed instead of giving dangerous and possibly lethal, doses of immunosuppressive agents. The gross functional survival of kidneys that have been transplanted has changed little in the past decade (Table 11.1).

Table 11.1   Kidney transplants — functioning grafts

	1 year	5 years
Sibling	75%	60%
Parent	70%	50%
Cadaver	50%	30%

Immunosuppression
Since 1961 clinical immunosuppression has rested on the two drugs, azathioprine, an antitumour drug, and corticosteroids. Other agents have been added but none has been proven to increase the safety and efficacy, that is the 'therapeutic index', of combined azathioprine and corticosteroids. Both these drugs have side effects. Azathioprine inhibits the bone marrow and can cause dangerously low levels of circulating white blood cells and also anaemia. The side effects of steroids that are most feared are stunting of growth and change of appearance but, in addition, steroids can lead to osteoporosis with crippling. Both agents increase the tendency to infection. It has been the policy of most transplant centres to attempt to reduce steroid dosage to a minimum and give a maximum tolerated dose of azathioprine as this is the

safer of the two. With kidneys transplanted from well-matched family donors, steroids can sometimes be stopped but this is seldom possible with kidneys transplanted from unrelated donors. Hundreds of agents have been investigated in the laboratory in the hope that they might prove to have immunosuppressive properties that were more effective than azathioprine and steroids. Until recently none has fulfilled this promise.

Borel (1976) working in the Sandoz Laboratories reported the immunosuppressive properties of a fungal peptide called cyclosporin A which had been investigated for its antifungal properties. His early experiments on a number of models included skin grafting in mice. The graft survival was prolonged, although eventually they were rejected. Kostakis, White & Calne (1977) working in Cambridge were the first to use cyclosporin A (CyA) in organ allografts — heterotopic heart allografts in rats. Following the demonstration of prolonged survival of the heart grafts they studied CyA in kidney grafting in dogs and orthotopic heart grafting in pigs. CyA proved to be more efficacious than azathioprine and steroids in these experiments and was particularly effective in pigs with heart grafts (Calne & White, 1977) (Calne et al, 1978). Green & Allison (1978) and Dunn, White & Wade (1978) showed that the agent also inhibited rejection of kidney grafts in rabbits and a very interesting property in this species was that a short course of treatment with CyA was often followed by prolonged acceptance of the kidney graft without any further drug being given. This, unfortunately, could not be reproduced in dogs with kidney grafts and only in a small number of pigs with heart grafts.

Because of these consistently good results in animal experiments the Cambridge group started a pilot study in patients receiving kidney grafts from mismatched cadaver donors where the sole initial immunosuppressive agent was CyA. To date 26 patients have been treated. Dosages varied between 10 and 25 mg/kg/day but is now initially 17 mg/kg/day. There are 20 life-sustaining functioning kidneys — 3 are more than a year post-operatively and 16 are not on steroids. This includes 14 of 15 given no additional immunosuppressive agents at any time. Acute rejection episodes were not seen in any of these patients. CyA can impair renal function, which is very worrying in kidney transplant patients. If, however, at the time of operation, patients are given large volumes of fluid and diuretic agents this nephrotoxicity can be avoided. Of the 15 patients who were only given CyA, 2 had self-limiting viral infections and 1 developed cytomegalovirus infection and had his immunosuppression changed.

The addition of other immunosuppressive drugs was followed by an increase in infection and deterioration of many of the patients' condition. Out of 6 patients given steroids and cytimun (a derivative of cyclophosphamide, a cytotoxic anticancer drug) 4 died of sepsis and 1 of these had a tumour of the lymphoid tissue. Of 4 patients given additional steroids, 1 died of sepsis and also had a lymphoma. Other side effects have been few. There has been mild impairment of liver function which tends to get better and most patients have had an increase in growth of hair. Tremor and gum hypertrophy have been observed but usually improve with time.

Other immunosuppressive agents should be avoided if possible when CyA is being used in patients with kidney grafts. Even at this early stage it is clear that CyA is the most effective immunosuppressive drug so far tried in organ grafting (Calne et al, 1979b). It is partially selective in its action, probably acting on a subpopulation of T-cells (White et al, 1979). One of its main advantages is sparing the patient the side effects of corticosteroids. It is relatively non-toxic to the bone marrow and it is well tolerated by patients.

LIVER TRANSPLANTATION

Liver transplantation was first performed in man by Starzl et al in 1963. In the intervening 16 years there have been more than 300 liver grafts, mostly in two centres, Dr Starzl's Department in Denver, Colorado (160 cases) and the University Department of Surgery in Cambridge collaborating with King's College Hospital, London (89 cases). The greatest hazard of liver grafting is the operation itself, which is a major undertaking usually on patients who are in a poor condition following long periods of severe liver disease. In the course of the operation half of the circulation returning to the heart has to be clamped and this has led to dangerous and sometimes fatal complications during surgery. Recently at Cambridge partial cardiopulmonary bypass using a heart–lung machine has been instituted to support the circulation in the lower part of the body and compensate the clamping of the venous return to the heart. This has produced a degree of control which has not previously been possible and early experience provides encouragement to continue with this technique in selected cases (Calne et al, 1979a).

Another major complication following surgery, has been blockage of the bile drainage reconstruction and leakage of bile. The gall bladder is now interposed between the bile ducts of the donor and recipient. This bridges the gap and allows a safer anastomosis than previous techniques with improved results.

One advantage that liver grafts have compared with those of heart and kidney is that the liver is less likely to be rejected, therefore the patient does not require such large doses of immunosuppressive drugs.

Liver transplantation has been used in many liver diseases but there appear to be only two main disorders which are suitable:
1. Terminal cirrhosis, whatever the cause of the cirrhosis.
2. Primary malignancy of the liver, which is rare in the United Kingdom and Europe, although very common in parts of Africa and the Far East (Balasegaram, 1975; Chan, 1967).

It is difficult to decide when to offer liver transplantation; it is frequently put off until it is too late. It is possible to preserve the liver removed from a dead person for up to 10 hours and transport it long distances in an ice-box (Wall et al, 1976). Two patients currently surviving after three and two years have livers that were removed in Holland and transported to Cambridge by plane.

The best results in terms of survival have been in Denver in children born with deficient bile ducts (primary biliary atresia). The many unpleasant investigations both in the pre- and postoperative phase and the complications of immunosuppressive drugs, particularly the corticosteroids producing, as they do, stunting of growth and a swollen 'moon face', have discouraged treating children at the Cambridge University Department of Surgery. A safer non-steroidal immunosuppressive drug would make the problem more tolerable. Currently four patients with orthotopically grafted livers are maintained on cyclosporin A as the only immunosuppressive drug.

All patients selected for liver grafting have fatal liver disease with short expectations of survival without liver transplantation. The results of liver grafting initially were extremely poor but now they are improving and approximately 50 per cent of the patients in Denver are surviving a year or more (personal communication). The longest has survived more than 10 years after operation and she is leading a normal life. Another woman has given birth to a normal child 2 years after liver transplantation. The results from Cambridge are summarized in Table 11.2. Eighteen patients survived a year or more and 10 of these are still alive, the longest for more than 5 years. Rehabilitation in many of the patients has been excellent and one patient has just completed a 70-mile camping and hiking holiday.

Table 11.2   89 orthotopic liver allografts

Year	No. of cases	Deaths				Alive
		1st week	1st week to 6 months	6 months to 1 year	More than 1 year	
1968–1979	89	17	43	9	8 (5 yr 3 months) (2 yr 1 month) (1 yr +)	12 (1:5 yr 8 months (1:3 yr 10 months) (5:2½ yr +) (1:2 yr +) (2:1½ yr +) (1:5 months) (1:1 month)
Total	89	17	43	9	8	12

When the operation becomes safer it will be justifiable to offer surgery a little earlier in the course of the patient's disease, and this should lead to improved results.

HEART TRANSPLANTATION

The heart seems more vulnerable to rejection than the kidney or perhaps a given immunological onslaught is less well tolerated by a life-sustaining heart than a kidney. Despite this disadvantage, Dr Shumway and his colleagues at Stanford have achieved outstanding results with an experience of nearly 200 heart grafts extending over a decade. Meticulous attention to detail and very careful monitoring of the patients after transplantation have been a feature of the Stanford series and their results are similar to those obtained in kidney grafting (Table 11.3).

Table 11.3   Heart transplants — expected survival rates (Shumway and Stinson, 1979)

1 year (over 40)	65%
1 year (40 and under)	66%
5 years	50%
1 year survival for whole series	50%

In addition to azathioprine and steroids the Stanford patients are given a powerful antithymocyte globulin prepared in rabbits against human thymocytes. One serious complication of this heavy immunosuppression has been an incidence of lymphoma of approximately 10 per cent and two of the Stanford cases developed lymphomas at the site of injection of the antithymocyte globulin. The two diseases most suitable for heart transplantation are severe myocardial ischaemia from coronary atherosclerosis in young people and cardio-myopathies. Rehabilitation of many of Shumway's cases has been excellent but the patients spend a long time in hospital after the operation in a semisterile environment and most of them have well developed stigmata of Cushing's syndrome due to the necessity for keeping up high corticosteroid doses.

Future prospects
From this brief survey of the three main organs that have been transplanted, it is clear that since more than 30 000 kidney transplants have been performed this is established throughout the world as a sensible and economical form of treatment.

Heart and liver transplantation remains confined to a few centres because of the immense organisation required for the present limited success. If cyclosporin A truly represents a new and improved class of immunosuppressant, then the results of heart transplantation should be much improved by this agent and many other organs that are not now transplanted may be grafted, especially, perhaps the pancreas. The young diabetic with severe angiopathy leading to renal failure is a bad risk for both dialysis and renal transplantation. His vessels may provide poor access for recurrent dialysis and he is prone to severe infection. If he is transplanted the steroids may aggravate the diabetes and infectious complications are frequent.

Much interest has been devoted to the possibility of transplanting pancreatic islets, which, if given in sufficient numbers, can maintain normoglycaemia in animals provided there is no immunological barrier between the donor and the recipient. Allografts, however, are rapidly rejected possibly being dealt with by macrophages prior to the initiation of the more usual immunological response. Whole organ pancreatic grafts are less aggressively rejected. One of the great difficulties has been dealing with the exocrine secretion. Dubernard et al (1978) working in Lyons, have obtained functioning grafts with a low morbidity by stopping the exocrine secretion with an intraduct injection of neoprene. It would be very attractive to consider using a non-steroidal immunosuppressive such as cyclosporin A, to control rejection of both kidney and pancreas in suitable diabetic cases and it will be of great interest to determine whether whole-organ pancreatic grafts would prevent the progress of microangiopathy, particularly in the retina. In Cambridge four patients with insulin-dependant diabetes are surviving with pancreatic allografts. Three have renal and one an orthotopic liver graft from the pancreas donors. All four no longer need insulin. Immunosuppression has been with cyclosporin A (Calne et al, 1979b).

If a safe effective immunosuppressant is found, then replacement surgery might be much extended. Other endocrine glands besides the pancreas could be grafted in deficiency states. Chronic pulmonary afflictions could be treated by lung grafts, and intestine transplants could be given to patients who suffered vascular disasters of their small bowel. This would initiate marked change in the pattern of surgical practice.

REFERENCES

Balasegaram M 1975 Management of primary liver cell carcinoma. American Journal of Surgery 130: 33–37
Borel J R 1976 Comparative study of in vitro and in vivo drug effects on cell-mediated cytotoxicity.
   Immunology 31: 631–641
Calne R Y, Farman J V, Lindop M, Bethune D W, Wheeldon D, Gill R, Smith D P, McMaster P,

Craddock G N, Rolles K, Williams R 1979a The use of partial cardio-pulmonary bypass during the anhepatic phase of orthotopic liver grafting. Lancet ii: 612–614

Calne R Y, Rolles K, White D J G, Thiru S, Evans D B, McMaster P, Dunn D C, Craddock G N, Henderson R G, Aziz S, Lewis P 1979b Cyclosporin A initially as the only immunosuppressant in 34 recipients of cadaveric organs — 32 kidneys, two pancreases and two livers. Lancet in press.

Calne R Y, White D J G 1977 Cyclosporin A — powerful immunosuppressant in dogs with renal allografts. IRCS Medical Science 5, 595

Calne R Y, White D J G, Evans D B, McMaster P, Dunn D C, Craddock G N, Pentlow B D, Rolles K 1978 Cyclosporin A in patients receiving renal allografts from cadaver donors. Lancet ii: 1323–1327

Chan K T 1967 The management of primary liver carcinoma. Annals of the Royal College of Surgeons of England. 41: 253–282

Dubernard J M, Traeger J, Neyra P, Touraine J L, Tranchant D, Blanc-Brunat N 1978 ga new method of preparation of segmental pancreatic grafts for transplantation: trials in dogs and in man. Surgery 84: 633

Dunn D C, White D J G, Wade J 1978 Survival of first and second kidney allogrants after withdrawal of cyclosporin A therapy. IRCS Medical Science 6: 464

Green C J, Allison A C 1978 Extensive prolongation of rabbit kidney allograft survival after short-term cyclosporin A treatment. Lancet i: 1182–1183

Kostakis A J, White D J G, Calne R Y 1977 Prolongation of the rat heart allograft survival by cyclosporin A. IRCS Medical Science 5: 280

Merrill J P, Murray J E, Harrison J H, Guild W R 1956 Successful homotransplantation of the human kidney between identical twins. Journal of the American Medical Association 160: 277–282

Shumway N E, Stinson E B 1979 Two decades of experimental and clinical orthotopic homotransplantation of the heart. Perspectives in Biology and Medicine 22: 81–88

Starzl T E, Marchioro T L, Von Kaulla K N, Hermann G, Brittain R S, Waddell W R 1963 Homotransplantation of the liver in humans. Surgery, Gynecology an Obstetrics 117: 659–676

Wall W J, Calne R Y, Herbertson B M, Smith D P, Underwood J, Kostakis A, Williams R 1977 Simple hypothermic preservation for transporting human livers long distances for transplantation. Transplantation 23: 210–216

White D J G, Plumb A M, Pawelec G, Brons G 1979 Cyclosporin A: An immunosuppressive agent preferentially active against proliferating T-cells. Transplantation 27: 55–58

12. Ectopic humoral syndromes

Lesley H. Rees

Tumours of non-endocrine tissues are capable of the production of hormones, hormone-related fragments and subunits and hormone precursors, a phenomenon known as ectopic hormone production. In recent years the application of hormone radioimmunoassays and radioreceptor assays to a wide variety of malignant tumours has lead to the recognition of the widespread distribution of polypeptide hormones in many tissues, formerly regarded as 'non-endocrine'. For example, immunoreactive and bioactive ACTH may be detected in significant amounts in most oat cell lung tumours (Knight, Ratcliffe & Besser, 1971; Bloomfield et al, 1977), and in other lung tumours (Gewirtz & Yalow, 1974) and human chorionic gonadotrophin (HCG) in cultures of human uterine cervix (HeLa cells) in vitro (Ghosh & Cox, 1976; Lieblich et al, 1976). Even more intriguing is the presence of HCG in non-malignant tissues such as normal liver, colon and testis (Yoshimoto, Wolfsen & Odell, 1977; Braunstein, Rasor & Wade, 1975).

Such observations have resulted in much controversy regarding the pathogenesis of ectopic hormone secretion, a subject thoroughly reviewed recently by Sherwood (1979). From a clinician's point of view, the impact of ectopic hormone secretion is twofold. Firstly, the metabolic sequelae of the ectopic secretion of some hormones may be far more malign than the histological nature of the underlying tumour itself. Secondly, the recognition of 'silent' peptide production without recognisable clinical syndromes, may provide 'tumour markers', occasionally of value to the clinician in diagnosis and during treatment.

THE ECTOPIC ACTH SYNDROME

History
Although the classical description of Cushing's syndrome was made in 1932 it is clear that ectopic ACTH secretion was described earlier, within reports associating non-endocrine tumours with skin pigmentation and adrenal hyperplasia. In 1952 Thorne suggested that such tumours might secrete ACTH-like peptides and subsequently adrenal-weight maintaining activity was detected in plasma from patients with the syndrome. Later a detailed study of ACTH levels in tumour tissues (Liddle et al, 1965) resulted in the introduction of the term 'ectopic hormone'.

In the last 15 years the ectopic ACTH syndrome has been extensively studied and reviewed (Liddle et al, 1969; Ratcliffe et al, 1972; Rees & Ratcliffe, 1974; Rees, 1975) and with increasing diagnostic awareness on the part of physicians and the availability of sensitive radioimmunoassay and bioassay techniques for measuring ACTH, the diagnosis is made more frequently. There is good biochemical evidence that ectopic ACTH secretion occurs in 30–50 per cent of all patients with oat cell carcinoma of the lung and that most if not all the remainder have the potential for ACTH synthesis (Gilby, Rees & Bondy, 1976).

The recognition that ectopic ACTH secretion is always associated with concomitant release of other related peptides soon followed and the presence of a melanocyte stimulating factor (called β-MSH at the time) was observed in tumour extracts from some patients (Island et al, 1965; Shimizu et al, 1965; Abe et al, 1967a). At the same time Abe and colleagues (1967b) described the ectopic secretion of α-MSH and we now recognise that multiple ectopic production of both related and non-related peptides may occur.

Clinical features

The clinical features of the ectopic ACTH syndrome are dominated by sustained high circulating glucocorticoid levels which cause myopathy, diabetes mellitus, acne, hypertension and oedema. Psychosis may be a prominent feature (Jeffcoate et al, 1979) but severe skin pigmentation is rare (Ratcliffe et al, 1972). The characteristic body habitus and facies of Cushing's syndrome is usually absent if the underlying tumour is an oat cell carcinoma of the lung and in this instance survival time is counted in weeks unless the hypercortisolaemia is relieved. In contrast, when the tumour is histologically benign or at least of a less malignant nature, the symptoms and appearance of the patient may be indistinguishable from that observed in pituitary dependent Cushing's disease.

Hypokalaemia is an invariable accompaniment of ectopic ACTH secretion and this important observation was first made by Thorne (1952). In the patients with Cushing's syndrome seen at St Bartholomew's Hospital during the last 10 years, hypokalaemia has been observed in all patients with proven ectopic ACTH secretion and is unusual in those with pituitary dependent disease or adrenal tumours.

The pathogenesis of hypokalaemia in the ectopic ACTH syndrome is unclear. Since an excellent correlation is observed between plasma cortisol and serum potassium in patients with Cushing's syndrome, hypokalaemia may be a reflection of the severity of the hypercortisolaema. However, excessive secretion of a more potent mineralocorticoid, deoxycorticosterone (DOC), in the ectopic ACTH syndrome has been implicated (Schambelan, Slaton & Biglieri, 1971).

Diagnosis

Ectopic ACTH secretion was previously thought to be a rare cause of Cushing's syndrome. However of 46 patients with Cushing's syndrome seen at St Bartholomew's Hospital from 1968–1978 20 per cent were ultimately proven to have ectopic ACTH production. In any patient with a tumour and hypokalaemia or with the clinical features of Cushing's syndrome and either high ACTH and cortisol levels or hypokalaemia, ectopic ACTH secretion should be seriously considered. In this latter group the tumour may be occult becoming clinically overt years after the initial presentation. The tests which are usually employed to try to prove the ectopic ACTH syndrome are:

1. *Plasma ACTH* levels are usually higher than those seen in pituitary dependent disease although overlap does occur (Ratcliffe & Rees, 1974; Himsworth et al, 1977) especially in those patients with clinically occult neoplasia (Rees, personal observa-

tions). Nonetheless, immunoreactive ACTH levels in excess of 200 pg/ml should be viewed with suspicion.

2. *During a 24 h metyrapone test (750 mg 4-hourly)* the majority of patients with the ectopic ACTH syndrome will not show a rise in urinary 17-OHCS or plasma ACTH in response to falling cortisol levels, since tumour ACTH secretion is autonomous. However, there are exceptions and a rise does not definitely exclude ectopic production (Meador et al, 1962; Strott et al, 1968; Upton and Amatruda, 1971; Drury et al, 1979).

3. *High dose dexamethasone (2 mg 6-hourly for 48 h)* will suppress ACTH and hence cortisol secretion by approximately 50 per cent (as measured by urinary 17OHCS) in the majority of patients with Cushing's disease, whilst only a small number (1 per cent) of the patients with ectopic production show such suppression (Liddle et al, 1969).

4. *Tumour localisation* can be made by the appropriate use of CAT scanning of organs known to harbour occult ACTH secreting tumours or by selective venous catheterisation with ACTH measurements to attempt biochemical localisation. In particular, in our own experience CAT scanning has proved invaluable for detecting occult thymic tumours (Thorner et al, 1979; Drury et al, 1979) not seen by conventional anterior mediastinal tomography, a non-catecholamine secreting adrenal phaechromocytoma and two islet cell tumours of the pancreas. Scanning of the anterior mediastinum seems particularly valuable, since the mediastinal adiposity of Cushing's syndrome (Santini & Williams, 1971) makes routine X-ray tomography difficult whereas a clear distinction between fat and tumour is seen on CAT scan (Bien et al, 1978; Drury et al, 1979).

ACTH measurements during selective venous catheterisation may be helpful. Documented successes include adrenal phaeochromocytomas (Schteingart et al, 1972; Rees et al, 1977) and thymic tumours (Rees et al, 1977). Obviously difficulties arise when the underlying neoplasm is in the lung because of the complexity of the venous drainage, although high azygos vein ACTH levels have been observed with pulmonary carcinoids secreting ACTH (L. H. Rees, personal communication). Other problems with this technique include rapidly fluctuating ACTH levels making interpretation of a single value difficult, and cyclical ectopic ACTH secretion when catheterisation may coincide with a quiescent phase (Drury et al, 1979). To try to obviate against fluctuant ACTH levels, ACTH measurements in blood taken from a peripheral vein simultaneously with particular 'high risk' site samples such as the thymic vein, may be helpful. Simultaneous ACTH measurements in high internal jugular vein samples and peripheral veins has been advocated as a diagnostic procedure to identify patients with pituitary ACTH dependent Cushing's disease rather than an ectopically secreting tumour by Corrigan and colleagues (1977), when the differential diagnosis of Cushing's disease and the ectopic ACTH syndrome has not been made by other non-invasive investigations. However, theoretically confusion could arise when a tumour is secreting substances capable of stimulating pituitary ACTH release such as corticotrophin releasing factors (Upton & Amatruda, 1971; Yamamoto et al, 1976).

Periodic or cyclical ACTH secretion is observed in patients with ectopic ACTH secretion but can occur in patients with Cushing's syndrome regardless of the underlying aetiology. Thus it is reported equally in patients with Cushing's disease (Brown et al, 1973; Liberman et al, 1976; Scott, Espiner & Donald, 1979) and the ectopic ACTH syndrome (Bailey, 1971; Thorner et al, 1979; Drury et al, 1979).

Treatment
The course of untreated ectopic ACTH secretion varies according to the nature of the underlying tumour. If an oat cell carcinoma of the lung is responsible then ACTH levels may be very high and the metabolic abnormality more severe with insulin-requiring diabetes mellitus and severe hypokalaemic alkalosis. The prognosis of this disease is appalling and the hypercortisolaemia constitutes a medical emergency requiring urgent treatment by medical or surgical adrenalectomy. Metyrapone either alone or in combination with op'DDD or aminoglutethimide (Liddle et al, 1969; Carey, Orth & Hartmann, 1973; Jeffcoate et al, 1977) may save the patient's life and allow conventional treatment with radiotherapy and/or chemotherapy to be directed at the tumour. During the initial stabilisation period, frequent plasma cortisol measurements are required until a mean plasma fluorigenic corticosteroid level of 300–400 nmol/l is achieved. This requires serial blood sampling throughout the day and calculation of a mean corticosteroid value obtained from eight plasma samples. Occasionally it may be necessary to completely inhibit cortisol biosynthesis using a blocking dose of metyrapone (1 to 1.5 g four times daily) with a replacement glucocorticoid such as prednisolone. It is important to remember that either a fluorimetric assay or a highly specific cortisol radioimmunoassay is required for measuring plasma cortisol in such patients, since the high circulating levels of 11-deoxycortisol achieved in patients on chronic metyrapone therapy will cause interference in competitive protein binding assays but this steroid does not fluoresce. Different patients vary in their requirements for metyrapone (2–8 g/day) and rapid resolution of both the clinical and biochemical abnormalities is usual on metyrapone alone and the addition of aminoglutethimide or op'DDD is not usually necessary, or desirable since with these drugs the incidence of undesirable side-effects such as skin rashes or nausea may be unacceptably high.

Using this combination of 'medical adrenalectomy' with more aggressive chemotherapy the prognosis for patients with oat cell carcinoma and ectopic ACTH secretion can be improved, with clinical remission and a good quality of life lasting for 6–18 months. Serial ACTH measurements may be helpful in monitoring the response to palliation with chemotherapy or radiotherapy (Rees et al, 1977).

In the other patients who have either a histologically less malignant or a benign tumour as the source of ACTH, treatment with metyrapone results in dramatic clinical improvement so that the source of the ACTH may be determined at a more leisurely pace. There is a resultant reduction in the morbidity and mortality associated with invasive investigations and ultimately with the operative removal of the tumour itself.

Biochemical characterisation of ectopic ACTH and related peptides
Studies of tumours associated with the ectopic ACTH syndrome have shown that some tumours (bronchial carcinoids, thymic and pancreatic tumours) may contain

ACTH in concentrations approaching those seen in the human pituitary gland ($10^{-3}\mu g/g$) whilst oat cell carcinomas may have much lower levels ($10^{-3}\,ng/g$). Hormone levels correlate well with the presence or absence of secretory granules on electron-microscopy, tumours with few granules (oat cell carcinomas) presumably secreting rather than storing hormone, accounting for the much higher circulating ACTH levels and the more severe nature of the subsequent biochemical abnormalities. In general ACTH levels measured by radioimmunoassay are higher than those detected by bioassay (Ratcliffe et al, 1972; Orth et al, 1973; Wolfsen & Odell, 1979) and there is evidence that this may be due to the presence of larger ACTH-like peptides (Yalow & Berson, 1973; Gewirtz & Yalow, 1974; Hirata et al, 1975), one of which may be the precursor hormone of ACTH and lipotrophin (LPH) (Bertagna et al, 1978; Orth et al, 1978; Pettingill, Mount & Orth, 1978; Pullan et al, 1980a). There is evidence for the presence in the plasma of patients with the ectopic ACTH syndrome, of a larger ACTH-related peptide with ACTH-immunoreactivity only, and this may sometimes be the only form of circulating immunoreactive ACTH (Ratter et al, 1979, 1980). Other ACTH and LPH related peptides that have been detected in extracts of tumour tissues and in the plasma of patients with the ectopic ACTH syndrome include β-LPH, γ-LPH, β-MSH, β-endorphin, corticotrophin-like intermediate lobe peptide (CLIP) and α-MSH (Scott et al, 1973; Bloomfield et al, 1974; Hirata et al, 1976a; Tanaka, Nicholson & Orth, 1978; Bertagna et al, 1978; McLoughlin et al, 1980; Pullan et al, 1980a; Ueda et al, 1980).

The clinical relevance of the elaboration of this wide array of peptides remains unclear at this time. However, although the production of β_h-LPH or its related peptides appears to invariably accompany either pituitary or ectopic ACTH secretion, the molar relationship of ACTH and β_h-LPH may not be constant, depending on the source. Thus the β_h-LPH: ACTH molar ratio tends to exceed 2, whereas in pituitary dependent disease it tends to be less (Gilkes, Rees & Besser, 1977). The demonstration of high levels of the opiate-like peptides β-endorphin and methionine enkephalin (Pullan et al, 1980a) in these tumours has considerable clinical implications. These opioid peptides have profound behavioural effects in laboratory animals, including the production of a catatonic-like state and it is tempting to speculate that their secretion may be responsible for some of the psychiatric disturbances observed in patients with malignancy but without brain metastases. Furthermore, both peptides possess potent analgesic activity and it is possible that their secretion could suppress some of the local clinical features including the generation of pain by the tumour, since in the patients studied in this report there was a considerable delay from the time of presentation of Cushing's syndrome to the time of localisation of the tumour (4.7 and 3.2 years). On a broader front, it is interesting to speculate that ectopic secretion of centrally active neuropeptides may combine to modify the clinical features of a wide variety of neoplasia.

MALIGNANT HYPERCALCAEMIA

Hypercalcaemia is a not infrequent accompaniment of cancer and is responsible for increased morbidity and mortality. Invariably the hypercalcaemia is associated with accelerated bone resorption, which is believed to be mediated by metabolic or humoral mechanisms. Cancer is the commonest cause of hypercalcaemia and hypercalcaemia develops in 10–20 per cent of all patients suffering from cancer. Although it may be associated with a wide variety of tumour types, it is most commonly associated with tumours of breast, lung, kidney and with multiple myeloma.

In 1941, Albright (1941) postulated that hypercalcaemia observed in a patient with a renal carcinoma without metastases might be due to elaboration by the tumour of parathyroid hormone (PTH) or another metabolically active substance. In the last decade this concept has received considerable support, although the exact biochemical nature of such substances remains highly controversial. However, it is agreed that if tumours do release such substances that they could exert their effects in two ways; (1) either by a direct local effect on surrounding normal tissues, e.g. skeletal metastases producing bone resorption and hypercalcaemia or (2) by the release of hormones or other metabolically active substances into the circulation which exert a systemic effect producing hypercalcaemia. The second mechanism is believed to operate in about 20 per cent of all hypercalcaemic patients who have cancer without bony metastases and in some of these patients removal of the tumour may relieve the hypercalcaemia. Readers are referred to current detailed reviews of the postulated mechanisms involved in the mediation of tumour-induced hypercalcaemia (Heath, 1976; Murray, Josse & Heersche, 1978; Martin & Atkins, 1979).

The roles of the possible contenders in the mediation of the hypercalcaemias of malignancy will be discussed briefly (Table 12.1) but it must be stated at the outset, that this is an area of considerable controversy. The frequency with which ectopic production of PTH, prostaglandins, osteoclast activating factors (OAFs) or other factors may be responsible for the hypercalcaemia in these patients remains unresolved.

Table 12.1   Possible mediators of tumour hypercalcaemia

1. Ectopic PTH (rare)
2. Prostaglandins and/or prostaglandin metabolites
3. Osteoclast activating factor(s) (OAF(s))
4. Vitamin-D-like sterols

Ectopic PTH secretion

Proven ectopic PTH secretion as a cause of cancer hypercalcaemia is rare (Rude et al, 1978). A material very similar to bovine PTH has been isolated from tumours obtained from patients with hypercalcaemia by Sherwood & colleagues (Sherwood et al, 1967) and raised immunoreactive PTH levels observed in the circulation of patients with increased urinary cyclic AMP (CAMP), resulting from the PTH (Shaw et al, 1977). However, others have observed immunochemical differences between ectopic PTH of tumour tissue or blood origin and native PTH (Benson et al, 1974), which may be due to release of hormonal precursors such as PreProPTH or ProPTH not normally secreted by the parathyroid glands (Martin et al, 1972; Greenberg, Martin & Sutcliffe, 1972), or C-terminal fragments of PTH secreted from the parathyroids during hypercalcaemia (Segre et al, 1972; Mayer et al, 1977; Yalow, 1978).

Ectopic PTH production has been implicated in the production of hypercalcaemia associated with a wide variety of different tumour types including squamous cell tumours of many different organs, carcinomas of breast, pancreas, liver and many others. However, the finding of raised or inappropriate levels of PTH in the plasma of patients with tumours and hypercalcaemia is not enough to justify a diagnosis of ectopic PTH production. Unfortunately, the criteria required for proof of ectopic hormone production (Table 12.2) are sorely lacking for PTH whereas the criteria have been adequately fulfilled for other hormones such as ACTH.

Table 12.2 Criteria required for proof of ectopic hormone production

1. Fall in circulating hormone level and/or regression of the clinical syndrome after tumour removal
2. No fall in circulating hormone level or regression of the clinical syndrome following removal of the normal gland of origin
3. Arteriovenous hormone gradient across the tumour bed
4. In vitro hormone secretion by the tumour tissue
5. Demonstration of hormone in the tumour tissue by biochemical, immunohistochemical and ultra-structural studies

However, the few conclusive data supporting ectopic PTH secretion are contained within single case reports and include demonstrations of an arterio-venous gradient of PTH across the tumour (Knill-Jones et al, 1970), in vitro PTH secretion by the tumour cells (Hamilton et al, 1977), high levels of PTH-like material in extracts of tumour tissue (Sherwood et al, 1967) and high circulating PTH levels and increased urinary CAMP in hypercalcaemic patients (Shaw et al, 1977). One patient developed high circulating PTH levels in the absence of parathyroid tissue (Licata, Guccion and Glowitz, 1978) which is of considerable interest. Normocalcaemia was maintained by ectopic PTH production in this parathyroidectomised patient whose requirement for calcium supplementation disappeared when he developed a lung tumour. Circulating PTH levels were increased and his serum calcium fell on irradiation of the tumour and returned with metastatic spread. At autopsy no bony metastases or parathyroid tissue was observed. More recently an animal model for ectopic PTH production has been described, since the metastasising rat carcinosarcoma (Walker tumour) will cause hypercalcaemia in transplanted parathyroidectomised rats by ectopic PTH secretion (Minne, Ziegler & Arnaud, 1978). Hopefully, studies with this animal model may answer some questions posed by human ectopic PTH secretion in relationship to basic mechanisms and therapy.

Whilst ectopic PTH production has been implicated for the hypercalcaemia of a wide variety of tumours it is probably the rarest cause of hypercalcaemia and in the majority of cancer patients the other mechanisms are operative. However, the finding of low or undetectable immunoreactive PTH levels and increased urinary CAMP in some hypercalcaemic patients with cancer, suggests the elaboration of a peptide with PTH-like bioactivity, but without immunoreactivity in conventional PTH assays. Finally, a note of caution, the finding of raised or inappropriate immunoreactive PTH levels in a patient with cancer does not necessarily diagnose ectopic PTH production since both cancer and primary hyperparathyroidism are common in the general population (cancer 1.4 per cent; hyperparathyroidism approximately 0.7 per cent) (Heath, Hodgson & Kennedy, 1980) so that the two may easily coexist (Boonstra & Jackson, 1965; Ackerman & Winer, 1975; Vichayanrat et al, 1976). In a review Heath (1976) noted 118 cases of the coexistence of these two diseases and Drezner & Lebovitz (1978) proved primary hyperparathyroidism in 6 of 11 patients referred with hypercalcaemia and cancer.

Prostaglandins
That prostaglandins may play an important role in the mediation of cancer hypercalcaemia owes much to studies using two animal models of human tumour hypercalcaemia, the HSDM fibrosarcoma in mice (Tashjian et al, 1972) and the VX_2 carcinoma in rabbits. However, the mechanisms by which prostaglandins cause hypercalcaemia in these models is complex. Thus, tumour production of prostaglandins has been demonstrated in vivo in the tumour effluent and in vitro from cultured tumour cells, some prostaglandins are powerful bone-resorbers in vitro and resolution of the hypercalcaemia can be achieved by treatment with prostaglandin synthesis inhibitors such as indomethacin. The exact nature of the prostaglandin(s) responsible is still a matter of controversy since some prostaglandin metabolites are more powerful bone resorbers in vitro than the parent compounds themselves (Raisz et al, 1977).

The evidence in man is conflicting; plasma prostaglandin levels are higher in some hypercalcaemic cancer patients than normocalcaemic cancer patients and raised levels of prostaglandin metabolites have been observed in the urine of hypercalcaemic cancer patients (mainly with bronchogenic carcinomas) (Seyberth, Raisz & Oates, 1978; Robertson et al, 1976; Demers et al, 1977). Clinical responsiveness with alleviation of hypercalcaemia has occurred in some patients treated with prostaglandin synthetase inhibitors such as aspirin and indomethacin (Seyberth et al, 1976). Thus Seyberth and colleagues (1976) studied 13 patients with hypercalcaemia and cancer and compared them with 12 patients with primary hyperparathyroidism, using measurements of urinary prostaglandin metabolites (PGE-M), urinary CAMP and plasma PTH. Patients with raised PGE-M and cancer responded to aspirin or indomethacin with a fall in serum calcium. The other group of patients with increased urinary CAMP, undetectable PTH levels and normal PGE-M excretion did not respond to prostaglandin synthetase inhibitors. Thus, it is possible that in this group there was production of a PTH-like peptide, not measured in their radioimmuno-assay. Similar observations have been made by others employing nephrogenous CAMP measurements (Rude et al, 1978). Apart from these postulated systemic effects, prostaglandins may be involved locally on the one hand causing the bone resorption associated with skeletal metastases (Galasko & Bennett, 1976) and on the other hand expediting the actual deposit of bony metastases. Support for the latter hypothesis was provided by Powles and his colleagues (1973) who showed in an animal model, that pretreatment of rats with aspirin or indomethacin prevented skeletal metastases occurring from transplanted carcinosarcoma cells. They demonstrated that patients whose breast tumour cells elaborated prostaglandins in vitro were more likely to develop bony metastases (Powles et al, 1976). However, prostaglandin activity only accounts for about half the bone resorbing activity of most breast tumours and recently Mundy and colleagues (1977) have identified a separate, distinct calcium mobilising substance which causes release of calcium without osteoclast stimulation. This substance appears to be distinct from the previously described osteoclast activating factors (OAF/s) which are large peptides, believed to be responsible for the hypercalcaemias associated with multiple myeloma and lymphoma (Mundy & Raisz, 1977).

Other mechanisms
One unique entity is the hypophosphataemic osteomalacia associated typically with

haemangiosarcomas producing profound renal phosphate wasting and mild hypercalcaemia which resolves on tumour removal (Stanbury, 1972; Daniels & Weisenfeld, 1979). The mechanism underlying this entity is unknown.

Diagnosis and treatment of malignant hypercalcaemias
The symptoms of hypercalcaemia are well known and will not be elaborated here. The severity of the hypercalcaemic syndrome usually relates directly to the serum calcium concentration and obviously to the extent of the underlying neoplasm. The serum calcium is usually over 4.0 mmol/l and the serum phosphate low (ectopic PTH production) or normal. If renal damage is severe then hypokalaemic alkalosis may ensue. The clinical features which help to distinguish this disorder from primary hyperparathyroidism include the rapid onset, absence of nephrocalcinosis, or subperiosteal bone resorption and ectopic tissue calcification. Although it is usually easy to differentiate malignant hypercalcaemia from primary hyperparathyroidism, the hydrocortisone suppression test (Dent & Watson, 1968) should be employed if there is any doubt. If this test is performed as originally described (120 mg hydrocortisone/day for 10 days, correcting the serum calcium for the haemodilution) then it provides excellent discrimination between the two causes of hypercalcaemia, since significant suppression of serum calcium does not occur in primary hyperparathyroidism whereas malignant hypercalcaemia is usually alleviated completely. The diagnosis and treatment of hypercalcaemia has been well reviewed (Watson, 1972; Leading Article, British Medical Journal, 1980).

Whilst treatment (tumour resection, irradiation, chemotherapy) must be directed where possible at the underlying tumour, in the acute stages hypercalcaemia may constitute a medical emergency. General measures that should be taken include rehydration with saline and administration of diuretics such as frusemide or ethacrynic acid. Attempts to reduce the serum calcium by a variety of manipulations include high dose glucocorticoids (hydrocortisone 400 mg/day or prednisolone 80 to 120 mg/day) which will relieve the hypercalcaemia in approximately 50 per cent of all patients, particularly in patients with breast carcinoma, by an unknown mechanism of action although corticosteroids will inhibit production of both prostaglandins and OAF(s) as well as having a direct antitumour effect. The administration of oral phosphate may be of value by precipitating calcium in the gut although it may not be well tolerated and may produce gastrointestinal symptoms. Intravenous phosphate has also been successfully employed as an emergency although extraskeletal calcification may occur; mithramycin and calcitonin both have their supporters. The use of prostaglandin synthetase inhibitors indomethacin and aspirin (Seyberth et al, 1976) whilst advocated by some has proved disappointing for others (Murray, Josse & Heersche, 1978).

Suffice it to say that all the above treatment regimens are of value only as short-term remedies. Although corticosteroids have been used for long periods of treatment they are by no means universally effective and if high doses are needed produce side effects and toxicity in their own right. More recently diphosphonates have been successfully used in the treatment of hypercalcaemia associated with multiple myeloma (Van Brenkelen, Bijvoet & Van Oosterom, 1979; Siris et al, 1980; Raisz, 1980). Only a correct understanding of the underlying aetiology of tumour hypercalcaemia will result in the availability of more specific, less toxic treatments. For example, peptides capable of inhibiting PTH action in vitro have been synthesised although their efficacy in patients with ectopic PTH secretion remains to be established (Rosenblatt et al, 1977).

INAPPROPRIATE ANTIDIURESIS

The association of hyponatraemia and bronchogenic carcinoma was first noted in 1938 (Winkler & Crankshaw, 1938) but it was not until 1957 that the hyponatraemia was attributed to the inappropriate sustained secretion of antidiuretic hormone (Schwartz et al, 1957). Raised vasopressin levels in urine (Thorn & Transbøl, 1963), plasma (Bower, Mason & Forsham, 1964) and tumour tissues (Amatruda et al, 1963) have been described in patients with the syndrome and cancer of the lung. In vitro synthesis of vasopressin by tumour tissue has been achieved (George, Caspan & Phillips, 1972) and chromatographic characterisation of tumour vasopressin studied (Morton, Kelly & Padfield, 1978). Ectopic vasopressin secretion is predominantly a feature only of oat cell lung cancer. Proven examples of its association with other malignancies are rare.

Clinical features

Inappropriate antidiuresis appears to be a common accompaniment of oat cell lung cancer (Table 12.3). Thus, in a series of 56 patients with this type of tumour studied by provocative water loading, at least 30 per cent showed clear evidence of inappropriate antidiuresis, and a further six patients probably also had this syndrome (Gilby, Rees & Bondy, 1976). Levels of bioactive arginine vasopressin (AVP) inappropriate for the plasma hypo-osmolality ($>2.0\,\mathrm{mU/ml}$) have been observed in such patients (Gilby, Rees & Bondy, 1976). In ten patients who could be evaluated after chemotherapy the syndrome completely resolved in three and partially in two. Furthermore, Padfield and colleagues (1976) detected raised AVP levels in patients with oat cell carcinoma without overt evidence of inappropriate antidiuresis and Odell and colleagues (1977) found raised AVP levels in 41 per cent and 43 per cent of patients with lung and colonic cancer respectively. AVP levels of about $2.0\,\mu\mathrm{U/ml}$ were observed in these patients whereas a mean value of $1.2\,\mu\mathrm{U/ml}$ was observed in 46 normal subjects after dehydration.

Table 12.3   The incidence of abnormal vasopressin secretion in patients with lung cancer

Author	Criterion	Histology	Incidence
Barjon et al (1972)	Water load	Oat cell	33%
Gilby, Rees & Bondy (1976)	Water load	Oat cell	32%
		Squamous	0%
Haefliger, Dubied & Vallotton (1977)	Urinary	Oat cell	65%
	Vasopressin	Squamous	16%
	(RIA)*	Adenocarcinoma	22%
Padfield et al (1976)			
Odell & Wolfsen (1978)	Plasma	Lung	
	Vasopressin	(unspecified)	41%
	(RIA)		
Kelly & Morton (1979)	Tumour	Oat cell	23%
	Vasopressin	Squamous	0%
	(RIA)	Adenocarcinoma	0%

*RIA = Radioimmunoassay

Whilst ectopic secretion of vasopressin may be the cause of the water retention in some patients, other mechanisms may be as, or more, important. Thus, Robertson (1978) studied osmoreceptor responsiveness in these patients using hypertonic saline infusions and delineated several different response patterns. He concluded that in about half the patients with lung cancer and inappropriate antidiuresis the posterior pituitary was the source of the vasopressin, stimulation occurring as a result of abnormal signals from an altered or defective osmoreceptor. He proposed several mechanisms for this defect (Table 12.4). Thus, hypovolaemia and/or hypotension of any aetiology, will stimulate vasopressin secretion by lowering the threshold set point of the osmoregulatory system, an effect that can also be achieved by tumour obstruction of the inferior vena cava. Carcinomatous involvement of the vagus nerve could interfere with baroregulatory input, a mechanism first postulated by Schwartz and his colleagues in their original paper; regulation of posterior pituitary vasopressin secretion might be disturbed by metastatic destruction of the hypothalamus or degenerative neuropathy. Finally, production by tumours of substances capable of stimulating pituitary vasopressin secretion is a possibility although this remains purely speculative.

Table 12.4 Cancer and inappropriate antidiuresis: possible causes of osmoreceptor dysfunction (after Robertson, 1978)

1. Hypovolaemia and/or hypotension
2. Obstruction of the vena cava (effective hypovolaemia)
3. Invasion of the vagus nerve (bone receptor afferents)
4. Hypothalamic metastases (regulatory defect)
5. Carcinomatous neuropathy (peripheral and/or central)
6. Ectopic secretion of a pituitary vasopressin releasing substance or other neurotransmitter

Vasopressin extracted from oat cell carcinomas associated with inappropriate antidiuresis has been studied by bioassay, radioimmunoassay and gel filtration (Rees et al, 1974; Hirata et al, 1976b; Morton, Kelly & Padfield, 1978; Pullan & Johnston, 1980). Ectopic vasopressin production is invariably accompanied by secretion of neurophysins I and II, specific proteins normally synthesized and secreted together with vasopressin and oxytocin in the neurohypophyseal system (Rees, 1974; Robinson et al, 1977). In a more recent study (Pullan & Johnston, 1980) a large number of patients with a variety of lung tumours were examined and ectopic vasopressin secretion found only in association with oat cell lung cancer and neurophysin was found as well. Since elevated levels of human neurophysin II are not seen in patients with non-cancerous causes for inappropriate antidiuresis (Pullan, Clappiston & Johnston, 1979), measurement of human neurophysin II might be employed as a tumour marker for oat cell lung cancer. A note of caution must be sounded since oestrogens (Robinson, 1977; Dax et al, 1979) and hepatic and renal disease (Robinson, 1977; Dax et al, 1979) may all elevate neurophysin II levels.

Whilst the consensus view is that ectopic vasopressin secretion in association with lung cancer appears confined solely to oat cell tumours other sporadic reports have appeared implicating ectopic vasopressin secretion in association with carcinomas of the duodenum, pancreas, bladder and prostate (Lebacq & Delaere, 1965; Vorherr et al, 1968; Kaye & Ross, 1977; Sacks et al, 1975).

Clinical management

Minor degrees of hyponatraemia are usually asymptomatic but severe hyponatraemia (Na less than 110 mEq/L) is associated with symptoms of water intoxication and may require urgent treatment. Water restriction alone (500–1000 ml/day) is remarkably effective and usually well tolerated by the patient. Before ectopic vasopressin secretion is assumed other causes of inappropriate antidiuresis must be excluded (De Troyer & Demanent, 1976).

The use of fluid restriction in combination with demethylchlortetracycline is more efficacious than fluid restriction alone (Cherrill et al, 1975; De Troyer, 1976), although the drug has a delayed onset of action. Demethylchloretetracycline produces nephrogenic diabetes insipidus resistant to vasopressin by interfering with the action of the hormone on the collecting duct and the generation of intracellular CAMP is inhibited. Demethylchlortetracycline has been compared with lithium in the management of the syndrome (White & Fetner, 1975; Forrest et al, 1978) and found to be equally efficacious and less toxic, although demethylchlortetracycline is associated with a high incidence of photosensitivity reactions. Earlier reports of nephrotoxicity associated with demethylchlortetracycline have not been confirmed.

Of course, whenever possible treatment, usually in the form of chemotherapy should be directed at the underlying tumour. Since this is invariably an oat cell carcinoma, cure is obviously unlikely.

ECTOPIC GONADOTROPHIN SECRETION

The glycoprotein hormone, human chorionic gonadotrophin (HCG) is normally synthesised and secreted by the trophoblastic cells of the human placenta and shares extensive structural, immunological and biological similarities to pituitary luteinising hormone (LH). Both share a common α-subunit whilst the amino acid sequence of their β-subunits differ markedly. The isolated subunits have no intrinsic biological activity.

It was hoped that HCG or its subunits secreted ectopically might be valuable as tumour markers since HCG should only be present in the circulation during pregnancy and in women with trophoblastic tumours or in males with testicular tumours containing trophoblastic elements. Using a sensitive radioimmunoassay capable of detecting HCG without measuring any circulating LH (Vaitukaitis, Braunstein & Ross, 1972) detectable HCG was first demonstrated in the circulation of 7 per cent of patients with non-gonadal neoplasia, including those arising in liver, stomach and pancreas. However, accumulating evidence suggests that, as with other tumour 'markers' such as carcinoembryonic antigen (CEA), specificity for malignancy is not present, since other diseases such as inflammatory bowel disease, peptic ulceration and cirrhosis may cause HCG secretion (Vaitukaitis et al, 1976). More recently, the specific use of radioimmunoassays for the α and/or β subunits of HCG has been investigated and Kahn and colleagues (1977) found increased levels of HCG or α or β subunits in 17 of 27 patients with islet cell carcinoma of the pancreas, with free α subunit production being the commonest occurrence; Odell and colleagues (1977) also observed that in 186 patients with a variety of malignancies 41 per cent exhibited raised α-subunit levels when compared with age-matched controls, whilst intact HCG was only detected in 6 per cent. These authors also studied tumour concentrations of HCG and HCG levels in control tissues. A material showing crossreaction in appropriate radioimmunoassays was detected in extracts of normal colon and liver as well as in the urine of non-pregnant women (Chen et al, 1976). However, subtle differences were detected by a variety of chemical manoeuvres, suggesting that tissue HCG differed from placental HCG, since normal tissues did not contain the enzymes necessary to add the carbohydrate residues (Yoshimoto, Wolfsen & Odell, 1979). Such desialated HCG-like peptides are known to have a reduced half-life and little biological activity (Van Hall et al, 1971; Tsuruhara et al, 1972), so that HCG produced in normal tissues or in some tumours would be expected to exhibit little biological activity in vivo.

Levels of HCG secreted ectopically may equal those seen in the first trimester of pregnancy without production of a recognisable clinical syndrome (Vaitukaitis, 1978). However, two clinical syndromes are recognised: precocious puberty may occur in male children and gynaecomastia and testicular interstitial cell hyperplasia may occur in adult males. However, it is not known if the gynaecomastia is related to the gonadotrophic stimulus to the testis causing increased oestrogen secretion or to steroid conversion within the tumour resulting in oestradiol production (Kirshner, Cohen & Jespersen, 1974; Kew et al, 1977), or whether the production of gynaeco-mastia depends on elaboration of some other peptide. The increasing recognition that many neoplasms which secrete HCG may also secrete human placental lactogen (HPL) (another placental protein not normally present in the circulation except in pregnancy) and that gynaecomastia occurs in these patients (Weintraub & Rosen, 1971; Rosen & Weintraub, 1978) has provoked controversy about the pathogenesis of gynaecomastia: thus, all patients with detectable HPL levels had elevated plasma oestrogen levels and whilst the HPL levels alone were not considered high enough to cause gynaecomastia, the associated ectopic gonadotrophin secretion stimulating testicular oestrogen secretion might in combination cause the breast enlargement. Recently, painful gynaecomastia associated with HCG production by a carcinoma of the lung was treated successfully by the antioestrogen, tamoxifen.

Isosexual precocious puberty has been reported in boys with hepatoma or hepatoblastoma (Root, Bongiovanni & Eberlein, 1968; McArthur et al, 1973) associated with HCG secretion. The clinical features are well known and include development of secondary sexual characteristics, advanced skeletal maturation, club-bing, Leydig cell hyperplasia and glandular prostatic cell hyperplasia. Treatment consists of tumour removal where possible and although chemotherapy has been used in the treatment of hepatoblastoma, the prognosis is poor. Whilst attempts have been made to use HCG and HPL as markers of response to therapeutic manoeuvres, discordance between tumour growth and circulating hormone levels and between levels of one hormone and another is often observed. This contrasts with the use of HCG in monitoring trophoblastic neoplasia in women and germ cell testicular tumours in men, where its role as a tumour marker is well established and excellent concordance between hormone level and malignant cell mass is usually observed.

ECTOPIC CALCITONIN SECRETION

Calcitonin is the normal product of the C cells of the thyroid. Although its value as a marker of medullary carcinoma of the thyroid is well established its ectopic production by non-thyroid cancers, particularly lung cancer, is less well known. In a recent prospective study of 61 patients with lung cancer, 52 per cent had raised circulating calcitonin levels, mean level 1250 pg/ml (normals under 250 pg/ml; Silva et al, 1979), and 78 per cent of these patients were normocalcaemic throughout the period of study. Venous sampling in a small group of patients with calcitonin measurements was carried out and two groups of patients were delineated; those with a thyroidal source of calcitonin and those with ectopic calcitonin production. The ectopic secretion was only associated with oat cell carcinomas. In 75 per cent of patients, raised calcitonin levels decreased during treatment directed at the primary neoplasm and in those patients available for continued evaluation, calcitonin levels reflected the clinical status 67 per cent of the time. Hypercalcaemia occurred approximately equally in the two groups with and without raised calcitonin levels. The authors state that with the exception of CEA, no other marker for lung cancer is elevated as often. Although hypercalcitoninaemia did not correlate with the presence of osseous metastases, it is possible that thyroidal calcitonin secretion in lung cancer patients represents a 'physiological' response to developing hypercalcaemia, associated with bone metastases. As with other tumour markers, immunoreactive calcitonin levels are raised in patients with non-malignant lung disease as well as in patients with other tumours such as breast cancer since Coombes and colleagues (1975) demonstrated that 23 of 28 patients with metastatic breast cancer had raised calcitonin levels and that monolayer cultures of breast cancer released calcitonin in vitro; similar in vitro studies with a lung tumour cell line are reported by others (Ellison et al, 1975).

ECTOPIC GROWTH HORMONE AND PROLACTIN SECRETION

The ectopic production of growth hormone (GH) is a rare event, but has been documented by the study of tumour extracts and in vitro GH release although none of the patients had clinical features of acromegaly (Beck & Burger, 1972; Greenberg et al, 1972). Of greater interest is the observation that some carcinoid tumours may release substances, as yet undefined, with pituitary growth-hormone-releasing activity which cause acromegaly (Beck et al, 1973; Dabek, 1974; Sönksen et al, 1976). Removal of these tumours is associated with a fall in circulating GH levels and regression of the clinical features of acromegaly. In two patients studied by Gomez-Pan and colleagues (1979) somatostatin suppressed circulating growth hormone levels but did not affect the associated hyperprolactinaemia which was present in one patient. In this patient, bromocriptine suppressed the elevated levels of both GH and prolactin. The biochemical nature of the GH-releasing substance has not been defined and it is not known whether it is a peptide or an amine neurotransmitter that is responsible.

Ectopic prolactin secretion is also a rare event associated with carcinomas of the lung and kidney (Turkington, 1971; Rees et al, 1974), although elevated prolactin levels are frequently observed in patients with lung cancer (Davis et al, 1979). This is probably due to 'stress' or possibly in some patients due to reflex neural stimulation of prolactin secretion in association with intrathoracid metastases.

ECTOPIC HUMAN PLACENTAL LACTOGEN SECRETION

Human placental lactogen (HPL) has been identified in a number of tumours, particularly of the lung, although the levels are low, and can sometimes only be detected after a concentration step has been employed (Weintraub & Rosen, 1971; Muggia et al, 1975). This peptide is structurally similar to GH and normally produced by the trophoblast. HPL has been studied in depth as a potential tumour 'marker' for carcinoma of the breast (Horne, Reid & Milne, 1976; Sheth et al, 1977), where it can be identified in the tumour tissues often in association with a pregnancy specific β_1-glycoprotein (Horne, Reid & Milne, 1976). These authors claim an improved prognosis associated with the absence of both these proteins from the tumour. In another study, Sheth and colleagues (1977) found low levels of detectable HPL in the serum of 10 of 72 women with breast carcinoma, without observing detectable levels in their controls (patients with mastitis, fibroadenosis and normal males and females). In males, ectopic HPL secretion is usually associated with lung cancer and may be associated with clinical evidence of gynaecomastia (Weintraub & Rosen, 1971) as discussed above (see ectopic HCG).

ECTOPIC THYROTROPHIN SECRETION

Hyperthyroidism can occur in two types of malignant disease. Firstly, it may occur in patients with trophoblastic neoplasia such as hydatidiform mole and choriocarcinoma and studies of the thyroid-stimulating substances isolated from the tumour tissues and sera of such patients have demonstrated differences from pituitary TSH. More recently it has been suggested that the thyroid stimulating material released from chorionic tumours, as well as in normal pregnancy, is HCG itself, since this glycoprotein has intrinsic thyroid stimulating activity. Secondly, ectopic TSH secretion has rarely been postulated to occur in association with lung cancer. Since ectopic HCG production is well recognised, this could be responsible for the production of hyperthyroidism in these patients, although the coexistence of Graves' disease with cancer remains the most likely diagnosis.

ECTOPIC GASTROINTESTINAL HORMONE SECRETION

With the rapid growth in interest and knowledge of the 'gut hormones' preliminary searches have been made for their ectopic production. This is complicated by the ever growing information about their normal sites of production outside the gastro-intestinal tract (Bloom, 1978). However, ectopic production of two peptides, vasoactive intestinal polypeptide (VIP) and somatostatin are reasonably well documented. Thus, Said & Faloona (1975) reported raised VIP levels in patients with a variety of tumours (pancreatic, lung, phaeochromocytoma and ganglioneuroblastoma) and associated chronic diarrhoea. Since the pancreatic tumours associated with watery diarrhoea are usually VIP secreting, a possible causal relationship between the two in non-pancreatic tumours seems likely.

Ectopic somastostatin secretion has rarely been reported (Mortimer, 1977; Bloom, Polak & West, 1978; Szabo et al, 1979). However, in a recent study by Penman and colleagues (1980) immunoreactive somatostatin secretion was observed in one patient with a thymic carcinoid and two patients with lung tumours. All three patients also had ectopic ACTH secretion. Peripheral somatostatin levels were increased and gradients of secretion observed in venous samples taken intraoperatively. Chromatographic studies of tumour extracts showed heterogeneity of tumour somatostatin, with two predominant molecular forms, one similar to synthetic cyclic somatostatin and one of higher molecular weight.

Whether ectopic somatostatin secretion will be associated with any clinical syndrome is unclear, although none of the patients described above exhibited the clinical syndrome observed with pancreatic somatostatin secreting tumours. It is however of interest that in the patient described by Mortimer (1977) circulatory immunoreactive GH levels temporarily rose into the acromegalic range following tumour removal and showed a paradoxical rise following oral glucose administration, possibly suggesting rebound GH release following removal of tonic inhibition mediated via somatostatin.

ECTOPIC INSULIN SECRETION

In a recent review (Skrabanek & Powell, 1978) the concept of ectopic insulin secretion was challenged using evidence based on 120 cases in the literature associating extrapancreatic tumours with hypoglycaemia in which insulin or insulin-like activity was measured. The authors rightly pointed out that no case met two or more of five criteria required to prove ectopic hormone production (Table 12.2). They conclude that the hypoglycaemia associated with extrapancreatic tumours cannot be attributed to insulin secretion and that in those cases in which circulating insulin levels were inappropriate or high, pancreatic beta cells could not be excluded as a primary source. The cause(s) of the hypoglycaemia in the other patients is (are) unknown.

MULTIPLE ECTOPIC HORMONE SECRETION

There are many well documented cases of neoplasms ectopically secreting more than one hormone. Common associations include ACTH with LPH, calcitonin and AVP, AVP with oxytocin, and HPL with HCG (Rees & Ratcliffe, 1974; Rees, 1975; Sherwood, 1979). However, these reports are biased and often reflect the interests and technical expertise available to the investigators, so that the true incidence of multiple ectopic hormone secretion is not known. Multiple ectopic hormone secretion has clinical implications since interaction between the biochemical hormonal effects may cause diagnostic confusion. A good example is the well known interaction between ectopic ACTH and AVP secretion. Raised corticosteroids and the associated hypokalaemia inhibit the action of AVP on the kidney so that inappropriate antidiuresis only becomes manifest when plasma cortisol levels are lowered and potassium levels corrected (Rees et al, 1974).

CONCLUSIONS

The basic mechanisms underlying the pathogenesis of ectopic hormone secretion are controversial and have not been discussed in this chapter. However, Sherwood (1979) has recently reviewed this subject concisely and readers are referred to his publication. To date no one hormone 'marker' or combination of 'markers' is of sufficient specificity to be used in population screening to detect an occult neoplasm (even if this were deemed desirable!). However, serial measurement of humoral 'markers' may be of value in monitoring the response to therapeutic manoeuvres in individual patients, although there are many documented instances of discordance between hormone level and clinical status of the patient (Rosen & Weintraub, 1978). Nevertheless, the recognition and understanding of the clinical manifestations of ectopic hormone secretion is of great importance, since although it may not always be possible to eradicate the tumour, correction of the metabolic derangements, be it hypercortisolaemia, hypercalcaemia or inappropriate antidiuresis may result in an improved prognosis or quality of life.

REFERENCES

Abe K, Nicholson W E, Liddle G W, Island D P, Orth D N 1967a Radioimmunoassay of β-MSH in human plasma and tissues. Journal of Clinical Investigation 46: 1609–1616

Abe K, Island D P, Liddle G W 1967b Radioimmunological evidence for α-MSH in human pituitary and tumour tissue. Journal of Clinical Endocrinology and Metabolism 27: 46–52

Ackerman N B, Winer N 1975 The differentiation of primary hyperparathyroidism from the hypercalcaemia of malignancy. Annals of Surgery 181: 266–231

Albright F 1941 Case records of the Massachusetts General Hospital, case 27461. New England Journal of Medicine 225: 789–794

Amatruda T T, Mulrow P J, Gallagher J C, Sawyer W H 1963 Carcinoma of the lung with inappropriate antidiuresis. New England Journal of Medicine 269: 544–549

Bailey R E 1971 Periodic hormonogenesis: a new phenomenon. Periodicity in function of a hormone producing tumour in man. Journal of Clinical Endocrinology and Metabolism 2: 317–327

Barjon P, Michel E B, Mion H, Vidal J 1972 Recherche systématique d'une sécrétion inappropriée d'hormone antidiurétique au cours du cancer bronchique primitif. Sem Hop Paris 48: 3305–3309

Beck C, Burger H G 1972 Evidence of the presence of immunoreactive growth hormone in cancers of the lung and stomach. Cancer 30: 75–79

Beck C, Larkins R G, Martin T J, Burger H G 1973 Stimulation of growth hormone release from superfused rat pituitary by extracts of hypothalamus and human bronchial tumours. Journal of Endocrinology 59: 325–333

Benson R C, Riggs B L, Pickard B M, Arnaud C D 1974 Immunoreactive forms of circulating parathyroid hormone in primary and ectopic hyperparathyroidism. Journal of Clinical Investigation 54: 175, 181

Bertagna X Y, Nicholson W E, Sorenson G D, Pettengill O F, Orth D N 1978 Endorphin (END), corticotrophin (ACTH) and lipotrophin (LPH) production by human non-pituitary tumor in tissue culture. Evidence for a common precursor. Clinical Research 25: 4089a

Bien M E, Mancuso A A, Mink M H, Hansen G C 1978 Computed tomography in the evaluation of mediastinal lipomatosis. Journal of Computer Assisted Tomography 2: 379–383

Bloom S R 1978 Gut hormones. Churchill-Livingston, Edinburgh

Bloom S R, Polak J M, West A M 1978 Somatostatin contained in pancreatic endocrine tumours. Metabolism 27: Suppl. 1, 1235–1238

Bloomfield G A, Scott A P. Lowry P J, Gilkes J J H, Rees L H 1974 A reappraisal of human β-MSH. Nature 252: 492–493

Bloomfield G A, Holdaway I M, Corrin B, Ratcliffe J G, Rees G M, Ellison M, Rees L H 1977 Lung tumours and ACTH production. Clinical Endocrinology 6: 95–104

Boonstra C E, Jackson C E 1976 Hyperparathyroidism detected by routine serum calcium analysis: prevalence in a clinic population. Annals of Internal Medicine 63: 468–474

Bower B F, Mason D M, Forsham P H 1964 Bronchogenic carcinoma with inappropriate anti-diuretic activity in plasma and tumour. New England Journal of Medicine 271: 934–938

Braunstein G D, Rasor J, Wade M E 1975 Presence in normal human testes of a chronic gonadotropin-like substance distinct from human lutenizing hormone. New England Journal of Medicine 293: 1339–1343

Brown R D, Van Loon G R, Orth D N, Liddle G W 1973 Cushing's disease with periodic hormonogenesis: one explanation for paradoxical response to dexamethasone. Journal of Clinical Endocrinology and Metabolism 32: 317–327

Buckle R 1974 Ectopic PTH syndrome, pseudohyperparathyroidism; hypercalcaemia of malignancy. Clinical Endocrinology and Metabolism 3: 237–251

Carey R W, Orth D N, Hartman W H 1973 Malignant melanoma with ectopic production of adrenocorticotropic hormone. Journal of Clinical Endocrinology and Metabolism 36: 482–487

Chen H C, Hodgen G D, Matsuura S, Lin J L, Gross E, Reichert L E, Birken S, Canfield R E, Ross G T 1976 Evidence for gonadotropin from nonpregnant subjects that has physical immunological and biological substances similar to human chorionic gonadotropin. Proceedings of the National Academy of Sciences 73: 2885–2889

Cherrill D A, Stote R M, Birge J R, Singer I 1975 Demeclocycline treatment in the syndrome of inappropriate anti-diuretic hormone secretion. Annals of Internal Medicine 831: 654–656

Coombes R C, Easty G C, Detre S I, Hillyard C J, Stevens U, Girgis S I, Galante L S, Heywood L, MacIntyre I, Neville A M 1975 Secretion of immunoreactive calcitonin by human breast carcinomas, British Medical Journal 4: 197–199

Corrigan D F, Schaaf M, Whaley R A, Czerwinski C L, Earll J M 1977 Selective venous sampling to differentiate colonic ACTH secretion from pituitary Cushing's syndrome. New England Journal of Medicine 296: 661

Dabek J T 1974 Bronchial carcinoid tumour with acromegaly in two patients. Journal of Clinical Endocrinology and Metabolism 38: 329–333

Daniels R A, Weisenfeld I 1979 Tumour phosphaturic osteomalacia. American Journal of Medicine 67: 155–159

Davis S, Proper S, May P B, Ertel N H, 1979 Elevated prolactin levels in bronchiogenic carcinoma. Cancer 44: 676–679

Dax E M, Clappison B H, Pullan P T, Pepperell R, Johnston C I 1979 Individual neurophysin concentrations in the pituitary and circulation of humans. Clinical Endocrinology 10: 253–263

Demers L M, Allegra J C, Harvey H A, Lipton A, Luderer J R, Mortel R, Brenner D E 1977 Plasma prostaglandins in hypercalcaemic patients with neoplastic disease. Cancer 39: 1559–1562

Dent C E, Watson L 1968 The hydrocortisone test in primary and tertiary hyperparathyroidism. Lancet ii: 662–664

De Troyer A, Demanet J C 1976 Clinical biological and pathogenic features of the syndrome of inappropriate secretion of antidiuretic hormone. Quarterly Journal of Medicine 45: 521–531

Drezner M K, Lebovitz H E 1978 Primary hyperparathyroidism in paraneophastic hypercalcaemia. Lancet i: 1004–1006

Drury P L, Pullan P T, Wass J, Clement-Jones V, Edwards C R W, Rees L H, Besser G M 1979 Variable weakness in a barmaid. Paper presented to the Endocrine Section of the Royal Society of Medicine.

Ellison M, Woodhouse D, Hillyard C, Dowsett M, Coombes R C, Gilby E D, Greenberg P B, Neville A M 1975 Immunoreactive calcitonin production by human lung carcinoma cells in culture. British Journal of Cancer 35: 777–784

Forrest J N, Cox M, Hong C, Morrison G, Bia M, Singer I 1978 Superiority of demeclocycline over lithium in the treatment of the chronic syndrome of inappropriate secretion of antidiuretic hormone. New England Journal of Medicine 298: 173–177

Galasko C S B, Bennett A 1976 Relationship of bone destruction in skeletal metastases to osteoclast activation and prostaglandins. Nature 263: 508–511

George J M, Capen C C, Phillips A S 1972 Biosynthesis of vasopressin in vitro and ultrastructure of a bronchogenic carcinoma. Journal of Clinical Investigation 51: 141–148

Gewirtz G, Yalow R A 1974 Ectopic ACTH production in carcinoma of the lung. Journal of Clinical Investigation 53: 1022–1032.

Ghosh N K, Cox R P 1976 Production of human chorionic gonadotrophins in HeLa cell cultures. Nature 259: 4161417

Gilby E D, Rees L H, Bondy P 1976 Ectopic hormones as markers of response to therapy in cancer. Excerpta Medica Series 375: 132–138

Gilkes J J H, Rees L H, Besser G M 1977 Plasma immunoreactive corticotrophin and lipotrophin in Cushing's syndrome and Addison's disease. British Medical Journal i: 996–997

Gomez-Pan A, Scanlon M E, Thorner M O, Rees L H, Schally A V, Hall R, Besser G M 1979 Effect of somatostatin on abnormal growth hormone and prolactin secretion in patients with the carcinoid syndrome. Clinical Endocrinology 10: 575–581

Greenberg P B, Martin T J, Beck C, Burger H G 1972 Synthesis and release of human growth hormone from lung carcinoma in cell culture. Lancet i: 350–352

Haefliger J M, Dubied M C, Vallotton M B 1971 Excrétion journalière de l'hormone antidurétique lors de carcinome bronchique. Schweiz. Med. Wochenschr 107: 726–732

Hamilton J W, Hartman C R, McGregor D H, Cohn D V 1977 Synthesis of parathyroid hormone-like peptides by a human squamous cell carcinoma. Journal of Clinical Endocrinology and Metabolism 45: 1023–1030

Heath D A 1976 Hypercalcaemia and malignancy. Annals of Clinical Biochemistry 13: 555–560
Heath H, Hodgson S F, Kennedy B S 1980 Primary hyperparathyroidism. Incidence, mortality and potential economic impact in a community. New England Journal of Medicine 302: 189–193
Himsworth R L, Bloomfield G A, Coombes R C, Ellison M, Gilkes J J H, Lowry P J, Setchell K D R, Slavin G, Rees L H 1977 Big ACTH and calcitonin in an ectopic hormone secreting tumour of the liver. Clinical Endocrinology 7: 45–62
Hirata Y, Yamamoto H, Matsukura S, Imura H 1975 In vitro release and biosynthesis of tumour ACTH in ectopic ACTH producing tumours. Journal of Clinical Endocrinology and Metabolism 41: 106–114
Hirata Y, Matsukura S, Imura H, Nakamura M, Tanaka A 1976a Size heterogeneity of beta MSH in ectopic ACTH-producing tumours. Presence of a β-LPH-like peptide. Journal of Clinical Endocrinology and Metabolism 42: 33–40
Hirata Y, Matsukura S, Imura H, Yakura T, Ihjiman S, Nagase E C, Itoh M 1976b Two cases of multiple-hormone producing small cell carcinoma of the lung. Cancer 38: 2575–2582
Horne C H W, Reid I N, Milne E D 1976 Prognostic significance of inappropriate production of pregnancy proteins by breast cancers. Lancet ii: 279–282
Island D P, Shimizu N, Nicholson W E, Abe K, Ogata E, Liddle G W 1965 A method of separating small quantities of MSH and ACTH with good recovery of each. Journal of Clinical Endocrinology and Metabolism 25: 975–983
Jeffcoate W J, Rees L H, Tomlin S, Jones A E, Edwards C R W, Besser G M 1977 Metyrapone in the long-term magnagement of Cushing's disease. British Medical Journal 2: 215–217
Jeffcoate W J, Silverstone J T, Edwards C R W, Besser G M 1979 Psychiatric manifestation of Cushing's syndrome: response to lowering of plasma cortisol. Quarterly Journal of Medicine 48: 465–472
Kahn C R, Rosen S W, Weintraub B D, Fajans S S, Gordon P 1977 Ectopic production of chorionic gonadotropin and its subunits by islet-cell tumors. New England Journal of Medicine 297: 565–569
Kaye S B, Ross E J 1977 Inappropriate anti-diuretic hormone (ADH) secretion in association with carcinoma of the bladder. Postgraduate Medical Journal 53: 274–276
Kelly P, Morton J J 1980 Antidiuretic hormone immunoreactivity in tumour tissue from patients with bronchogenic carcinoma: with and without hyponatraemia. Clinical Endocrinology 12: 99–101
Kew M, Kirschner M A, Abrahams G E, Katz M 1977 Mechanisms of feminisation in primary liver cancer. New England Journal of Medicine 296: 1084–1088
Kirshner M A, Cohen F B, Jespersen D 1974 Estrogen production and its origin in man with gonadotropin producing neoplasms. Journal of Clinical Endocrinology and Metabolism 39: 112–118
Knight R A, Ratcliffe J G, Besser G M 1971 Tumour ACTH concentrations in the ectopic ACTH syndrome and in control tissues. Proceedings of the Royal Society of Medicine 64: 1266
Knill-Jones R T, Buckle R M, Parsons V, Calne R Y, Williams R 1970 Hypercalcaemia and increased parathyroid-hormone activity in primary hepatoma: studies before and after hepatic transplantation. New England Journal of Medicine 282: 704–708
Leading Article 1980 Management of severe hypercalcaemia, British Medical Journal i: 204–205
Lebacq E, Delaere J 1965 Origine des substances antidiuretiques et explication de l'hypernatriume dans le syndrome de Schwartz-Bartter. Annales d'Endocrinologic 26: 375–382
Liberman B, Wajchenberg B L, Tambascia M A, Mesquita C H 1976 Periodic remission in Cushing's disease with paradoxical dexamethasone response: an expression of periodic hormonogenesis. Journal of Clinical Endocrinology and Metabolism 43: 913–918
Licata A A, Guccion J G, Glowitz R J 1978 Spontaneous return of normocalcaemia. Journal of the American Medical Association 240: 468–469
Liddle G W, Givens J R, Nicholson W E, Island D P 1965 The ectopic ACTH syndrome. Cancer Research 25: 1057–1061
Liddle G W, Nicholson W E, Island D P, Orth D N, Abe K, Lowder S C 1969 Clinical and laboratory studies of ectopic humoral syndromes. Recent Progress in Hormone Research 25: 283–314
Lieblich J M, Weintraub B D, Rosen S W, Chou J Y, Robinson J C 1976 HeLa cells produce α-subunit of glycoprotein tropic hormones. Nature 260: 530–532
McArthur J, Toll G D, Russfield A B, Reiss A M, Quinby W C, Baker W H 1973 Sexual precocity attributable to ectopic gonadotrophin secretion by hepatoblastoma. American Journal of Medicine 54: 390–403
McLoughlin L, Lowry P J, Ratter S, Besser G M, Rees L H 1980 β-endorphin and β-MSH in human plasma. Clinical Endocrinology 12: 287–292
Martin T J, Greenberg P B, Beck C, Johnston C I 1972 Peptide hormone synthesis by human tumours in cell culture. In: Proceedings of 4th International Congress of Endocrinology. Excerpta Medica, Amsterdam
Martin T J, Atkins D 1979 Biochemical regulators of bone resorption and their significance in cancer. Essays in Medical Biochemistry 5: 49–82
Mayer G P, Keaton J A, Hurst J G, Habener J F 1977 Effects of plasma calcium concentration on the

relative proportion of hormone and carboxyl fragment in parathyroid venous blood. Abstract of the 59th Meeting of the Endocrine Society, p 234

Meador C K, Liddle G W, Island D P, Nicholson W E, Lucas C P, Nuckton J G, Luetscher J A 1962 Cause of Cushing's syndrome in patients with tumors arising from non-endocrine tissue. Journal of Clinical Endocrinology and Metabolism 22: 693–703

Minne H, Ziegler R, Arnaud C D 1978 Paraneoplastic parathyroid hormone production by the hypercalcaemic Walker carcinosarcoma of the rat. In Copp D H, Talmage R V (eds) The Endocrinology of Calcium Metabolism: Proceedings of the 6th Parathyroid Conference, Vancouver, Canada, June 12–14, 1977. Excerpta Medica, Amsterdam

Mortimer C H 1977 Clinical applications of the gonadotrophin releasing hormone. Clinics in Endocrinology & Metabolism 6: 167–179

Morton J J, Kelly P, Padfield P L 1978 Antidiuretic hormone in bronchogenic carcinoma. Clinical Endocrinology 1: 357–370

Muggia F M, Rosen S W, Weintraub P D, Hansen H H 1975 Ectopic placental proteins in nontrophoblastic tumours. Cancer 36: 1327–1337

Mundy G R, Eilon G, Altman A J 1977 Direct resorption of bone by cultured exogenous cells. In: Endocrinology of Calcium Metabolism, Proceedings of the 6th Parathyroid Conference, p 374

Mundy G R, Raisz L G 1977 Big and little forms of osteoclast activating factor. Journal of Clinical Investigation 60: 122–128

Murray T M, Josse R G, Heersche J N M 1978 Hypercalcaemia and cancer: an update. Canadian Medical Association Journal 111: 915–920

Odell W, Wolfsen A, Yoshimoto Y, Wertzinan R, Fisher D, Hirose F 1977 Ectopic peptide synthesis: a universal concommitant of neoplasia. Transactions of the Association of American Physicians 90: 204–227

Odell W D, Wolfsen A 1978 Humoral syndromes associated with cancer. Annual Review of Medicine 29: 379–406

Odell W D, Wolfsen A, Bachelot I, Hirase F M 1979 Ectopic production of lipotropin by cancer. The American Journal of Medicine 66: 631–638

Orth D N, Nicholson W E, Mitchell W M, Island D P, Liddle G W 1973 Biologic and immunologic characterization and physical separation of ACTH and ACTH fragments in the ectopic ACTH syndrome. Journal of Clinical Investigation 52: 1756–1769

Orth D N, Nicholson W E 1977 Higher molecular weight forms of human ACTH are glycoproteins. Journal of Clinical Endocrinology & Metabolism 44: 214–217

Orth D N, Guillemin R, Ling N, Nicholson W E 1978 Immunoreactive endorphins, lipotrophins and corticotropins in a human nonpituitary tumor: Evidence for a common precursor. Journal of Clinical Endocrinology & Metabolism 46: 849

Padfield P L, Morton J J, Brown J J, Lever A F, Robertson J I S, Wood M, Fox R 1976 Plasma arginine vasopressin in the syndrome of antidiuretic hormone excess associated with bronchogenic carcinoma. American Journal of Medicine 61: 825–831

Penman E, Wass J A H, Lowry P J, Dawson A M, Besser G M, Rees L H 1980 Somatostatin secretion from non-endocrine tumours. Clinical Endocrinology, in press

Pettengill O F, Mount C D, Orth D N 1978 Corticotropin, lipotropin and endorphin production by a human non-pituitary tumor in culture: evidence for a common precursor. Proceedings of the National Academy of Sciences 75: 5160–5164

Powles T J, Dowsett M, Easty D M, Easty G C, Neville A M 1973 The inhibition by aspirin and indomethacin of osteolytic tumour deposits and hypercalcaemia in rats with Walker tumour and its possible application to human breast cancer. British Journal of Cancer 28: 316–321

Powles T J, Dowsett M, Easty D M, Easty G C, Neville A M 1976 Breast cancer osteolysis, bone metastases and the antiosteolytic effect of aspirin. Lancet i: 608–610

Pullan P T, Clappison B H, Johnston C I 1979 Plasma vasopressin and human neurophysins in physiological and pathological states associated with changes in vasopressin secretion. Journal of Clinical Endocrinology and Metabolism 49: 580–587

Pullan P T, Clement-Jones V, Corder R, Lowry P J, Rees G M, Rees L H, Besser G M, Macedo M M, Galvao-Teles A 1980a Ectopic production of methionine enkephalin and β-endorphin. British Medical Journal i: 758–763

Pullan P T, Johnston C I 1980b Ectopic production of vasopressin and human neurophysins by lung tumours. Clinical Endocrinology, in press

Raisz L G 1980 New diphosphonates to block bone resorption. New England Journal of Medicine 302: 347–348

Raisz L G, Dietrich J W, Simmons H A, Seyberth H W, Habbard W, Oates J A 1977 Effects of prostaglandin endoperoxides and metabolites on bone resorption in vitro. Nature 267: 532–535

Ratcliffe J G, Knight R A, Besser G M, Landon J, Stansfeld A G 1972 Tumour and plasma ACTH concentrations in patients with and without the ectopic ACTH syndrome. Clinical Endocrinology 1: 27–44

Ratcliffe J G, Rees L H 1974 Clinical manifestations of ectopic hormone production. British Journal of Hospital Medicine, May 1974, 685–689

Ratter S J, Lowry P J, Besser G M, Rees L H 1979 Characterisation of ACTH in human plasma by chromatography and radioimmunoassay. Abstract of the 61st Annual Meeting of the Endocrine Society, p 134

Ratter S J, Lowry P J, Besser G M, Rees L H 1980 Chromatographic characterisation of adrenocorticotrophin in human plasma. Journal of Endocrinology 85: 359–369

Rees L H, Bloomfield G A, Rees G M, Corrin B, Franks L M, Ratcliffe J G 1974 Multiple hormones in a bronchial tumor. Journal of Clinical Endocrinology and Metabolism 38: 1090–1097

Rees L H, Ratcliffe J G 1974 Ectopic hormone production by nonendocrine tumours. Clinical Endocrinology 3: 263–299

Rees L H 1975 The biosynthesis of hormones by non-endocrine tumours — a review. Journal of Endocrinology 67: 143–175

Rees L H, Bloomfield G A, Gilkes J J H, Besser G M 1977 ACTH as a tumor marker. Annals of the New York Academy of Sciences 297: 603–620

Robertson R P, Baylink D J, Metz S A, Cummings K B 1976 Plasma prostaglandin E in patients with cancer with and without hypercalcaemia. Journal of Clinical Endocrinology and Metabolism 43: 1330–1335

Robertson G L 1978 Cancer and inappropriate antidiuresis. In: Biological Markers of Neoplasia: Basic and Applied Aspects, Ruddon R W (ed). Elsevier, New York

Robinson A G, Haluszczak C, Wilkins J A, Huellmantel A B, Watson C G 1977 Physiological control of two neurophysins in humans. Journal of Clinical Endocrinology and Metabolism 44: 330–339

Root A W, Bongiovanni A M, Eberlein W R 1968 A testicular-interstitial-cell stimulating gonadotrophin in a child with hepatoblastoma and sexual precocity. Journal of Clinical Endocrinology and Metabolism 28: 1317–1322

Rosen S W, Weintraub B D 1978 Ectopic placental lactogen. In Ruddon R W (ed) Biological markers of neoplasia. Elsevier, New York

Rosenblatt M, Callahan E N, Maheffez J E 1977 Parathyroid hormone inhibitors. Design, synthesis and biologic evaluation of hormone analogues. Journal of Biological Chemistry 252: 5847–5851

Rude R K, Sharp C J, Oldham S D, Singer F R 1978 Plasma cyclic AMP (PcAMP) urinary cyclic AMP (UcAMP) and nephrogenic cyclic AMP (NcAMP) in the hypercalcaemia of malignancy. Clinical Research 26: 427A

Sacks S A, Rhodes D B, Malkasian D R, Rosenbloom A A 1975 Prostatic carcinoma producing syndrome of inappropriate secretion of anti-diuretic hormone. Urology 6: 489–492

Said S T, Faloona G R 1975 Elevated plasma and tissue levels of vasoactive intestinal polypeptide in the watery diarrhoea syndrome due to pancreatic, bronchogenic and other tumors. New England Journal of Medicine 293: 155–160

Santini L C, Williams J L 1971 Mediastinal widening (presumably lipomatosis) in Cushing's syndrome. New England Journal of Medicine 284: 1357–9

Schambelan M, Slaton P E, Biglieri E G 1971 Mineralocorticoid production in hyperadrencorticism. American Journal of Medicine 51: 299–303

Schteingart D E, Conn J W, Orth D N, Harrison T S, Fox J E, Bookstein J J 1972 Secretion of ACTH and β-MSH by an adrenal medullary parganglioma. Journal of Clinical Endocrinology and Metabolism 34: 676–683

Schwartz W B, Bennett W, Curelop S, Bartter F C 1957 A syndrome of renal sodium loss and hyponatraemia probably resulting from inappropriate secretion of antidiuretic hormone. American Journal of Medicine 23: 529–542

Scott A P, Ratcliffe J G, Rees L H, Landon J, Bennett H P J, Lowry P J, McMartin C 1973 Pituitary peptide. Nature 244: 65–67

Scott R S, Espiner E A, Donald R A 1979 Intermittent Cushing's syndrome with spontaneous remission. Clinical Endocrinology 11: 561–566

Segre G U, Habener J F, Powell D, Tregear G W, Potts J T 1972 Parathyroid hormone in human plasma: immunochemical characterization and biological implications. Journal of Clinical Investigation 51: 3163–3172

Seyberth H W, Raisz L G, Oates J A 1978 Prostaglandins and hypercalcaemic states. Annual Revue of Medicine 29: 23–29

Seyberth H W, Segre C V, Hamet P, Sweetman B J, Potts J T Jr, Oates J A 1976 Characterization of a group of patients with hypercalcaemia of cancer who respond to treatment with prostaglandin synthesis inhibitors. Transactions of the Association of American Physicians 89: 92–104

Shaw J W, Oldham S B, Rosoff L, Beltune J E, Fichman M T 1977 Urinary cyclic AMP analyzed as a function of the serum calcium and parathyroid hormone in the differential diagnosis of hypercalcaemia. Journal of Clinical Investigation 59: 14–21

Sherwood L M, O'Riordan J L H, Aurbach G D, Potts J T 1967 Production of parathyroid hormone by non-parathyroid tumors. Journal of Clinical Endocrinology and Metabolism 27: 140–146

Sherwood L M 1979 Ectopic hormone syndromes. In: Ingbar S H (ed) Contemporary endocrinology. Plenum Publishing Corporation, New York

Sheth N A, Suraiyz J N, Sheth A R, Randive K G, Jussawalla D J 1977 Ectopic production of human placental lactogen by human breast tumors. Cancer 39: 1693–1699

Shimizu N, Ogata E, Nicholson W E, Island D P, Ney R L, Liddle G W 1965 Studies on the melanotropic activity of human plasma and tissues. Journal of Clinical Endocrinology and Metabolism 25: 984–990

Silva O L, Broder L E, Doppman J L, Snider R H, Moore C F, Cohen M H, Becker K L 1979 Calcitonin as a marker for bronchogenic cancer. Cancer 44: 680–684

Sivis E S, Sherman W H, Baquiran D C, Schlafferer J P, Osserman E F, Canfield R E 1980 Effect of dichloromethylene diphosphonate on skeletal mobilisation of calcium in multiple myeloma. New England Journal of Medicine 302: 310–315

Skrabanek P, Powell D 1978 Ectopic insulin and Occam's razor: reappraisal of the riddle of tumour hypoglycaemia. Clinical Endocrinology I: 141–154

Sönksen P H, Ayres A B, Braimbridge M, Corrin B, Davies D R, Jeremiah G M, Oaten S W, Lowy C, West T E T 1976 Acromegaly caused by pulmonary carcinoid tumours. Clinical Endocrinology 5: 503–513

Stanbury S W 1972 Tumour-associated hypophosphataemic osteomalacia and rickets. Clinics in Endocrinology and Metabolism I: 256

Strott C A, Nugent C A, Taylor F H 1968 Cushing's syndrome caused by bronchial adenomas. American Journal of Medicine 44: 97–104

Szabo M, Berelowitz M, Pettengill O F, Sorenson G D, Frohman L A 1979 Somatostatin (SRIF) secretion by cultured human small cell carcinoma of the lung. Abstract of the 61st Meeting of the Endocrine Society, p 144

Tanaka K, Nicholson W E, Orth D N 1978 The nature of the immunoreactive lipotropins in human plasma and tissue extracts. Journal of Clinical Investigation 62: 94–104

Tashjian A H, Voelkel E F, Levine L, Goldhaber P 1972 Evidence that the bone-resorption-stimulating factor produced by mouse fibrosarcoma cells is prostaglandin E_2: A new model for the hypercalcaemia of cancer. Journal of Experimental Medicine 136: 1329–1342

Thorn N A, Transbøl I 1963 Hyponatraemia and bronchogenic carcinoma associated with renal excretion of large amounts of antidiuretic material. American Journal of Medicine 35: 257–268

Thorne M G 1952 Cushing's syndrome associated with bronchial carcinoma: enquiry into the relationship of this syndrome to neoplastic disease. Guy's Hospital Reports 101: 251

Thorner M O, Ragan G, Ortt B, Swgert N, Williamson B R J, MacLeod R M, Orth D N 1979 Thymic carcinoid tumour secreting ACTH intermittently and identified by CAT scan. Abstract of the 61st Annual Meeting of the Endocrine Society, p 155

Tsuruhara T, Dufau M L, Hickman J, Catt K J 1972 Biological properties of HCG after removal of terminal sialic acid and galactose residues. Endocrinology 91: 296–301

Turkington R W 1971 Ectopic production of prolactin. New England Journal of Medicine 285: 1455–1458

Ueda M, Takeuchi T, Abe K, Miyakawa S, Ohnami S, Yanaihara N 1980 β-MSH immunoreactivity in human pituitaries and ectopic ACTH-producing tumors. Journal of Clinical Endocrinology and Metabolism 50: 550–556

Upton G V, Amatruda T T 1971 Evidence for the presence of peptides with corticotropin-releasing-factor-like activity in ectopic ACTH-producing tumors. New England Journal of Medicine 285: 419–424

Vaitukaitis J L 1978 Tumors and human chorionic gonadotropin. In: Ruddon R W (ed) Biological markers of neoplasia. Elsevier, New York

Vaitukaitis J L, Braunstein G D, Ross G T 1972 A radioimmunoassay which specifically measures human chorionic gonadotropin in the presence of luteinizing hormone. American Journal of Obstetrics and Gynaecology 113: 751–758

Vaitukaitis J L, Ross G T, Braunstein G D, Rayford P L 1976 Gonadotropins and their subunits: basic and clinical studies. Recent Progress in Hormone Research 32: 289–331

Van Brenkelen, F J M, Bijvoet O L M, Van Oosterom A T 1979 Inhibition of osteolytic bone lesions by (3-amino-1-hydroxypropylidene)-1,1-biphosphonate (A.P.D.). Lancet i: 803–805

Van Hall E V, Vaitukaitis J L, Ross G T, Hickman J W, Ashwell G 1971 Immunological and biological activity of HCG following progressive desialylation. Endocrinology 88: 456–464

Vichayanrat A, Avramides A, Gardner B, Wallach S, Carter A C 1976 Primary hyperparathyroidism and breast cancer. American Journal of Medicine 61: 136–139

Vorherr H, Massry S G, Utiger R D, Kleema C R 1968 Antidiuretic principle in malignant tumor extracts from patients with inappropriate ADH syndrome. Journal of Clinical Endocrinology and Metabolism 28: 162–168

Watson L 1972 Diagnosis and treatment of hypercalcaemia. British Medical Journal 2: 150–152
Weintraub B D, Rosen S W 1971 Ectopic production of human chorionic somatomammotropin by nontrophoblastic cancers. Journal of Clinical Endocrinology and Metabolism 32: 94–101
White M G, Fetner C D 1975 Treatment of the syndrome of inappropriate secretion of antiduretic hormone with lithium carbonate. New England Journal of Medicine 292: 390–392
Winkler W A, Crankshaw O F 1938 Chloride depletion in conditions other than Addison's disease. Journal of Clinical Investigation 17: 1–6
Wolfsen A R, Odell W D 1979 ProACTH: use for early detection of lung cancer. American Journal of Medicine 66: 765–772
Yalow R S, Berson S A 1973 Characteristics of 'big ACTH' in human plasma and pituitary extracts. Journal of Clinical Endocrinology and Metabolism 36: 415–423
Yalow R S 1978 Significance of the heterogeneity of parathyroid hormone. In: Tolmage R V, Copp D H (eds) Endocrinology of calcium metabolism. Excepts Medica, Amsterdam
Yamamoto H, Hirata Y, Matsukura S, Imura H, Nakamura N, Tanaka A 1976 Studies on ectopic ACTH-producing tumors. IV CRF-like activity in tumor tissue. Acta Endocrinologica 82: 183–192
Yoshimoto Y, Wolfsen A R, Odell W D 1977 Human chorionic gonadotropin-like substance in nonendocrine tissues of normal subjects. Science 197: 575–577
Yoshimoto Y, Wolfsen A R, Odell W D 1979 Glycosylation, a variable in the production of hCG by cancers. American Journal of Medicine 67: 414–420

13. Exotic fevers: viral haemorrhagic fevers and Legionnaires' disease

Ronald T. D. Emond

Before World War II air travel was a privilege of the wealthy and most travellers from the tropics came by sea to Europe and North America. The duration of the voyage exceeded the incubation period of most infectious diseases thus providing effective quarantine against the introduction of disease. This protective barrier of the oceans has now been completely removed by the speed of modern aircraft while the risks of infection have been greatly enhanced by the vast increase in the number of travellers.

Between 1945 and 1976 there was a 50-fold increase in passengers using scheduled air services throughout the world from 9 million to 475 million and countless millions more now use charter flights (International Civil Aviation Organisation 1972, 1977). London airport at Heathrow alone in 1976 dealt with 23 million passengers (Civil Aviation Authority 1977) and the three airports serving London now receive over 700 arrivals a day from tropical Africa. Meanwhile the continuing increase in world population has brought pressure on land and other resources in the tropics. The resulting agricultural and economic expansion has encroached upon previously remote areas thus exposing man to hazard from strange zoonoses. It is ironic that the tremendous social and technological changes of the post-war era, which contributed to the decline of serious epidemic diseases in Europe and North America, have opened the door to dangerous virus infections from the underdeveloped world. It is unlikely that these diseases are really new for it is probable that they have passed unrecognised until submitted to scientific scrutiny in modern virus research institutes.

VIRAL HAEMORRHAGIC FEVERS OF THE TROPICS

The Oxford English Dictionary defines exotic as alien or barbarous, a very apt description for the many viral haemorrhagic fevers (VHF) which have caused so much concern in many parts of the world. These fevers have in common a dramatic tendency to haemorrhage and a very high mortality. Some are borne by arthropods, others are transmitted directly, many have an animal reservoir. The viral haemorrhagic fevers of African origin are particularly important to Europe because of the close political and economic ties with tropical African countries where these infections are endemic.

Geographic distribution of viral haemorrhagic fevers

Africa   Lassa fever
                       Marburg disease
                       Ebola virus disease
                       Yellow fever
                       Crimea-Congo haemorrhagic fever — virus
                             detected in several countries but disease rare

Asia   Korean haemorrhagic fever
                Crimea-Congo haemorrhagic fever
                Kyasanur Forest disease
                Dengue
Europe   Crimea-Congo haemorrhagic fever
South America Argentinian haemorrhagic fever
                Bolivian haemorrhagic fever

Lassa fever

History

In 1969 an American nurse in the mission hospital of the little town of Lassa in the north east corner of Nigeria became ill with a strange fever. Her condition deteriorated alarmingly so she was transferred along 300 miles of dirt road to the parent hospital at Jos, where she later died. A second nurse in the Bingham Hospital at Jos, who had cared for the first, also succumbed to the infection. When a third nurse became ill she was evacuated by air to the United States of America, where she eventually recovered after a stormy course. Dr Jordi Casals at Yale University succeeded in isolating a hitherto unknown virus from this nurse, before he too fell victim. Fortunately he survived but a second scientist working in the same building succumbed, whereupon all futher work on the virus in the United States was transferred to the maximum security laboratory at Atlanta (Fuller 1974).

Lassa virus was found to be indistinguishable morphologically from lymphocytic choriomeningitis virus, Machupo, Junin and other arenaviruses spread from rodents so it seemed likely that the newcomer would have a rodent host. Investigation at Jos eliminated *Rattus rattus* and *Mus musculus* but in 1972, following an outbreak of Lassa fever in Sierra Leone, virus was detected in the common multimammate rat, *Mastomys natalensis* (Monath et al, 1974). This finding was later confirmed in Nigeria (Wulff, Fabiyi & Monath 1975).

Lassa fever was identified in hospitals in Liberia (Monath et al, 1973) and Sierra Leone (Fraser et al, 1974). Subsequently serosurveys have demonstrated that infection with Lassa virus is widespread in the human population of many countries in West Africa, including Nigeria, Sierra Leone, Ivory Coast, Ghana, Senegal, Guinea, Gambia, Upper Volta, Mali and the Central African Empire (Frame 1975, Monath 1975).

Epidemiology

Although the multimammate rat is widely distributed throughout Africa south of the Sahara, Lassa fever appears to be confined to West Africa. The reasons for this remain obscure though it may be related to variations in the *Mastomys* population for it has been noted that West African rodents have 32 and 38 chromosomes while those living in Southern Africa have either 32 or 36 (Bellier 1975, Green, Gordon & Lyons 1978). *Mastomys* is a prolific breeder and is found in both fields and houses. In the rainy season it may desert the open countryside and seek shelter within dwellings, spreading infection to the occupants. Primary infection in man is either acquired directly from infected rodent urine or indirectly from foodstuffs or dust contaminated by urine. Secondary spread from person to person may occur in overcrowded village houses but has been especially important within country hospitals in West Africa. All the hospital-acquired infections have arisen from patients suffering from Lassa fever. The route of transmission has been accidental inoculation from needles or surgical instruments, direct personal contact and close exposure to pharyngeal secretions. There has been little evidence of airborne spread in hospital outbreaks in Sierra Leone (Keane & Gilles 1977) and no evidence of airborne transmission of virus from patients evacuated by aircraft to Europe and North America (Galbraith et al, 1978). However, in the Jos outbreak airborne spread from a pregnant woman with severe lung involvement was thought to be the mode of transmission to secondary cases in the ward (Carey et al, 1972). Subclinical infection or mild attacks of Lassa fever appear to be common in Sierra Leone, where surveys of villagers have revealed antibody against the virus in 6–13 per cent of the population. In Panguma Catholic Hospital in Sierra Leone, where 156 clinically diagnosed cases of Lassa fever were admitted over a period of three years, 2 out of the 75 hospital staff died, 13 were infected but recovered and the remainder showed no serological evidence of recent active infection (Keane & Gilles 1977). Galbraith and his colleagues (1978) reviewed the eight episodes when patients with Lassa fever were evacuated to Europe and North America without spread of infection and concluded that the risks of community spread have been exaggerated and that the risks of hospital and laboratory spread require emphasis.

Virology
Lassa virus has been classified as an arenavirus. This group of RNA viruses have a granular appearance on electron microscopy due to incorporation of host-cell ribosomes (arenosus — sandy) and include amongst others:

Lymphocytic choriomeningitis virus
Junin virus of Argentinian haemorrhagic fever
Machupo virus causing Bolivian haemorrhagic fever

The virus particles measure 70–150 nm and have surface projections (Fig. 13.1). The entrapped ribosomes form electron-dense granules, 20–30 nm in diameter. The *arenaviridae* share a specific group antigen revealed by immunofluorescence and in some cases by complement fixation (Rowe et al, 1970).

Lassa virus grows well in African green monkey kidney cells (Vero) and produces a cytopathogenic effect within 4–5 days. When adult mice are inoculated intracerebrally some succumb. Newborn mice usually survive but may continue to shed virus in the urine for long periods (Buckley & Casals 1970).

The virus in human infections may be recovered from the throat, blood and urine during the acute stage of the illness and may persist in urine for as long as 42 days (Emond 1978). In the second week of the illness both virus and antibodies may be detected in the blood (Monath et al, 1974).

Pathology
In fatal cases of Lassa fever there is evidence of widespread capillary damage with increased permeability leading to interstitial oedema and haemorrhages. Necrotic foci are found in many organs. It is uncertain if the damage is caused directly by the virus or by the immunological responses to infection.

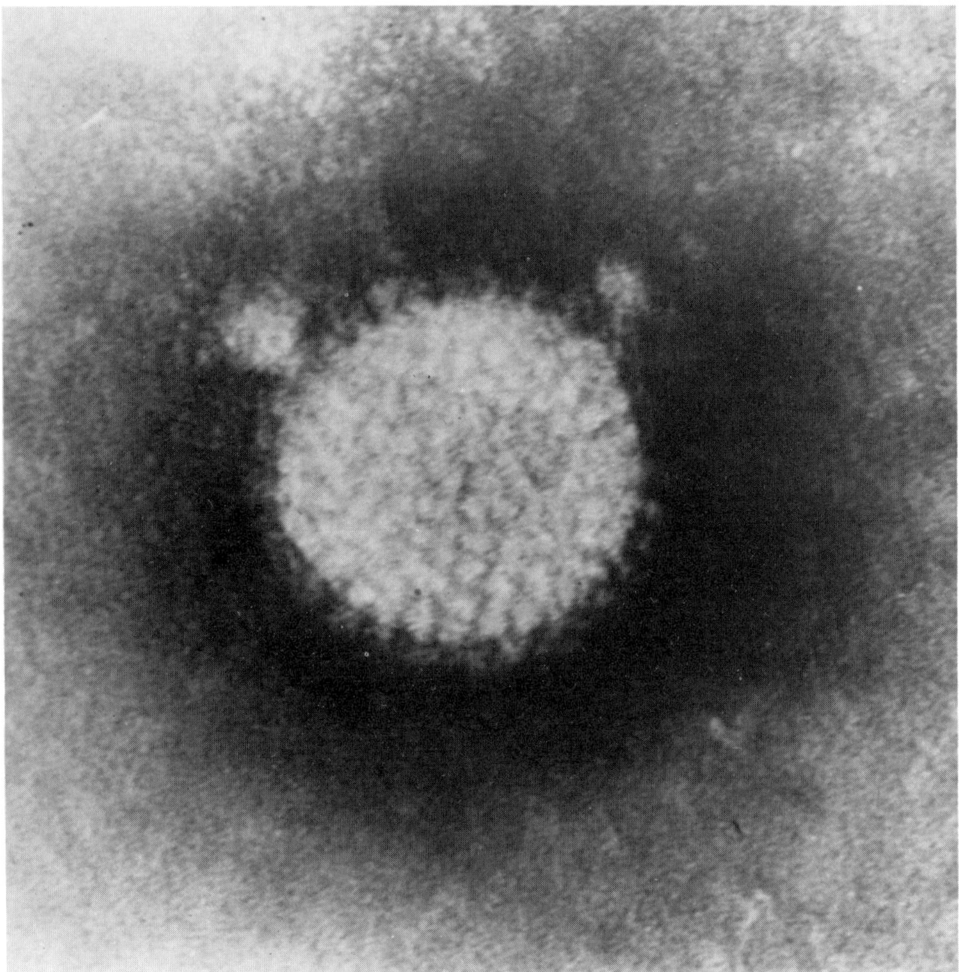

Fig. 13.1   Electron micrograph of Lassa virus × 220 000.

The heart muscle is congested and oedematous with numerous small haemorrhages. There may be evidence of interstitial pneumonitis with infiltration by histiocytes and megakaryocytes. The liver is severely affected with diffuse and widespread focal eosinophilic necrosis and the Küpffer cells are full of necrotic material. In the spleen the Malpighian bodies are depleted of cells and are surrounded by areas of coagulation necrosis. Follicles in lymph nodes are similarly depleted. The submucosa of the small bowel is oedematous and there may be bleeding into the mucosa and submucosa. Morphological changes in the kidneys are minimal and in striking contrast to the functional impairment. The medulla is congested and there may be small haemorrhages. Hyaline casts may be present in the tubules (Frame et al, 1970; Edington & White 1972).

Clinical features (Table 13.1)
Serological surveys in endemic areas have disclosed a pattern of infection varying widely in severity from the trivial to the fatal. In most instances only the more severe cases are recognised and even these are seldom suspected unless there is a focal outbreak.

Table 13.1   Symptoms and signs in 156 clinical cases of Lassa fever, Panguma Hospital 1973–76 (Keane & Gilles, 1977)

Major symptoms	No (%) of cases	Minor symptoms	No (%) of cases
Fever	98 (63)	Nausea of vomiting	62 (40)
Pharyngitis (with patchy		Abdominal or chest	
exudates	89 (57)	pain	58 (37)
Leucopenia	88 (56)	Headache	55 (35)
Proteinuria	68 (44)	Cough	52 (33)
Lethargy	66 (42)	Myalgia	47 (30)
Abnormal bleeding (bleeding		Diarrhoea	31 (20)
from mouth, petechiae,		Lymphadenopathy	11 (7)
etc.)	11 (7)	Arthralgia	6 (4)
Hypotension	11 (7)	Conjunctivitis	3 (2)
Puffiness of face and neck	11 (7)	Jaundice	2 (1.3)
Pleural effusion	3 (2)	Pericardial effusion	2 (1.3)

The incubation period is usually 7–10 days but may extend from 3–17. The onset is insidious with feverishness and shivering accompanied by malaise, headache and myalgia. Soreness of the throat is a common early symptom and examination may reveal inflammation of the pharynx and tonsils with raised patches of whitish or yellowish exudate. Occasionally small vesicles or shallow ulcers may be detected on the tonsils or adjacent areas of the palate. As the illness progresses the temperature may rise as high as 41°C with daily fluctuation of 2–3°. There may be occasional rigors. The severity and duration of the fever are very variable. The average duration is 16 days but extremes of 6–30 days have been reported (Keane & Gilles, 1977). A constant feature in severe attacks is lethargy or even prostration out of proportion to the fever.

During the second week of illness fluid may leak into the tissues and the body cavities through the damaged capillary blood vessels producing oedema of the face and neck, pleural effusion and ascites. Vomiting, diarrhoea and renal failure aggravate the circulatory failure. In the severest cases bleeding into the skin, mucosae and internal organs presage death. The terminal phase may be marked by coma and accompanied by myoclonic twitching.

As the fever subsides the patient's condition rapidly improves though tiredness may persist for several weeks. There may be temporary loss of hair and a few patients may have residual deafness.

Diagnosis
The absence of characteristic symptoms or signs makes clinical diagnosis extremely difficult in the early stages unless there is a history of contact or there is a local outbreak. The possibility of Lassa fever should be considered whenever a patient

from an endemic area presents with an unexplained fever and strict barrier nursing should be enforced until a diagnosis has been established. In the early acute stage the differential diagnosis would include malaria, typhoid fever, typhus, septicaemia and severe virus infections, such as yellow fever, dengue, influenza and enterovirus infections.

Laboratory investigations
Investigation of a suspected case of Lassa fever should only be undertaken in an approved maximum security laboratory. A throat swab, blood and urine should be sent for virus culture. Great care must be taken in collecting and packing the specimens for despatch to the laboratory because all specimens are highly infectious and dangerous.

Paired sera should be obtained for antibody studies. A four-fold or greater rise in antibody level or an initial titre of at least 1/1024 by the indirect immunofluorescence technique is evidence of active infection (Wulff & Lange, 1975). Complement-fixing antibodies develop slowly, are rarely present before the fourteenth day and may fail to develop in half the cases confirmed by virus culture (WHO, 1974). It may be possible to make an early diagnosis by detecting Lassa-specific antigen in epithelial cells by the indirect fluorescent antibody technique. The cells are obtained by curetting the conjunctiva (McCormick & Johnson, 1978).

Relatively few routine investigations have been conducted in cases of Lassa fever because of the lack of facilities in endemic areas and because of the inherent dangers. There is usually a leucopenia and there may be a reduction in the platelet count. The prothrombin level may be normal or low. Other blood clotting studies have been normal. Lactic dehydrogenase, serum glutamic-oxaloacetic transaminase and creatinine phosphokinase may be elevated. Serum bilirubin and protein levels are not altered. Proteinuria is a common finding and there may be an occasional granular cast. The blood urea is usually raised (Leifer, Gocke & Bourne, 1970).

Prognosis
Mortality rates have varied considerably in different outbreaks. In Africa between 1969–77 there have been 386 reported cases with 105 deaths, an overall mortality of 27 per cent. Death rates of 40–50 per cent have been reported from hospital outbreaks in Nigeria while much lower rates of about 20 per cent have been recorded in Sierra Leone. It is not clear why there should be this difference though there is some evidence that the strain of Lassa virus may vary (Monath, 1974). Pregnancy adversely affects the prognosis as does bleeding and circulatory collapse.

Treatment
Treatment is largely symptomatic for there is no specific chemotherapy of proven value. An antiviral drug, ribavivin, has been shown to be beneficial in treatment of rhesus monkeys experimentally infected with Lassa virus but has not been assessed in human infection (Jahrling et al, 1980). Convalescent serum has been advocated but there is no conclusive evidence that it is beneficial (Leifer, Gocke & Bourne, 1970; Woodruff et al, 1975; Keane & Gilles, 1977). Care should be taken to maintain water and electrolyte balance. In the event of renal failure peritoneal dialysis may be required.

Prevention
No vaccine is available for active immunisation so control measures are directed at the rodent reservoir. A benign arenavirus, Mozambique virus, has been isolated from *Mastomys natalensis* in South-east Africa. This virus is closely related to Lassa virus and confers cross-immunity, suggesting the possibility that it may be used for preparation of a vaccine (Kiley et al, 1979). Strict isolation of suspect cases and careful handling of laboratory specimens are essential to prevent direct spread.

Marburg and Ebola virus infections

History
In the summer of 1967 consignments of African green monkeys, captured round Lake Kyoga in central Uganda, were flown to West Germany and Yugoslavia, where their tissues were used for the preparation of cell cultures. A strange new infectious disease broke out amongst the laboratory workers handling the monkeys and their tissues. Subsequently infection spread to hospital staff and to the wives of two of the primary cases. A total of 31 people were affected and 7 of the primary cases died (Stille et al, 1968; Martini & Siegert, 1971). The route of infection in the primary cases was not established. Four of the secondary cases had intimate contact with blood from the primary cases and another appeared to have acquired infection by sexual intercourse.

A bizarre virus was isolated from the patients and from the blood and tissues of a few of the monkeys. Further investigations in Uganda failed to reveal evidence of infection with the virus in the wild monkeys or the trappers so the source of the virus remained a mystery. Although large numbers of African green monkeys had been used throughout the world for virological work in laboratories there had been no previous outbreaks. Experimental infection of African green monkeys and other primates proved uniformly fatal and caused illness similar to that in man. It seemed unlikely, therefore, that the unfortunate monkey was the primary host.

No further cases were recognised until 1975, when a young Australian died from the disease in Johannesburg. His travelling companion and a nurse from the hospital also became infected but survived. Prior to the onset of illness the Australian had been hitchhiking through Rhodesia and South Africa. The source of the infection in the young man was never discovered. His companion had been in close contact and the nursing sister had attended him during the final stages of his illness. After his death she had attempted to console his friend and had touched several wet facial tissues with her bare hands (Gear et al, 1975) (Fig. 13.2).

All remained quiet until the beginning of July 1976 when a catastrophic outbreak began in the Western Equatoria Province of the Sudan followed shortly afterwards by a similar outbreak in the Equateur Region of Zaire about 1000 km away. The severity of the illness and the high mortality justifiably caused great alarm. By the time the epidemics terminated towards the end of November over 280 cases had been recognised in the Sudan and 151 people had died (Francis et al, 1978); in Zaire the outbreak proved to be an even greater disaster for only 38 survived out of 318 documented patients (Breman et al, 1978). The cause of the epidemics was quickly identified as a virus, morphologically identical to Marburg virus but antigenically distinct. This has been named Ebola virus after a small river in Zaire. Ebola virus infection is likely to be a zoonosis but the animal reservoir has yet to be discovered

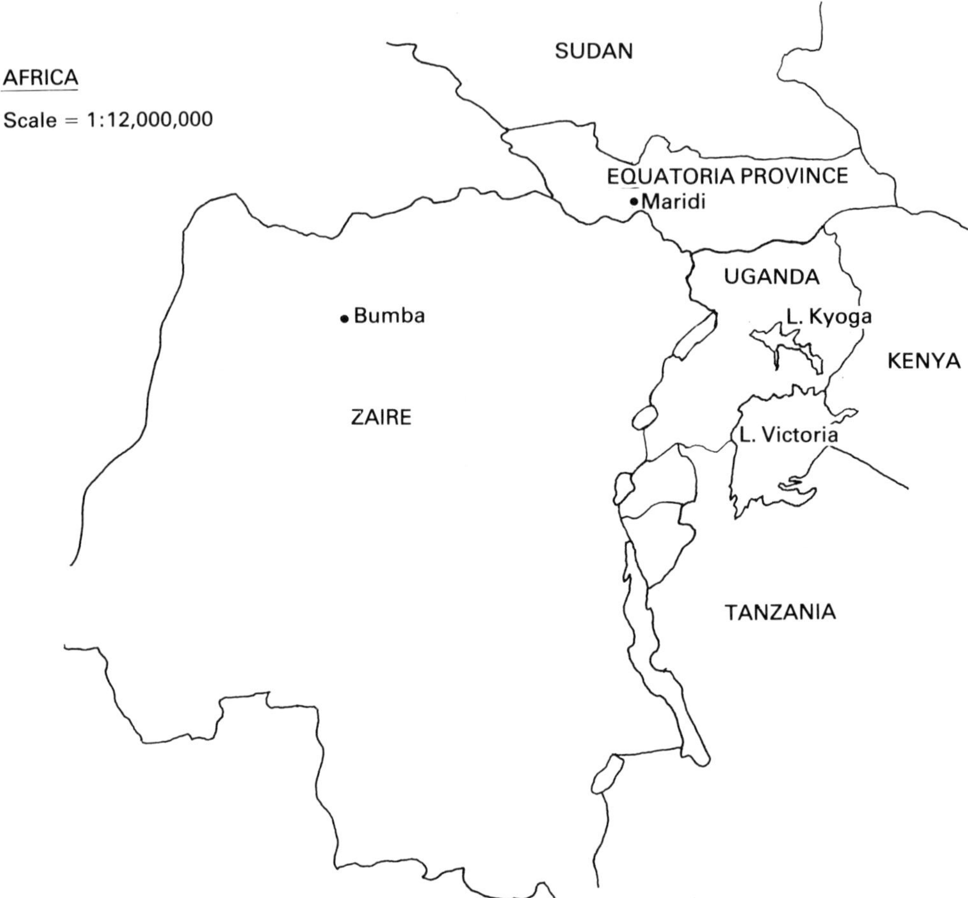

Fig. 13.2   Map of central Africa showing sources of Marburg and Ebola virus infection. The monkeys captured around Lake Kyoga in Uganda gave rise to the episodes of Marburg disease in Europe. Ebola virus infection broke out in the Equatoria Province of the Sudan around Maridi and in the Bumba zone of northern Zaire.

(Germain, 1978; Arata & Johnson, 1978). Three years later a further outbreak was reported from the same district in the Southern Sudan (WHO, 1979).

Epidemiology
In the original Marburg outbreak the primary cases acquired the virus from blood and organs of the green monkey or from cell-culture material. The monkeys themselves had been exposed to animals from 48 other species en route from Uganda to West Germany and Yugoslavia. The secondary cases gave a history of accidental exposure to patient's blood. One man, who had recovered from the disease, continued to harbour virus in his semen despite the presence of specific antibody and infected his wife after 83 days. The source of infection and mode of spread was not established in the South African outbreak.

Marburg virus was isolated from blood throughout the acute stage of the illness and from throat secretions during the early stages. It was also isolated from the liver of fatal cases and from the semen of one man during late convalescence (Siegert, 1972). In South Africa, virus was recovered from the anterior chamber of the eye 80 days after the onset of illness (Gear et al, 1975).

The original source of the infection in the Ebola virus outbreaks was never discovered. Once infected patients had been admitted into the local hospitals infection spread rapidly to the staff and to other patients. In one Sudanese hospital with 230 employees at least one-third were infected and 41 died. Virus appeared to be readily transmitted by blood or close personal contact with a patient. Delivery of a pregnant woman was particularly hazardous. Airborne transmission did not appear to be common. The outbreaks seemed to be amplified by the hospital and terminated shortly after the hospitals closed (Breman et al, 1978; Francis et al, 1978).

Ebola virus was isolated from the blood of patients in Africa during the acute illness. Accidental infection of a scientific worker in England provided an opportunity to study the infection (Emond et al, 1977). Virus was detected in blood throughout the acute illness. No virus was isolated from faeces, urine and throat swabs collected between days 14 and 27 though virus was isolated from seminal fluid collected on days 39 and 61 but not subsequently.

Virology
Marburg and Ebola viruses have a similar appearance on electron microscopy (Fig. 13.3). In negative contrast preparations they are pleomorphic with long filamentous, U-shaped, crook-shaped and circular forms. They measure 80 nm in diameter and are extremely variable in length. The length of the basic unit appears to be 665 nm but giant particles may be formed from multiple units and reach a length of 8000 nm in Marburg virus and 14 000 nm in Ebola virus. The viruses contain RNA. The morphology of Marburg and Ebola viruses resembles that of rabies, vesicular stomatitis and other rhabdoviruses.

African green, rhesus and squirrel monkeys are highly susceptible but unsuitable for routine work. Guinea pigs are easily infected and are suitable for isolation of virus from heavily contaminated specimens. Vero cells have been extensively used for isolation of both viruses and many other cell lines are susceptible. Biochemical studies have been restricted by the hazards to laboratory staff (Siegert, 1972; Bowen et al, 1977; Johnson et al, 1977; Pattyn et al, 1977).

Pathology
The effects of Marburg and Ebola viruses are very similar. Necrotic foci and haemorrhages are found in nearly all organs but especially in the liver, spleen, lymph nodes, testes and ovaries. In experimental infections of monkeys high concentrations of virus are consistently found in the liver, spleen and lungs. Virus may also be detected in the kidneys, adrenals, testes, lymph nodes and pancreas.

The liver is severely affected in man and animals with widespread degeneration and necrosis. The sinusoids are full of cellular debris and the Küpffer cells packed with debris and red cells. Eosinophilic intracytoplasmic inclusion bodies may be detected in a proportion of hepatocytes on light microscopy while electron microscopy may reveal virus particles in the extracellular spaces. Lymphoid tissue is severely

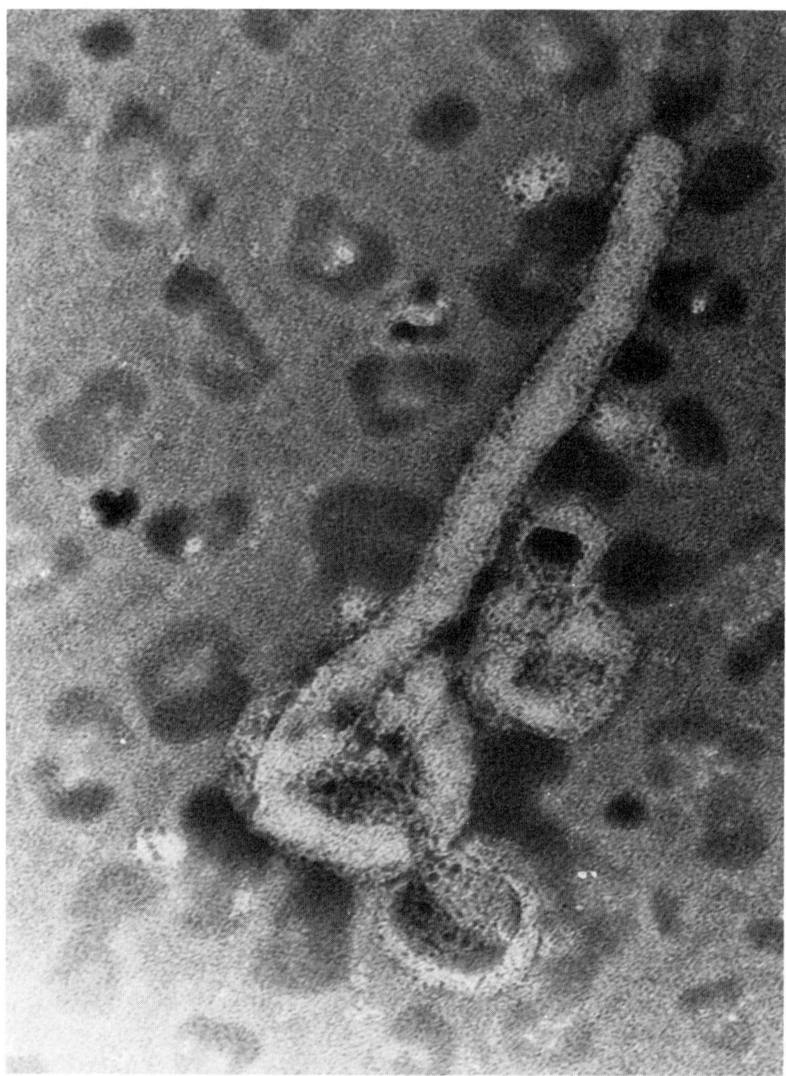

Fig. 13.3 Ebola virus. The virus particles are composed of an internal helical structure presumed to be the nucleocapsid, an envelope derived from host-cell membrane, and surface spikes about 10 nm long. ×73 000.

degenerated. Fibrin clots may be found in the small blood vessels of the renal cortex and outer medulla and there may be areas of tubular necrosis accompanied by interstitial haemorrhages and microscopy may show proliferative or degenerative glial lesions (Gedigk, Bechtelsheimer & Korb, 1971; Baskerville et al, 1978; Bowen et al, 1978; Dietrich et al, 1978).

Clinical features
The course of the illness in both Marburg and Ebola virus outbreaks was very similar though epidemics of Ebola virus infection tended to be more severe and had a much higher death rate.

The incubation period of Marburg disease in the European outbreak was 3–9 days while the incubation period of Ebola virus infection in Africa ranged from 4–16 days and was commonly around 7 days.

In contrast to Lassa fever the onset of Marburg and Ebola virus infection was abrupt with shivering and a rapid rise in temperature accompanied by severe headache, backache, generalised aching in muscles and joints, and malaise. Central abdominal pain and nausea were presenting features in some cases but gastrointestinal disturbance commonly commenced about the third day of illness with anorexia, nausea, vomiting and diarrhoea. The stools were watery and sometimes contained mucus and blood. Profuse diarrhoea might continue for several days and lead to dehydration.

After 3–8 days an erythematous maculopapular rash appeared on the trunk and quickly spread to other parts of the body ultimately becoming confluent. The rash faded after 3 or 4 days and was followed by fine desquamation. The erythematous stage of the rash was easily overlooked in dark-skinned patients though the desquamation was obvious. Swallowing was often painful; the throat was reddened and small transparent lesions resembling tapioca granules were present on the soft palate. About half of the patients had inflammation of the conjunctivae and some complained of photophobia.

The fever reached a peak after 3–4 days and continued at a high level for at least a week before falling by lysis (Fig. 13.4) The duration of the febrile phase varied from 10–20 days and was commonly between 14–16 days. Some patients had a secondary rise in temperature. Within 4–5 days from the onset of illness the patient's condition usually became critical with extreme lethargy and alteration in the mental state.

COURSE OF ILLNESS IN EBOLA VIRUS INFECTION

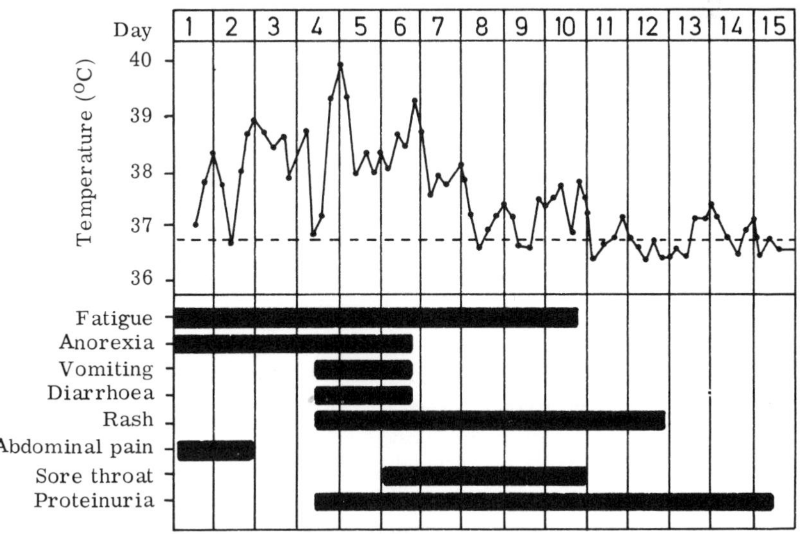

Fig. 13.4   Course of illness in Ebola virus infection.

Nearly all patients in the German outbreak became sullen and had aggressive or negativistic behaviour, while those who died became restless and confused before sinking into deep coma. Two had convulsions. Others complained of paraesthesia and one developed Guillain-Barré syndrome.

About half of the patients with Marburg disease had spontaneous bleeding, which was particularly troublesome at needle puncture sites. A very high proportion of patients with Ebola virus infection had severe bleeding especially from the respiratory and gastrointestinal tracts. Abortion with massive haemorrhage was common in pregnant women with Ebola virus infection in Zaire. Spontaneous bleeding usually commenced towards the end of the first week and was a striking feature in fatal attacks. The cause of the bleeding remains obscure. In many cases the platelet count was low and the prothrombin time prolonged. A few had evidence of disseminated intravascular coagulation with increase in fibrin degradation products.

Liver function tests showed evidence of hepatocellular damage in the South African cases and in some of the German cases but frank jaundice was rare. Several patients with Marburg disease had elevated serum amylase levels pointing to pancreatic involvement. Electrocardiography showed evidence of myocardial disturbances. Many patients had proteinuria and oliguria and most of the fatal cases had acute renal failure.

Death commonly occurred between the 8th and 17th day, very often on day 8 or 9. Those who survived faced a prolonged period of convalescence with anorexia, fatigue and loss of hair. Some patients had testicular atrophy and some had persistent psychological problems. One patient developed uveitis and virus was recovered from the anterior chamber after 83 days (Martini, 1973; Gear et al, 1975; Piot et al, 1978; Isaäcson et al, 1978; Smith, Francis & Simpson, 1978; Emond et al, 1977).

Laboratory investigations
Laboratory examination of specimens from a patient with Marburg or Ebola virus infection is extremely dangerous and should only be undertaken in a designated high-security laboratory. The greatest care must be taken in collecting and despatching samples. For details see Simpson (1977). Blood, urine and a throat swab should be sent for virus culture during the acute stage and paired sera obtained for antibody studies. The following investigations may help to establish an accurate diagnosis:

1. Electron microscopy of patient's serum may sometimes reveal the characteristic virus particles during the first few days of illness and provide a rapid diagnosis.

2. Blood, urine and throat secretions should be inoculated into Vero cells and incubated for 5–7 days. The virus does not usually produce a cytopathogenic effect but may be detected by electron microscopy of the supernatant fluid. Viral antigen may be demonstrated in the cells by immunofluorescence and histopathological staining.

3. Guinea-pig inoculation is particularly useful for isolating virus from contaminated specimens. The animal develops a severe febrile illness and virus may be detected by electron microscopy in the blood and liver.

4. A four-fold rise in specific antibodies between an acute and convalescent samples of serum provides convincing evidence of active infection. Indirect immunofluorescence tests are the most reliable. They are performed by layering the patient's serum on a prepared lawn of cells known to be infected with Marburg or Ebola virus.

Complement fixation tests are less reliable, for antibody appears late and does not persist for more than two years. Neutralisation tests are not satisfactory.

5. The diagnosis may be established after death with minimal risk by removing a sample of liver with a liver-biopsy needle. Part of the specimen should be placed in 10 per cent buffered formalin and the remainder in a sterile dry container. Virus may be detected by electron microscopy or by immunofluorescence.

The white blood cell count may be very low and the blood film show atypical plasmacytoid lymphocytes and polymorphonuclear cells with an acquired Pelger-Huet anomaly. Thrombocytopenia is a common finding. The ESR is usually low. The raised serum enzyme levels have already been mentioned. The blood urea is high, the protein low and the serum potassium levels low. The prothrombin time may be prolonged and there may be evidence of disseminated intravascular coagulation. Unfortunately because of the risks to laboratory staff it is seldom possible or justified to undertake extensive biochemical studies.

Differential diagnosis
It is not possible to make a clinical diagnosis of Marburg or Ebola virus infection until the characteristic rash emerges. Malaria, typhoid fever, typhus, septicaemia, Lassa fever, yellow fever and other arbovirus infections should be considered and appropriate tests performed. Sophisticated investigations are seldom possible in rural Africa so therapeutic trials with chloroquine and chloramphenicol may serve to differentiate malaria, typhoid fever and typhus from the virus infections.

Prognosis
The case fatality of Marburg fever in Germany was 22 per cent. Mortality in the Ebola virus infections in Africa was much greater and was almost 90 per cent throughout the whole of the Zaire outbreak and during the earlier stages of the Sudanese epidemic. Severe bleeding, renal and circulatory failure, and pronounced cerebral disturbance were prominent features in fatal attacks. The illness was exceptionally severe in pregnant women.

Treatment
Convalescent serum has been advocated for the treatment of both Marburg and Ebola virus infections. There has been no controlled trial to establish its value and very little scientific evidence to support its use. In one patient with Ebola virus infection, who was treated with a combination of interferon and convalescent serum, there was a striking fall in the quantity of virus in the blood but no obvious change in the clinical condition though the patient survived (Emond et al, 1977). Interferon appeared to delay the onset of viraemia in rhesus monkeys experimentally infected with Ebola virus but had no effect on the outcome (Bowen et al, 1978).

Treatment is otherwise directed to the relief of symptoms and the maintenance of water and electrolyte balance. The use of heparin has been recommended to diminish damage caused by disseminated intravascular coagulation but its use is controversial and great care must be taken to monitor its effects (Gear et al, 1975).

Prevention
No vaccine is available for active immunisation. Until the animal reservoirs of the

viruses have been identified it is not possible to institute control measures. Man-to-man spread can be prevented by identifying and isolating suspect cases, and by taking the greatest care in handling laboratory specimens. High standards of hygiene and scrupulous care in sterilising syringes and needle would lessen the risk of nosocomial infection in African rural hospitals where further outbreaks are likely to occur. Simpson (1977) has recommended containment measures for outbreaks in under-developed countries.

Assessment of patients with exotic fever

By 1970 the decline of serious epidemic disease within the British Isles and the impending demise of smallpox throughout the world had engendered a false sense of security and the significance of the tremendous social and technicological changes of the post-war era had been overlooked. The recognition of dangerous viral haemorrhagic fevers (VHF) in many tropic countries and the importation of a few well-publicised cases of Lassa fever from Africa into Europe and North America brushed aside all complacency and threw the spotlight of public opinion on to the hazards from imported disease. The new problems were entirely different from those posed by smallpox, where the characteristic rash usually permitted accurate clinical assessment and active immunisation limited spread of infection. The new diseases had no distinguishing features, at least in the early stages, and vaccines were not available to protect the community.

The initial response to these infections was one of blind panic followed by overreaction to the possibility of spread. With increasing knowledge of the diseases and greater experience in managing suspected cases a more rational approach has prevailed. Analysis of the 15 episodes of Lassa fever reported between 1969 and 1977 indicates that community spread is rare unless there is severe pulmonary involvement. Similarly person-to-person spread of Marburg and Ebola virus infection has involved close and prolonged household contact or contact with blood and other secretions. Moreover, there has been no evidence of spread of infection prior to onset of illness (Galbraith et al, 1978).

It is common for travellers, who have recently arrived from Africa, to develop feverish illnesses and the possibility of a viral haemorrhagic fever should always be considered. Nevertheless, most of these patients will have minor respiratory infections or malaria and very few will have VHF. During a two-year period more than 500 000 travellers arrived from tropical Africa and only 40 had an illness sufficiently suspicious to warrant admission to the high-security unit designated to serve the south-east of England with a population of 11 million. Two suspects were found to be positive, one with Lassa virus and another with Ebola virus. It is obviously impracticable and unnecessary to take stringent precautions with all who have become ill before or immediately after arrival from tropical Africa. Nevertheless, some may be suffering from VHF and constitute a threat to hospital and laboratory staff.

Because it is so difficult to make a firm diagnosis on clinical grounds it is necessary to pay particular attention to the epidemiological evidence when assessing a patient from tropical Africa with unexplained fever. Emond, Smith & Welsby (1978) have suggested that travellers who develop a fever within three weeks after arrival should be classified in three categories according to the degree of risk and be dealt with accordingly.

Minimal risk. Those who have come from major cities, where the risk of VHF is negligible, should be admitted to standard isolation rooms with routine barrier nursing. Specimens for investigation may be sent to routine laboratories. When there is no immediate threat to life patients in this category may be nursed at home, while appropriate investigations are being carried out.

Moderate risk. Patients from small towns or country districts in tropical Africa should be regarded with more suspicion, especially if the onset and course of the illness is consistent with VHF, and should be admitted to an isolation room with filtered negative-pressure ventilation and separate facilities. Malaria is the commonest and most urgent diagnosis to be excluded so specimens of blood should be despatched to a laboratory for processing in a high-security cabinet. If no parasites are found and fever continues these patients should be transferred to a designated unit and admitted to a Trexler isolator for further observation and investigation (Fig. 13.5).

High risk. The last and potentially the most dangerous group of patients are those who have been working in rural areas where VHF is known to be endemic; medical and nursing staff from country hospitals; contacts of confirmed cases; and laboratory workers handling dangerous material. Patients in this category should be admitted directly into a Trexler isolator and specimens sent to an approved maximum-security laboratory.

Malaria is the most common diagnosis in patients admitted with suspected VHF and was found to be the cause of fever in 29 out of 65 patients admitted to a high-security unit over a period of three years. It cannot be stressed too strongly that a history of regular chemoprophylaxis with proguanil or pyrimethamine does not preclude a diagnosis of falciparum malaria and should not influence the decision to search for parasites (Emond, Smith & Welsby, 1978; 1979).

In many instances the fever settles uneventfully within 48 hours, and simple observation under strict isolation is all that is required. In a few cases, however, where symptoms persist, more elaborate studies are necessary, and these can be performed only in suitably equipped and staffed laboratories. A throat swab and specimens of blood and urine should be despatched to a laboratory approved for handling Lassa, Marburg and Ebola viruses so that tests can be performed for VHF. Blood for haematology, bacteriological culture and serology should be sent to a laboratory approved for dealing with category A pathogens. Very few patients will prove to have a VHF; many others will have arbovirus infections, Coxsackie virus infections, influenza, typhus, typhoid fever or septicaemia. Woodruff, Bowen & Platt (1978) examined sera from 86 patients at the Hospital for Tropical Diseases in London, who gave a history of feverish illness while in tropical Africa, and found that 15 had antibodies against arboviruses but none against Lassa virus. Although this indicates that arbovirus infections are important causes of fever in Africa comprehensive serological screening involves a very large number of tests and is not feasible as a routine when investigating patients with suspected viral haemorrhagic fever. Although a diagnosis of VHF may be excluded the precise cause of the illness may not be identified in many patients.

Isolation of patients

Standard isolation accommodation and barrier nursing techniques are satisfactory for containing the spread of infection from infectious diseases endemic in the United Kingdom but are unsuitable for dealing with the more dangerous haemorrhagic fevers against which there is no effective immunisation (Emond, 1976). Spread of infection to the community can be prevented by nursing patients with VHF in a negative-pressure room with filtered ventilation; all waste material must be heat-treated or destroyed by incineration. Members of the staff coming into direct contact with the patient must wear full protective clothing including visor, mask and rubber gloves. In some circumstances it may be necessary to wear a suitable respirator or ventilated helmet. Protective clothing is cumbersome and uncomfortable to wear for any length of time, and probably does not afford the same degree of protection as a flexible film isolator.

Flexible film isolators have been shown to be effective in maintaining microbial isolation of laboratory animals (Trexler, 1971) and have been used to protect neutropenic patients (Trexler, Spiers & Gaya, 1975). Negative-pressure plastic isolators have proved successful in containing infection under laboratory conditions (Hutchison et al, 1978) and have been demonstrated to be effective in dealing with patients suffering from dangerous infections (Trexler, Emond & Evans, 1977). They have now been accepted as standard equipment in many high-security units dealing with suspected VHF (Fig. 13.5).

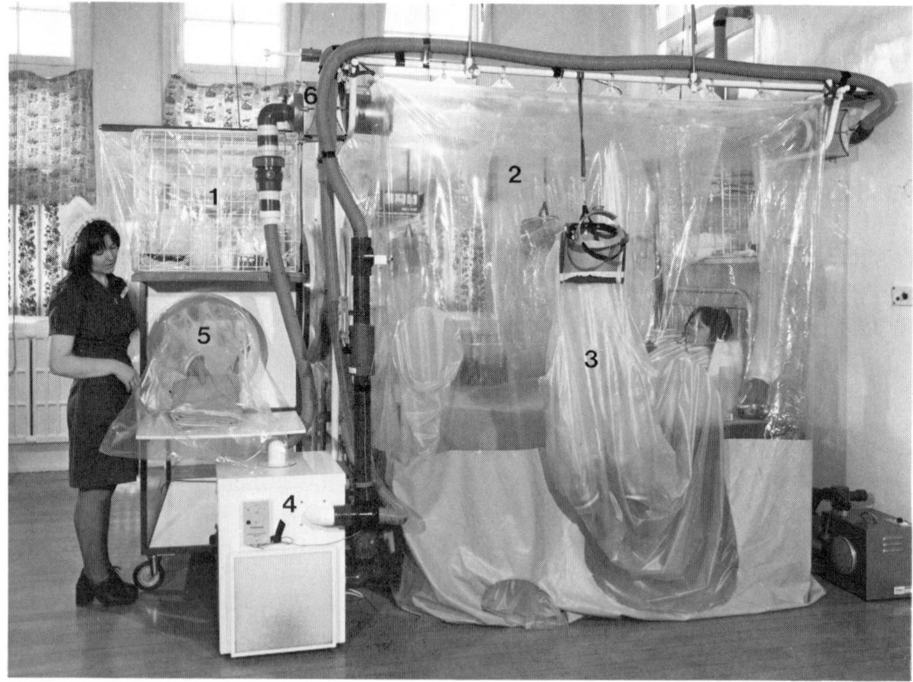

Fig. 13.5   Trexler Bed Isolator.
1. Supply isolator. 2. Patient isolator. 3. Half suit. 4. Air pump. 5. Supply port. 6. High-efficiency filter. The supply isolator is connected to the patient isolator by a plastic sleeve thus forming the bed isolator. The patient is physically separated from the attendants and a negative pressure is maintained within the isolator to prevent escape of infected particles.

The medical and nursing staff are separated from the patient by a barrier of plastic film forming the envelopes and by rubber gloves attached to the half suits welded to the side-walls of the envelopes. Air entering and leaving the isolator envelopes is filtered and a negative pressure is maintained within the isolator to ensure that there is no escape of contaminated air to the surroundings. All supplies are taken into the isolator through an entry port in the supply envelope and all waste material is removed by the same route for disposal by sterilisation and incineration. The seal on the entry port is maintained by a tightly fitting polythene bag held in position by a stout rubber band. All routine nursing and medical procedures can be carried out with minimal interference by the physical barrier, though it is not practicable to undertake artificial respiration or haemodialysis. The isolator should be sited in a large room in a high-security unit to ensure safety should there be a major failure of equipment. Stretcher and aircraft-transit isolators may be used to transfer patients safely from one hospital to another. They work on the same principles and can be docked with the bed-isolator so that the patient can be transferred without coming into direct contact with the attendants.

Public health control
In 1976 the Department of Health and Social Security published a Memorandum on Lassa Fever giving advice on the management of a suspected case of Lassa fever and measures to be taken to prevent spread of infection. A small number of hospitals and laboratories were made responsible for the care of patients and the handling of specimens. The Department also made Lassa fever, Marburg disease and viral haemorrhagic fever notifiable, thus providing Medical Officers for Environmental Health with statutory powers for disease control.

Surveillance of contacts of confirmed and suspected cases of VHF has thrown a considerable workload on local environmental health services, especially during the initial period when little was known about the spread of the diseases and their infectivity. After reviewing the known outbreaks of Lassa fever, Marburg and Ebola virus diseases Galbraith and his colleagues (1978) at the Communicable Diseases Surveillance Centre have concluded that the difficulties arising from VHF could be reduced by making surveillance more selective, by establishing a panel of clinical specialists, by regularly drawing the attention of hospital and laboratory staff to the potential risks when caring for febrile patients arriving from West and Central Africa, and by forming a central emergency control team to assist in management of outbreaks. They have suggested that contacts of patients in the minimum risk category should not be placed under surveillance and recommended that only close contacts of those in the other two categories should be placed under surveillance unless the patient is seriously ill with pulmonary involvement, in which event more remote contacts should be traced. The Department of Health has recommended that close contacts be kept under surveillance with daily visits to check the state of health, record temperature and inspect the throat for evidence of pharyngitis. It is very doubtful if throat examination is of any value in detecting the onset of illness and may increase the slight risk to the physician so should be omitted as a routine.

A patient who has recovered from the acute stage of the illness may continue to shed virus during convalescence. Blood, throat secretions, and urine should be cultured for virus at weekly intervals until three consecutive sets of specimens have proved negative. Semen from patients with Marburg or Ebola virus infection may remain positive for several weeks and should be tested at regular intervals.

LEGIONNAIRES' DISEASE

History

In 1976, at a time when interest in developed countries was focused on Lassa fever and other exotic diseases from the tropics, complacency was rudely shattered by a mysterious outbreak of severe respiratory illness afflicting members of the American Legion, who had attended the annual convention in Philadelphia. One hundred and eighty two people fell victim, 147 were admitted to hospital and 29 died. As usual, fear of the unknown caused great alarm in the community and led to irrational behaviour more in keeping with the Middle Ages than the 20th century (Hudson 1979). The disease inevitably became known as Legionnaires' disease (Fraser et al, 1977) and was soon found to be caused by a previously unrecognised bacterium (McDade et al, 1977; Chandler et al, 1977).

Subsequently, at least 10 epidemics of Legionnaires' disease and the closely related Pontiac fever have been identified (Eickhoff, 1979) and more than a thousand cases reported in the United States of America over a period of five years (Center for Disease Control, 1978a). Sporadic cases have also been discovered in many other countries (Broome & Faser, 1979).

Bacteriology

Scientists investigating the original outbreak of Legionnaires' disease isolated a bacterium from pulmonary tissue of four out of six patients by inoculating guinea pigs intraperitoneally and passaging the animal tissues through yolk sacs of embryonated eggs (McDade et al, 1977). This organism has subsequently been examined in great detail and has provisionally been classified in a new genus and species, *Legionella pneumophila* belonging to a new family, *Legionellaceae* (Brenner et al, 1979).

The bacterium commonly exists as short rods, 2–3 μm in length, and may form filaments exceeding 20 μm. The bacillus is fimbriated and may possess a single polar flagellum (Thomason et al, 1979). *L. pneumonia* stains faintly with Gram stains and is weakly Gram-negative. It can be demonstrated more definitely by Dieterle's silver-impregnation technique and can be detected in tissues by direct immunofluorescence. On electron microscopy it has the structure of a typical Gram-negative bacillus (Chandler et al, 1979).

L. pneumophila can be cultured aerobically on enriched Mueller-Hinton chocolate agar and on charcoal yeast-extract agar. It grows slowly over a period of several days on Mueller-Hinton medium forming tiny ground-glass colonies and producing brown pigment. Analysis of the colonies by gas liquid chromatography has revealed a unique composition with a very high proportion of branched-chain fatty acids (Moss et al, 1977). A distinct lipopolysaccharide has been detected in the bacillus and may be responsible for endotoxicity (Wong et al, 1979). A specific bacterial antigen has been found in urine of experimentally infected guinea pigs and in urine from three out of five of the Philadelphia patients by means of an ezyme-linked immunosorbent assay (ELISA) (Tilton, 1979). A test of this type may provide a quick and easy means of establishing an early diagnosis of Legionnaires' disease. Four serogroups have already been distinguished by direct fluorescence and the recognition of antigen variants within the established groups suggests that the number of serogroups will be extended (Taylor & Harrison, 1979).

The bacterium of Legionnaires' disease has been detected in lungs, pleural fluid, respiratory secretions, blood and placenta in human cases. It has also been found in the water used in cooling towers and evaporative condensers of air-conditioning plants, in the water from a stream and mud from its bank (Center for Disease Control, 1978b; Dondero, 1978; Cordes, 1978; Politi et al, 1979).

Epidemiology

Once the cause of the Philadelphia epidemic had been discovered and a specific antibody test developed, serological surveys were undertaken to establish the incidence and distribution of the disease. Retrospective investigation of previously inexplicable epidemics of febrile or respiratory illness in the United States revealed two distinct clinical syndromes associated with *L. pneumophila.* These are Pontiac fever, a benign feverish illness with minimal respiratory involvement (Glick et al, 1978; Fraser et al, 1979), and Legionnaires' disease, a severe pneumonic illness with high mortality (Eickhoff, 1979; Broome & Fraser, 1979). More than 1000 cases of Legionnaires' disease have been reported in the United States over a period of five years (Center for Disease Control, 1978c) and sporadic cases have been indentified in many other parts of the world, including Canada, Great Britain, Denmark, Sweden, the Netherlands, Spain, Israel and Australia (Center for Disease Control, 1979). Legionnaires' disease has been diagnosed retrospectively by culturing the organism from blood obtained in 1947 from a patient with a respiratory illness (McDade, Brenner & Bozeman, 1979).

The prevalence of infection appears to vary greatly from one part of the United States to another. In serological surveys of patients with unexplained pneumonia the incidence of Legionnaires' disease has varied between 0.3 and 4.4 per cent and the incidence of antibody in control populations has ranged between 1.3 and 24.8 per cent in different states (Broome & Fraser, 1979). Such a large variation in these surveys implies that hyperendemic foci of infection may be present within the United States (Storch et al, 1979). Although a considerable number of sporadic cases have been recognised in Great Britain, particularly in Nottingham, there has been no evidence of a similar epidemiological pattern (Bartlett, 1974). In Nottingham Legionnaires' disease has been found to be as common as proven pneumococcal or mycoplasma pneumonia, though rather unexpectedly a serological survey of 2023 people revealed only 31 with antibody (Macrae et al, 1979). The Nottingham investigators have estimated that 1 case of Legionnaires' disease occurs in every 50 000 of the population each year.

Epidemics of Legionnaires' disease in the United States have occurred during the months of July, August and September and sporadic cases have also tended to occur at that time of year. Hospital outbreaks have had no seasonal prevalence (Center for Disease Control 1978d).

TRANSMISSION

Infection is thought to be spread by the airborne route from sources in the environment. Focal epidemics have been associated with infected airconditioning plants in public buildings (Center for Disease Control 1978) but there has been no evidence to incriminate home air-conditioning units (Storch et al, 1979). Water used in cooling towers and evaporative condensers may be contaminated by infected dust in the atmosphere and continue to harbour the organism for a very long time. Under laboratory conditions the bacterium has survived for over a year in tap water (Skaliy & McEachern 1979). It is believed that infection is disseminated through the ventilation system from aerosols generated in the air-conditioning plant. *L. pneumophila* has been isolated from soil, although there have been great technical difficulties (Eickhoff 1979, Broome & Fraser 1979), and it would seem likely that soil is its natural habitat. Outbreaks have been related to soil excavation (Thacker et al, 1978) and sporadic cases have been found more frequently in people living near excavation or construction sites than in other groups. Moreover, there has been a slight, but significant, excess of construction workers among the sporadic cases (Storch et al, 1979).

Immune-deficient patients in hospital have been particularly susceptible. In an prospective study by Haley and others (1979) at the Wadsworth Medical Center in California 15 patients were found to have a fourfold rise in antibody titre to *L. pneumophila* within six weeks from admission and 7 of these patients had developed pneumonia. There has been very little evidence of spread of infection from patients to hospital staff, either in the United States (Broome & Fraser, 1979) or in the United Kingdom (Morgan et al, 1979). Employees of hotels, where outbreaks have occurred, have been found to have serological evidence of subclinical or mild infection (Fraser et al, 1977). Case-to-case spread appears to be rare though three instances have been reported. A pathologist conducting a post-mortem examination on a fatal case in the Netherlands contracted the disease (Meenhorst et al, 1979), a microbiologist working with infected lung samples in Philadelphia developed Legionnaires' disease (Katz, 1978) and a general practitioner in Glasgow appeared to contracted the infection from a patient (Love et al, 1978).

ASSOCIATED FACTORS

Legionnaires' disease has been diagnosed in a wide range of ages from 10 months to 84 years but is particularly common in later life. The mean age of confirmed cases is 55–60 years. Pontiac fever or non-pneumonic legionellosis has affected a much younger group between 18 and 39 years but this may reflect the age range of the population exposed to risk (see Table 13.2). Males are involved three times more frequently than females. Cigarette smoking and possibly the consumption of alcohol predispose to Legionnaires' disease.

Eight out of 15 patients in the Netherlands had recently returned from countries bordering the Mediterranean Sea (Meenhorst et al, 1979), while the outbreak among Scottish tourists was centered on Benidorm in Spain (Reid et al, 1978). Bartlett (1979), analysing 84 sporadic cases reported in Great Britain, found that 18 had recently returned from holiday abroad but Macrae and his colleagues (1979) in Nottingham did not find any convincing link with overseas travel in 41 confirmed cases.

Pathology

The lungs in a fatal case of Legionnaires' disease are congested but not haemorrhagic. They are greyish in colour and have a friable granular structure. The appearance is that of an acute fibrinopurulent bronchopneumonia affecting any part of the lungs. In many cases the areas of consolidation may become confluent and involve one or more lobes. Abscesses may form but are not a prominent feature of Legionnaires' disease and are sometimes associated with secondary invasion by other bacteria, such as klebsiella (Saravolatz et al, 1979; Venkatachalam et al, 1979). Fibrinous pleurisy is a common finding and there may be small amounts of serous or serosanguineous fluid in the pleural cavity. Extensive organising pneumonia has been reported by Schoenhaum & Mark (1978).

On histological examination there is evidence of acute diffuse alveolar damage. The alveoli contain many neutrophil polymorphonuclear leucocytes and macrophages, and a large amount of fibrin. Lysis of the inflammatory cells is a prominent feature in some cases. Many epithelial cells separate from the alveolar walls but the capillary and epithelial basement membranes remain intact. The small bronchioles are always involved in the inflammatory reaction but the large air passages escape. The histological appearances are not sufficiently characteristic to establish a diagnosis of Legionnaires' disease, which must be confirmed by other means.

Large numbers of short pleomorphic rods may be demonstrated in lung sections stained by Dieterle's method. The bacteria are present within the leucocytes and macrophages, and in the extracellular fluid. Failure to detect the organism by Dieterle's method does not exclude the diagnosis. Final assessment depends on isolating legionella on culture, demonstrating bacterial antigen by direct immuno-fluorescence or detecting specific antibody in serum (Carrington, 1979).

No consistent abnormalities have been found in other organs. Renal failure has been a prominent feature in some cases and rhabdomyolysis has been suggested as a possible cause but no evidence has been found on histological examination of the kidney to support this hypothesis (Relman & McCluskey, 1978). Acute tubulointer-stitial nephritis has been reported in one case but there was a possibility that it might have been induced by a drug hypersensitivity reaction (McCluskey, 1978).

Clinical Features

Legionnaires' disease. The incubation period of Legionnaires' disease is usually 2–10 days but may extend to 18 days. With the onset of illness there is a slight rise in temperature accompanied by malaise, headache and widespread aching in muscles. During the next day or two the patient becomes progressively more ill with frequent bouts of shivering and occasional rigors leading to an impressive fever of 40°C or more. Relative bradycardia is noted in 50 per cent of cases (Terranova et al, 1978; Kirby et al, 1978).

Coryza or a sore throat are uncommon but most patients develop a dry cough, which may later become productive with clear mucoid or purulent sputum. In 20–40 per cent of patients this may be streaked with blood. About one-third of patients complain of chest pain, usually of pleuritic character. Clinical examination in the early stages may reveal little more than a few fine inspiratory crepitations; later there may be evidence of consolidation. Diarrhoea is a prominent early feature and is present in 50 per cent of cases. The stools are watery and do not contain blood or excessive mucus. Abdominal pain is seldom troublesome (Swartz, 1979). Nausea and vomiting were reported in 20 per cent of cases in the Vermont outbreak (Beaty et al, 1978).

After four or five days the patients are toxic and acutely ill with a continuous high fever. Most are severely prostrated and many have obvious mental disturbance with sommnolence, confusion and delirium. Breathing is rapid and laboured. When the outcome is favourable the symptoms begin to abate after 8–10 days and the temperature falls by lysis. Recovery is slow and convalescence prolonged. Many patients have amnesia and cannot remember the acute stage of the illness. In fatal cases death may result from respiratory failure, circulatory collapse or renal failure.

Radiological examination is helpful but the lung changes are not characteristic and the diagnosis must be established by other means. In 70 per cent of cases the lesions are confined to one lung and consist of ill-defined nodular opacities or more diffuse patchy shadowing consistent with bronchopneumonia. As the illness progresses the shadows enlarge and tend to become lobar with a ground-glass or uniformly dense appearance (Dietrich et al, 1978). After admission to hospital there is extension of the shadowing to involve another lobe in more than 40 per cent of cases (Fig. 13.6). Small pleural effusions can be detected in more than a third of patients and may precede

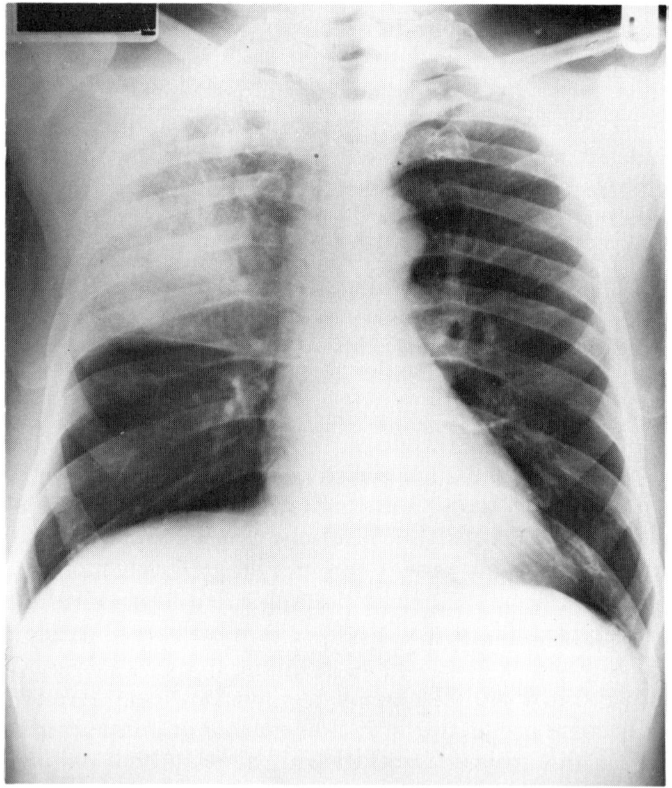

Fig. 13.6 Chest radiograph from 61-year-old patient with confirmed Legionnaires' disease. The radiograph taken on the fifth day of illness shows extensive patchy shadowing in the right upper and mid-zones.
WBC 8.2×10^9/L
ESR 90 mm in first hour
Serum Na^+ 121 mmol/L
Urine contained protein, bilirubin and excess urobilinogen.

signs of lung infiltration. Large effusions have been reported in patients receiving corticosteroid therapy. Cavitation has been noted but is not a common occurrence. Radiological changes may persist for several months.

The white blood cell count varies between $10–20 \times 10^9/1$ and shows a shift to the left. The erythrocyte sedimentation rate is increased and exceeded 70 mm in one hour in 12 out of 15 cases (Helms et al, 1979). Liver function tests frequently reveal slightly elevated levels of serum bilirubin, glutamicoxalacetic transaminase, lactic dehydro genase and alkaline phosphatase. Hyponatraemia is a common finding (Helms et al, 1979) and is probably related to inappropriate secretion of antidiuretic hormone as in other pneumonias. Hypophosphataemia has been reported by Kirby and others (1978) but its significance is not known. A low serum albumin level is a helpful diagnostic finding (Miller 1979). Sixty-three per cent of patients with Legionnaires' disease in the series reported by Helms and his colleagues (1979) had serum albumin levels below 32 g/1. Moderate proteinuria and microscopic haematuria are commonly found. The cerebrospinal fluid has been reported to be normal (Kirby et al, 1978).

Pontiac fever. Two unusual outbreaks of non-pneumonic legionellosis have been reported from the United States. The first involved 144 people at Pontiac in Michigan (Glick et al, 1978) and the second a small group of 10 people working in a condenser at James River in Virginia (Fraser et al, 1979). The illnesses were characterised by a very high attack rate and a short incubation period of 5–66 hours (median 36–37 hours). The initial symptoms were very similar to those of Legionnaires' disease with headache, myalgia, shivering and a high fever. However, the acute stage subsided within 2–5 days with no deaths. In striking contrast to Legionnaires' disease none of the patients with Pontiac fever developed pneumonia. Moderate leucocytosis was the only consistent laboratory finding. So far there has been no satisfactory explanation to account for the sharp contrast between the two clinical syndromes.

Diagnosis

The early diagnosis of Legionnaires' disease in sporadic cases is very difficult because many clinical features of the illness are also found in viral and mycoplasmal pneumonias, in psittacosis and in Q fever. During epidemics the clinical diagnosis is usually suspected because of the characteristic overall pattern of the illnesses (Swartz, 1979). The diagnosis is usually made retrospectively by serological tests or at autopsy by demonstrating legionella in lung tissue by special staining techniques. Since treatment with erythromycin appears to reduce mortality, it is important to consider the possibility of Legionnaires' disease in any patient with a severe pneumonia.

Miller (1979) has analysed the clinical features of Legionnaires' disease in 17 patients admitted to hospital in Nottingham and has suggested the following diagnostic criteria.

Within 24 hours of admission. Legionnaires' disease is very likely if any three of these are present:
1. Prodromal toxic illness with pyrexia of 39°C or more for at least four days before admission.
2. Mental confusion or diarrhoea or non-productive cough, or a combination of these.

3. Lymphopenia less than $1 \times 10^9/1$ only if the total leucocyte count is less than $15 \times 10^9/1$.
4. Hyponatraemia less than 130 mmol/1.

Within the next 2 to 4 days. If blood cultures are sterile and no relevant pathogen has been isolated from sputum the presence of one of the following is highly suggestive diagnostically:
1. Radiological extension of consolidation in spite of conventional antibiotic therapy.
2. Serum bilirubin or transaminase levels more than twice the upper limit of normal in the absence of known liver disease.
3. Serum albumin less than 26 g/1.

Helms and his colleagues (1979) have suggested that unexplained encephalopathy, haematuria and elevated serum transaminase at presentation may be useful in differentiating Legionnaires' disease from pneumonoccal and mycoplasmal pneumonias but advised caution until prospective studies have confirmed the value of these observations.

Laboratory investigations
The diagnosis may be suspected on epidemiological or clinical evidence but should be confirmed by demonstrating the organism or detecting specific antibodies in the patient's serum.

Culture of *L. pneumophila* from lung tissue, pleural fluid, respiratory secretions or blood is technically too difficult for routine practice. The organism may be demonstrated in sputum or transtracheal aspirate by direct fluorescent-antibody staining (Lattimer et al, 1978). However, it should be appreciated that at least one strain of *Pseudomonas fluorescens* has been shown to cross-react and may be mistaken for legionella (Tsai & Fraser, 1978). After death the diagnosis may be confirmed by demonstrating the agent in lung sections by Dieterle's stain or by direct immunofluorescence.

In view of the practical difficulties in demonstrating the presence of *L. pneumophila* the diagnosis is usually established retrospectively by antibody tests. A fourfold rise in antibody in paired sera taken 3–6 weeks apart or a single titre of 1:128 by an indirect fluorescent-antibody test may be accepted as evidence of recent active infection. False-positive reactions have been found in patients with psittacosis, plague, tularaemia and leptospirosis (McDade et al, 1977; Tsai & Fraser, 1978), and possibly in mycoplasmal infections (Grady & Gilfillan, 1979). Antibodies form slowly over a period of six weeks (Kirby et al, 1978). A microagglutination test has been developed and is simpler to use but does not appear to be as sensitive as the indirect fluorescent-antibody test (Farshy et al, 1978; Farshy et al, 1979).

Prognosis
An attack of Legionnaires' disease may vary in severity from mild to overwhelming infection resulting in death from respiratory failure. Mortality in the original Philadelphia outbreak was 16 per cent (Fraser et al, 1977) but recognition of milder attacks and more effective treatment has reduced mortality considerably. In the Vermont epidemic mortality in cases treated with erythromycin was 4 per cent as opposed to 17 per cent in other cases (Broome et al, 1979). Non-pneumonic legionellosis or Pontiac fever is a benign illness and has not proved fatal.

After an acute attack of Legionnaires' disease general weakness and shortness of breath on exertion may persist for several weeks. Radiological resolution lags behind clinical recovery and may be delayed for several months (Miller et al, 1978; Jenkins et al, 1979). Diminished diffusing capacity for carbon monoxide has been shown two years after the acute illness (Lattimer et al, 1979).

Treatment

Erythromycin and rifampicin have been shown in laboratory experiments to be active against *L. pneumophila* (Lewis et al, 1978; Fraser et al, 1978). Although no control trials have been conducted in the treatment of Legionnaires' disease with erythromycin, experience in the Philadelphia and Vermont outbreaks suggests that it is effective in reducing mortality (Fraser et al, 1977; Broome et al, 1979). The recommended dosage is 0.5–1.0 g six-hourly by mouth for adults and 15 mg/kg six-hourly for children (Center for Disease Control 1978e). Fever usually subsides within 24–48 hours of commencing treatment. In severe cases treatment should be continued for two or three weeks otherwise there is a danger of relapse. When a patient is critically ill the antibiotic should be given intravenously in a dosage of 2–4 g daily. If the response is unsatisfactory rifampicin should be prescribed in addition to erythromycin.

Oxygen or mechanical ventilation may be required for patients with respiratory failure. Dialysis may be necessary if renal failure supervenes.

ACKNOWLEDGEMENTS

I wish to thank Dr E. T. W. Bowen of the Centre of Applied Microbiology and Research, Porton Down, for permission to publish the electron micrograph of Ebola virus, Dr G. Lloyd and Dr D S. Ellis for permission to publish the electron micrograph of Lassa virus, and also Vickers Medical Ltd, for permission to publish the photograph of the Trexler Isolator.

REFERENCES

Viral haemorrhagic diseases of the tropics

Arata A A, Johnson B 1978 Approaches towards studies on potential reservoirs of viral haemorrhagic fever in Southern Sudan (1977). In: Ebola virus haemorrhagic fever. Elsevier, North Holland, p 191–200

Baskerville A, Bowen E T W, Platt G S, McArdell L B, Simpson D I H 1978 The pathology of experimental Ebola virus infection in monkeys. Journal of Pathology 125: 131–138

Bellier L 1975 The genus Mastomys in the Ivory Coast. Bulletin, World Health Organisation 52: 665

Bowen E T W, Platt G S, Lloyd G, Baskerville A, Harris W J, Vella E E 1977 Viral haemorrhagic fever in Southern Sudan and Northern Zaire. Preliminary studies on the aetiological agent. Lancet 1: 571–573

Bowen E T W, Baskerville A, Cantell K, Mann G F, Simpson D I H, Zuckerman A J 1978 The effect of interferon on experimental Ebola virus infection in Rhesus monkeys. In: Ebola virus haemorrhagic fever. Elsevier, North Holland, p 245–252

Bowen E T W, Platt G S, Simpson D I H, McArdell L B, Raymond R T 1978 Ebola haemorrhagic fever: experimental infection in monkeys. Transactions of the Royal Society of Tropical Medicine and Hygiene 72: 188–191

Bremen, J A, Piot P, Johnson K M, White M K, Mbuyi M, Sureau P, Heyman D L, Van Nieuwenhove S, McCormick J B, Ruppol J P, Kintoki V, Isaäcson M, Van der Groen G, Webb P A, Ngvete K 1978 The epidemiology of Ebola haemorrhagic fever in Zaire 1976. In: Ebola virus haemorrhagic fever. Elsevier, North Holland, p 103–121

Buckley S M, Casals J 1970 Lassa fever, a new virus disease of man in West Africa. III. Isolation and characterization of the virus. American Journal of Tropical Medicine and Hygiene 19: 680–691

Carey D E, Kemp G E, White H A, Pinneo L, Addy R E 1972 Lasa Fever. Epidemiological aspect of the 1970 epidemic, Jos, Nigeria. Transactions of the Royal Society of Tropical Medicine and Hygiene 66: 402

Civil Aviation Authority 1977 Annual Statistics, Civil Aviation Authority, London

Department of Health and Social Security 1976 Memorandum on Lassa Fever. HMSO, London

Dietrich M, Schumacher H H, Peters D, Knobloch J 1978 Human pathology of Ebola (Maridi) virus infection in the Sudan. In: Ebola virus haemorrhagic fever, Elsevier, North Holland, p 37–41

Edington G M, White H A 1972 The pathology of Lassa fever. Transactions of the Royal Society of Tropical Medicine and Hygiene 66: 381–389

Emond R T D 1976 Isolation for high-risk patients. Postgraduate Medical Journal 52: 563–566

Emond R T D 1978 Hospitalisation of patients suspected of highly infectious disease. In: Ebola virus haemorrhagic fever. Elsevier, North Holland, p 396

Emond R T D, Evans B, Bowen E T W, Lloyd G 1977 A case of Ebola virus infection. British Medical Journal 2: 541–544

Emond R T D, Smith H, Welsby P D 1978 Assessment of patients with suspected viral haemorrhagic fever. British Medical Journal 1: 966–967

Emond R T D, Smith H Welsby P D 1979 Management of viral haemorrhagic fever suspects: a further year's experience. Communicable Disease Report 79/8

Frame J D 1975 Surveillance of Lassa fever in missionaries stationed in West Africa. Bulletin, World Health Organisation 52: 593–598

Frame J D, Baldwin J M, Gocke D J, Troup J M 1970 Lassa fever, a new virus disease of man from West Africa. I. Clinical description and pathological findings. American Journal of Tropical Medicine and Hygiene 19: 670–676

Francis D P, Smith D H, Highton R B, Simpson D I H, Lolik P, Deng I M., Gillo A L, Idris A A, El Tahir B 1978 Ebola fever in the Sudan, 1976: Epidemiological aspects of the disease. In: Ebola virus haemorrhagic fever. Elsevier, North Holland, p 129–135

Fraser D W, Campbell C C, Monath T P 1974 Lassa fever in the Eastern Province of Sierra Leone, 1970–1972 1. Epidemiologic studies. American Journal of Tropical Medicine and Hygiene 23: 1131–1139

Fuller J G 1974 Fever. The hunt for a new killer virus. Hart-Davis, MacGibbon, London

Galbraith N S, Berrie J R H, Forbes P, Young S 1978 Public health aspects of viral haemorrhagic fevers. Journal of the Royal Society of Health 98: 152–160

Gear J S S, Cassel G A, Gear A J, Tappler B, Clausen L, Myers A M, Kew M C, Bothwell T H, Sher R, Miller G B, Schneider J, Koornhof H J, Gompeters E D, Isaäcson M, Gear J H S 1975 Outbreak of Marburg virus disease in Johannesburg. British Medical Journal 4: 489–493

Gedigk P, Bechtelsheimer H, Korb G 1971 Pathologic anatomy of the Marburg virus disease. In: Marburg virus disease. Springer, Berlin, Heidelberg, New York, p 50–53

Germain M 1978 Collection of mammals and arthropods during the epidemic of haemorrhagic fever in Zaire. In: Ebola virus haemorrhagic fever. Elsevier, North Holland, p 185–190

Green C A, Gordon D H, Lyons N F 1978 Biological aspects in Praomys (Mastomys) natalensis (Smith), a rodent carrier of Lassa virus and bubonic plague in Africa. American Journal of Tropical Medicine and Hygiene 27: 627–629

Hutchison J G P, Gray J, Flewett T H, Emond R T D, Evans B, Trexler P C 1978 The safety of the Trexler isolator as judged by some physical and biological criteria: a report of experimental work at two centres. Journal of Hygiene, Cambridge 81: 311–319

International Civil Aviation Organisation 1972 Airline traffic 1961–1971. Digest of statistics No. 169. International Civil Aviation Organisation, Montreal

International Civil Aviation Organisation 1977 Airline traffic 1972–1976. Digest of statistics No. 218B, International Civil Aviation Organisation, Montreal

Isaäcson M, Sureau P, Courteille G, Pattyn S R 1978 Clinical aspects of Ebola virus infection at the Ngaliema Hospital, Kinshasa, Zaire 1976. In: Ebola virus haemorrhagic fever. Elsevier, North Holland, p 15–20

Jahrling P B, Hesse R A, Eddy G A, Johnson K M, Callis R T, Stephen E L 1980 Lassa virus infection of rhesus monkeys: pathogenesis and treatment with ribavivin. The Journal of Infectious Disease 141: 580–589

Johnson K M, Webb P A, Larige V E, Murphy F A 1977 Isolation and partial characterisation of a new virus causing acute haemorrhagic fever in Zaire. Lancet 1: 569–571

Keane E, Gilles H M 1977 Lassa fever in Panguma Hospital, Sierra Leone 1973–6. British Medical Journal, 1: 1399–1402

Kiley M P, Lange J V, Johnson K M 1979 Protection of rhesus monkeys from Lassa virus by immunisation with closely related arenavirus. Lancet 2: 738

Leifer E, Gocke D J, Bourne H 1970 Lassa fever, a new virus disease of man from West Africa II. Report of a laboratory acquired infection treated with plasma from a person recently recovered from the disease. American Journal of Tropical Medicine and Hygiene 19: 677–679

Martini G A 1973 Marburg virus disease. Postgraduate Medical Journal 49: 542–546
Martini G A, Siegert R 1972 Marburg virus disease. Springer Verlag, Berlin, Heidelberg, New York
McCormick J B, Johnson K M 1978 Lassa fever: historical review and contemporary investigation. In: Ebola virus haemorrhagic fever. Elsevier, North Holland, p 279–283
Monath T P 1975 Lassa fever: Review of epidemiology and epizootiology. Bulletin, World Health Organisation 52: 577–592
Monath T P, Maher M, Casals J, et al (1974) Lassa fever in the Eastern Province of Sierra Leone. II. Clinical and virological studies in selected hospitalized patients. American Journal of Tropical Medicine and Hygiene 23: 1140–1149
Monath T P, Mertens P E, Patton R, Gary G W, Kissling R E 1973 A hospital epidemic of Lassa fever in Zorzor, Liberia, March–April 1972. American Journal of Tropical Medicine and Hygiene 22: 773–779
Monath T P, Newhouse V F, Kemp G E et al 1974 Lassa virus isolation from Mastomys natalensis rodents during an epidemic in Sierra Leone. Science 185: 263–265
Pattyn S R, Jacob W, Van der Groen G, Piot P, Courteille G 1977 Isolation of Marburg-like virus from a case of haemorrhagic fever in Zaire. Lancet 1: 573–574
Piot P, Sureau P, Breman J G, Heymann D L, Kintoki V, Masamba M, Mbuyi M, Miatudila M, Ruppol J F, van Nieuwenhove S, White M K, van der Groen G, Webb P A, Wulff H, Johnson K M 1978 Clinical aspects of Ebola virus infection in Yambuku area, Zaire 1976. In: Ebola virus haemorrhagic fever. Elsevier, North Holland, p 7–14
Rowe W P, Murphy F A, Bergold G H et al 1970 Arenaviruses: proposed name for a newly defined virus group. Journal of Virology 5: 651–652
Siegert R 1972 Marburg virus. Virology Monographs 11: 97–154. Springer Velag, Berlin, Heidelberg, New York
Simpson D I H 1977 Marburg and Ebola virus infections: a guide for their diagnosis, management, and control. WHO Offset Publication No. 36, World Health Organisation, Geneva
Smith D H, Francis D P, Simpson D I H 1978 African haemorrhagic fever in the Southern Sudan 1976: the clinical manifestations. Ebola virus haemorrhagic fever. Elsevier, North Holland, p 21–26
Stille W, Bohle E, Helm E, von Rey W, Siede W 1968 Über eine durch Ceropithecus aethiops übertragene Infektionskrankheit. Deutsche Medizinische Wochenschrift 12a: 572–582
Trexler P C 1971 Microbiological isolation of large animals. Veterinary Record 88: 15
Trexler P C, Emond R T D, Evans B 1977 Negative-pressure plastic isolator for patients with dangerous infections. British Medical Journal 2: 559–561
Trexler P C, Spiers A S D, Gaya H 1975 Plastic isolators for treatment of acute leukaemia patients under 'germ-free' conditions. British Medical Journal 4: 949
Woodruff A W, Bowen E T W, Platt G S 1978 Viral infections in travellers from tropical Africa. British Medical Journal 1: 956–1958
World Health Organisation 1974 Lassa Fever. Weekly Epidemiological Record 49: 341–343
World Health Organisation 1979 Viral haemorrhagic fever surveillance. Weekly Epidemiological Record 54: 319
Wulff H, Fabiyi A, Monath T P 1975 Recent isolations of Lassa Virus from Nigerian rodents. Bulletin, World Health Organisation 52: 609–613
Wulff H, Lange J V 1975 Indirect immunofluorescence for the diagnosis of Lassa fever infection. Bulletin of the World Health Organisation 52: 429–36

Legionnaires' disease

Bartlett C L R 1979 Sporadic cases of Legionnaires' disease in Great Britain. Annals of Internal Medicine 90: 592–595
Beaty H N, Miller A A, Broome C V, Goings S, Phillips C A 1978 Legionnaires' disease in Vermont, May to October 1977. Journal of the American Medical Association 240: 127–131
Brenner D J, Steigerwalt B S, McDade J E 1979 Classification of the Legionnaires' disease bacillus: Legionella pneumophila, genus novum, species nova, of the family Legionellaceae, family nova. Annals of Internal Medicine 90: 656–658
Broome C V, Fraser D W 1979 Epidemiologic aspects of legionellosis. Epidemiologic Reviews 1: 1–16
Carrington C B 1979 Pathology of Legionnaires' disease. Annals of Internal Medicine 90: 496–499
Center for Disease Control 1978a Isolation of organisms resembling Legionnaires' disease bacterium—Tennessee. Morbidity and Mortality Weekly Report 27: 368–369
Center for Disease Control 1978b Isolation of organisms resembling Legionnaires' disease bacterium — Georgia. Morbidity and Mortality Weekly Report 27: 415–416
Center for Disease Control 1978c Legionnaires' disease — United States. Morbidity and Mortality Weekly Report 27: 439–441
Center for Disease Control 1978d Isolates of organisms resembling Legionnaires' disease bacterium from environmental sources — Bloomington, Indiana. Morbidity and Mortality Weekly Report 27: 283–285

Center for Disease Control 1978e Legionnaires' disease: diagnosis and management. Annals of Internal Medicine 88: 363–365

Center for Disease Control 1979 Legionnaires' disease — Australia. Morbidity and Mortality Weekly Report 27: 523

Chandler F W, Hicklin M D, Blackmon J A 1977 Demonstration of the agent of Legionnaires' disease in tissue. New England Journal of Medicine 297: 1218–1220

Chandler F W, Cole R M, Hicklin M D 1979 Ultra-structure of the Legionnaires' disease bacterium: a study using transmission electron microscopy. Annals of Internal Medicine 90: 642–647

Cordes L G 1978 Legionnaires' disease outbreak at an Atlanta country club: evidence for spread from an evaporative condenser. Paper presented at the International Symposium on Legionnaires' Disease, Atlanta, Georgia, 13–15 Nov. 1978

Dietrich P A, Johnson R D, Fairbank J T, Walke J S 1978 The chest radiograph in Legionnaires' disease. Radiology 127: 577–582

Dondero T J 1978 Legionnaires' disease outbreak temporally associated with contaminated cooling tower. Paper presented at the International Symposium on Legionnaires' Disease, Atlanta, Georgia, 13–15 Nov. 1978

Eickhoff, T C 1979 Epidemiology of Legionnaires' disease. Annals of Internal Medicine 90: 499–502

Farshy C E, Klein G C, Feeley J C 1978 Detection of antibodies to Legionnaires' disease or organism by microagglutination and micro-enzyme-linked immunosorbent assay tests. Journal of Clinical Microbiology 7: 327–331

Farshy C E, Cruce D D, Klein G C, Wilkinson H, Feeley J C 1979 Immunoglobulin specificity of microagglutination test for the Legionnaires' disease bacterium. Annals of Internal Medicine 90: 690

Fraser D W, Wachsmuth I K, Bopp C, Feeley J C, Tsai T F 1978 Antibiotic treatment of guinea-pigs infected with agent of Legionnaires' disease. Lancet 1: 175

Fraser D F, Tsai T R, Orenstein W, Parkin W E, Beecham H J, Sharrar R G, Harris J, Mallison G F, Martin S M, McDade J E, Shepard C C, Brachman P S and the Field Investigation Team 1977 Legionnaires' Disease. Description of an epidemic of pneumonia. New England Journal of Medicine 297: 1189–1197

Fraser D W, Deubner D C, Hill D L, Gilliam D K 1979 Non-pneumonic, short-incubation-period legionellosis (Pontiac fever) in men who cleaned a steam turbine condenser. Science 205: 690–691

Glick T H, Gregg M B, Berman B, Mallison G, Rhodes W W, Kassanoff I 1978 Pontiac fever: an epidemic of unknown etiology in a health department. I. Clinical and epidemiologic aspects. American Journal of Epidemiology 107 (2): 149–160

Grady G F, Gilfillan R F 1979 Relation of *Mycoplasma pneumoniae* sero-activity, immunosuppression and chronic disease to Legionnaires' disease. A twelve-month prospective study of sporadic cases in Massachusetts. Annals of Internal Medicine 90: 607–610

Haley C E, Cohen M L, Halter J, Meyer R D 1979 Nosocomial Legionnaires' disease: a continuing common-scource epidemic at Wadsworth Medical Center. Annals of Internal Medicine 90: 583–586

Helms C M, Viner J P, Sturm R H, Renner E D, Johnson W 1979 Comparative features of pneumococcal, mycoplasmal and Legionnaires' disease pneumonias. Annals of Internal Medicine 90: 543–547

Jenkins P, Miller A C, Osman J, Pearson S B, Rowley J M 1979 Legionnaires' disease: a clinical description of thirteen cases. British Journal of Chest Diseases 73: 31–38

Katz S M 1978 Examination of sputum in Legionnaires' disease. Lancet 2: 987–988

Kirby B D, Snyder K M, Meyer R D, Finegold S M 1978 Legionnaires' disease: clinical features of 24 cases. Annals of Internal Medicine 89: 297–309

Lattimer G L, Rodes III L V, Salventi J S, Stonebraker V, Boley S, Haas G 1979 The Philadelphia epidemic of Legionnaires' disease: Clinical, pulmonary, and serologic findings two years later. Annals of Internal Medicine 90: 522–525

Lewis V J, Thacker W L, Shephard C C, McDade J E 1978 In vivo susceptibility of the Legionnaires' disease bacterium to 10 antimicrobial agents. Antimicrobial Agents and Chemotherapy 13: 419

Love W C, Chaudhuri A K R, Chin K C, Fallon R 1978 Possible case-to-case transmission of Legionnaires' disease. Lancet 2: 1249

McDade J E, Brenner D J, Bozeman F M 1979 Legionnaires' disease bacterium isolated in 1947. Annals of Internal Medicine 90: 659–661

McDade J E, Shepard C C, Fraser D W, Tsai T R, Redus M A, Dowdle W R and the Laboratory Investigation Team 1977 New England Journal of Medicine 297: 1197–1203

McCluskey R T 1978 Cause of renal failure in Legionnaires' disease. New England Journal of Medicine 299: 362

Macrae A D, Appleton P N, Laverick A 1979 Legionnaires' disease in Nottingham, England. Annals of Internal Medicine 90: 580–583

Meenhorst P L, van der Meer, J W M, Borst J 1979 Sporadic cases of Legionnaires' disease in the Netherlands. Annals of Internal Medicine 90: 529–532

Miller A C 1979 Early clinical differentiation between Legionnaires' disease and other specific pneumonias. Annals of Internal Medicine 90: 526–528

Miller A C, Pearson S B, Roderick Smith W H 1978 Legionnaires' disease: radiological resolution and bronchoscopy. Lancet 2: 570

Morgan J R, Ryder R, Paull P, Thomas J P 1979 Antibodies in hospital staff exposed to Legionnaires' disease. Lancet I: 1083

Moss C W, Weaver R E, Dees S B, Cherry W B 1977 Cellular fatty acid composition of isolates from Legionnaires' disease. Journal of Clinical Microbiology 6: 140–143

Politi B D, Fraser D W, Mallison G F, Mohatt J V, Morris G K, Patton C M, Feeley J C, Telle R D, Bennett J V 1979 A major focus of Legionnaires' disease in Bloomington, Indiana. Annals of Internal Medicine 90: 587–591

Reid D, Grist N R, Najera R 1978 Illness associated with 'package tours': a combined Spanish-Scottish study. Bulletin of the World Health Organisation 56: 117–122

Relman A S, McCluskey R T 1978 Case records of the Massachusetts General Hospital. Acute renal failure and hemoptysis in a 44-year old man. New England Journal of Medicine 298: 1014–1021

Saravolatz L D, Burch K H, Fisher E, Madhaven T, Kiani D, Neblett T, Quinn E L 1979 The compromised host and Legionnaires' disease. Annals of Internal Medicine 90: 533–537

Schoenhaum S C, Mark E J 1978 Case records of the Massachusetts General Hospital. Rapidly progressing pulmonary consolidation in a 31-year-old man. New England Journal of Medicine 299: 347–354

Skaliy P, McEachern H V 1979 Survival of the Legionnaires' disease bacterium in water. Annals of Internal Medicine 90: 662–663

Storch G, Baine W B, Fraser W D, Broome C V, Clegg II, H W, Cohen M L, Goings S A J, Politi B D, Terranova W A, Tsai T F, Plikaytis B D, Shepard C C, Bennett J V 1979 Sporadic community-acquired Legionnaires' disease in the United States. A case-control study. Annals of Internal Medicine 90: 596–600

Swartz M N 1979 Clinical aspects of Legionnaires' disease. Annals of Internal Medicine 90: 492–495

Taylor A G, Harrison T G 1979 Legionnaires' disease caused by Legionella pneumophila serogroup 3. Lancet 2: 47

Terranova W, Cohen M L, Fraser D W 1978 1974 outbreak of Legionnaires' disease diagnosed in 1977: clinical and epidemiological features. Lancet 2: 122–124

Thacker S B, Bennett J V, Tsai T F, Fraser D W, McDade J E, Shepard C C, Williams K H, Stuart W H, Dull H B, Eickhoff T C 1978 An outbreak in 1965 of severe respiratory illness caused by Legionnaires' disease bacterium. Journal of Infectious Diseases 138: 512

Thomason B M, Chandler F W, Hollis D G 1979 Flagella in Legionnaires' disease bacterium: an interim report. Annals of Internal Medicine 91: 224–246

Tilton R P 1979 Legionnaires' disease antigen detected by enzyme-linked immunosorbent assay. Annals of Internal Medicine 90: 697–698

Tsai T F, Fraser D W 1978 The diagnosis of Legionnaires' disease. Annals of Internal Medicine 89: 413–414

Ventatachalam K K, Saravoletz L D, Christopher K L 1979 Legionnaires' disease. A cause of lung abscess. Journal of the American Medical Association 241: 597–598

Wong K H, Moss C W, Hochsten D H, Arko R J, Schalla W O 1979 'Endotoxicity' of the Legionnaires' disease bacterium. Annals of Internal Medicine 90: 624–627

14. Diabetes and its complications

P. H. Sönksen   P. M. Brown

INTRODUCTION

Diabetes, whether insulin requiring (type I) or non-insulin requiring (type II), is characterised by an absolute or relative deficiency of insulin. In other hormone-deficiency states replacement of the missing hormone results in return to complete clinical and biochemical normality (e.g. myxoedema treated with thyroxine). However, the current treatment of diabetes with insulin often fails to prevent the morbidity of specific long-term complications and premature death. The prognosis of a group of 370 diabetic patients who developed diabetes before 1933 has been described by Deckert, Poulsen & Larsen (1978a). The fate of 289 was recorded after more than 40 years of diabetes. Sixty per cent had died, a mortality rate two to six times that in an age and sex-matched non-diabetic population. Renal failure was the cause of death in 31 per cent. The development of persistent proteinuria was associated with a three- to four-fold increased mortality when compared with those who did not develop proteinuria. Of the survivors, 22 per cent had impaired renal function, 16 per cent of the group became blind and an additional 14 per cent had severely impaired vision. Twenty-one per cent had had a myocardial infarction, 10 per cent a stroke and 12 per cent either gangrene or had undergone amputation. Deckert also investigated the factors influencing prognosis in this group of long standing diabetic patients (Deckert, Poulsen & Larsen, 1978b). It seemed that survival was longest in those who had:

1. Frequent contact with a specialised diabetes clinic from an early stage of their disease.
2. Good blood glucose control (assessed 'blind' from out patient records).
3. Low insulin dose.
4. Low body weight.
5. Mean blood pressure below 100 mmHg.

Diabetes is therefore clearly associated with considerably increased mortality and morbidity both of which can result from either the diabetes-specific microangiopathy or the non-specific but premature macroangiopathic complications. Effective innovations in diabetic care should therefore be aimed at either preventing the development of the disease or reducing or eliminating diabetic complications.

DEFINITION

A prerequisite for studying a disease is a workable definition. Although there is no problem of diagnosis in diabetic patients with classical signs and symptoms and marked hyperglycaemia there is considerable uncertainty about the use of the diagnosis 'diabetes' in patients with minor glucose intolerance. This uncertainty occurs because population studies have generally shown a continuous spectrum of both fasting glycaemia and glucose tolerance with no obvious division of the results into 'normal' and 'abnormal'. Prospective studies have tended to show that the microvascular complications of diabetes develop in those subjects whose blood glucose was greater than 11.1 mmol/l two hours after 50 grams of oral glucose (Jarrett & Keen, 1976; Jarrett & Al Sayegh, 1978). It has therefore been suggested that the label diabetes be applied only to those subjects with a fasting blood glucose over 7.0 mmol/l and blood glucose two hours after oral glucose over 10.0 mmol/l (Keen, Jarrett & Alberti, 1979). Subjects with lesser degrees of glucose intolerance previously called 'borderline diabetes' with fasting blood glucose under 7.0 mmol/l but two-hour glucoses during oral glucose tolerance test above 7.0 mmol/l appear to have relatively little risk of developing specific microvascular complications but do have an increased risk of cardiovascular mortality, particularly if female. Only 2.3 per cent per year of patients in this 'borderline' group show worsening of glucose tolerance to overt diabetes and a large proportion reverted spontaneously to normal glucose tolerance (Jarrett, et al, 1979). It has therefore been suggested that this group be described as having Impaired Glucose Tolerance (IGT) since there is little clinical benefit from defining such patients 'diabetic' while the sociological problems generated are substantial. Although these suggested definitions are still being debated it seems likely that a more liberal definition will soon become accepted.

THE AETIOLOGY OF DIABETES

The aetiology of non-insulin requiring diabetes remain obscure but the 'classical' twin studies of Pyke (1977) which showed very high concordance in identical twins with onset of diabetes after 40 years demonstrated a strong genetic basis. Obesity and diet also seem to be predisposing factors though recent population studies showing an inverse correlation between calorie intake and body weight suggest that the role of diet may require reassessment (Keen et al, 1979). The concept of the 'thrifty genotype' that is very efficient at conserving calories and therefore, prone to obesity and diabetes may provide a link between genetic make-up and food intake.

Insulin-dependent (type I) diabetes is also undoubtedly genetically determined but since only 50 per cent of such identical twins are concordant for diabetes, environmental factors must play a very important part in precipitating the disease. Recent developments have cast light on the possible interplay between genetic make up and environmental triggers in causing diabetes.

Studies of the major histocompatability (HLA) system in diabetes has shown that inheritance of certain HLA antigens is associated with an increased or decreased risk of developing type I diabetes, though none of the associations approach the frequency with which HLA B27 occurs in patients with ankylosing spondylitis. The interpretation of these findings involves careful statistical methods since certain antigens tend to be inherited together and an excess of one antigen may be produced by the rarity of another. This association with certain HLA types occurs whatever the age of onset of insulin-dependent diabetes. This subject is reviewed by Cudworth (1978). Studies of families with more than one sibling with type I diabetes have shown that certain HLA antigens occur together in the affected subjects. The susceptibility to diabetes within families may therefore be enhanced when 'high risk' HLA-linked genes occur together.

The importance of these studies is two fold: (1) They have been interpreted as concrete evidence of genetic heterogeneity in diabetes, since no HLA antigen type has been found associated with insulin independent (type II) diabetes, with the corollary that type I and type II diabetes are different diseases and not variations in severity of the same disease. (2) They have suggested a mechanism for the genetic predisposition to type I diabetes. In mice and rats the major histocompatibility genes are closely associated with genes concerned with immunological responses. If this association also occurs in man then interaction between HLA genes and immune-response genes could determine an individual's susceptibility to infection with a pancreas-damaging virus. Such an interplay of HLA genes and immune-response has been suggested by the finding that antibodies to pancreatic islet cells five years after the development of type I diabetes occur more commonly in patients with particular HLA types (Bottazzo et al, 1978a; Bottazzo et al, 1978b). An increase in antibody titres to Coxsackie B virus types soon after developing type I diabetes also occurred more commonly in patients with certain HLA types (Cudworth et al, 1977).

Another link with virus infection comes from the isolation of a Coxsackie B4 virus from the pancreas of a child who died soon after the onset of type I diabetes (Yoon et al, 1979). When the virus was inoculated into a susceptible strain of mice they developed diabetes and Coxsackie B4 associated antibodies were demonstrated in their β cells. The passive transfer of diabetes to immunologically incompetent athymic nude mice by injection of lymphocytes from newly diagnosed type I diabetics suggest the importance of immune mechanisms (Buxhard, Madshad & Rygaard, 1979) although others have been unable to repeat these results. If a viral infection is important in type I diabetes then prevention by prophylactic immunisation of genetically suspectible individuals may soon become possible.

THE AETIOLOGY OF THE COMPLICATIONS OF DIABETES

The prevention of the microvascular and macroangiopathic complications of diabetes presents a major challenge. Siperstein has claimed that thickening of the capillary basement membrane in muscle characteristic of diabetic macroangiopathy occurs at a very early stage of diabetes and also in prediabetes. This suggests that diabetic complications can occur in the absence of hyperglycaemia and imply that complications will develop in diabetics independently of the degree of control of the metabolic abnormalities. Siperstein's results have not been confirmed by others and considerable controversy continues (Gundersen, Østerby & Lundback, 1978; Siperstein, Feingold & Bennet, 1978; Williamson & Rito 1979). A large number of clinical and animal studies indicate that there is a relationship between diabetic control and the development of microvascular complications. The evidence has recently been reviewed by Tchobroutsky (1978). Of 14 prospective studies designed to show any relationship between the incidence of retinopathy or glomerulopathy and the quality of diabetic control only 4 have failed to show a positive relationship. Such studies are hampered by imperfect methods of assessing control and the impossibility of achieving perfect control means that they compare varying degrees of imperfection. It has also been argued that patients in whom good control has been achieved have a milder form of diabetes and therefore develop fewer complications. A prospective study has been reported (Eschwege et al, 1979) in which randomly assigned groups of diabetic patients were treated with either: (1) One injection of a long-acting insulin, or (2) two or three injections of shorter-acting insulins. After four years the increase in the number of retinal microaneurysms and mean fasting blood glucose were significantly lower in the group treated with multiple injections. In another study (Viberti et al, 1979) improvement in diabetic control reduced urinary excretion of albumin and β_2 microglobulin in insulin-dependant diabetics.

Animals with experimentally induced diabetes develop similar microvascular changes and many well-controlled prospective studies have found that diabetic control reduces these changes. The glomerular capillary basement membrane thickening (BMT) correlated closely with average plasma glucose concentrations in experimentally diabetic rats (Fox et al, 1977), normalisation of blood glucose preventing BMT thickening (Fig. 14.1). Retinal lesions in alloxan-diabetic dogs were less in animals with good diabetic control with twice daily insulin than in intentionally poorly controlled animals (Engerman, Bloodworth & Nelson, 1977).

Both clinical and animal studies have indicated the importance of blood glucose control in diabetes and this evidence has resulted in a statement from the American Diabetes Association (American Diabetes Association — Policy Statement, 1976) emphasising the importance of attempting to achieve normal blood glucose values in diabetic patients, an approach which is now followed by the majority of physicians caring for diabetics.

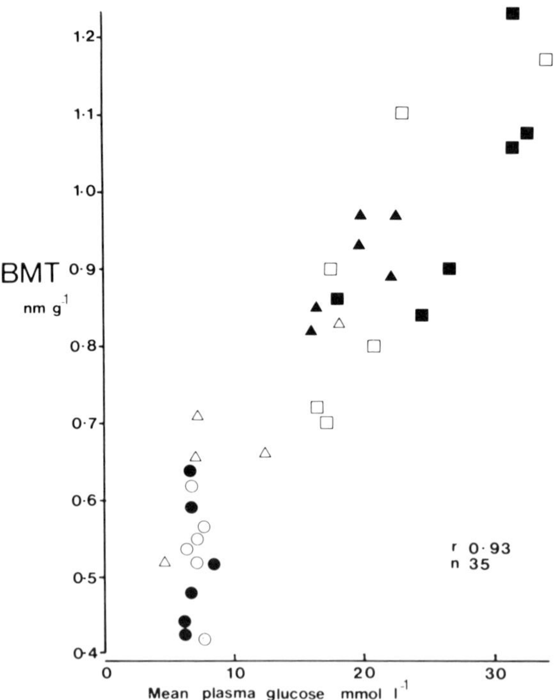

Fig. 14.1   Relation between glomerular capillary basement membrane thickness (BMT) corrected for body weight and mean plasma glucose (MPG) in 35 rats. Rats on normal diet: ● = non-diabetic; ▲ = diabetic with insulin; ■ = diabetic without insulin. Rats on low carbohydrate diet: ○ = non-diabetic; △ = diabetic with insulin; □ = diabetic without insulin.
Conversion of SI to traditional units — Glucose: 1 mmol/l = 18 mg/100 ml

Tchobroutsky pointed out that, 'The definite demonstration that the microvascular complications of diabetes can be prevented by normalisation of blood glucose concentrations in man cannot be made since normoglycaemia cannot be sustained from the beginning of the disease with our current methods of treatment'. Nevertheless available evidence has encouraged the development of many innovations to improve use of currently available modes of treatment i.e. insulin, diet and drugs.

Insulin

New insulins

Ordinary crystalline insulin also contains pro-insulin, dimeric forms of insulin and large molecular weight pancreatic peptides. These impurities can be removed by gel filtration chromatography producing highly purified insulins ('monocomponent' or 'rarely immunogenic'). These insulins have now been available for eight years and their use in the treatment of diabetes has steadily increased. The advantages claimed for highly purified insulins relate to their freedom from impurities causing local reactions and their lower immunogenicity. All insulin-treated diabetic patients develop antibodies to insulin. It has been shown that antibodies develop more slowly and to lower titres in patients treated with highly purified insulins (Yue & Turtle, 1975). It has been suggested that the development of insulin antibodies predisposes to the development of basement membrane changes in diabetes but this is very unlikely as the changes in insulin treated diabetes are identical to those in non-insulin treated patients. Changing from conventional to highly purified insulins may reduce the patients' insulin requirements (Mustaffa, Daggett & Nabarro, 1977). There may be an immediate reduction which is probably due to a species difference in the binding by the circulating antibodies of pork and beef insulin since most highly purified insulins are porcine. A further fall in insulin requirements usually occurs over the ensuing two to three months, particularly in those previously requiring a large dose, which parallels a reduction in insulin-binding antibodies. Although many studies have reported an improvement in diabetic control on changing to highly purified insulins no controlled studies have been performed and any improvement may have been due to the increased attention given to patients participating in such studies.

Highly purified insulins very rarely produce the local insulin allergy with red patches and irritation which occurs frequently with conventional insulins. Lipoatrophy which can cause considerable disfigurement occurs less frequently with highly purified insulins, but whether these advantages outweigh the increased cost of these insulins can only be decided by individual physicians. There is, at present, no firm evidence that diabetic control is improved or complications avoided by the use of highly purified insulins (Editorial, Lancet, 1979a; Alberti & Natrass, 1978).

The use of highly purified insulins is absolutely indicated in certain groups of patients: (1) those with either local or general insulin allergy, (2) those in whom insulin treatment is likely to be intermittent, e.g. type II diabetes, during pregnancy or surgical operations and for subjects undergoing insulin tolerance tests since such intermittent administration of insulin is more likely to lead to general allergy or anaphylaxis. (At a recent British Diabetic Association meeting, a show of hands suggested that a substantial majority of diabetologists were starting all new patients on highly purified insulin.)

One field of research which may result in improved diabetic care in the future is the study of analogues of insulin with altered peptide structure and biological properties. A similar approach led to the introduction of an analogue of antidiuretic hormone, DDAVP, with greater potency and duration of action than the native hormone. Alteration of the molecular structure of insulin may produce advantageous biological properties. A semisynthetic insulin analogue A1 B29 dodecoyl insulin has been shown to have a predominant hepatic action in normal dogs and a prolonged plasma half-life and duration of action in diabetic patients (Brown et al, 1980) and such molecules may have therapeutic advantages in man, e.g. they may overcome the problems of variable absorption which occur with conventional zinc or protamine complexed insulins.

Treatment of diabetic ketoacidosis
In the past the treatment of diabetic ketoacidosis has emphasised the use of large intermittent doses of insulin given intravenously and intramuscularly. Studies of the kinetics of insulin which demonstrated that its plasma half-life is three to five minutes, led to the development of continuous low-dose infusions of 4 to 8 units per hour of insulin for the treatment of diabetic ketoacidosis (Sönksen et al, 1972). These new methods (Page et al, 1974) met with considerable resistance particularly in the United States but two recent studies have compared the effects of low and high-dose insulin therapies in diabetic ketoacidosis (Lutterman, Adriansen, van't Laar, 1979; Gonzalez-Villalpanelo et al, 1979). Low dose insulin was infused continuously at 6 to 12 units per hour. High dose insulin was given either as an hourly intravenous injection of 100 units or as 40 to 80 units per hour both intravenously and intramuscularly. In both studies the rates of fall of blood glucose and rate of rise of arterial pH were similar with both methods. Hypoglycaemia occurred in four out of twelve patients on high dose insulin due to delay in starting glucose infusion but in no patients on low dose. Plasma potassium was significantly lower after three hours treatment with high dose insulin despite similar potassium replacement in both groups. However, there was no difference in plasma potassium concentrations in the Dutch study (Lutterman et al, 1979). The two groups of investigations concluded that low-dose continuous intravenous methods are as safe and effective as conventional treatments and in addition are much simpler to use and have less risk of producing hypoglycaemia or hypokalaemia.

These conclusions are in keeping with recent studies on the mechanism of action of insulin in diabetic patients. The conventional view is that the hyperglycaemia of uncontrolled diabetes is due to failure of glucose utilisation by tissues and that insulin produces its hypoglycaemic effect by increasing glucose transport into muscle. The rate of glucose production can be measured by following the decay curve of plasma specific activity following the injection of a tracer of ^{3}H-3-glucose. This method has shown that glucose production is consistently elevated in untreated diabetic patients when compared with non-diabetics and that insulin treatment results in a lowering of glucose production (Hall, Saunders & Sönksen, 1979). In the same study free fatty acid (FFA) turnover was measured by a similar technique and it was found that the elevation of FFA concentrations in the diabetic subjects was associated with an increased production of FFA's from increased lipolysis. This increased FFA concentration results in increased FFA utilisation part of which is by hepatic ketogenesis.

A study using a constant infusion of tracer ^{3}H-3-glucose has compared the effects of infusions of insulin at 2.4 and 10.6 units per hour on hepatic glucose production and peripheral glucose utilisation (Brown et al, 1978). It was found that the low-dose infusion (2.4 units per hour) lowered plasma glucose concentrations entirely by reducing hepatic glucose production (Ra) with no effect on glucose utilisation (Rd) (Fig. 14.2). The higher infusion rate had a similar effect on glucose production and in addition increased glucose utilisation. The liver is, therefore, the main site of action of the hypoglycaemic effects of physiological insulin concentrations. This suggests that intraportal insulin concentrations are of major importance in glucose homeostasis. In this study the reduction of ketone body and FFA concentrations were similar with both rates of insulin infusion indicating that lipolysis and ketogenesis can be inhibited by low insulin concentrations.

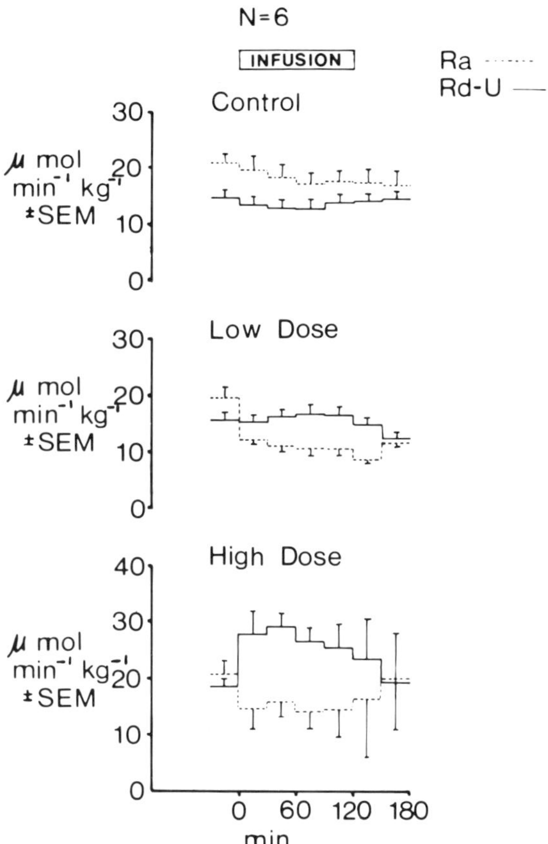

Fig. 14.2 Mean rates of appearance (Ra) and disappearance of glucose corrected for urinary losses (Rd–U) (± SE of mean) for six diabetic patients during saline infusion (control) and low dose 2.6 units/hour and high dose 10.6 units/hour insulin infusions.

Insulin infusion systems

Measurement of the day profile of blood glucose and other metabolites have shown that subcutaneously administered insulin fails to 'normalise' the metabolic abnormalities associated with insulin lack. This failure is due to the difficulty of mimicking the rapid response of endogenous insulin secretion with subcutaneously administered insulin. Attempts have been made to mimic the action of the β cell with so called 'closed loop' insulin delivery systems which continuously monitor the patient's blood glucose and infuse an appropriate dose of insulin or glucose. Such devices can be used only as research tools as they are large (the size of a washing machine) and expensive. It has been demonstrated that it is possible to achieve and maintain normal blood glucose, amino acid and other metabolic concentrations with such systems (Buckle et al, 1977). The other abnormalities of diabetes can therefore be corrected solely by the administration of an appropriate dose of insulin. This finding has led to the development of simpler systems which infuse insulin intravenously at a predetermined rate and are suitable for ambulatory patients (Irsigler & Kritz, 1979). It has been shown that the subcutaneous infusion of insulin (which avoids the risk of infection inherent with intravenous infusions) will produce near normal glucose, lipid and amino acid metabolism (Pickup et al, 1979; Tamborlane et al, 1979a; Tamborlane et al, 1979b). Patients receiving such treatment are closely supervised and it has not yet been shown that the results with such infusion pumps are superior to those obtained with intermittent insulin administrations and similar monitoring. Infusion methods may however, produce interesting further developments.

Pancreatic transplantation (Editorial Lancet, 1979b)
The injection of isolated islets from normal rats into an inbred diabetic rat results in permanent amelioration of diabetes and also prevents the development of glomerular changes associated with diabetes (Gray & Watkins, 1976). Such studies indicate that successful transplantation of islet tissue in diabetic patients would completely reverse the metabolic abnormalities of diabetes and also prevent diabetic complications. Experience with human pancreatic transplantation has so far been disappointing, partly because of rejection but also because of surgical problems with anastomosis and autodigestion of the pancreas associated with secretion of proteolytic enzymes by the exocrine tissue. Recent evidence suggests that this may be controllable by injecting resin up the pancreatic duct before transplantation. It has also been suggested that the use of human fetal islet preparations might avoid these problems.

Home monitoring of blood glucose
Even if pancreatic transplantation or portable artificial pancreases are successfully developed they would be available to only a fraction of the diabetic population. Improvement in the treatment of insulin requiring diabetics must therefore come from better use of subcutaneously administered insulin. It is now widely accepted that the aim of treatment of diabetics should be to achieve blood glucose levels as close to those of the non-diabetic state as possible. If the patient is to achieve this without frequent episodes of hypoglycaemia then he must have some means of measuring his diabetic control. Measurements of urinary glucose concentration although traditionally a cornerstone of diabetic care rarely provide useful information for the insulin treated diabetic since a negative urine test can occur with either a blood glucose value of 10 mmol/l i.e. above the range for non-diabetics or with a low blood glucose producing hypoglycaemic symptoms. Direct measurement of blood glucose would, however provide the patient with information as to how successfully he is maintaining normoglycaemia and whether changes of insulin administration are necessary.

Although the methodology for such self-measurement of blood glucose by patients has been available for more than 10 years (using an enzyme reagent strip and reflectance meter) it is only with the recent renewal of emphasis on strict diabetic control that these methods have been used by patients. Several reports (Sönksen, Judd & Lowy, 1979; Walford et al, 1979) have shown that the method is acceptable to most patients and that the measurement of blood glucose has resulted in improvement in control in the majority of patients. Figure 14.3 shows the use of urine tests and blood glucose measurements in a group of diabetic teenagers on a diabetic camp. They were given a free choice of urine test or self-blood tests and it can be seen that blood testing was preferred and maintained by the majority of this group of usually uncooperative diabetics.

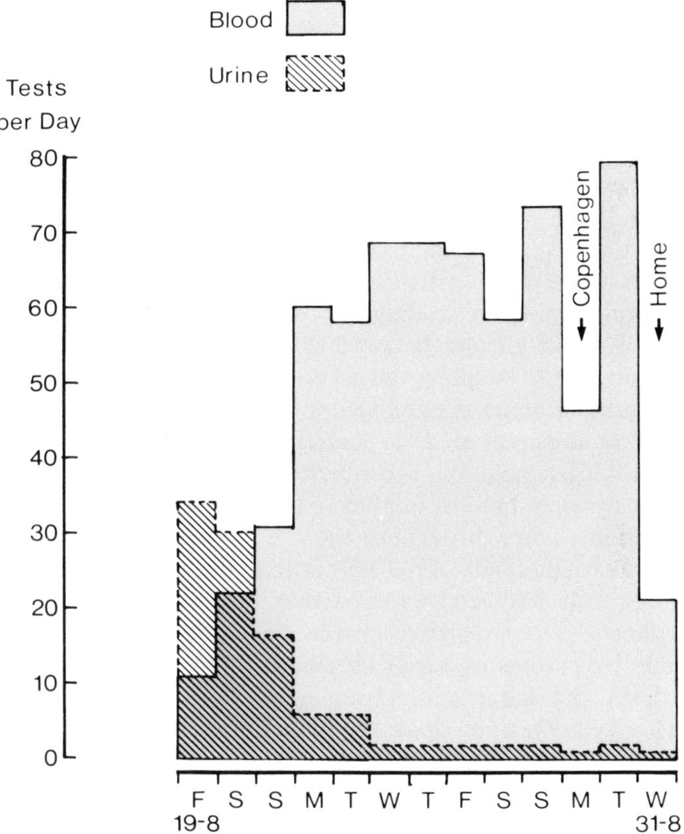

Fig. 14.3 Number of urine (cross-hatched) and blood (grey) estimations performed per day by 20 diabetic children at a summer camp over a 13-day period given the choice between the two assessment methods. Copenhagen indicates a day visit to that city.

Despite lowering of blood glucose levels hypoglycaemic symptoms were not increased. This is probably because severe hypoglycaemia is more likely to occur in patients with large fluctuations of blood glucose and it was these fluctuations which were improved by self-monitoring. Most patients reported an increase in self-confidence, and a feeling that they had greater control over their diabetic condition.

The method is also quicker and socially more acceptable than urine testing. The results of home monitoring in pregnant diabetics has shown that near-normoglycaemia can be achieved in this well motivated group with resultant normal birth weight infants despite allowing mothers to go to term before delivery (West, Hunter & Lowy, 1980).

Good fetal outcome can therefore be achieved without the conventional policy of admitting such patients to hospital for the last eight weeks of gestation. Small portable reflectance meters (Glucochek obtainable from Medistron Ltd, Alpine Works, Oak Road, Southgate, Crawley, Sussex or Hypocount from Hypoguard Limited, 49 Grimston Lane, Trimley, Ipswich, Suffolk) are now available and it seems likely that in view of the undoubted preference by patients and efficacy in improving diabetic control that increasing numbers of insulin-treated diabetics will adopt home blood glucose monitoring and abandon urine testing (Tattersall, 1979).

Glycosylated haemoglobins
An accurate independent method for assessing diabetic control would be useful for both long-term studies of the effect of blood glucose control on complications and also for recognising those patients whose control could be improved. Current methods of control are often based on random clinic blood glucose measurements which are inadequate due to the infrequency of measurement and unreliable because the patient's activities on the day he attends clinic are different from his usual ones. Urine glucose estimations are often misleading due to high or low renal threshold and do not reflect changes of blood glucose below that patient's renal threshold. The recent discovery that the size of a minor glycosylated haemoglobin fraction (HbAlC) is determined by ambient blood glucose values over several weeks (Spicer et al, 1969; Hoenig et al, 1976; Gonen et al, 1977) has therefore aroused considerable interest. HbA the major adult haemoglobin is converted to a glycosylated derivative, HbAlC, by a non-enzymic covalent binding of glucose to the N terminal valine residue of the β chain. This reaction occurs throughout the life of the red cell and the amount of HbAlC formed in a haemolysate of red cells reflects the average glucose concentration to which the red cell has been exposed over the average life of that red cell. Glycosylation increases the negative charge on haemoglobin and HbAlC can be measured readily by cationic exchange chromatography. The complete separation of HbAlC from HbA and other minor haemoglobins i.e. AlA, AlB requires a long column and a long elution time. Separation HbAlC together with haemoglobins AlA and AlB from HbA, that is the total HbAl, can be accomplished quickly with short columns and this is the method usually employed. Many studies have shown that the percentage of HbAl is increased in diabetic patients and that the concentration correlates with fasting plasma glucose concentrations, mean daily glucose levels and the physician's assessment of the degree of diabetic control achieved (Hoenig et al, 1976; Gonen et al, 1977). HbAlC fell progressively over about two months (the normal half life of circulating erythrocytes) when diabetic control was improved in a group of patients (Peterson et al, 1977). The current view is that the concentration of HbAlC is the best independent index of diabetic control for both individual patients and for making comparisons between groups of patients and is likely to be very useful in assessing the effect of diabetic control on the development of complications (Gonen & Rubenstein, 1978).

The measurement of HbAlC may alert the physician to the need for improved control in a particular patient but will not indicate how to achieve this. Home blood glucose monitoring can provide the patient with this information and the two methods of assessing control can be complementary.

One major problem is using measurements of glycosylated haemoglobin to assess control is that different centres using the same, or different methods of separation have different normal values and at present there is no quality control between laboratories. Comparisons of different groups may therefore be misleading. In addition haemolytic processes, e.g. uraemia (Dandona, Freedman & Moorhead, 1979) which shorten red cell survival will lower the concentration of glycosylated haemoglobin and may lead to misleading results. The presence of abnormal haemoglobins will also invalidate the measurement of HbAl since they may elute from the columns atypically due to altered charge.

Diet

The diet prescribed to both insulin-requiring and non-insulin requiring diabetics is usually based on a reduction and limitation of carbohydrate intake to about 40 per cent of total calories. This advice probably dates from the pre-insulin era when rigid dietary carbohydrate restriction was the only treatment available for diabetics. Recent studies have suggested that it may not be the amount of carbohydrate which needs to be changed but the source of the carbohydrate. Maturity onset diabetics (Simpson et al, 1979) were prescribed either a high carbohydrate diet (60 per cent of total calories) containing carbohydrate as wholemeal bread and tuberous vegetables or a lower carbohydrate diet (34 per cent of total calories). After six weeks on the diets, fasting and preprandial blood glucose concentrations and glycosylated haemoglobin were lower in the high carbohydrate diet group. The authors conclude that carbohydrate restricted diets are no longer justified in maturity onset non-insulin requiring diabetics. The improvement may have been due to the increased fibre in the high carbohydrate diet. The role of dietary fibre in diabetes has produced much interest. It has been suggested that Western diets with low fibre content predispose to the development of diabetes (Trowell, 1975). This suggestion is based on the rarity of diabetes in Africans who consume a diet containing about four times the fibre content of a Western diet. Although this hypothesis lacks experimental evidence and may be based on low ascertainment rather than low prevalence of diabetes, much interest has been generated about the effect of fibre in patients with established diabetes. Kiehm, Anderson & Ward (1976) have shown that feeding a high fibre, high carbohydrate diet for two weeks to patients on sulphonylureas or low doses of insulin (<28 units per day) improved carbohydrate tolerance so that all five drug-treated and four out of five insulin-treated patients could stop medication. However, in three patients on higher doses of insulin no improvement occurred. The source of fibre is clearly important: oral glucose tolerance was improved in normal subjects after one month of diets containing 25 g of corn brans, soy hulls or carrot powder but not by diets supplemented with wheat bran (Munoz, Sandstead & Jacobs, 1979). In another study guar had the greatest effect in flattening glucose tolerance curves in normal subjects (Jenkins et al, 1978a; Jenkins et al, 1978b). Guar is not well tolerated at therapeutic doses and often causes considerable flatus. Much work, therefore, remains to be done on the relative effects of different fibre components and the development of palatable fibre supplements (Gouldo & Alberti, 1978). There can be no doubt, however, that the concept of 10 g carbohydrate exchanges ('portions') is 'dead'. From now on we will have to pay more attention to the form of the carbohydrate. Patients who monitor their own blood glucose are finding that the postprandial hyperglycaemia is as much dependent on the type of carbohydrate as the amount. This allows them to learn from their experience and the information that they gather should prove most valuable.

Sulphonylureas

Sulphonylurea drugs have an established place in the treatment of those maturity onset diabetics in whom dietary advice fails to achieve normoglycaemia. The use of these drugs was questioned by the reports from the University Group Diabetes Programme (University Group Diabetes Programme, 1971) study which were widely reported in both the medical and lay press. The UGDP study reported that there was an excess of cardiovascular mortality, particularly myocardial infarction in maturity onset diabetic patients treated with tolbutamide compared with patients treated with diet alone. This resulted in the Federal Drug Administration issuing a warning on the use of sulphonylurea drugs and restrictions on the use of these drugs in many centres in the United States. The effect of the UDGP report on the prescribing of sulphonylureas in Europe was much less dramatic. Recently reassessment of the UGDP study data has revealed anomalies in patient selection and drop out rates, and have indicated a need for more critical review of the data and have also raised doubts over the original conclusions of the study (Policy Statement, 1979). Follow up of sulphonylurea treated patients in several other studies have revealed no excess mortality (Keen, Jarrett & Fuller, 1974) and the general view (at least outside the United States) is that the drugs retain an important place in management of the maturity onset diabetic.

Although sulphonylureas are generally believed to act mainly by stimulating further insulin secretion from the diabetic pancreas, there are those who believe they have important other actions such as an increase in insulin sensitivity due to increase in the number of insulin receptors since. Nattrass et al (1978a; 1978b) have found that increasing the dose of sulphonylurea can increase the hypoglycaemic effect without change in plasma insulin concentrations. However, it is generally agreed that they are ineffective in insulin-dependent patients. A recent cross-over study of sulphonyl-ureas and placebo in a group of patients who had failed to respond to dietary restriction alone, reaffirmed the importance of increased insulin secretion with sulphonylureas (Perkins et al, 1980). In this study treatment with active drug improved fasting blood glucose, glucose tolerance, insulin secretion as well as fatty acid or ketone body concentrations. The patients relapsed after four months on placebo but remitted with reintroduction of active drug. This study found chlorpropamide and glibenclamide to have similar effects.

Biguanides

The value of biguanides in the treatment of diabetes has been debated for several years and recently the use of phenformin in the United States has been restricted. The main reason for concern over the use of biguanides is the risk of development of lactic acidosis in biguanide-treated diabetic patients. Luft (1978) has reviewed 330 case reports of biguanide associated lactic acidosis. Published reports undoubtedly underestimate the true incidence since with more than 300 reported cases there is little cause to publish single observations. The majority, 281 of the 330 cases, were treated with phenformin at an average dose of 123 mg per day. Thirty were treated with buformin and 12 with metformin. Lactic acidosis occurred in older patients (average age 64 years) and it is therefore not surprising that many patients had additional cardiovascular and renal disease. The overall mortality was 50 per cent indicating that present treatment is unsatisfactory and that every effort should be made to avoid lactic acidosis.

Are all biguanides equally dangerous? It appears that metformin is less likely to produce lactic acidosis than phenformin since in France, where 76 per cent of biguanide treated patients receive metformin, only 14 per cent of reported cases of lactic acidosis occurred in metformin treated patients, the majority occurring during phenformin therapy.

The relative safety of metformin is also supported by the finding that blood lactate and pyruvate levels were higher during phenformin than in metformin therapy during both clinical use (Waters, Morgan, Wales, 1978) and during 12-hour metabolic studies in diabetic patients (Nattrass et al, 1977). The combination of sulphonylurea and biguanide produces similar abnormalities of lactate metabolism as biguanide alone (Nattrass et al, 1978a; 1978b). However, in studies in non-diabetic subjects the increase of blood lactate after alcohol, fructose and exercise was augmented to a similar degree by phenformin, metformin or buformin (Czyzyk et al, 1978). In conclusion some people feel that biguanides may still have a role in the treatment of certain maturity onset diabetics in whom sulphonylurea drugs are either ineffective or contraindicated. However, in the majority of such patients treatment with insulin may be a safer and more effective alternative to biguanide therapy. If a biguanide is to be used then metformin appears to be a safer drug but since it is excreted unchanged by the kidneys, renal function should be assessed before and during therapy. The use of phenformin is not justified as even with careful screening of patients for renal, cardiovascular and hepatic disease lactic acidosis may still occur.

Photocoagulation
Diabetic retinopathy is the most common cause of blindness in patients aged 30 to 64 years in Great Britain and as a cause of blindness in newly registered blind persons has risen from 7 per cent in 1955–1962 to 16 per cent in the years 1963–1968. Diabetic retinopathy can be divided into two types, background and proliferative. Background retinopathy occurs in 80 per cent of patients whose duration of diabetes exceeds 15 years and is characterised by microaneurysms, dot and blot haemorrhages, and hard exudates. This form of retinopathy may lead to visual deterioration when exudates and, or oedema occur in the area of the macula (maculopathy). Such changes have been found in 6 per cent of patients in a survey in a diabetic clinic (Donovan, 1978). Proliferative retinopathy characterised by the development of retinal new vessels was found in 4.4 per cent of patients in the same survey. The presence of new vessels heralds a poor prognosis, visual loss developing in 50 per cent of such patients over five years due to vitreous haemorrhage and retinal detachment.

The early recognition of patients with either maculopathy or proliferative retino-pathy has become very important since treatment of these conditions with Xenon-arc or Argon Laser photocoagulation has been shown to result in a better visual prognosis.

Two studies have compared the effects of photocoagulation in patients with maculopathy in whom only one of two similarly affected eyes in the same patient was treated (Patz, Schatz & Berkow, 1973; Multicentre study group, 1975). Both studies showed a significantly better visual acuity in the treated eye after an average of two years. However, this difference only occurred if the initial visual acuity was better than 6/24 in the British study and 6/36 in the American. These results emphasise the importance of regular assessment of visual acuity in all diabetics and referral to those patients whose visual acuity beings to deteriorate since the changes of macular oedema cannot be seen on indirect ophthalmoscopy. The results of photocoagulation of patients with proliferative retinopathy is even more impressive. Again two studies, American (Diabetic Retinopathy Study Research Group, 1976) and British (Multi-centre Study Group, 1977), compared treated and untreated eyes in the same patients. Both studies showed that treated eyes retained significantly better vision particularly when there were new vessels arising from around the optic disc when vitreous haemorrhage had occurred. These results imply that physicians caring for diabetic patients should be aware of the symptoms of vitreous haemorrhage (complaints of floaters or sudden deterioration of vision) and that regular ophthalmoscopic examination of the fundus should be carried out to detect early proliferation. Those patients with new vessels arising from the disc will probably benefit from treatment and those with peripheral new vessels require careful follow-up. Such careful examination of eyes must now become a routine for all those accepting the responsibility for long-term diabetic care. It requires regular measurement of visual acuity and indirect ophthalmoscopy usually with a dilated pupil. It is perhaps easiest to make the patient responsible for ensuring that someone competent does this at least once a year. The person performing the test will vary from place to place. The diabetic clinic probably providing the major service but ophthalmologists, general physicians, general practitioners and ophthalmic opticians need to be encouraged to participate in this daunting task.

REFERENCES

Alberti K G M M, Nattrass M 1978 Highly purified insulins. Diabetologia 15: 77–80
American Diabetes Association 1976 Policy statement — blood glucose control in diabetes. Diabetes 25: 237–239
Bottazzo G F, Mann J I, Thorogood M, Baum J D, Doniach D 1978a Autoimmunity in juvenile diabetics and their families. British Medical Journal ii: 165–167
Bottazzo G F, Cudworth A G, Moul D J, Doniach D, Fenenstein H 1978b Evidence for a primary autoimmune type of diabetes mellitus. British Medical Journal ii: 1253–1256
Brown P M, Tompkins C V, Juul S, Sönksen P H 1978 Mechanism of action of insulin in diabetic patients: a dose related effect on glucose production and utilisation. British Medical Journal i: 1239–1242
Brown P M, Juul S, Prestwich S, Sönksen P H 1980 The metabolic effects of infusions of a semisymethetic insulin, A_1-B_{29} dodecoyl insulin and native insulin in diabetic patients: In: Diabetes: Proceedings of the 10th Congress of the International Diabetes Federation. Excerpta Medica Amsterdam, in press
Buckle A L J, Nattrass M, Cluett B E, Stubbs W A, Walton R J, Alberti K G M M, Clemens A H 1977 Blood metabolite concentrations in diabetes: Effect of normalisation of blood glucose using a glucose controlled insulin infusion system (GCIIS). Diabetologia 13: 385 abstract p 385
Buxhard K, Madshad S, Rygaard J 1979 Passive transfer of diabetes mellitus from man to mouse. Lancet i: 908–910
Cudworth A G, Gamble D R, White G B B, Lendrum R, Woodrow J C, Bloom A 1977 Aetiology of diabetes. A prospective study. Lancet 1: 385–388
Cudworth A G 1978 Type I Diabetes Mellitus. Diabetologia 14: 281–291

Czyzk A, Lao B, Baitosiewicz W, Szcepanik Z, Orlowska K 1978 The effect of short term administration of antidiabetic biguanide derivatives on the blood lactate levels in healthy subjects. Diabetologia 14: 89–94

Dandona P, Freedman D, Moorhead J F 1979 Glycosylated haemoglobin in chronic renal failure. British Medical Journal 1: 1183–1184

Deckert T, Poulsen J E, Larsen M 1978a Prognosis of diabetes with diabetes onset before the age of thirty-one. I Survival, causes of death and complications. Diabetologia 14: 363–370

Deckert T, Poulsen J E, Larsen M 1978b Prognosis of diabetes with diabetes onset before the age of thirty one. II Factors influencing the prognosis. Diabetologia 14: 371–377

Diabetic Retinopathy Study Research Group 1976 Preliminary report on the effects of photocoagulation therapy. American Journal of Ophthalmology 81: 383–396

Donovan R J 1978 Prevalence of retinopathy in a diabetic clinic. British Medical Journal 1: 1441–1442

Editorial: 1979a Highly purified insulins. Lancet 1: 363–364

Editorial: 1979b New insulin infusion systems for diabetics. Lancet 1: 1275–77

Engerman R, Bloodworth J M B, Nelson S 1977 Relationship of microvascular disease in diabetes to metabolic control. Diabetes 26: 760–769

Eschwege E, Job D, Goyot-Argenton C, Aubry J P, Tchobroutsky C 1979 Delayed progression of diabetic retinopathy by divided insulin administration a further follow up. Diabetologia 16: 13–16

Fox C J, Darby S C, Ireland J T, Sönksen P H 1977 Blood glucose control and glomerular capillary basement membrane thickening in experimental diabetes. British Medical Journal 2: 605–607

Gonzalez-Villalpando C, Blackley J D, Vaughan G M, Smith J D 1979 Low and high dose intravenous insulin therapy for diabetic ketoacidosis. Journal of the American Medical Association 241: 925–927

Gonen B, Rubenstein A H, Rochamn H, Tanega S, Horwitz D L 1977 Haemoglobin Al: an indicator of the metabolic control of diabetic patients. Lancet ii: 734–737

Gonen B, Rubenstein A H 1978 Haemoglobin Al and diabetes mellitus. Diabetologia 15: 1–8

Gouldo T J, Alberti K G M M 1978 Dietary fibre and diabetes. Diabetologia 15: 285–288

Gray B N, Watkins E 1976 Prevention of vascular complications of diabetes by pancreatic islet transplantation. Archives of Surgery 111: 254–257

Gundersen H J G, Osterby R, Lundbaek K 1978 The basement membrane controversy. Diabetologia 15: 361–363

Hall S E H, Saunders J, Sönksen P H 1979 Glucose and free fatty acid turnover in normal subjects and in diabetic patients before and after treatment. Diabetologia 16: 297–306

Hoenig R J, Paterson C M V, Jones R L, Sandek C, Lehrmann M, Cerami A 1976 The correlation of glucose regulation and haemoglobin AlC in diabetes mellitus. New England Journal of Medicine 295: 417–420

Hung Cheng 1979 Photocoagulation and diabetic retinopathy. British Medical Journal i: 365–366

Irsigler K, Kritz H 1979 Long term continuous intravenous insulin therapy with a portable insulin dosage-regulating apparatus. Diabetes 28: 196–203

Jarrett R J, Keen H 1976 Hyperglycaemia and diabetes mellitus. Lancet ii: 1009–1012

Jarrett R J, Al Sayegh H 1978 Impaired glucose tolerance defining those at risk of diabetic complications. Diabetologia 15: 243 abstract p 243

Jarrett R J, Keen H, Fuller J H, McCartney M 1979 Worsening to diabetes in men with impaired glucose tolerance ('Borderline diabetics'). Diabetologia 16: 25–30

Jenkins D J A, Wolever T M S, Leeds A R, Gassull M A, Haisman P, Dilawari J, Goff D V, Metz G L, Alberti K G M M 1978a Dietary fibre, fibre analogues and glucose tolerance: importance of viscosity. British Medical Journal 2: 1392–1394

Jenkins D J A, Wolever T M S, Nineham R, Taylor R, Metz G L, Bacon S, Hockaday T D R 1978b. Guar crispbread in the diabetic diet. British Medical Journal 11: 1744–1746

Keen H, Jarrett R J, Fuller J H 1974 Tolbutamide and arterial disease in borderline diabetics: In: Diabetes Proceedings of the Eighth Congress of the International Diabetes Federation. Excerpta Medica Amsterdam, p 588

Keen H, Jarrett R J, Alberti K G M M 1979 (ed) Diabetes mellitus: a new look at diagnostic criteria. Diabetologia 16: 283–285

Keen H, Thomas B J, Jarrett R J, Fuller J H 1979 Energy intake adiposity and diabetes. British Medical Journal 1: 655–658

Kiehm T G, Anderson J W, Ward K 1976 Beneficial effect of a high carbohydrate high fibre diet on hyperglycaemic diabetic man. American Journal of Clinical Nutrition 29: 895–899

Luft D, Schmulling R M, Eggstein M 1978 Lactic acidosis in biguanide-treated diabetics. A review of 330 cases. Diabetologia 14: 75–87

Lutterman J A, Adriaansen A A J, van't Laar A 1979 Treatment of semi diabetic ketoacidosis. A comparative study of two methods. Diabetologia 17: 17–22

Multicentre study group 1975 Photocoagulation in treatment of diabetic maculopathy. Lancet 2: 1110–1113

Multicentre study group 1977 Proliferative diabetic retinopathy: treatment with Xenon-arc photocoagulation. British Medical Journal 1: 739–741

Munoz J M, Sandstead H H, Jacob R A 1979 Effects of dietary fibre on glucose tolerance of normal man. Diabetes 28: 496–502
Mustaffa B E, Daggett P R, Nabarro J D N 1977 Insulin binding capacity in patients changed from conventional to highly purified insulins. An indication of likely response. Diabetologia 13: 311–315
Nattrass M, Todd P G, Hinks L, Lloyd B, Alberti K G M M 1977 Comparative effects of phenformin, metformin and glibenclamide on metabolic rhythms in maturity onset diabetics. Diabetologia 13: 145–152
Nattrass M, Hinks L, Smythe P, Todd P G, Alberti K G M M 1978a Comparative effects of 2 doses of glibenclamide upon metabolic rhythms in maturity-onset diabetes. Diabete et Metabolisme 4: 175–180
Nattrass M, Todd P G, Turnell D, Alberti K G M M 1978b Metabolic abnormalities during combined sulphonylurea and phenformin therapy in maturity onset diabetics. Diabetologia 14: 389–395
Page M M, Alberti K G M M, Greenwood R, Gumaa K A, Hockaday T D R, Lowy C, Nabarro J D N, Pyke D A, Sönksen P H, Watkins P J, West T E T 1974 Treatment of daibetic coma with continuous low dose infusion of insulin. British Medical Journal 2: 687–690
Patz A, Schatz H, Berkow J W 1973 Macula oedema — an overlooked complication of diabetic retinopathy. Transactions of the American Academy of Ophthalmology and Otolaryngology 77: 34–42
Perkins J R, West T E T, Lowy C, Sönksen P H 1980 Hormonal and metabolic effects of chlorpropamide, glibenclamide and placebo in a cross-over study in diabetics not controlled by diet alone. Diabetologia, in press
Peterson C M, Jones R L, Koenig R J, Melvin E T, Lehrman M L 1977 Reversible haematologic sequelae of diabetes mellitus. Annals of Internal Medicine 86: 425–429
Pickup J C, Keen H, Parsons J A V, Alberti K G M M, Rowe A S 1979 Continuous subcutaneous insulin infusions: improved blood glucose and intermediary metabolic control in diabetes. Lancet i: 1255–58
Policy Statement 1979 The UDGP controversy. Diabetes 28: 165–170
Pyke D A 1977 Genetics of diabetes. In: Clinics in endocrinology and metabolism, vol 6, p 285–303
Simpson R W, Mann J I, Eaton J, Moore R A, Carter R, Hockaday T D R 1979 Improved glucose control in maturity onset diabetes treated with high carbohydrate modified fat diet. British Medical Journal 1: 1753–1756
Siperstein M D, Feingold K R, Bennet P H 1978 Hyperglycaemia and diabetic microaniography. Diabetologia 15 365–367
Sönksen P H, Srivastava M C, Tompkins C V, Nabarro J D N 1972 Growth hormone and cortisol responses to insulin infusion in patients with diabetes mellitus. Lancet ii: 155–159
Sönksen P H, Judd S L, Lowy C 1978 Home monitoring of blood glucose: Method for improving diabetic control. Lancet i: 729–732
Spicer K M, Allen R C, Hallett D, Buse M G 1969 Synthesis of haemoglobin AlC and related minor haemoglobins by erythrocytes. In vitro study of regulation. Journal of Clinical Investigation 64: 40–48
Tamberlane W V, Sherwin R S, Genel M, Felig P 1979a Restoration of normal lipid and amino acid metabolism in diabetic patients treated with a portable insulin-infusion pump. Lancet i: 1258–1261
Tamberlane W V, Sherwin R S, Genel M, Felig P 1979b Reduction to normal of plasma glucose in juvenile diabetes by subcutaneous administration of insulin with a portable infusion pump. New England Journal of Medicine 300: 573–578
Tattersall R B 1979 Home blood glucose monitoring. Diabetologia 16: 71–74
Tchobroutsky C 1978 Relation of diabetic control to development of microvascular complications. Diabetologia 15: 143–152
Trowell H C 1975 Dietary fibre hypothesis of the aetiology of diabetes mellitus. Diabetes 24: 762–764
University Group Diabetes Programme 1971 Effects of hypoglycaemic agents on vascular complications in patients with adult-onset diabetes. 111. Clinical implications of UGDP results. Journal of the American Medical Association 218: 1400–1410
Viberti G C, Pickup J C, Jarrett R J, Keen H 1979 Diabetic control and renal function. New England Journal of Medicine 300: 638–641
Walford S, Gale E A M, Allison S P, Tattersall R B 1979 Self monitoring of blood glucose: Improvement of diabetic control. Lancet i: 732–735
Waters A K, Morgan D B, Wales J K 1978 Blood lactate and pyruvate levels in diabetic patients treated with biguanides with and without sulphonylureas. Diabetologia 14: 95–98
West T E T, Hunter P R, Lowy C 1980 Self-monitoring of blood glucose during pregnancy. In: Diabetes: Proceedings of the 10th Congress of the International Diabetes Federation. Excerpta Medica, Amsterdam
Williamson J R, Kito C 1979 A common sense approach makes the basement membrane. Diabetologia 17, 129–132
Yoon J, Austin M, Onodera T, Al Notkins 1979 Virus-induced diabetes mellitus: insulation of a virus from the pancreas of a child with diabetic ketoacidosis. New England Journal of Medicine 300: 1173–1179
Yue D R, Turtle J R A 1975 Antigenicity of 'monocomponent' pork insulin in diabetic subjects. Diabetes 24: 625–32

15. Crohn's disease

D. P. O'Donoghue

Patients faced with a disease will invariably ask of it two questions: 'What is its cause?' and, 'What is the "cure"?' Regretably, as regards Crohn's disease, despite almost 50 years of worldwide attention and research, the answer to both questions is unknown. Advances in our knowledge of Crohn's disease have involved what might be called the periphery. For example, recent epidemiological studies have clearly documented the increasing incidence of Crohn's disease; the occurrence and presentation of the disease in the very young and old is now recognised; and the very limitation of present-day medical and surgical treatment is better understood. These features and a number of other related topics discussed in this chapter may be of little consolation to the patient with Crohn's disease today, but they nevertheless represent advances in our understanding of this troublesome disease and merit attention in the hope that the extension of one or more of these ideas may lead to the vital clue(s) and an answer to the patient's questions.

The classical presenting symptoms, radiological findings and pathological features of Crohn's disease are well described in a number of major textbooks and are beyond the scope of this chapter.

DEFINITION

Crohn's disease may be defined as a chronic inflammatory condition, classically remitting and relapsing, involving any part of the gastrointestinal tract from mouth to anus. Histologically, the chronic inflammatory response is characteristically submucosal or transmural and may be patchy or focal. The presence of non-caseating granulomata or fissure ulcers are considered pathognomonic, but not essential for the diagnosis. Crohn's disease, thus defined, relies heavily on histological criteria, yet often a diagnosis must be entertained in the absence of suitable biopsy material. Although there are a number of clinical and radiological 'pointers' in Crohn's disease, no clinician enjoys making a 'diagnosis of faith'.

The definition of a disease whose cause is unknown is, of its nature, arbitrary and limiting. These limitations apply not only to the categorisation of disease complexes but to the very thought processes behind them. Crohn's disease provides a perfect example of this problem: Crohn, Ginzburg & Oppenheimer (1932) in their initial paper established the terminal ileum as the epicentre of the disease and this was to blinker for years the views of many workers in this field. Although Crohn's disease involving parts of the small bowel other than the terminal ileum was quickly recognised, it was almost 30 years before Crohn's disease of the colon achieved recognition (Lockhart-Mummery & Morson, 1960). Crohn's colitis had been well described long before this but, by definition, could not exist (Dalziel, 1913; Wells, 1952). The problems of definition are well reviewed by Scadding (1959).

NOMENCLATURE

Eponyms do not find favour in medicine today, but Crohn's disease is worthy to be an exception to the rule. Terminal ileitis, regional enteritis, transmural colitis and granulomatous colitis are but a number of terms used to describe Crohn's disease, yet none are adequate. Terminal ileitis has causes other than Crohn's disease and regional enteritis is a term generally regarded as being confined to the small bowel. Transmural or granulomatous colitis are misleading terms in that it implies the disease must invariably be accompanied by specific histological features. The simple use of the words 'Crohn's disease —' followed by a brief anatomical description of the involved areas is preferable, e.g. Crohn's disease of the terminal ileum and anorectal region. Such a descriptive term is neither restrictive to any part of the gastrointestinal tract nor presumptive of a certain pathological process. This eponym has long found favour in the United Kingdom and it is hoped is now achieving similar recognition in the United States (Schachter & Kirsner, 1975).

EPIDEMIOLOGY

Crohn's disease occurs on a worldwide basis but is most commonly seen and reported from Western Europe, Scandinavia and the North Eastern United States. Although still a relatively rare disorder, recent European surveys indicate an alarming increase in the incidence of this disorder (Miller, Keighley & Langman, 1974; Brahme Lindstrom & Wenckert, 1975; Smith et al, 1975; Mayberry, Rhodes & Hughes, 1979). Thus the study in the Nottingham area showed a 5-fold increase over a 13-year period (Miller et al, 1974) whilst the most recent of these reports from Cardiff tells of a 25-fold increase over a longer period of time. An incidence rate of approximately 5 from the Nottingham and Cardiff studies means that there are 2500 new cases of Crohn's disease each year in England and Wales assuming a population of 50 000 000. Working with a prevalence rate of 20 per 100 000 (probably a modest estimate) there are approximately 10 000 patients with this disease at any one time in England and Wales.

Crohn's disease occurs in both sexes and most studies show a bimodal distribution with the first peak occurring in the 20s and 30s and a later one in the 60–70 year old age group. An interesting feature to emerge from many recent studies and one first noted by Kyle (1971) in his epidemiological work in north-east Scotland is that this later peak is largely composed of females with Crohn's colitis. The inference of this is as yet unknown.

Variations in the incidence of a disease in different racial or ethnic groups within a defined population are difficult to assess, not least because the availability of medical services may differ within the groups. Even allowing for this it appears that Crohn's disease is more common amongst Jews than non-Jewish whites in the United States (Acheson, 1960) and similarly it is more common amongst non-Jewish whites compared to non-whites in the same country (Monk et al, 1969). The fact that racial or ethnic groupings is not the sole determinant of this disease is well demonstrated by a recent survey of Crohn's disease in Israel (Rozen et al, 1979). Contrary to expectations (though not those of the author's) the incidence of Crohn's disease was less than 2 per 100 000 in Tel-Aviv. Within this group, the disease was seen more frequently in Ashkenazi (mostly immigrants and their descendents from the United

States or Europe) than in the non-Ashkenazi Jew. Similarly, Crohn's disease has only been recently recognised among the West Indian population in Britain (O'Donoghue & Clarke, 1976) and further studies comparing the incidence rates of this disease in immigrants and the indigenous population of the UK might be rewarding. Miller and colleagues (1974) have pointed out that the true value of epidemiological studies may not be discovered until extensive work is carried out in areas of low disease frequency. Similar epidemiological work on multiple sclerosis has led to the present intensive search for an infective cause.

HISTOLOGY

Two histological features of Crohn's disease, one new and one old, have received considerable attention over the past decade, namely the aphthoid ulcer and the granuloma.

Aphthoid ulcer

Recent years have seen the addition of the aphthoid ulcer to the classical histological description of Crohn's disease (Blackburn, Hadfield & Hunt, 1939). These ulcers, widely but not universally accepted as part of the disease, represents minute areas of inflammation over lymph follicles and may be the earliest histological feature of Crohn's disease (Morson, 1972). The significance of these ulcers as regards the pathogenesis of the disease is not clear, but they can, as will be discussed, be a useful diagnostic marker.

The granuloma

The cause and significance of granuloma formation remain as puzzling as the disease. Spector & Heesom (1968) have shown that antigen-antibody complexes formed in the presence of antibody excess may lead to granuloma formation; but although immune complexes are found in the sera of some patients with Crohn's disease (Doe, Booth & Brown, 1973) the exact conditions of Spector & Heesom's work have not yet been shown to exist. Ward (1977) has proposed that the granuloma, and Crohn's disease itself, result from defective macrophage function and that this may be the final common pathway to a number of agents capable of triggering Crohn's disease in susceptible individuals. Defective migration of neutrophils has been shown in Crohn's disease (Segal & Loewi, 1976), but whether this is cause or effect is unknown.

Does granuloma formation affect the course and prognosis of Crohn's disease? Although Assarsson & Raf (1974) could find no difference between patients with or without granuloma formation, two recent reports have suggested that the occurrence of granuloma is beneficial as regards prognosis. (Glass & Baker, 1976; Chambers & Morson, 1979). These last named authors feel that the granuloma may represent 'an adaptive mechanism for the removal or localisation of the causative agent of Crohn's disease'. Further studies on granuloma formation may well prove rewarding.

AETIOLOGY

Although the cause of Crohn's disease remains unknown, the 1970s have seen a veritable explosion in the interest paid to a number of possible aetiological factors, some of which deserve closer attention.

1. A transmissible agent

The possibility that Crohn's disease might be caused by a transmissible agent received renewed interest over the past decade following the works of Mitchell & Rees (1970) who induced granuloma formation in the foot pads of eight mice inoculated with homogenates of Crohn's disease tissue. Two of these mice later developed granulomatous change in the bowel wall of the terminal ileum. The same workers then managed to induce granulomata in mice inoculated with homogenates prepared from the original foot pad granulomata and this 'passage' suggested a transmissible agent. Cave and his colleagues in 1973, produced similar granulomatous changes in the bowel wall of a number of New Zealand white rabbits by the intraileal inoculation of the same Crohn's disease homogenate. These transmission experiments were supported by the work of Sachar, Taub & Janowitz (1976). Cave, Mitchell & Brooke (1975) then managed to induce ileal granulomata by the intravenous inoculation of the homogenate. The agent in all these experiments survived passage through an $0.2\,\mu$ filter but was destroyed by autoclaving. What is this 'transmissible agent'? There are currently two popular theories:

A. VIRAL

Support for a viral theory came from Los Angeles where Gitnick, Arthur & Shibata (1976), using continuous rabbit ileum as a sensitive tissue culture line, isolated cytopathic agents from each of four Crohn's disease specimens. Electronmicroscopic appearances suggested a small RNA virus. In 1977, Whorwell et al in Vermont isolated a reovirus-like agent from 6 of 10 resected Crohn's disease specimens. This isolation, as the authors point out, does not necessarily imply a causal relationship.

B. CELL WALL DEFICIENT (CWD) BACTERIA

Cell wall deficient (CWD) bacteria, by their nature, are also able to squeeze through a $0.2\,\mu$ filter. This knowledge has led to an intensive search in very recent times for such organisms. Using hypertonic culture media (conventional isotonic media are unsuitable) Parent & Mitchell (1978) isolated CWD bacteria from homogenised tissues of all eight Crohn's disease patients they studied. These bacteria reverted to their 'parent form' on subculture and were identified as pseudomonas-like organisms. Burnham and his colleagues in London (1978) have also queried a role for CWD bacteria in Crohn's disease. These workers, in a search for mycobacteria, isolated a strain of *Mycobacterium Kansasii* from a mesenteric lymph node of one of 27 patients undergoing bowel resection for Crohn's disease — in isolation an unexciting finding. However, skin testing with an extract prepared from this mycobacterium showed that whereas only 20 per cent of a control population gave a positive result, almost 50 per cent of patients with Crohn's disease reacted, a difference not mirrored by a large number of other mycobacteria so tested. Although no other mycobacteria were isolated, Burnham and his colleagues, using hypertonic media, isolated organisms that appeared under the electron microscope to be cell wall deficient from 22 of 27 Crohn's cultures, 7 of 13 ulcerative colitis cultures and just one of 11 control samples.

On this evidence, the case for a transmissible agent would appear to be very strong. The drawbacks in these experiments, however, are well outlined by Sachar & Auslander (1978). The fact that not all workers can reproduce the findings of those in London and New York is perhaps worrying (Heatley et al, 1975), but the ability of others to do so using diseased *or normal* tissues and to prevent this with antibiotics is more alarming (Donnelly, Delaney & Healy, 1977) and must cast some doubt on the interpretation of transmission experiments.

2. *Tuberculosis*

Tuberculosis ought to be mentioned among the list of possible infective causes, not because of any new or exciting evidence, but because as long as the aetiology of Crohn's disease is unknown, this ubiquitous organism should not be forgotten. Fielding (1972), noting that Crohn's disease followed in the wake of intestinal tuberculosis in much the same way that sarcoidosis followed the decline in respiratory tuberculosis, put forward the hypothesis that 'host resistant' was the deciding factor on whether an individual got Crohn's disease, intestinal tuberculosis or no disease at all following exposure of the intestinal tract to the bacillus. Although there is no evidence to support this hypothesis a precedent exists in our knowledge of leprosy where in the tuberculous variety of the disease it is often very difficult to isolate the mycobacterium leprae. Despite Hansen's discovery of the bacillus a century ago it still cannot be grown on artificial media. The tubercle bacillus cannot, by definition, be found in Crohn's disease as this would change the diagnostic label.

If Crohn's disease has an infective aetiology, one might expect to find evidence of clustering of cases in time and space. Miller and colleagues have looked in vain for such evidence using both the time — space clustering analysis of Knox & Pike and the case contagion method of Pike & Smith (Miller et al, 1975 and 1976). However, these methods as the authors point out, would not exclude a disease with a long incubation period or a condition that is a rare response to a common infection.

3. *Genetic factors*

Almy & Sherlock (1966) have calculated that the probability of a chance familial occurrence of inflammatory bowel disease is one in a 1 000 000 for ulcerative colitis and one in 25 000 000 for Crohn's disease. Yet familial inflammatory bowel disease is not rare and in a prospective study from Chicago a positive family history was documented in 113 of 646 patients (17.5 per cent), the highest familial incidence so far recorded (Singer et al, 1971). In this study, first degree relatives were more commonly affected than second or third degree relatives, a pattern fitting the theory of polygenic inheritance. Similar findings have been noted by others (Goligher et al, 1968).

Usually one proband has the disease. Numberous reports exist, however, where two or more members of the same family are affected (Kirsner & Spencer, 1963; Sherlock et al, 1963) and indeed a recent report has recorded mixed inflammatory bowel disease in *all* three members of one family (Rosenberg, Kraft & Kirsner, 1976). This last mentioned study is one of only two documented reports of the disease occurring in both husband and wife (Whorwell et al, 1978) and the rarity of this situation is a strong argument against those who believe that familial occurrences could be explained by an environmental factor alone.

The problem of genes versus the environment is well reviewed by Lewkonia & McConnell (1976) who list four possible explanations for familial aggregation of cases: (1) random chance, (2) the effect of shared environment, (3) the effects of shared genes, and (4) the effects of shared genes controlling the response to shared environmental influences. While disposing of the first two possibilities on the grounds of the extreme rarity of the disease in the spouse of an affected patient, the authors feel that 'environmental factors . . . must be envoked to account for the apparent increase in the incidence of inflammatory bowel disease in the last few decades: the genes in a population would not change to any appreciable extent during such a short time'. In summary, it would appear that genetic factors must be invoked to explain the frequency which familial inflammatory bowel disease is noted and the rarity of its occurrence in the spouse of a patient while environmental factors must be invoked to explain the increasing incidence of the disease in recent years.

4. Immunological aspects

A major criticism of all reported immunological studies in Crohn's disease is the absence of suitable controls: none of the publications have included appreciable numbers of 'sick controls', e.g. patients with *specific* inflammatory bowel disease such as amoebic dysentery or diverticulitis. Those studies that have included small numbers of these patients have yielded results not dissimilar from patients with Crohn's disease or ulcerative colitis (Lagercrantz et al, 1966; Watson, Quigley & Bolt, 1966a). Thus, even the most elegant study leaves one with a question — Is the result cause or effect?

Immunological studies in Crohn's disease are plagued with inconsistencies but one aspect that has been readily reproducible in a number of centres involves cell cytotoxicity. In 1963, Pearlmann & Broberger showed that the circulating leucocytes from patients with inflammatory bowel disease were cytotoxic for human colonic cells grown in tissue culture. This work was confirmed by Watson and colleagues, who showed that the likely effector cell was the lymphocyte (Watson, Quigley & Bolt, 1966b). In 1970, workers in the Mayo Clinic made the fascinating observation that 'normal' lymphocytes could be made cytotoxic for colonic epithelial cells by incubating them with serum from patients with inflammatory bowel disease (Shorter et al, 1970). Stobo and colleagues have suggested that the non-T, non-B killer cell is the effector lymphocyte in this system (Stobo et al, 1976) and Thayer (1976) has postulated that immune complexes are the triggering mechanism. Although it may be difficult to implicate these mechanisms in the aetiology of Crohn's disease because of the problems mentioned above they may, nevertheless, be of importance in the pathogenesis of the disease and further work in this area of cell cytotoxicity might lead to a more rational form of treatment.

5. Diet

The possible role of diet in the aetiology or pathogenesis of Crohn's disease has received little attention considering the disorder involves the gastrointestinal tract. No doubt the bewildering variety of foodstuffs ingested wittingly and unwittingly in society today deters many workers. Recent studies from Bristol may help fill this void and, if confirmed, lighten the gloom that surrounds the present treatment of the disease: Thornton, Emmett & Heaton (1979) analysed the pre-illness diet of 30 newly diagnosed patients with Crohn's disease and prepared them with 30 well-matched controls. They found that the patients had a diet that was high in refined sugar and low in raw fruit and vegetables and they suggested that this may favour the development of the disease. In a second study, the same group of workers showed that patients placed on a fibre-rich, unrefined-carbohydrate diet in addition to conventional treatment faired significantly better than matched patients who were given similar treatment but no dietary instruction (Heaton, Thornton & Emmett, 1979). Confirmation of this work will be eagerly awaited.

CLINICAL ASPECTS

Investigations
Recent advances in the investigation of the patient with Crohn's disease are confined to improvements or extensions of existing traditional methods.

Sigmoidoscopy and rectal biopsy
Sigmoidoscopy remains a vital procedure in the investigation of any patient with suspected Crohn's disase, and a rectal biopsy may be diagnostic even in the presence of normal sigmoidoscopic appearances (Dyer, Stansfeld & Dawson, 1970). Although proximity to the rectum improves the yield of diagnostic histology in these circumstances, 5 per cent of patients with isolated small bowel disease will have proof of Crohn's disease on a random rectal biopsy (Hill, Kent & Hansen, 1979). This low pick-up rate must be weighed against the ease of the procedure and the difficult differential diagnosis that small bowel Crohn's disease may present (see below).

Colonoscopy
Colonoscopy, the most useful of the new endoscopic procedures, can play a definite but defined role in the investigation of patients with inflammatory bowel disease. Classification and extent of disease is best outlined by sigmoidoscopy, rectal biopsy and barium enema and the colonoscope should be reserved for those few patients with convincing symptoms, but negative investigations. The ability to take biopsies from the caecum and terminal ileum via colonscopy may be of considerable value in the differential diagnosis of patients with predominantly ileocaecal disease (see below).

Barium studies

Small bowel. The barium follow-through examination remains the most important means of assessing the small bowel. Intubation and direct installation of barium and air into the small bowel (small bowel enema) is a useful procedure if short strictures, often missed by routine methods, are suspected. Definition of the terminal ileum may be improved by the inflation of air per rectum at the barium follow-through examination.

Large bowel. However, it is the barium enema that has undergone greatest change in recent years. The use of air contrast, the double contrast barium enema (D.C.B.E.) has greatly increased the diagnostic yield of this procedure as is well shown in Figure 15.1. This barium enema shows numerous aphthous ulcers which, as was discussed above, may be a characteristic of Crohn's disease. Note also that in the lower half of this X-ray, one can see through three overlapping layers of large bowel. It is likely that this colon would have been adjudged normal if inspected with a single contrast enema. The D.C.B.E. is now a routine procedure in most major centres within the UK and is better tolerated by patients than the older version, presumably because of the smaller

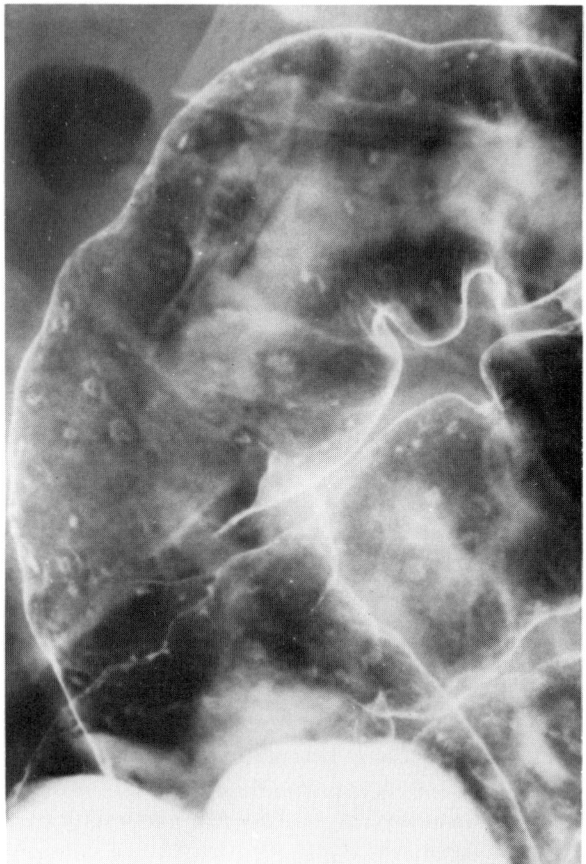

Fig. 15.1 D.C.B.E. — numerous aphthous ulcers in Crohn's colitis.

amounts of barium used. The single contrast barium enema is dead and deserves to be buried.

Patients with severe diarrhoea will usually have an empty colon and it is both dangerous and unnecessary to prepare the bowel for contrast studies. The careful introduction of a little barium and the subsequent rotation of the patient on the X-ray table can give considerable information as regards the extent of the inflammatory process (the unprepared or 'instant' enema).

The plain abdominal X-ray
This procedure is simple, safe, but often forgotten yet the amount of information it yields may be considerable. Inspection of the gas pattern may show a thickened and irregular wall in a bowel that is devoid of faecal material. Conversely, it can be assumed that in areas where faeces are seen the bowel wall is not severely involved in the inflammatory process. Repeated plain abdominal X-rays are imperative for all patients with severe 'colitic' symptoms in order to detect perforation (often masked by corticosteroid treatment) and to look for the development of a toxic megacolon.

Differential diagnosis
The differential diagnosis of Crohn's disease is potentially enormous given that the disease may present with any of its extraintestinal manifestations. This chapter will consider only gastrointestinal disorders that may be confused with Crohn's disease and these are listed in Table 15.1. Apart from the ubiquitous tubercle bacillus, there is probably no other condition that need be considered in the patient with *discontinuous* small *and* large bowel disease.

Table 15.1 Differential diagnosis of Crohn's disease according to site of involvement

Small bowel	Ileocaecal	Large bowel	
Lymphoma	Tuberculosis	Ulc. colitis	
Tuberculosis	Amoebiasis	Ischaemia	Important
	Neoplasia	Diverticulitis	
		Amoebiasis	
Radiation damage	Yersinia	Tuberculosis	
Chronic ulceration		Yersinia	Uncommon
Jejunoileitis		Behçet's	
Scleroderma		Salmonella	

Small bowel disease
The radiological features of small bowel Crohn's disease may be divided into stenotic and non-stenotic. The differential diagnosis of the former type includes tuberculosis, carcinoid tumour, radiation damage and chronic ulcerative jejunoileitis. A laparotomy may be required occasionally before a definite diagnosis can be established and this is particularly advisable in patients coming from areas where intestinal tuberculosis is endemic. Figure 15.2 shows a typical example of the non-stenotic variety of small bowel Crohn's disease and must be distinguished from an intestinal lymphoma. A peroral jejunal biopsy may be helpful in diagnosing the latter, but here again, a diagnostic laparotomy may be required.

Ileocaecal disease
Tuberculosis, amoebiasis and carcinoma of the caecum are the three conditions that may readily mimic Crohn's disease in this area. Again, tuberculosis must be the first condition considered in the immigrant population in the United Kingdom. The problem of amoebiasis is discussed below. As mentioned above, colonscopy may be reassuring both for patient and doctor in those cases not requiring surgery.

Large bowel disease

CROHN'S DISEASE VS ULCERATIVE COLITIS
The differentiation of ulcerative colitis from Crohn's disease *confined* to the large bowel may at times prove impossible (Lennard-Jones, Lockhart-Mummery & Morson, 1968; Schachter et al, 1970). To assess the value of various clinical parameters O'Donoghue and colleagues studied 54 consecutive patients with non-specific inflammatory disease of the large bowel and found that 11 patients with a final diagnosis of Crohn's disease had sigmoidoscopic appearances 'typical' of ulcerative colitis, while 7 had radiological features indistinguishable from ulcerative colitis

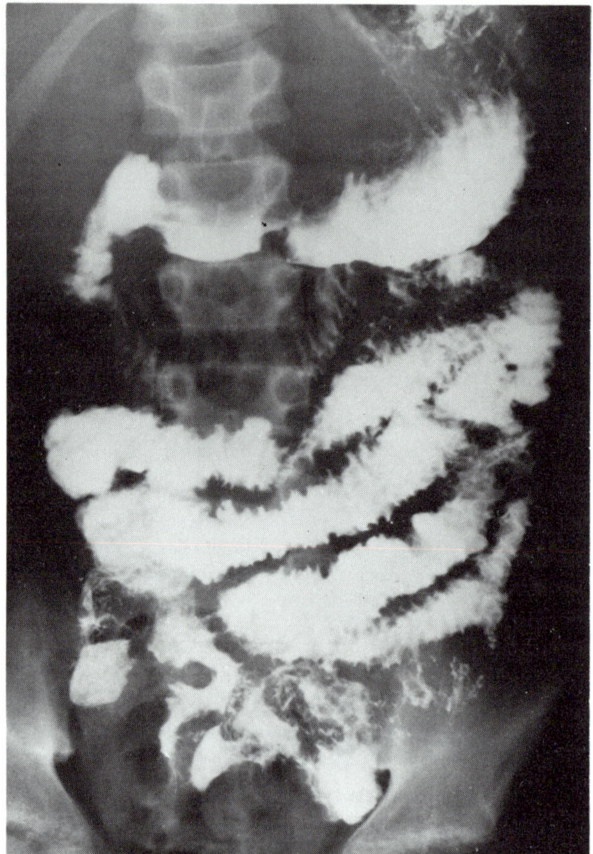

Fig. 15.2   Barium follow-through — non-stenotic Crohn's disease of the entire small bowel.

(O'Donoghue et al, 1979). Because of these findings, the authors concluded that the diagnosis of ulcerative colitis ought to be based on histological criteria. A positive diagnosis of Crohn's colitis is more easily made and those features which are strongly suggestive of the disorder are listed in Table 15.2.

Table 15.2   Clinical or radiological features suggestive of Crohn's disease

1. Enterocutaneous or enteroenteric fistulae

2. Chronic destructive anal lesions

3. Skip lesions

4. Deep ulceration ($>3\,\mathrm{mm}$)

5. Aphthous ulceration

6. Rectal sparing

CROHN'S DISEASE VS DIVERTICULAR DISEASE
Diverticular disease is common in the western world and diverticulitis may present not only with abdominal pain and diarrhoea, but may also produce stricture formation and fistulae. The problem in differentiation arises when Crohn's disease is largely confined to the sigmoid colon. Because of the increasing incidence of Crohn's disease in the elderly it is not surprising to find that the two diseases can coexist. Meyers and colleagues have recently reviewed the problems that may arise when these two conditions concur (Meyers et al, 1978).

CROHN'S DISEASE VS ISCHAEMIC COLITIS
Ischaemic colitis may mimic Crohn's disease but its presentation is usually more acute and blood loss more profound. In the acute phase thumb printing may be seen on plain abdominal X-rays or on a barium enema and in the chronic phase smooth stricture formation, often of considerable length, may develop.

CROHN'S DISEASE VS SPECIFIC INFECTIONS

Amoebiasis. Amoebiasis may present in an identical fashion to Crohn's colitis and the finding of ulcers on proctoscopy may appear to confirm the latter diagnosis. Although this disease is seen mainly in people living or visiting the tropics or subtropics sporadic cases have occurred in the UK in which there was no history of travel. Diagnosis is made by finding the trophozoites in a fresh stool specimen or a rectal swab or biopsy. It is vital to examine all specimens rapidly as the organisms lose their motility when cooled below body temperature. Ingestion of red blood cells by the trophozoites confirms the invasiveness of the amoeba. Fluorescent antibody tests in serum are available, but, unfortunately, are of more use in cases of amoeboma or amoebic liver abscess.

Salmonella. Inflammation of the colon due to salmonella infection may be impossible to distinguish by sigmoidoscopy, radiology or histology from non-specific inflammatory bowel disease. Schofield, Mandal & Ironside (1979) in a recent report remind us of the importance of stool cultures in all patients with a diarrhoeal illness *even* if they are known to have ulcerative colitis or Crohn's disease. These authors report four patients with salmonella colitis presenting as an acute toxic dilatation of the colon. Travel abroad may alert one to the possibility of infection but two of the four cases they report had no such history.

Yersinia. It has recently been recognised that yersinia infections may, in addition to acute terminal ileitis, cause a colitis that presents with aphthoid ulcers (Vantrappen et al, 1977). There is no evidence that yersinia infections are being misdiagnosed as acute Crohn's colitis within the UK (Swarbrick et al, 1979).
    The importance of searching for specific infections cannot be stressed too much. Most of these infections will respond well to appropriate antibiotics whereas corticosteroid treatment of surgery is dangerous and inappropriate.

Crohn's disease in children
Increasing numbers of children with Crohn's disease is the inevitable outcome of the epidemiological trends mentioned above. Atypical presentations add to a diagnostic

problem that is relatively new to paediatricians and physicians. Unexplained fever and retardation of growth and sexual development are not uncommon manifestations of the disease in children (Burbige, Huang & Bayliss, 1975; O'Donoghue & Dawson, 1977; Gryboski & Spiro, 1978). It comes as little surprise therefore that a disorder which has many diagnostic pitfalls in adults (Dyer & Dawson, 1970) should prove even more troublesome in children. In a recent British study of childhood Crohn's disease the mean time from onset of symptoms to diagnosis was almost three years and failure to consider the diagnosis was the principal cause for this delay (O'Donoghue & Dawson, 1977).

The response of Crohn's disease in children to medical and surgical treatment is depicted in Figure 15.3, taken from O'Donoghue & Dawson's study. This shows cumulative relapse rates for children treated medically or surgically of approximately 80 per cent and 60 per cent respectively at 6 years. Thus the natural history is disappointingly similar to that seen in adults (see below). Further analysis of Figure 15.3 reveals one very important point that may be particularly relevant to children. This concerns the median relapse time (MRT) which is the time taken for 50 per cent of the group to relapse. The MRT in these children was a mere 16 months following medical treatment but was 48 months following surgery. This time 'bought' by surgery will get many of these young people through the growth spurt of puberty and the formative years of their education, factors which far outweight the inevitability of a recurrence.

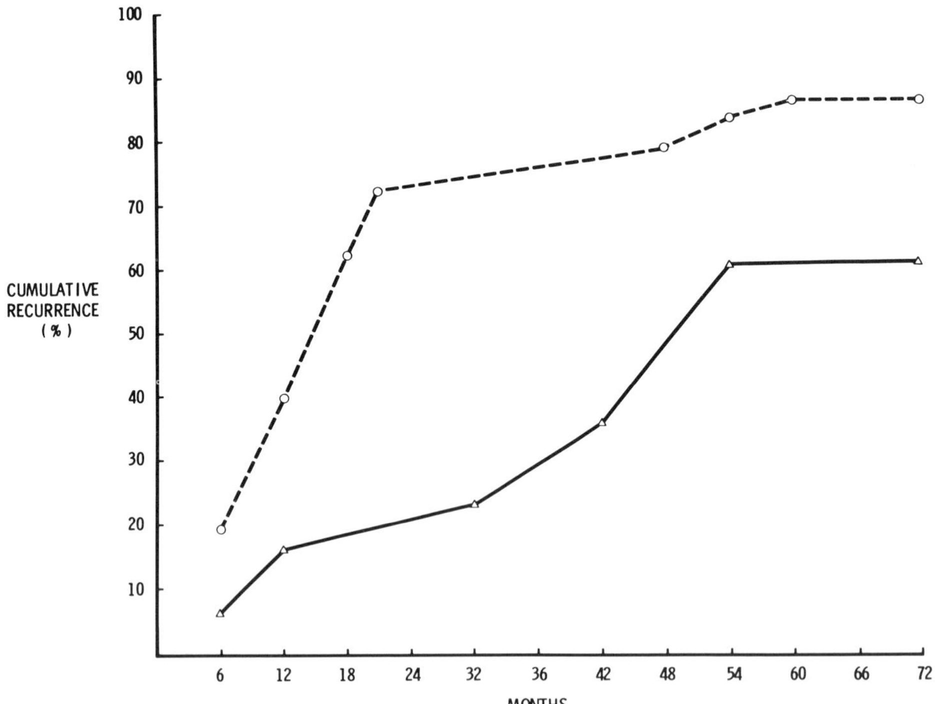

Fig. 15.3   Relapse rate after medical treatment. MRT 16 months O----O, relapse rate after surgery, MRT 48 months △———△. (Reproduced by kind permission of The Archives of Diseases in Childhood.)

Growth retardation

The realisation that growth retardation is a frequent complication of childhood Crohn's disease has stimulated considerable interest in its cause and treatment. The site of disease involvement is irrelevant as growth stunting is seen with equal frequency whether the small or large bowel is affected (Farmer, Hawk & Turnbull, 1975). Initial impressions that the problem resulted from inadequate growth hormone release has been discounted by recent detailed endocrine studies (Gryboski & Spiro, 1978; Kirschner, Voinchet & Rosenberg, 1978). Corticosteroid therapy may contribute to growth retardation in a few individuals, but clearly is not the major cause of this complication which is often present by the time the patient first presents. Indeed suppression of disease activity with corticosteroids may be followed by a growth spurt. Malabsorption is a rare occurrence of Crohn's disease and does not explain this failure of growth. Malnutrition, however, occurs more frequently and may be a major contributing factor in many children with this problem.

Kelts and colleagues (1979), using parenteral nutrition as a supplement to oral intake, markedly increased the growth velocity in six of seven children with growth retardation secondary to Crohn's disease. However, all seven children had inactive disease at the time of entry into the study and it is by no means certain whether children with active disease would respond in a similar manner. Nevertheless studies such as this emphasise the importance of an adequate calorie intake both before and after suppression of disease by routine methods.

Growth retardation is a problem that must be actively sought in childhood Crohn's disease by the use of sensitive indices such as growth velocity curves and when found attention must be paid to the provision of an adequate calorie intake and the suppression of disease activity by medical or surgical means as appropriate. If these methods fail or prove inappropriate (e.g. extensive small bowel disease) supplemental or parenteral nutrition ought to be considered.

Natural history and management

Natural history

The remitting and relapsing nature of Crohn's disease is now well established and is emphasised by the examination of the placebo-treated patients in a recent large American study. Mekhjian and colleagues have shown that 32 per cent of untreated patients might be expected to achieve a spontaneous remission within four months and half of these will remain well over a two-year period (Mekhjian et al, 1979). The same study showed that patients with inactive Crohn's disease who were treated with placebo experienced a 28 per cent relapse rate at one year and 41 per cent at the end of two years. It is against figures such as these that the effects of treatment must be compared.

Medical management

General. Bed rest, nutritional support, and the replacement of fluid and blood loss are important in the general management of any patient with severe inflammatory bowel disease. Antidiarrhoeal agents may be useful in mild disease and sedation can be helpful for the frightened patient. Analgesia is sometimes necessary but the use of strong analgesia should question the need for a surgical opinion: severe pain in Crohn's disease may indicate a perforation or intestinal obstruction.

Corticosteroids. Retrospective studies had shown that corticosteroids were of use in inducing a remission in Crohn's disease but were of little benefit in maintaining one (Hywel-Jones & Lennard-Jones, 1966; Cooke & Fielding, 1970) and this has now been confirmed in a large prospective study (Summers et al, 1979). The failure of corticosteroids to maintain a remission has led to a search for other drugs and it is here that the controversy begins.

Sulphasalazine. Sulphasalazine is of undoubted value as a prophylactic measure in ulcerative colitis, but its use in Crohn's disease has never been adequately proven. This however may be partly explained by the *misuse* of the drug in Crohn's disease. There is now evidence that sulphasalazine is split by colonic bacteria into sulphapyridine and 5-aminosalicylic acid (Goldman & Peppercorn, 1975) and the latter ingredient might be the active constituent of the drug (Azad Khan, Piris & Truelove, 1977). Thus it is possible that sulphasalazine is inactive until it reaches the colon and this may explain the negative results from earlier studies in Crohn's disease where the vast majority of the patients had predominently small bowel disease (Anthonisen et al, 1974; Bergman & Krause, 1976; a Multicentre Trial, 1977). Thus it is interesting that the recent American report suggested a role for the drug in the acute stage of large bowel Crohn's disease but, surprisingly, the same study failed to show any benefit when the drug was used as maintenance treatment (Summers et al, 1979). This drug deserves further study in Crohn's colitis.

Azathioprine. The value of this drug in the management of patients with Crohn's disease is also controversal but, as with corticosteroids, recent studies have helped define its role in this condition. Control studies have consistently failed to show any value for the drug when used alone in the acute condition despite earlier uncontrolled reports to the contrary. However, recent studies have indicated that azathioprine (2 mg/kg body wt/day) may be effective maintenance treatment for certain patients with Crohn's disease but as yet there is no way of predicting which patients will benefit (Willoughby et al, 1971; Rosenberg et al, 1975; O'Donoghue et al, 1978).

Nutritional

The use of 'bowel rest' by means of elemental (no-residue) diets or total parenteral nutrition (TPN) is attractive and, although early reports are encouraging, the numbers involved are very small. Elemental diets are still unpalatable and patients already anorectic because of their disease, often have difficulty in taking them. TPN is not without serious risk and this hazardous procedure should only be carried out by experienced clinicians with an interest in this field (Powell-Tuck et al, 1978). Some unfortunate patients with extensive small bowel Crohn's disease or with a short bowel syndrome following repeated resections may require elemental diets or TPN on a long-term basis and in these selected cases parenteral nutrition may be organised within the home (Fleming, McGill & Berkner, 1977).

Surgery and its indications

The surgeon, like the physician cannot cure Crohn's disease and recent years have seen the use of more conservative surgery. Nowadays microscopic clearance of diseased bowel is no longer advocated and this policy ought to reduce the number of iatrogenic short bowel syndromes. Bypass surgery is another procedure in Crohn's disease that is rarely practised today. One important exception to this rule is when the disease involves the duodenum. Here bypass surgery is not only followed by excellent results but saves the patient from difficult and dangerous surgery (Warren Nugent, Richmond & Park, 1977). The limitations of surgery are well depicted by Greenstein and his colleagues (1975) who have shown a cumulative reoperation rate of 89 per cent by the 15th year after the initial operation and an overall clinical recurrence rate of 94 per cent 15 years on. Thus surgery in Crohn's disease is reserved for patients who have been failed by medical treatment or who have developed the classical complications of strictures, fistulae, toxic megacolon (not the prerogative of ulcerative colitis) or perforation. Severe bleeding is a rare cause for surgical intervention. Occasionally, as discussed earlier, surgery will be required to control the extra intestinal manifestations of the disease such as stunting of growth.

REFERENCES

Acheson A D 1960 The distribution of ulcerative colitis and regional enteritis in United States veterans with particular reference to the Jewish religion. Gut 1: 291–293

Almy T P, Sherlock P 1966 Genetic aspects of ulcerative colitis and regional enteritis. Gastroenterology 51: 757–763

Anthonisen P, Barany F, Fokenborg O, Holtz A, Jarnum S, Kristensen M, Riis P, Walan A, Worning H 1974 The clinical effect of salazo-sulphapyridine (Salazopyrin) in Crohn's disease. A controlled double-blind study. Scandinavian Journal of Gastroenterology 9: 549–554

Assarsson L, Räf L 1974 Incidence of granuloma in Crohn's disease. Acta Chirurgica Scandinavica 140: 249–251

Azad Khan A K, Piris J, Trulove S C 1977 An experiment to determine the active therapeutic moiety of sulphasalazine. Lancet 2: 892–895

Bergman L, Krause U 1976 Postoperative treatment with corticosteroids and salazosulphapyridine (Salazopyrin) after radical resection for Crohn's disease. Scandinavian Journal of Gastroenterology 11: 651–656

Blackburn G, Hadfield G, Hunt A H 1939 Regional Ileitis. St Bartholomew's Hospital Reports 72: 181–224

Brahme F, Lindstrom C, Wenckert A 1975 Crohn's disease in a defined population. Gastroenterology 69: 342–351

Burbige E J, Huang S S, Bayliss T M 1975 Clinical manifestations of Crohn's disease in children and adolescents. Paediatrics 55: 866–871

Burnham W R, Lennard-Jones J E, Stanford J L, Bird R G 1978 Mycobacteria as a possible cause of inflammatory bowel disease. Lancet 2: 693–696

Cave D R, Mitchell D N, Brooke B N 1975 Experimental animal studies of the aetiology and pathogenesis of Crohn's disease. Gastroenterology 69: 618–624

Cave D R, Mitchell D N, Kane S P, Brooke B N 1973 Further animal evidence of a transmissible agent in Crohn's disease. Lancet 2: 1120–1122.

Chambers T J, Morson B C 1979 The granuloma in Crohn's disease. Gut 1979, 20: 269–274

Cooke W T, Fielding J F 1970 Corticosteroid or corticotrophin therapy in Crohn's disease (regional enteritis). Gut 11: 921–927

Crohn B D, Ginzburg L, Oppenheimer G D 1932 Regional ileitis. A pathological and clinical entity. Journal of American Medical Association 99: 1323–1329

Dalziel T K 1913 Chronic interstitial enteritis. British Medical Journal 2: 1068–1070

Doe W F, Booth C C, Brown D L 1973 Evidence for complement — binding immune complexes in adult coeliac disease, Crohn's disease, and ulcerative colitis. Lancet 1: 402–403

Donnelly B J, Delaney P V, Healy T M 1977 Evidence for a transmissible factor in Crohn's disease. Gut 18: 360–363

Dyer N H, Dawson A M 1970 Diagnosis of Crohn's disease. A continuing source of error. British Medical Journal 1: 735–737

Dyer N H, Stansfeld A G, Dawson A M 1970 The value of rectal biopsy in the diagnosis of Crohn's disease. Scandinavian Journal of Gastroenterology 5: 491–496

Farmer R G, Hawk W A, Turnbull J R B 1975 Clinical patterns in Crohn's disease. A statistical study of 615 cases. Gastroenterology 68: 627–635

Fielding J F 1972 Aetiology of Crohn's disease. In: Badenock J, Brooke B N (eds) Recent advances in gastroenterology. Churchill Livingstone, Edinburgh, p 276–284

Fleming C R, McGill D B, Berkner S 1977 Home parenteral nutrition as primary therapy in patients with extensive Crohn's disease of the small bowel and malnutrition. Gastroenterology 73: 1077–1081

Gitnick G L, Arthur M H, Shibata I 1976 Cultivation of viral agents from Crohn's disease — a new sensitive system. Lancet 2: 215–217

Glass R E, Baker W N W 1976 Role of granuloma in recurrent Crohn's disease. Gut 17: 75–77

Goldman P, Peppercorn M A 1975 Drug therapy. Sulphasalazine. New England Journal of Medicine 293: 20–23

Goligher J C, deDombal F G, Watts J Mc K, Watkinson G 1968 Familial incidence of ulcerative colitis. In: Ulcerative colitis. Williams & Wilkins, Baltimore, p 58–61

Greenstein A J, Sachar D B, Pasternak B S, Janowitz H D 1975 Re-operation and recurrence in Crohn's colitis and ileocolitis. New England Journal of Medicine 293: 685–690

Gryboski J D, Spiro H M 1978 Prognosis in children with Crohn's disease. Gastroenterology 74: 807–817

Heatley R V, Bolton P M, Owen E, Jones Williams W, Hughes L E 1975 A search for a transmissible agent in Crohn's disease. Gut 16: 528–532

Heaton K W, Thornton J R, Emmett P M 1979 Treatment of Crohn's disease with an unrefined carbohydrate, fibre-rich diet. British Medical Journal 2: 764–765

Hill R B, Kent T H, Hansen R N 1979 Clinical usefulness of rectal biopsy in Crohn's disease. Gastroenterology 77: 938–944

Hywel-Jones J, Lennard-Jones J E 1966 Corticosteroids and corticotrophin in the treatment of Crohn's disease. Gut 7: 181–187

Kelts D G, Grand R J, Shen G, Watkins J B, Werlin S L, Boehme C 1979 Nutritional basis of growth failure in children and adolescents with Crohn's disease. Gastroenterology 76: 720–727

Kirschner B S, Voinchet O, Rosenberg I H 1978 Growth retardation in inflammatory bowel disease. Gastroenterology 75: 504–511

Kirsner J B, Spencer J A 1963 Familial occurrences of ulcerative colitis, regional enteritis, and ileocolitis. Annals of Internal Medicine 59: 133–144

Kyle J 1971 An epidemiological study of Crohn's disease in N.E. Scotland. Gastroenterology 61: 826–833

Lagercrantz R, Hammarstrom S, Perlmann P, Gustafson B E 1966 Immunological studies in ulcerative colitis, III. Incidence of antibody to colon antigen in ulcerative colitis and other gastrointestinal diseases. Clinical and Experimental Immunology 1: 263–276

Lennard-Jones J E, Lockhart-Mummery H E, Morson B C 1968 Clinical and pathological differentiation of Crohn's disease and proctocolitis. Gastroenterology 54: 1162–1170

Lewkonia R M, McConnell R B 1976 Progress report. Familial inflammatory bowel disease — hereditary or environment? Gut 17, 235–243

Lockhart-Mummery H E, Morson B C 1960 Crohn's disease (regional enteritis) of the large intestine and its distinction from ulcerative colitis. Gut, 1: 87–105

Mayberry J, Rhodes J, Hughes L E 1979 Incidence of Crohn's disease in Cardiff between 1934 and 1977. Gut 20: 602–608

Mekhjian H S, Switz D M, Melnyk C S, Roukin G B, Brooks R K 1979 Clinical features and natural history of Crohn's disease. Gastroenterology 77: 898–906

Meyers M A, Alonso D R, Morson B C, Bartram C 1978 Pathogenesis of diverticulitis complicating granulomatous colitis. Gastroenterology 74: 24–31

Miller D S, Keighley A C, Langman M J S 1974 Changing patterns in epidemiology of Crohn's disease. Lancet II: 691–693

Miller D S, Keighley A, Smith P G, Hughes A O, Langman M J S 1975 Crohn's disease in Nottingham: a search for time-space clustering. Gut 16: 454–457

Miller D S, Keighley A, Smith P G, Hughes A O, Langman M J S 1976 A case-control method for seeking evidence of contagion in Crohn's disease. Gastroenterology 71: 385–387

Mitchell D N, Rees R J W 1970 Agent transmissible from Crohn's disease tissue. Lancet 2; 168–171

Monk M, Mendeloft A I, Siegel C I, Lilienfield A 1969 An epidemiological study of ulcerative colitis and regional enteritis among adults in Baltimore. II. Social and demographic factors. Gastroenterology 56: 847–857

Morson B D 1972 The pathology of Crohn's disease In: Brooke B N, (ed) Clinics in gastroenterology. Saunders, p 265–277

A Multicentre Trial 1977 Sulphasalazine in asymptomatic Crohn's disease. Gut 18: 69–72

O'Donoghue D P, Bartram C I, Blackshaw A J, Simmons M, Dawson A M 1979 Paper in preparation

O'Donoghue D P, Clark M L 1976 Inflammatory bowel disease in West Indians. British Medical Journal 2: 796

O'Donoghue D P, Dawson A M 1977 Crohn's disease in childhood. Archives of Diseases in Childhood 52: 627–632

O'Donoghue D P, Dawson A M, Powell-Tuck J, Bown R H, Lennard-Jones J E 1978 Double-blind withdrawal trial of azathioprine as maintenance treatment for Crohn's disease. Lancet 2: 954–957

Parent K, Mitchell P 1978 Cell wall-defective variants of pseudomonas-like (group Va) bacteria in Crohn's disease. Gastroenterology 75: 368–372

Perlmann P, Broberger O 1963 In vitro studies of ulcerative colitis. II Cytotoxic action of white blood cells from patients on human fetal colon cells. The Journal of Experimental Medicine 177: 717–733

Powell-Tuck J, Farwell J A, Nielsen T, Lennard-Jones J E 1978 Team approach to long-term intravenous feeding in patients with gastrointestinal disorders. Lancet 2: 825–828

Rosenberg J L, Kraft, S C, Kirsner J B 1976 Inflammatory bowel disease in all three members of one family. Gastroenterology 70: 759–760

Rosenberg J L, Levin B, Wall A J, Kirsner J B 1975 Controlled trial of azathioprine in Crohn's disease. American Journal of Digestive Diseases 20: 721–726

Rozen P, Zonis J, Yekutiel P, Gilat T 1979 Crohn's diease in the Jewish populations of Tel-Aviv-Yafo. Gastroenterology 76: 25–30

Sachar D B, Auslander M O 1978 Missing pieces in the puzzle of Crohn's disease. Gastroenterology 75: 745–748

Sachar D B, Taub R N, Janowitz H D 1976 A transmissible agent in Crohn's disease? New pursuit of an old concept. New England Journal of Medicine 293: 354

Scadding 1959 Principles of definition in medicine with special reference to chronic bronchitis and emphysema. Lancet 1: 323–325

Schachter H, Goldstein M J, Rappaport H, Fennessy J J, Kirsner J B 1970 Ulcerative and 'granulomatous' colitis — validity of differential diagnostic criteria. Annals of Internal Medicine 72: 841–851

Schachter H, Kirsner J B 1975 Definitions of inflammatory bowel disease of unknown aetiology. Gastroenterology 68: 591–600

Scholfield P F, Mandal B K, Ironside A G 1979 Toxic dilatation of the colon in Salmonella colitis and inflammatory bowel disease. British Journal of Surgery 66: 5–8

Segal A W, Loewi G 1976 Neutrophil dysfunction in Crohn's disease. Lancet 2: 219–221

Sherlock P, Bell B M, Steinberg H, Almy T P 1963 Familial occurrence of regional enteritis and ulcerative colitis. Gastroenterology 45: 413–420

Shorter R B, Huizenga J A, Re Mine S G, Spencer R J 1970 Effects of preliminary incubation of lymphocytes with serum on their cytotoxicity for colonic epithelial cells. Gastroenterology 58: 843–850

Singer H C, Anderson J G D, Frischer H, Kirsner J B 1971 Familial aspects of inflammatory bowel disease. Gastroenterology 61: 423–430

Smith I S, Young S, Gillespie G, O'Connor J, Bell J R 1975 Epidemiological aspects of Crohn's disease in Clydesdale 1961–1970. Gut 16: 62–67

Spector W G, Heesom N 1968 The production of granulomata by antigen-antibody complexes. Journal of Pathology 98: 31–39

Stobo J D, Tomasi T B, Huizenga K A, Shorter R G 1976 In vivo studies in inflammatory bowel disease. Gastroenterology 70: 171–176

Summers R W, Switz D M, Sessions J T, Becktal J M, Best W R, Kern Jr F, Singleton J W 1979 National co-operative Crohn's disease study: results of drug treatment. Gastroenterology 77: 847–869

Swarbrick E T, Kingham J G C, Price H L, Blackshaw A J, Griffiths P D, Darougar S, Buckall N A 1979 Chlamydia cytomegalovirus and yersinia in inflammatory bowel disease. Lancet 2: 11–12

Thayer W R 1976 Are the inflammatory bowel diseases immune complex diseases? Gastroenterology 70: 136–137

Thornton J R, Emmett P M, Heaton J W 1979 Diet and Crohn's disease: characteristics of the pre-illness diet. British Medical Journal 2: 762–764

Vantrappen G, Agg, H O, Ponette E, Geboes K, Bertrand P L 1977 Yersinia enteritis and entercolitis: Gastroenterological aspects. Gastroenterology 72: 220–227

Ward M 1977 The pathogenesis of Crohn's disease. Lancet 2: 902–905

Warren Nugent F, Richmond M, Park S K 1977 Crohn's disease of the duodenum. Gut, 18: 115–120

Watson D W, Quigley A, Bolt R J 1966a The cytotoxicity of circulating lymphocytes from patients with ulcerative colitis for human colonic epithelial cells: Disease specificity and relationship to disease activity. Gastroenterology 50: 886–887

Watson D W, Quigley A, Bolt R J 1966b Effect of lymphocytes from patients with ulcerative colitis on human adult colon epithelial cells. Gastroenterology 51: 985–993

Wells C 1952 Ulcerative colitis and Crohn's disease. Annals of the Royal College of Surgeons 11: 105–120

Whorwell P J, Phillips, C A, Beeken W L, Little P K, Roessner K D 1977 Isolation of reovirus-like agents from patients with Crohn's disease. Lancet 1: 1169–1171

Whorwell P J, Eade O E, Hossenbocus A, Bamforth J 1978 Crohn's disease in a husband and wife. Lancet 2: 186–187

Willoughby J M T, Kumar P J, Beckett J, Dawson A M 1971 Controlled trial of azathioprine in Crohn's disease. Lancet ii: 944–947

16. Medical aspects of diseases of the optic nerve and retina

R. W. Ross Russell   J. S. Shilling

The retina may be only the first small step in the visual pathway but its visibility and the frequency with which it is involved in disease give it a unique importance. This chapter considers a number of common disorders which affect this region and which fall into two main groups: vascular lesions of the retina and optic nerve, and demyelinating lesions of the nerve.

These conditions share a common symptom, uniocular visual loss of rapid onset and present as a rule to an ophthalmologist but the underlying causes are often remote from the eye itself and more in the province of the general physician or neurologist. The basic research on pathogenesis, much of which has appeared in the past few years, is derived from such diverse sources as the study of platelet aggregation on damaged vascular endothelium, the effects of temperature on nervous conduction across demyelinated segments of axon, or the interplay of environmental and genetic factors in the immune response to virus infection.

Just as the range of clinical symptoms in ophthalmology is small so the range of pathological reactions of retinal neurones and vasculature is also limited. An attempt is made to define these reactions in some of the common types of vascular and inflammatory eye disease.

TRANSIENT RETINAL ISCHAEMIA

Pathogenesis

Transient loss of vision (amaurosis fugax) is a painless symptom but an alarming one both to patient and physician. The onset is characteristically abrupt, the vision of one eye is wholly or partially obscured but returns to normal within a few minutes. The attacks, which often recur, are caused by a reduction in ocular blood supply and one important mechanism is arterial embolism (Fisher, 1959). The onset of the attack coincides with a blockage of the opthalmic or central retinal artery by a fibrin-platelet embolus; after a few minutes this breaks up and is carried into smaller vessels eventually dissolving completely with restoration of the circulation (Fig. 16.1). In other patients amaurosis fugax may be caused by the impaction of a cholesterol embolus which produces a less drastic though more prolonged obstruction of blood flow (Russell 1968) (Fig. 16.2). On rare occasions other circulatory disturbances are responsible as when systemic hypotension occurs in a patient whose ocular circulation is already compromised by local arterial narrowing, or when amaurosis fugax is a premonitory symptom to a migrainous attack. Raised intracranial pressure or raised intraocular tension may also reduce blood flow by obstructing venous drainage and result in transient impairment of vision.

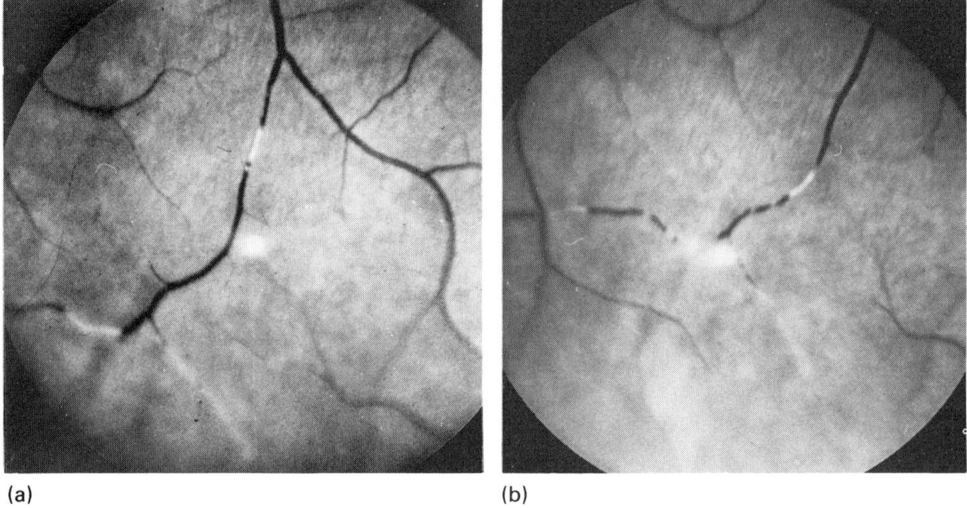

(a)   (b)

Fig. 16.1 (a) and (b) Retinal platelet embolism. Passage of a white platelet embolus along a branch retinal artery during an attack of anaurosis fugax. Interval between a and b approximately one minute. The patient was a young woman in whom no definite source for embolism was discovered.

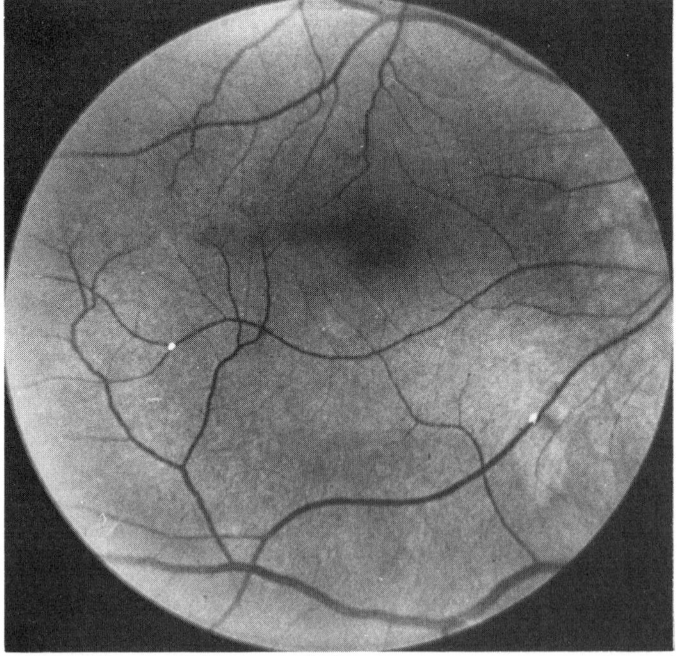

Fig. 16.2 Cholesterol emboli in branches of the retinal artery. The source of the emboli was an atheromatous lesion of the carotid artery.

Angiography
Fisher (1954) first drew attention to the association of amaurosis fugax, transient cerebral ischaemic attacks (TIAs) and atheromatous narrowing of the internal carotid artery suggesting that this artery was the source of thrombo-embolism to brain and retina. This, together with the advent of vascular surgery, stimulated an active policy of investigation by carotid arteriography. It was discovered that localised carotid stenosis suitable for surgical treatment was present in some but not all patients. Some had atheromatous lesions without significant narrowing of the lumen and others showed no abnormality (Harrison & Marshall, 1975). A recent study has attempted to determine which patients should be investigated by arteriography (Wilson & Russell, 1977). In a prospective study of 60 patients with amaurosis fugax, but without overt cardiac or haematological abnormality, carotid arteriography was performed. One-third were found to have internal carotid artery narrowing or a local atheromatous plaque suitable for surgery. The remainder showed either no abnormality, complete carotid occlusion or widespread disease unsuitable for surgery. Clinical features indicating a high probability of arterial disease suitable for surgery were a localised carotid bruit, a history of TIAs, systemic hypertension, intermittent claudication and an age of over 50. In the absence of all these features angiography only occasionally revealed a surgically treatable lesion. It is suggested, therefore, that the use of angiography should be restricted to those patients who show at least one of the above features.

Other investigations
The cause of symptoms remains a problem in those patients with negative angiography. There is recent evidence that cardiac disease may be responsible for transient ischaemia and amaurosis fugax more often than was previously thought. Certain types of cardiac arrhythmia such as isolated atrial fibrillation or atrial fibrillation in association with hyperthyroidism, at one time considered to be benign, have been shown to carry a definite risk of systemic embolism (Hinton et al, 1978). Furthermore, the use of continuous cardiac monitoring has shown that significant unsuspected arrhythmias are relatively common and may be responsible either for episodes of generalised cerebral ischaemia or for the dislodgement of microemboli (Figures 16.3, 16.4). In a recent study (Luxon et al, 1979) 60 unselected patients with transient cerebral symptoms underwent 24-hour ambulatory e.c.g. monitoring. Significant arrhythmias including supraventricular and ventricular tachycardia, atrial fibrillation with block, rapid atrial fibrillation (over 110/minute), and complete atrioventricular dissociation were observed in 32 per cent of patients but in only 3 per cent of a control group. Nine patients were treated for their arrythmia with marked improvement in all cases. The possibility of a cardiac source of embolism can be investigated by the non-invasive technique of echocardiography which may reveal lesions such as prolapse of the mitral valve leaflet, ventricular aneurysm, valvular vegetations or atrial myxoma.

Platelets and amaurosis fugax
Platelet adhesion and aggregation have long been known to be the initial event in the formation of thrombus on the wall of arteries and they are thought to be especially important in the genesis of thrombi and emboli in the ophthalmic circulation. This

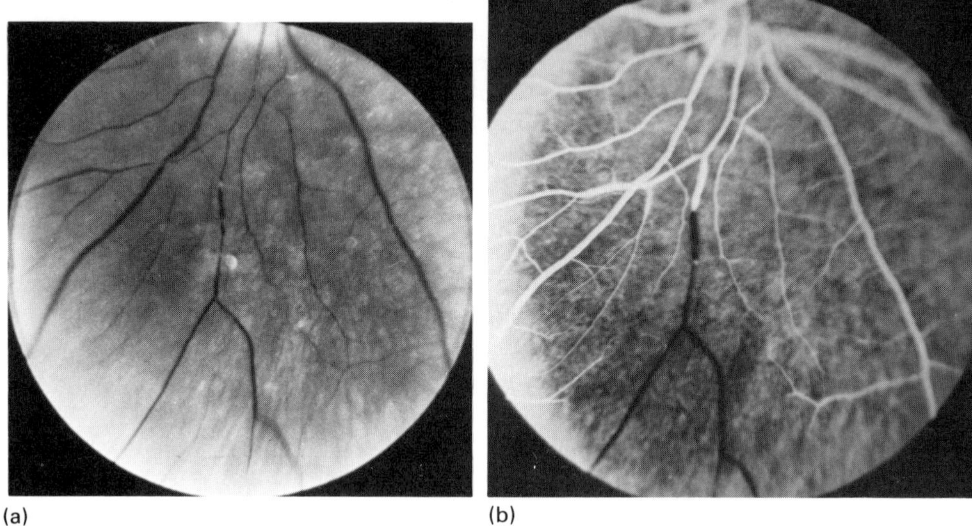

(a)   (b)

Fig. 16.3 (a) Red thrombus occluding a retinal arteriole of a young woman with atrial septal defect. Visual defect lasted 48 hours and circulation was restored. (b) Fluorescein angiogram showing complete occlusion and region of impaired perfusion.

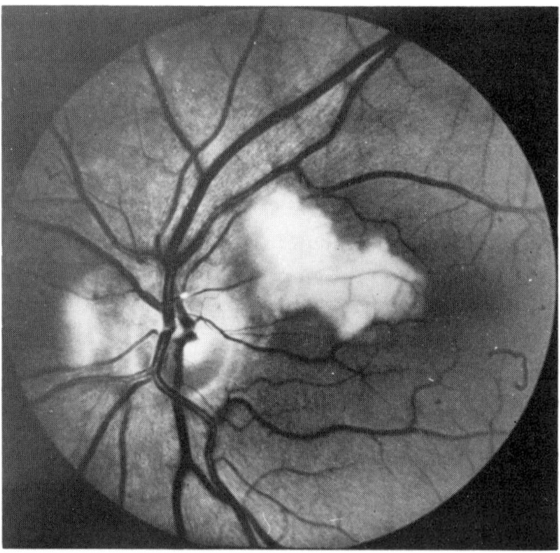

Fig. 16.4 Cardiac embolus to retina. In this patient with aortic stenosis a single small embolus has occluded a retinal branch vessel producing micro-infarction.

view gains support because the descriptions of white fragmenting emboli traversing the retinal circulation closely resemble those of platelet aggregates (Fisher, 1959), the finding of platelet thrombus on the inner surface of the carotid artery at endarterectomy suggesting that this may be the source of platelet emboli (Gunning et al, 1964), and the occurrence of amaurosis fugax in platelet disorders such as thrombocythaemia (Mundall et al, 1972).

Early studies revealed increased platelet adhesiveness in cerebral vascular disease but the proportion of patients with abnormal findings varied with different techniques and also included some with non-vascular conditions. More recently isotopic methods have been developed which enable the life span of platelets in the circulation to be measured. In a study of patients with amaurosis fugax, all with normal total platelet counts, Wilson (1978) has found two distinct groups, one in which platelet life span is shortened and another in which it is normal. In the first group there is a high prevalence of carotid stenosis and cardiac valvular lesions while in the second group these abnormalities are not found. In patients with cardiac or degenerative arterial disease the presence of an abnormality or atheromatous plaque may lead to local deposition and an increased turnover of platelets. The finding of a reduced platelet life span may be a useful indication that further cardiac or angiographic investigations should be undertaken.

Medical treatment

In spite of two decades of study the place of anticoagulants or antiplatelet drugs in patients with amaurosis fugax or other transient ischaemic attacks is still far from clear. There is good evidence and general agreement that patients with TIAs caused by systemic embolism from chronic heart disease (e.g. mitral stenosis and atrial fibrillation) should be on permanent anticoagulant treatment (Carter, 1965). In patients with TIAs but without heart disease the benefits of anticoagulants are more doubtful. They reduce the frequency of TIA and lessen the chance of developing a permanent stroke within one year but fail to have any effect on mortality (Whisnant, Metsumoto & Elveback, 1973). This and the vagaries of anticoagulant control has led to the search for other drugs, principally those acting on platelets. Two of these drugs have attracted particular attention, aspirin and dipyridamole.

Aspirin

Aspirin influences the biosynthesis of the various prostaglandins from platelet lipoproteins by inhibiting the breakdown of arachidonic acid, the first step in the metabolic pathway. Its antithrombotic effects are thought to be due to the consequent fall in the amounts of prostaglandin endoperoxides and thromboxane A2 which are powerful platelet-aggregating agents. Aspirin has been found to be active in vitro and in vivo, is known to prolong bleeding time and to inhibit the second phase of platelet aggregation induced by collagen and ADP. Many reports on the value of aspirin in clinical thrombosis have appeared although few deal specifically with amaurosis fugax. Some years ago individual case reports of patients with very frequent amaurosis fugax appeared to show a striking effect from aspirin in some instances, the attacks ceasing within a few hours (Harrison et al, 1976). A retrospective study on a small number of patients with transient cerebral ischaemia indicated that treatment with 600 mg aspirin daily lessened the number of subsequent attacks (Dyken et al, 1973) but the two groups differed in the duration of follow up. In a limited but well-conducted trial of carotid TIAs which continued over two years aspirin was found to improve the outcome as judged by a reduction in the frequency of further TIAs (Fields et al, 1977) and cerebral or retinal infarction. The number of patients was insufficient for each feature to be assessed separately. Patients with multiple attacks seemed to benefit most. There was a significant effect even after carotid endarterectomy.

In the recent large Canadian study of patients with minor strokes, transient cerebral ischaemia and amaurosis fugax, aspirin was found to reduce the incidence of ischaemic episodes and strokes and also reduced mortality by 19 per cent (Canadian Co-operative Study Group, 1978). This beneficial effect, however, was only found in men and follow up was sometimes only one year so that long-term efficacy, toxicity and the optimum effective dose of aspirin are still uncertain.

The evaluation of aspirin therapy is made more difficult by the fact that low and high doses may have different effects. It has been suggested that low dose aspirin may selectively inhibit only the thromboxane pathway and so cause decreased platelet aggregation. On the other hand larger doses may have lesser antithrombotic properties since they also inhibit prostacyclin which protects the vessel wall from platelet deposition (Moncada & Vane, 1979).

DIPYRIDAMOLE
Dipyridamole has also been used extensively as an antithrombotic agent although its mode of action is still uncertain. Its effect may be via prostacyclin, another derivative of arachnidonic acid which is produced by vessel walls and has both vasodilatator and platelet antiaggregation properties. Inhibition of the platelet enzyme phosphodiesterase by dipyridamole potentiates the effect of prostacyclin on platelets. This may explain why its antiaggregate properties are more marked in vivo than in vitro. The strongest clinical evidence in favour of dipyridamole is its use in combination with anticoagulants in preventing thromboembolic events in patients who have had a mitral or aortic valve prosthesis (Sullivan, Harken & Gorlin, 1968). A controlled trial in patients with transient cerebral ischaemia showed no significant effect on natural history (Acheson, Danta & Hutchinson, 1969). In the future it may find a use as adjunct to low dose aspirin.

Surgical treatment

The value of surgery in patients with lesions of the internal carotid artery is also unclear. Trials have shown an improved prognosis in surgically over medically treated patients but the difference between the two groups has been small and has not taken into account the morbidity of the operation or of the angiogram which preceded it (Fields et al, 1970). However, those patients who have survived carotid endarterectomy without complications have a better outlook than those undergoing any form of medical treatment including aspirin.

In the best hands and in suitable patients carotid surgery carries a very small operative risk with a mortality of under one per cent, but increasing age, hypertension and the presence of residual neurological signs all have an adverse affect on the prognosis.

What advice should therefore be given to the individual patient with recurrent amaurosis fugax? If the patient is middle-aged or elderly and has evidence of generalised arterial disease, especially if he also has transient cerebral symptoms or a carotid bruit, carotid artery stenosis is a strong possibility. In such a patient, if he is fit for surgery, an angiogram should be done. Should localised disease be found, and if experienced vascular surgery is available, carotid endarterectomy is recommended.

For all other patients, except those intolerant to the drug, aspirin is the treatment of choice at a dose of 300–600 mg/day.

OCCLUSIONS OF THE RETINAL ARTERIES

Retinal branch occlusion (see Table 16.1)

When a retinal branch artery is totally occluded over a short segment blood may bypass the obstruction by flowing from surrounding vascular territories into the surviving capillary bed of the occluded vessel. The amount of collateral supply, however, is insufficient to sustain the viability of the inner retinal neurones and as a result cloudy swelling develops over the affected area due to oedema of axons. At the periphery of the ischaemic area a dense white exudate may signify the arrest of axoplasmic transport from intact ganglion cells. Branch occlusions usually cause permanent visual loss; the field defect, which is altitudinal or fibre bundle in type, depends on the size of the vessel involved.

As with amaurosis fugax there is pathological evidence that most retinal branch occlusions are due to embolism. In contrast to the frail platelet plugs which fragment in the circulation, these emboli are more stable. There are three main types, those derived from cholesterol, from mural thrombus or from cardiac valves. Flakes of cholesterol-containing material derived from atheromatous lesions in large arteries such as the internal carotid comprise the majority of emboli. These appear in the retinal circulation as multiple refractile plaques often lodged at arterial bifurcations. Some cause no obstruction to blood flow and the majority disappear in a few weeks often leaving behind a white sheathed segment of artery.

Fragments of organised mural thrombus originating from the heart or from the walls of arteries are less commonly seen. These emboli are dark red in colour, occupy a length of retinal artery and cause more complete arrest of the circulation and more severe ischaemia. Small emboli of this type may undergo lysis or the artery may recanalise but in the majority of patients the vessel remains permanently occluded appearing as a white solid cord.

The third type is the single white calcareous embolus derived from a cardiac valve. These patients usually prove on investigation to have calcific aortic or mitral stenosis of rheumatic origin, and the occurrence of retinal embolism often coincides with a period of deterioration of cardiac function culminating in the need for valve replacement.

The occurrence of a branch retinal occlusion with a visible retinal embolus is thus a strong indication for full cardiac and carotid investigation with the object of discovering a source of the embolus. If a localised carotid lesion is found the most satisfactory treatment is endarterectomy while in the case of cardiac embolus it may be possible to correct the cardiac defect by surgical means or to administer long term anticoagulant treatment.

In a recent series of 68 patients with branch retinal artery occlusion cardiovascular investigations gave the following results: carotid bruit 18 per cent, cardiac valvular abnormality 34 per cent, visible retinal emboli 68 per cent, hypertension 25 per cent. A localised carotid bruit is a valuable physical sign reliably indicating the presence of operable stenosis of the carotid artery but unfortunately the absence of a murmur does not exclude minor atheromatous lesion or ulcers which may also act as a source of emboli. However, no operable lesions were found in patients under 50 years of age who did not also have a bruit or cholesterol embolus (Wilson, Warlow & Russell, 1979).

Table 16.1   Principal arterial diseases causing uniocular visual loss

	Vascular abnormality	Associated features	Clinical effects	Retinal appearances
Amaurosis Fugax	Transient platelet embolism	Carotid atheroma TIAs	Brief attacks uniocular loss	Normal White platelet emboli during attacks
	Cholesterol embolism	Valvular heart disease	Half or whole field	Refractile plaques in vessels
Retinal branch occlusion	Complete occlusion Retinal branch artery (embolic)	Carotid atheroma Cardiac valvular disease	Permanent sector or fibre bundle defect Central vision often spared	Visible embolus Focal cloudy swelling Axoplasmic exudates
Central retinal artery occlusion	Thrombotic occlusion Ophthalmic or central retinal artery (rarely embolic)	Hypertension, diabetes, ischaemic heart disease	Permanent severe visual loss Usually complete	Cloudy swelling posterior Macular red spot, visible stasis
Microvascular retinopathy	Progressive obstruction Retinal arterioles, capillaries Lipohyaline change, fibrinoid necrosis	Diabetes, hypertension, vasculitis, sickle cell disease	Cumulative episodes of visual loss Often bilateral	Retinal haemorrhage, soft exudates, microaneurysm, capillary closure, neo-vascularisation, vitreous haemorrhage
Ischaemic papillopathy (non-arteritic)	Progressive obliteration ciliary arteries	Chronic hypertension, diabetes, atheroma	Rapid visual loss lower field, some recovery Central vision often spared	Swollen discs, some pallor, radiating haemorrhage, sector disc atrophy
Ischaemic papillitis (arteritis)	Inflammatory occlusion ciliary arteries	Over 60 age-group Temporal arteritis Polymyalgia	Severe visual loss Often bilateral	Swollen pale disc, radiating haemorrhages, secondary atrophy

Central retinal artery occlusion (see Table 16.1)
Occlusion of the central retinal artery may occur at the level of the optic disc or at a more proximal point in the artery. Since there are no effective collateral channels in either event this results in a drastic reduction in blood supply to the inner retina at the posterior pole and to immediate and profound visual loss. The condition is painless and previous attacks of amaurosis fugax occur in only the minority of patients.

Pale cloudy swelling envelops the posterior pole of the retina with a red spot at the macula. The arteries are reduced in calibre and dark red in colour and in the veins blood flow may be seen to be retarded with aggregation of the corpuscles. The disc capillaries are engorged and axoplasmic exudates are not seen.

There are some important aetiological differences between central and branch occlusions. In contrast to branch occlusions which are usually embolic, central retinal artery occlusion is most often due to local thrombosis arising either in the ophthalmic artery as a result of atheroma or following extension of thrombosis from the internal carotid artery in the skull. Central retinal artery occlusion occurs in older patients who show a higher prevalence of hypertension and complete carotid thrombosis than those with branch occlusion but have a lower prevalence of cardiac valvular disease and carotid stenosis (Wilson, Warlow & Russell, 1979).

Consequently there is no necessity to subject these patients to detailed cardiac and carotid angiographic investigation. The treatment of hypertension and diabetes and the avoidance of smoking are the most important measures available to minimise the risk of further thrombotic lesions in other arteries.

ISCHAEMIC OPTIC NEUROPATHY AND GIANT CELL ARTERITIS

Pathogenesis

It has been known for some time that giant cell arteritis is not confined to branches of the external carotid system or to the temporal artery but affects particularly vessels with large amounts of elastic tissue. These include the aorta and its major branches in the chest and neck, the coronary, visceral and limb arteries.

The intracranial arteries and the branches of the central retinal artery within the globe itself are rarely affected. This is probably because of the small content of elastic tissue in these vessels. The vertebral artery for instance is frequently involved by arteritis in its cervical portion but once it has pierced the dura the amount of elastic tissue in the wall decreases markedly and no arteritis can be found beyond this point (Wilkinson, 1972). Although ischaemic infarction in the vertebrobasilar territory may occur in the course of the disease it results from embolism of thrombus formed in the vertebral arteries rather than from inflammatory changes in the intracranial basilar system (Wilkinson & Russell, 1972).

The particular risk of blindness from retinal or optic nerve ischaemia has been shown to be the result of arteritis involving the ophthalmic artery and its branches within the orbit, including both the central retinal and ciliary arteries (Crompton, 1959). This is still a major cause of preventable blindness in the elderly which is too often overlooked until vision has been irretrievably lost.

Diagnosis

The recognition of the disease before the onset of visual symptoms is of the greatest importance. The classical features of temporal arteritis are well known; less familiar are the symptoms of ischaemia in other parts of the external carotid system — pain in the jaw on eating, difficulty in opening the mouth, painful induration of the tongue, pain in the throat and tenderness in the neck over the carotid arteries. Systemic manifestations such as pain, stiffness and weakness in the proximal limb muscles, weight loss and anaemia are present in only a proportion of patients but the sedimentation rate is a most valuable indication of generalised disease and is seldom normal. Biopsy of a scalp or facial artery in the region of the pain is essential but should not delay the initiation of steroid treatment. False negative results are not uncommon, the biopsy should consist of at least 1 cm of artery and must be examined at a number of sites.

Painless rapidly progressive visual loss in one or both eyes is usually the first indication of orbital arteritis. Occasionally there may be attacks of transient loss of vision with full recovery but more commonly visual acuity progressively fails over a few hours. The central and nasal fields are lost early but perception of finger counting is often retained in the temporal field. Ophthalmoscopic examination at an early stage sometimes shows cotton wool spots but more often the retina is normal and remains so even in the first few hours after visual loss. Subsequently pallor and swelling of the optic disc becomes apparent with radiating linear haemorrhages — the classical features of ischaemic papillopathy (Fig. 16.5). A few patients show the more familiar appearance of central retinal artery occlusion with pallor and cloudy swelling of the posterior pole of the retina, attenuation of retinal vessels, slowing of blood flow, corpuscular aggregation and a macular cherry red spot.

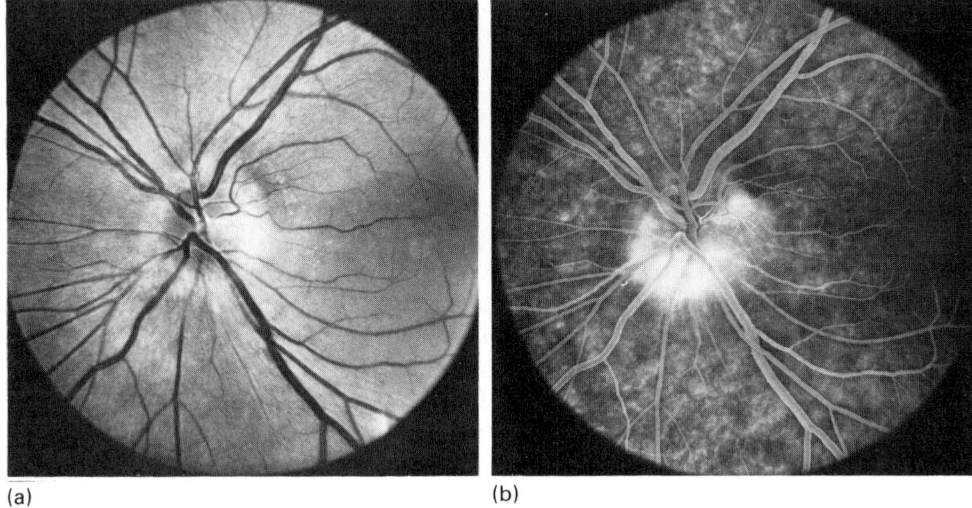

(a)   (b)

Fig. 16.5   (a) and (b) Ischaemic papillopathy. In this elderly patient with giant cell arteritis there is a recent infarction and swelling of the optic disc due to occlusion of the ciliary arteries. (b) Leakage of fluorescein.

Treatment
Once oedema has developed there is little that can be done to restore vision. However in patients with unilateral loss of vision the high risk of involvement of the second eye within a few days demands the most urgent treatment, as does fluctuating or episodic visual loss. Of first importance is the control of arteritis by prednisone, initially at a daily dosage of 60 mg and subsequently reducing this to a maintenance level of 20–40 mg. This should be combined with intravenous low molecular-weight dextran (500 ml per 24 hours). By its plasma expanding property dextran reduces blood viscosity and in addition has an inhibitory effect on platelet aggregation. A careful check is kept for signs of cardiac failure or raised intraocular tension and the latter may be treated with acetozolamide. In addition to systemic steroid treatment retrobular steroids are sometimes recommended (Glaser, 1978). The blood supply to the optic nerve may be at a critical level and in some patients the small difference in perfusion pressure between the lying and sitting position may be enough to cause loss of vision. In uncomplicated cases of giant cell arteritis without visual involvement only steroid treatment is necessary.

In spite of these vigorous measures it is unusual to achieve any improvement in the vision of an eye already affected and the second eye may occasionally become involved within two or three days in spite of treatment. However once arteritis is suppressed and the sedimentation rate reduced to 30 mm or less, the risk to sight is greatly diminished.

Natural history
The late effects and duration of treatment of giant cell arteritis are difficult to determine. In some patients the disease appears to regress within a few months and steroids can be withdrawn. Pulsation may return in affected scalp arteries. A few

patients later develop a severe generalised disease resembling polyarteritis nodosa with multiple vascular occlusions in visceral, coronary and muscular arteries. This tends to progress despite large doses of corticosteroids and may prove fatal. The histology of the arteries at autopsy may resemble acute polyarteritis nodosa rather than giant cell arteritis (Russell, 1959). A larger number of patients continue to suffer a subacute type of arteritis for many years which can be easily controlled by a small dose of corticosteroids, sometimes as little as 2.5 to 5 mg daily. Any attempt to withdraw steroids may provoke polymyalgia but seldom headache. Patients of this type may show progressive aortic enlargement but the expectation of life appears to be unaffected.

NON-ARTERITIC OPTIC NERVE ISCHAEMIA (ATHEROMATOUS)

Idiopathic ischaemic papillopathy which, like giant cell arteritis, may impair the blood supply to the optic nerve head is now becoming increasingly familiar to ophthalmologists and physicians. Although few reports have appeared the underlying pathology is probably obliterative disease of small arteries of the ciliary system which supply the prelaminar portion of the optic nerve. The majority of patients are middle-aged men, often hypertensive or diabetic; occasionally the condition may result from carotid atheroma or may follow an episode of severe systemic hypotension. It has also been reported in association with migraine, neurosyphilis, polyarteritis nodosa and polycythaemia rubra vera (Eagling, Sanders & Miller, 1974).

There are some important differences between this condition and giant cell arteritis (see Table 16.1). Initial visual loss is less severe and the long-term prognosis is better. Visual field impairment is usually altitudinal beginning in the lower field and tending to spare central vision. Ischaemic swelling of the optic disc may be confined to the upper or lower halves of the disc and sector atrophy may be obvious. Atrophic cupping of the disc does not occur. Head pains and systemic symptoms do not occur, the ESR is not raised but, as with giant cell arteritis, there is a tendency for involvement of the second eye at an interval of months rather than days. When the second eye is affected the finding of disc swelling combined with optic atrophy in the other eye may raise the suspicion of a frontal lobe tumour (pseudo Foster–Kennedy sign).

Although steroids are often used the benefits are doubtful (Boghen & Glaser, 1975). It is rare to find any improvement in acuity or in visual fields and high steroid treatment presents difficulties in diabetic or hypertensive patients. Optimal control of diabetes or hypertension in the hope of retarding further microvascular change is the mainstay of treatment.

MACULAR OEDEMA AND NEOVASCULARISATION — AN APPROACH TO THERAPY

There are many pathological conditions that affect the retinal blood vessels and may cause visual loss. Systemic diseases such as degenerative vascular or inflammatory conditions are often implicated, but in other cases local ocular disease is responsible. The responses of the retinal vasculature to disease are limited, and are non-specific.

Vascular diseases may be classified according to these responses rather than to the underlying diseases. Such a classification is useful not only because it gives some understanding of the mechanism of visual loss, but also because it is relevant to therapy.

There are two basic retinal vascular responses which will be discussed separately. The first is the abnormal vascular permeability response and, the second the ischaemic/neovascular response due to reduced or absent retinal capillary perfusion (Shilling, 1976).

Abnormal vascular permeability

Abnormal vascular permeability leads to an increase in the passage of intravascular substances through the vessel wall into the extravascular spaces of the retina and often subsequently into the vitreous. The most important consequence of this response is macular oedema which is a significant cause of visual loss in many of the vascular retinopathies (ffytche & Blach, 1970). This may be due to changes in the intravascular pressure or disease of the vessel walls. These factors may occur together, but will be discussed separately.

Increased intravascular pressure

A change in the intravascular pressure may be due to increased arterial pressure as in arterial hypertension, or to increased venous pressure obstructing the outflow.

Systemic hypertension increases the intravascular pressure but autoregulatory mechanisms in the healthy retinal vascular tree compensate for this with arteriolar constriction; this protects the capillaries and therefore there is no increased accumulation of fluid in the extravascular space. However in accelerated hypertension this mechanism breaks down and the retina is often oedematous. Multiple factors contribute to the lesions of accelerated hypertension but the exact pathogenesis remains controversial, (Garner & Ashton, 1979).

The rapid improvement in the oedematous response which follows reduction in blood pressure supports the view that increased extravasation of fluid from capillaries due to raised intracapillary pressure is contributary.

Obstructed venous return from the eye is a common cause of increased vascular permeability. Occlusion of branch and central retinal veins often presents as retinal oedema. This may involve the macula, reducing central visual acuity, (Clemett, Kohner & Hamilton, 1973; ffytche & Blach, 1970; Laatikainen & Kohner 1976). Both capillaries and veins leak fluid in these conditions, and this is well demonstrated by fluorescein angiography (Kohner & Shilling, 1976; Shilling, 1976).

The site of venous obstruction determines the area of retina involved. Central vein occlusion occurs within the optic nerve in the region of the lamina and therefore affects the whole retina, whereas occlusion of tributaries involves localised areas. Occlusion of venous tributaries occurs most commonly at arteriovenous crossings especially in hypertensive patients and the position of these crossings determines the pattern of branch venous occlusion (Archer, Ernest & Newell, 1974). Occlusion at other sites in the venous tree are observed in glaucoma — at the edge of the optic disc cup, in diabetes, along main veins (Kohner, Shilling & Clemett, 1974) and in periphlebitis (Sanders & Shilling, 1976).

Disease of the vessel walls
Damage to the vessel walls may be the cause of increased vascular permeability. This may either be primary as in retinal vasculitis or secondary to changes in the surrounding retina as a response to intraocular inflammation or to retinal ischaemia.

Retinal vasculitis remains an enigma. The pathogenesis is not fully understood and the treatment is controversial. It most commonly affects the retinal veins (periphlebitis) although occasionally retinal arteritis is seen, e.g. in systemic lupus erythematosis and syphilis (ffytche, 1977). Periphlebitis often has no known cause but a number of associated conditions have been identified. In sarcoidosis and Behcet's disease there is good pathological evidence of inflammatory cells surrounding the retinal veins (Gass & Olson, 1973; Shikano, 1966).

The retinal blood vessels respond to generalised intraocular inflammation with increased vascular permeability well demonstrated by fluorescein leakage. This has been studied in a group of patients with uveitis (O'Day, Shilling & ffytche, 1979). Most of the abnormalities are limited to the capillaries and veins, and leakage from arterioles is rare. Abnormal permeability may also affect the optic disc vessels with subsequent disc oedema.

Damage to vessel walls with leakage may occur in the absence of inflammation at the arteriovenous crossings following branch retinal vein occlusion when it is presumably due to intimal damage at the site of occlusion (Clemett, 1974). Leakage may also occur as arteries or veins pass through areas of retinal ischaemia, i.e. areas of capillary non-perfusion. This finding has sometimes been mistakenly used as evidence for inflammation when discussing the aetiology of retinal vascular syndromes.

The pathogenesis of abnormal vascular permeability may be multifactorial. For example, in diabetes mellitus the abnormal permeability response, which causes the odematous maculopathy is partly due to primary vascular abnormalities but there may be an occlusive element with raised intravascular pressure, and associated systemic hypertension.

The ischaemic/neovascular response
Closure of retinal capillaries if sufficiently extensive is followed by new vessels proliferating on the optic disc, in the peripheral retina or on the iris (rubeosis iridis) (Fig. 16.6). This neovascular response is a serious threat to vision.

The new vessels in the posterior segment cause vitreous haemorrhage, and progression of the response leads to fibrovascular tissue growing onto the posterior vitreous face. This may result in retinal detachment due to traction which develops either because of increasing traction or because of retinal tears which are secondary to the traction. Detachment of the posterior vitreous is an essential part of this process although the exact sequence of events is not completely understood (Shilling, McLeod & Restori, 1978).

Neovascularisation in the anterior segment of the eye is a cause of severe and often untreatable glaucoma. In this condition (rubeotic or thrombotic glaucoma) new vessels grow on the surface of the iris and into the drainage angle. The trabecular meshwork is occluded with fibrovascular tissue, resulting in closure of the angle, and therefore raised intraocular pressure because of reduced aqueous drainage.

The ischaemic/neovascular response occurs in many of the vascular retinopathies. Diabetes mellitus is the most common cause and it is this response in the retina which

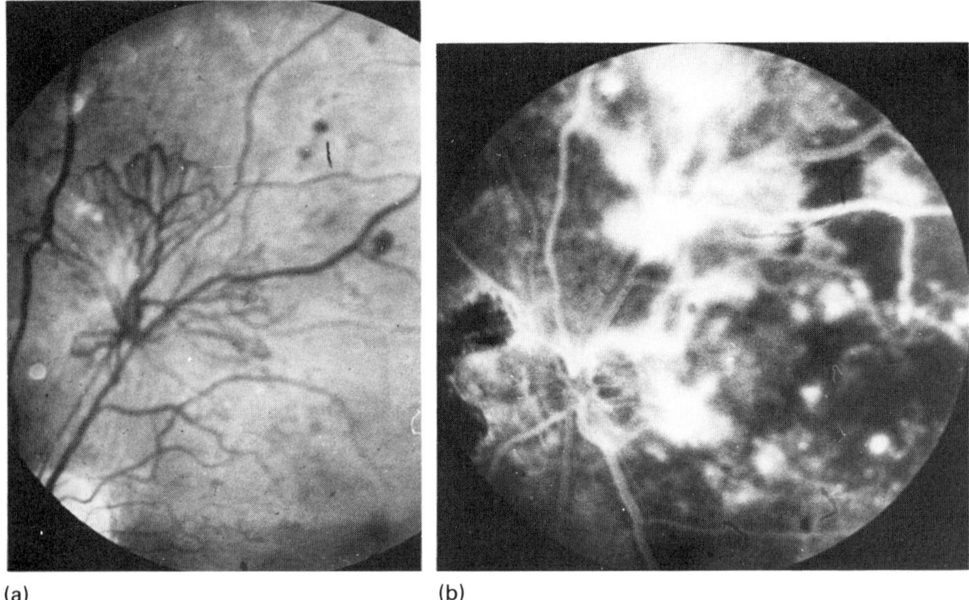

(a) (b)

Fig. 16.6 (a) From a retinal colour photograph of a diabetic patient showing a frond of pre-retinal new vessels. (b) Fluorescein angiogram of (a) in the late phase showing leakage of dye from the neovascular complex, and associated areas of capillary closure.

accounts for much of the serious visual loss in this disease. It is particularly important because it affects young adults and at this age it comprises the commonest cause of new blind registration.

In diabetes the neovascular response affects both the anterior segment of the eye and the retina, and both rubeotic glaucoma and vitreous haemorrhage or retinal detachment are seen. In most of the other vascular retinopathies in which neovascularisation occurs the response predominantly affects either the retina or the iris. In central retinal vein occlusion, for example, anterior segment new vessels are the rule while posterior segment new vessels are less common. In retinal branch vein occlusion the neovascular response predominantly affects the retina (Shilling & Kohner, 1976) and iris new vessels are much less frequent.

The incidence of neovascularisation
The chance of a patient with a vascular retinopathy developing new vessels is related to the amount of retina affected by capillary closure. This is independent of the underlying cause of the retinopathy. This has been shown particularly in branch vein occlusion in which new vessels only develop in eyes with large areas of non-perfusion and are not seen when only small areas of retina are involved (Shilling & Kohner, 1976).

Table 16.2 gives some indication of the frequency of the retinal responses in retinal vascular diseases.

Table 16.2 Indication of frequency of retinal responses in retinal vascular disease

Disease	Abnormal permeability response	Neovascular response
Diabetes mellitus	+++	+++
Central vein occlusion	++	++
Branch vein occlusion	++	++
Peripheral vein occlusion	0	++
Sarcoidosis	++	+
Behcets disease	+++	+
Retrolental fibroplasia	+	+++
Sickle cell disease	0	+++
Eales syndrome	0	+++
Retinal vasculitis	++	++
Syphilis	++	0
Uveitis/pars plantis	+++	+
Systemic lupus erythematosis	±	+
Systemic hypertension	++	0

THERAPY OF RETINAL VASCULAR DISEASE

Understanding the processes leading to visual loss provides a rational approach to the treatment of retinal vascular disease. This can be broadly directed at relieving the underlying systemic disease or on the other hand treating the resulting eye lesions for which photocoagulation is the mainstay of treatment.

Systemic disease
The systemic treatment of degenerative retinal vascular disease is difficult and often unsatisfactory. Hypertension has been shown to be an important underlying cause of some ocular vascular conditions and must be treated effectively. Many of the changes of hypertensive retinopathy are reversible, particularly the dramatic vascular and disc changes of accelerated hypertension with hypotensive therapy. It may also be possible to prevent retinal vascular occlusion by this treatment. Established arterial occlusions are doubtfully influenced by antihypertensive therapy, and there is little evidence that the retinal responses which follow a venous occlusion, whether oedematous or neovascular are in any way changed by treating high blood pressure once occlusion has occurred.

Similarly there is controversy as to the effect of careful diabetic control in diabetic retinopathy. It is a clinical impression that patients with severe proliferative retinopathy tend to be those whose diabetic control is less than excellent but it is also well known that severe retinopathy occurs in some patients with either mild diabetes or a well controlled diabetic state. Animal experiments provide evidence that strict control has a beneficial effect on retinopathy. Clinical studies have supported this finding (Coldwell, 1966; Kohner et al, 1969) but have involved only small numbers of patients and more work is urgently required in this field. As strict control as possible should be maintained in these patients.

Clofibrate
The cholesterol-lowering property of clofibrate has been advocated for exudative retinopathies, particularly for diabetic retinopathy. There is no doubt that the drug

promotes the absorption of exudate. This was shown in a control study (Cullen, Town & Campbell, 1974) but there was no significant difference in the visual acuities in the treated and control groups and therefore this therapy is not routinely advised.

Anticoagulants

These have been advocated for retinal venous occlusion (Vannas & Orma, 1957). There is however no real evidence of their value and they may sometimes do harm in that further retinal haemorrhage may occur during treatment. The situation in regard to fibrinolytic therapy is similar. Trials in central retinal vein occlusion have failed to indicate significant visual benefit. The incidence of rubeotic glaucoma was reduced but vitreous haemorrhages were a serious complication in those patients who received the drug (Kohner et al, 1974).

Corticosteroids

Systemic steroids have a place in the treatment of intraocular inflammation particularly when there is involvement of the retinal vasculature and oedema or progressive vascular occlusions. The place of treatment is not certain, but corticosteroids in high doses are often used. It is very difficult to assess the long-term benefits of treatment in this group of diseases which have a very variable natural history and in which there have been no adequate clinical trials of treatment.

In the absence of inflammatory signs it is difficult to justify the use of steroids for retinal vascular disease.

Immunosuppressive agents

There is no doubt that some intraocular inflammations have an immunological basis. Immunosuppression with azathioprine is advocated for retinal vasculitis especially in cases where intolerably high doses of systemic corticosteroids might otherwise be required. It is however difficult to evaluate the effectiveness of this treatment, as no controlled clinical studies are yet available. A number of papers have been published advocating the use of immunosuppressives in Behcet's disease (Tricoulis, 1976). The long-term benefit to vision from this treatment however remains questionable.

Local treatment

Local treatment of retinal vascular disease may be divided into the therapy of the retinal responses and the treatment of associated ocular conditions. Photocoagulation has become a standard method of treatment for retinal vascular disease. It is used to influence both macular oedema and neovascularisation. The Xenon arc photocoagulator has been used for a number of years, but more recently the Argon laser has become the instrument of choice. The slit-lamp delivery system makes the laser application easy and safe, particularly when close to the macula where accuracy is essential.

The clinical effects of the laser and xenon arc are nevertheless similar in experienced hands. Studies in proliferative diabetic retinopathy have shown that the two sources have similar therapeutic effects on new vessels, and that there is little difference in side effects or patient acceptance (Crick, Chignell & Shilling, 1978). There is however, experimental evidence in animals that the two sources of energy have different effects on the retinal circulation (Hill and Atherton, 1979).

Macular oedema

Photocoagulation of the abnormal permeability response is aimed at reducing the amount of leakage from the involved vasculature by destroying the capillaries involved, and thereby allowing the remaining normal vessels to absorb the oedema fluid. The best example of this treatment is in diabetic exudative maculopathy in which photocoagulation is applied to the centres of circinate exudate rings where the main vascular leaks occur (Figure 16.7). This method is now standard and its efficacy has been proved in clinical trials (British Diabetic Study, 1975).

Recently three types of diabetic maculopathy have been defined, and studies have shown differing therapeutic responses (Whitelocke et al, 1979). The three types are exudative (focal), cystoid maculopathy and ischaemic maculopathy. Differentiation is important because only in the first type can consistently good results be anticipated. Careful slit-lamp biomicroscopy and fluorescein angiography is necessary to identify the type of disease.

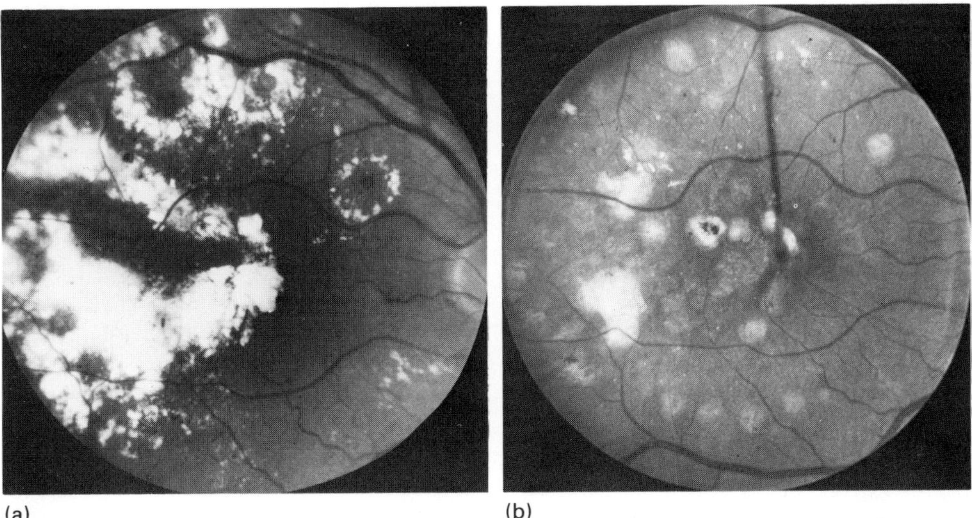

(a)   (b)

Fig. 16.7   (a) From a retinal colour photograph of a diabetic patient with exudative macular oedema. (b) The same eye following absorption of exudate achieved by the use of paramacular photocoagulation.

Clinical trials have been important in assessing the effects of this treatment in different diseases. For example, in branch vein occlusion where macular oedema is a significant cause of visual impairment photocoagulation has been shown to have little effect on the visual prognosis (Shilling, 1976); there are similar findings in central retinal vein occlusion (Laatikainen, 1977). This result is disappointing in view of the improvement in the appearance of the retina seen after treatment.

By comparison it has been shown that the oedematous response caused by retinal arterial microaneurysms is often improved by photocoagulation with a beneficial effect on vision (Cleary et al, 1975).

There are a number of rare causes of macular oedema for which photocoagulation is often useful. The lesion of Coat's disease for example, which may be either in the retinal periphery or in the paramacular area, may benefit greatly from photocoagulation (Cleary, 1976).

It is important to diagnose accurately the underlying cause of the oedematous response when considering photocoagulation. It would be wrong, for example to use this treatment for inflammatory macular oedema for which anti-inflammatory drugs are indicated. Similarly there is no place for photocoagulation in aphakic macular oedema.

Neovascularisation

Photocoagulation for the neovascular response is in many ways more rewarding than in the treatment of oedema.

Preretinal new vessels which threaten vision because of vitreous haemorrhage may be destroyed by direct photocoagulation (Figure 16.8). New vessels on the disc

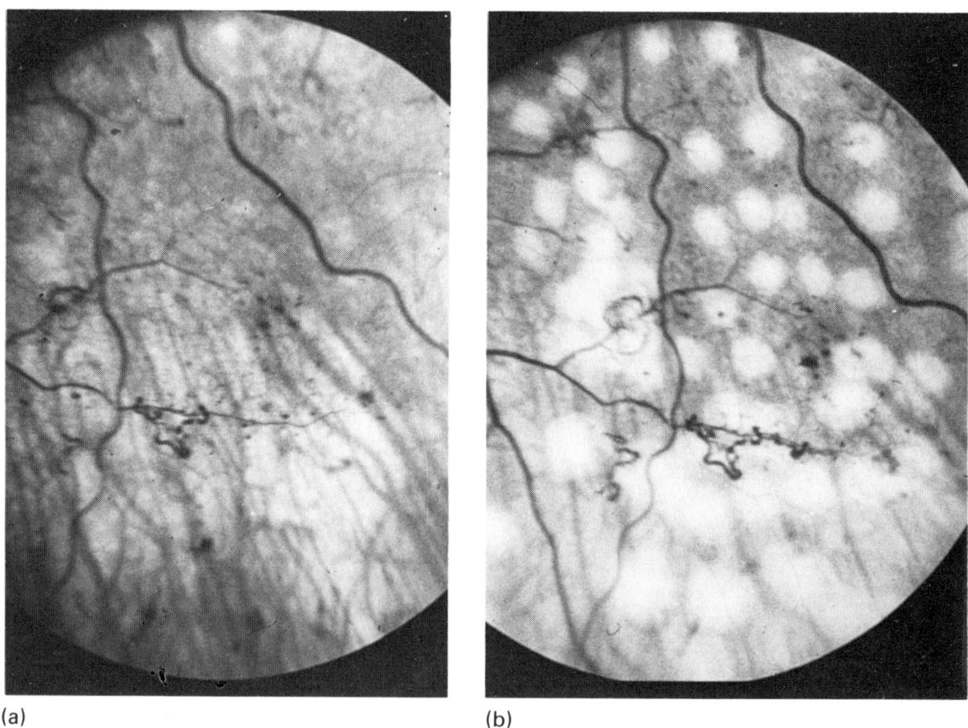

(a)   (b)

Fig. 16.8   (a) From a retinal colour photograph of a diabetic patient showing small areas of neovascularisation. (b) The same area of retina shortly following treatment showing laser burns applied to the new vessels and associated areas of capillary closure.

although not amenable to direct treatment may often respond to an indirect approach in which areas of capillary closure are coagulated (peripheral retinal ablation). This reduces the neovascular stimulus and new disc vessels usually regress although to a variable extent (Figure 16.9).

New vessels in diabetics constitute the classical example of this and clinical trials have confirmed the place of this therapy (American Diabetic Study, 1976; British Diabetic Study, 1975). Similar good results are seen in retinal vein occlusions (Shilling, 1976) and it is only in the neovascular response to retinal vascular

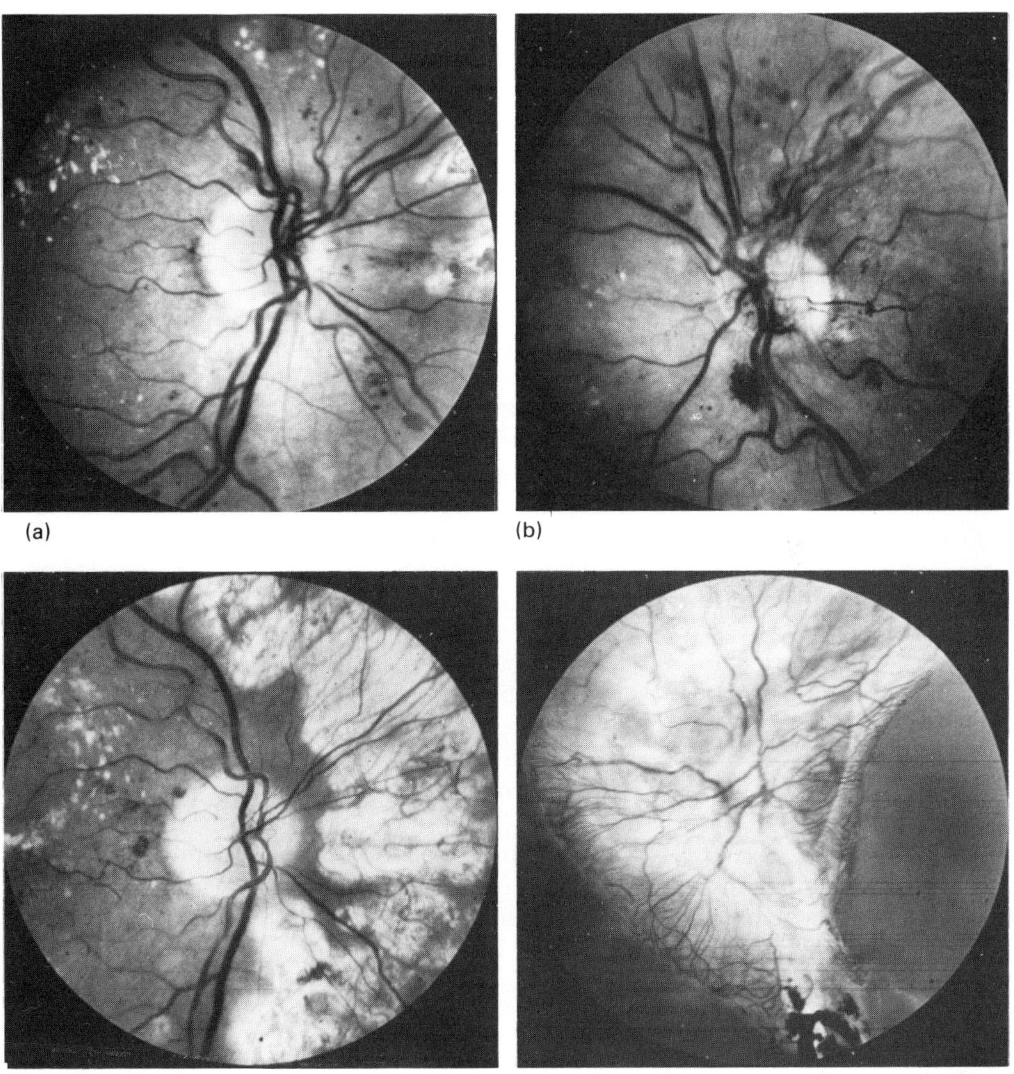

Fig. 16.9   (a) and (b) From colour photographs of the optic discs of a diabetic showing early neovascularisation. (c) and (d) From colour photographs of the same patient two years later. The right eye had been treated with peripheral photocoagulation and maintains good vision. The left eye has progressed to blindness because of extensive neovascularisation.

inflammatory disease that doubt still exists as to the efficacy of this treatment, (Sanders & Shilling, 1976).

Rubeosis iridis is also treated by pan-photocoagulation of the retina. This treatment was first suggested in 1961 (Smith, 1961). Studies in patients with central retinal vein occlusion have recently confirmed that painful thrombotic glaucoma may be prevented by this therapy (Blach, Hitchings & Laatikainen, 1977). Vision in this condition is poor and is very rarely improved, but resolution of the neovascularisation is undoubtedly a worthwhile result of this treatment. It is best carried out in the early stages of rubeosis before there is permanent damage to the drainage angle because when this has developed treatment becomes much more difficult and alternative therapy is required to control the intraocular pressure.

In addition to photocoagulation, diathermy and cryotherapy have been used to ablate areas of retina, but diathermy is now rarely used. Cryotherapy is however sometimes useful for peripheral retinal ablation particularly when the clarity of the ocular media is reduced so that photocoagulation is impossible to apply.

Treatment of the late complications of retinal vascular diseases
The most severe sequeleae of retinal vascular disease leading to blindness are neovascular glaucoma, vitreous haemorrhage and vitreous traction, causing either macular traction or retinal detachment. Photocoagulation unquestionably has a place in their prevention but once these late complications have occurred it is unhelpful.

The treatment of established neovascular glaucoma remains very difficult; cyclocrotherapy is sometimes helpful in reducing the intraocular pressure, and occasionally glaucoma drainage surgery is used (Molteno, Van Rooyen & Bartholomew, 1977). Blind painful eyes due to this cause have in the past often required enucleation, but the necessity for this has been reduced by a regimé of intensive local steroids and atropine which often relieves discomfort but does not restore vision (Blach, Hitchings & Laatikainen, 1977).

Vitreous haemorrhages and traction retinal detachments are now treatable by vitrectomy using techniques which have been developed recently. Opaque vitreous may be removed by microsurgical instruments inserted through small incisions in the pars plana ciliaris. It is also possible with this method to cut vitreoretinal traction bands which are causing retinal detachment allowing the retina to reattach (Aaberg, 1974; Michael, 1978).

It is interesting that following the removal of the vitreous scaffold previously forward-growing neovascular tissue often resolves and this has lead to theories as to the role of the vitreous in the neovascular response; these are as yet incompletely formulated (Shilling, McLeod & Restori, 1978).

GLAUCOMA AND RETINAL VASCULAR DISEASE

Chronic glaucoma is an important cause of visual loss because of optic nerve damage. There is in addition a link between raised intraocular pressure and retinal vascular occlusive disease. Patients with central retinal vein occlusion have a high incidence of glaucoma (Kohner, 1964) and the reverse is also true (Hitchings & Spaith, 1976). There is little relationship between branch vein occlusion and glaucoma. Hemisphere occlusions may occur at the margin of a glaucomatous optic disc, but most studies fail to show any relationship between the more peripheral vein occlusions and glaucoma. Recently it has been found, however, that patients with either central or branch vein occlusion show a greater rise in intraocular pressure when changing from the sitting to the lying position than controls (Williams & Peart, 1978) and this mechanism has been suggested as an aetiological factor.

Retinal arteriolar occlusions may follow very high intraocular pressure particularly in patients whose ocular circulation is also compromised by other causes. Acute closed angle glaucoma is the commonest condition in which the intraocular pressure is high enough to cause this type of occlusion but it may also occur after external pressure on the globe.

The effect of raised intraocular pressure on ocular perfusion has been demonstrated in normal subjects by fluorescein angiogram studies, which have confirmed reduction in the perfusion of both choroid and retina with increasing intraocular pressure (Blumenthal et al, 1971). Similar studies in patients with chronic glaucoma have demonstrated reduced peripapillary choroidal perfusion (Best et al, 1972). The significance of these findings in the pathogenesis of glaucomatous visual loss remains controversial.

Reduction of the intraocular pressure to normal is essential when there is evidence of optic nerve or retinal vascular occlusion. This may require medical or surgical treatment, the latter being usually reserved for those cases in which non-operative methods have failed to lower the intraocular pressure sufficiently.

OPTIC NEURITIS

Natural history

Few clinical problems have as many medical and social implications for the future as a young woman with retrobulbar neuritis. The diagnosis can usually be made with certainty on clinical grounds and the prospects of satisfactory return of vision are good. However, the gravest uncertainty exists in predicting the long-term outcome in terms of the development of multiple sclerosis.

That multiple sclerosis can begin as a retrobulbar neuritis is undoubted; approximately 20 per cent of patients are said to present in this way (Liebowitz & Alter, 1973). Furthermore, 50 per cent of patients with multiple sclerosis have a clinical episode involving the optic nerve at some time during the course of their illness and many more have clinical evidence of optic nerve involvement in the form of pallor of the optic disc or delayed conduction in the visual pathways detectable by electro-physological testing (Halliday, McDonald & Mushin, 1973). At autopsy in fatal cases of multiple sclerosis pathological changes in the optic nerve are constantly found (Lumsden, 1970). On the other hand, some patients after a typical attack of retrobulbar neuritis remain free of symptoms and signs and apparently never develop multiple sclerosis.

What is at present uncertain is whether patients who suffer only from retrobulbar neuritis have a mild form of multiple sclerosis or whether isolated retrobulbar neuritis is a distinct disease entity perhaps with a different cause.

Factors influencing prognosis

Previous studies on the proportion of patients with optic neuritis who develop multiple sclerosis have given conflicting results. Recently Compston et al (1978) have investigated the relative importance of genetic and environmental factors in forecasting the prognosis of patients presenting with isolated optic neuritis. Of 146 patients reassessed clinically one month to 23 years after presentation, 58 (40 per cent) had developed multiple sclerosis. All patients were tissue typed. Three factors were found to be significantly associated with the development of multiple sclerosis. These were recurrent attacks of optic neuritis, the presence of HLA antigen, BT 101 (now equivalent to HLA-DRw2) and the occurrence of the attack during the winter months. Using an actuarial analysis it was calculated that 73 per cent of patients with optic neuritis with the BT 101 antigen would develop the disease within 8 years compared with 34 per cent in those in whom it was not found.

Although the practical value of these findings in individual patients is limited, the results go some way to reconciling the differences between environmental and genetic theories of causation, and indicate that both may be important. Previous observations emphasising genetic influences (such as those showing an increased incidence in first degree relatives) are not necessarily at varience with those linking the development of multiple sclerosis to virus infection or to environmental factors such as latitude. It had previously been shown that patients who move in adult life from a region of high prevalence (such as northern Europe) to one of low prevalence (such as South Africa) continue to show the same susceptibility to multiple sclerosis as those in their country of origin whereas children who emigrate before the age of 15 show the lower incidence levels similar to those of their new environment (Dean, 1967).

Compston et al conclude that there are at least two forms of optic neuritis each having a different aetiology and the subsequent development of multiple sclerosis is due to the interaction between an environmental agent and a genetically susceptible host. Multiple sclerosis does not manifest itself unless both factors are present. The environmental agent may possibly be a virus — there are certainly many reports of virus particles resembling myxoviruses present in the brains of multiple sclerosis patients and of transmission of a cytopathic factor in the cell free extract of brains from multiple sclerosis patients to animals (Carp, 1972). However there is as yet no agreement as to the identity of such an agent.

A single hypothesis is now beginning to emerge from the various apparently separate approaches to the aetiology of this baffling disease. It is that a genetically determined immunological deficiency allows the persistence of a virus infection acquired during the early years of life and that the virus periodically becomes reactivated and produces myelin breakdown, the products of which are themselves antigenic and lead to an autoimmune reaction and further damage.

The practical lessons from recent epidemiological work are clear. Young patients with an isolated first attack of optic neuritis who are negative for BT 101 can be reassured not only that full symptomatic recovery is likely but also that there is a reasonable prospect (approximately 65 per cent) that they will remain free of further episodes; the chance of a relapse decreases with time but there is no fixed period beyond which a relapse may not occur.

On the other hand, in patients with optic neuritis who are found to carry the antigen BT 101 and have the onset during the winter months then the prognosis should be more guarded, for the chances of developing multiple sclerosis are high.

Detection of minor degrees of optic neuritis
It is an old observation that optic neuritis may be followed by pallor of the optic disc although visions has apparently completely recovered. The sign is of limited value because minor degrees of optic disc pallor are difficult to detect with confidence. There are, however, a number of clinical features which may enable the physician to detect mild unilateral impairment of the optic nerve function even when corrected visual acuity and conventional field testing are equal and normal in each eye. The

testing of colour vision is often rewarding either employing pseudoisochromatic plates or relying on subjective differences reported by the patient in brightness or in the degree of saturation of coloured objects when comparison is made between the two eyes. Subjective deterioration in visual acuity after a hot bath or after exercise are also highly characteristic of optic neuritis; this may relate to an alteration in the electrophysiological characteristics of segmentally demyelinated nerve fibres as a result of a small rise in central body temperature.

Other subjective abnormalities occasionally helpful in assessing progression and recovery are the visual illusions affecting binocular perception of moving objects (particularly when two images are moving relative to one another as when a patient is in a vehicle). This again is probably an expression of slight differences in the velocity of conduction between the two eyes and can be demonstrated in the pendulum test devised by Pulfrich. To the patient with unilateral optic neuritis the pathway described by the pendulum may appear as an ellipse rather than a straight line.

Subjective methods of analysis may also be applied to field testing. Small arcuate partial defects in the field of vision above or below the fixation point caused by fall out of bundles of nerve fibres may be detected by the alert patient as a flickering effect when a small test object is moved along the vertical meridian. The slit like grooves left in the superficial nerve fibre layer of the retina by the disappearance of groups of nerve fibres may also be seen ophthalmoscopically, especially with the aid of red free light (Hoyt, 1976). This requires considerable practice and the appearances are difficult to distinguish from the normal crescentic opacities seen above and below the papillomacular bundle. When nerve fibre fall out is extensive the retinal blood vessels become unduly prominent, standing out in sharp relief from the shrunken nerve fibre layer.

Visual evoked potentials
Electrophysiological recording of the potential generated at the occipital cortex by a visual stimulus applied separately to each eye has also proved a most valuable tool in detecting optic nerve damage especially when a pattern reversal stimulus is used.

Experimental work has shown that demyelination in the central nervous system may have various effects; there may be complete conduction block, there may be a partial block with failure of transmission of trains of impulses or there may be slowing of conduction through the demyelinated segment. These effects can be shown in the optic nerve in clinical optic neuritis using either a flash or a pattern reversed stimulus but in practice the latter shows the least variation and enables an abnormality to be recognised more easily in an individual patient. The delay in conduction is established early in the disease and persists after clinical recovery whereas the amplitude of the response tends to reflect the visual acuity and returns to normal as the acute attack subsides. The changes are not specific for multiple sclerosis since similar delays have been found in patients with toxic or ischaemic damage to the optic nerves. However, it remains the most sensitive test currently available and is particularly valuable when used to detect asymptomatic lesions of the optic nerve in patients with spinal cord disease thus establishing the diagnosis of multiple sclerosis. Abnormal latencies are found in 95 per cent of patients with definite multiple sclerosis irrespective of the presence or absence of visual impairment (Halliday, McDonald & Mushin, 1973).

OPTIC NEURITIS AND PUPILLARY CHANGES

Clinical observations relating visual acuity to impairment in the pupillary light reflex go back for hundreds of years but the recording of pupillary responses has always presented technical difficulty. The recent introduction of infra-red pupillography and computer assisted analysis of the results has confirmed and refined some old observations. The comparison of amplitude of the pupillary response from each eye shows a reduction in amplitude on the side of the optic nerve lesion and this is the principal feature of the afferent pupillary defect ascribed to Marcus Gunn. Pupillography has shown that in normal subjects the amplitude, latency and velocity of contraction are all dependent to some extent on the intensity of the light stimulus. In optic neuritis the response of the pupil on the affected side is not only smaller but is also delayed and would be appropriate to a lesser light stimulus (Ellis, 1979). The abnormality which can be detected in pupillary function is less marked than that in the visual evoked potential and the responses from an affected eye may fall within the normal range. Comparison between the two eyes, however, shows consistent differences in pupillary response which persist even after the attack has subsided and normal visual acuity has been regained (Ellis, 1979). Even without the aid of pupillometer the detection of a relative afferent pupillary defect by the swinging light test is a constant and valuable sign of unilateral optic neuritis, past or present, especially if carefully performed under optimal conditions with attention to details such as the degree of pupillary escape (failure to sustain contraction).

REFERENCES

Aaberg T M 1974 Diabetic traction retinal detachment. American Journal of Ophthalmology 88: 246–253

Acheson J, Danta G, Hutchinson E C 1969 Controlled trial of dipyridamole in cerebral vascular disease. British Medical Journal 1: 614

Archer D B, Ernest J T, Newell F V 1974 Classification of branch retinal obstruction. Transactions of the American Academy of Ophthalmology and Otolarynology 78: 148–165

Best M, Blumenthal M, Galin M A, Toyofuku H 1972 Fluorescein angiography during induced ocular hypertension in glaucoma. British Journal of Ophthalmology 56: 6–12

Blach R K, Hitchings R A, Laatikainen L 1977 Thrombotic glaucoma. Transactions of the Ophthalmological Society of the United Kingdom 97: 275–279

Blumental M, Best M, Galin M A, Gitter K A 1971 Ocular circulation: analysis of the effect of induced ocular hypertension on retinal and choroidal blood flow in man. American Journal of Ophthalmology 71: 819–825

Boghen D, Glaser J S 1975 Iachaemic optic neuropathy — clinical profile and natural history. Brain 98: 689

British Diabetic Retinopathy Study 1975 Photocoagulation in the treatment of diabetic maculopathy. Lancet ii: 1110–1113

Canadian Co-operative Study Group 1978 A randomised trial of asprin and sulphinpyrazone in threatened stroke. New England Journal of Medicine 299: 53–59

Carp R I, Licursi P C, Merz P A, Merz G S 1972 Decreased percentage of polymorphonuclear neutrophils in mouse peripheral blood after inoculation with material from multiple sclerosis patients. Journal of Experimental Medicine 136: 618–629

Carter A B 1965 Prognosis of cerebral embolism. Lancet ii: 514

Cleary P E 1976 Retina-vascular malformations. Transactions of the Ophthalmological Society of the United Kingdom 96: 213–215

Cleary P E, Kohner E M, Hamilton A M, Bird A C 1975 Retinal Macroaneurysms. British Journal of Ophthalmology 59: 355–361

Clemett R S 1974 Retinal branch vein occlusion. British Journal of Ophthalmology 58: 548–554

Clemett R S, Kohner E M, Hamilton A M 1973 Visual prognosis in retinal branch vein occlusion. Transactions of the Ophthalmological Society of the United Kingdom 93: 523–535

Coldwell J S 1966 Effect of diabetic control on retinopathy. Diabetes 15: 497–499

Compston D A S, Batchelor J R, Earl C J, McDonald W I 1978 Factors influencing the risk of multiple sclerosis developing in patients with optic neuritis. Brain 101: 495–511

Crick M D P, Chignell A H, Shilling J S 1978 Argon laser v. xenon arc photocoagulation in proliferative diabetic retinopathy. Transactions of the Ophthalmological Society of the United Kingdom: 98: 170–171

Crompton M R 1959 Visual changes in temporal arteritis. Brain 82: 377

Cullen J F, Town S M, Campbell C J 1974 Double-blind trial of Atromid S in exudative diabetic retinopathy. Transactions of the Ophthalmological Society of the United Kingdom 94: 554–562

Diabetic Retinopathy Study Research Group 1976 Preliminary report on effects of photocoagulation therapy. American Journal of Ophthalmology 81: 1–14

Dyken M L, Kolar O J, Jones F H 1973 Differences in the occurrence of carotid transient ischaemic attacks associated with antiplatelet aggregation therapy. Stroke 4: 732–736

Dean G 1967 Annual incidence, prevalence and mortality of multiple sclerosis in white South-African-born and in white immigrants to South Africa. British Medical Journal i: 724–730

Eagling E M, Sanders M D, Miller S J H 1974 Ischaemic papillopathy. British Journal of Ophthalmology 58: 990

Ellis C J K 1979 The afferent pupillary defect in acute optic neuritis. Journal of Neurology, Neurosurgery and Psychiatry 42: 1008–1017

ffytche T J 1977 Retinal vasculitis. Transactions of the Ophthalmological Society of the United Kingdom 97: 457–461

ffytche T J, Blach R K 1970 The aetiology of macular oedema. Transactions of the Ophthalmological Society of the United Kingdom 90: 637–656

Fields W S, Lemak M A, Frankowski R F, Hardy R J 1977 Controlled trial of asprin in cerebral ischaemia. Stroke 8: 301–316

Fields W S, Maslenikov V, Meyer J S et al 1970 Joint study of extracranial arterial occlusion. Journal of American Medical Association 211: 1933

Fisher C M 1954 Occlusion of the carotid arteries. Archives of Neurology and Psychiatry 72: 187

Fisher C M 1959 Observations on the retinal blood vessels in monocular blindness. Neurology 9: 333

Garner A, Ashton N 1979 Pathogenesis of hypertensive retinopathy — a review. Journal of the Royal Society of Medicine 72: 362–365

Gass J D M, Olson C L 1973 Sarcoidosis with optic nerve and retinal involvement — a clinicopathological case. Transactions of the American Academy of Ophthalmology and Otolaryngology 77 Op: 739–750

Glaser J 1978 Neuro-ophthalmology. Harper & Row, New York

Gunning A, Pickering G, Robb Smith A H T et al 1964 Mural thrombosis of the internal carotid-artery and subsequent embolism. Quarterly Journal of Medicine 33: 155

Halliday A M, McDonald W I, Mushin J 1973 Visual evoked response in diagnosis of multiple sclerosis. British Medical Journal iv: 661–664

Harrison M J G, Marshall J 1975 Indications for angiography and surgery in carotid artery disease. British Medical Journal i: 616

Harrison M J G, Marshall J, Meadows J C, Russell R W R 1971 The effect of asprin in amaurosis fugax. Lancet ii: 743–744

Hill D W, Atherton H 1979 Experimental studies of the retinal circulation relating to diabetic retinopathy. Transactions of the Ophthalmological Society of the United Kingdom (in press)

Hinton R C, Kistler J P, Fallon J T et al 1977 Influence of aetiology of atrial fibrillation on incidence of systemic embolism. American Journal of Cardiology 40: 509–513

Hitchings R A, Spaeth G. L. 1976 Chronic retinal vein occlusion in glaucoma. British Journal of Ophthalmology 60: 694–699

Hoyt W F 1976 Fundoscopic changes in the retinal nerve fibre layer in chronic and active optic neuropathies. Transactions of the Ophthalmological Society of the United Kingdom 71: 368

Kohner E M 1964 Retinal vein occlusion. Proceedings of the Royal Society of Medicine 57: 816

Kohner E M, Fraser T R, Joplin G F, Oakley N W 1969 In: The affect of diabetic control on diabetic retinopathy in treatment of diabetic retinopathy. Goldberg & Fine (eds) US Dept of Health Education and Welfare, p 119–128

Kohner E M, Hamilton A M, Bulpitt C J, Dollery C T 1974 Streptokinase in the treatment of central retinal vein occlusion. Transactions of the Ophthalmological Society of the United Kingdom 94: 599–603

Kohner E M, Shilling J S 1976 Retinal vein occlusion. In: Clifford Rose F (ed) Medical ophthalmology. Chapman and Hall, Ch 28, p 393–429

Kohner E M, Shilling J S, Clemett R S 1974 Clinical aspects of retinal branch vein occlusion signficant for the understanding of its pathogenesis and preventive therapy. World Congress of Ophthalmology. Document Ophthal. Cong. Series No. 5

Laatikainen L. 1977 Preliminary report on effect of retinal pan-photocoagulation on rubeosis and new vessel glaucoma. British Journal of Ophthalmology 61: 278–284

Laatikainen L, Kohner E M 1976 Fluorescein angiography and its prognostic significances in central retinal vein occlusion. British Journal of Ophthalmology 60: 411–418

Liebowtiz U, Alter M 1973 Multiple sclerosis — clues to its cause. Amsterdam, Holland

Lumsden C E 1970 Neuropathology of multiple sclerosis. In: Vinken P J, Bruyn G W (eds) Handbook of clinical neurology. Amsterdam, vol 9, p 217–309

Luxon L M, Crowther A, Harrison M J G, Coltart D J 1979 A controlled study of 24-hour ambulatory electrocardiographic monitoring in patients with transient neurological symptoms. British Medical Journal (in press)

Moncada S, Vane J R 1979 Arachidonic acid metabolites and the interactions between platelets and blood vessel walls. New England Journal of Medicine 300: 1142–1147

Michaels R G 1978 Vitrectomy for complications of diabetic retinopathy. Archives of Ophthalmology 96: 237–246

Molteno A C B, Van Rooyen M M B, Bartholomew R S 1977 Implants for draining neovascular glaucoma. British Journal of Ophthalmology 61: 120–125

Mundall J, Quintero P, v Kualla K N, Harmon R, Austin J 1972 Transient monocular blindness and increased platelet aggregability treated with asprin. Neurology 22: 280–285

O'Day J, Shilling J S, ffytche T J 1979 Retinal vasculitis. Transactions of the Ophthalmological Society of the United Kingdom (in press)

Russell R W R 1959 Giant cell arteritis: a review of 35 cases. Quarterly Journal of Medicine, 28: 471

Russell R W R 1968 The source of retinal emboli. Lancet ii: 789

Sanders M D, Shilling J S 1976 Retinal, choroidal and optic disc involvement in sarcoidosis. Transactions of the Ophthalmological Society of the United Kingdom 96: 140–144

Shikano S 1966 In: Monacelli & Nassaro (eds) International symposium on Behcets disease. Kargel, Basel, New York p 111

Shilling J S 1976 Retinal haemorrhages — a specific example — retinal vein occlusion. In: 5th Congress of European Ophthalmology. Ferdinand Enke Verlag, Stuttgart, p 164–166

Shilling J S 1976 Vascular changes after retinal branch vein occlusion. Transactions of the Ophthalmological Society of the United Kingdom 96: 193–196

Shilling J S, Kohner E M 1976 New vessel formation in retinal branch vein occlusion. British Journal of Ophthalmology 60: 810–815

Shilling J S, McLeod D, Restori M 1978 The control of intraocular neovascularisation. Excerpta Medica International Congress Series No. 450: 822–825

Smith R J H 1961 Neovascularisation in ocular disease. Transactions of the Ophthalmological Society of the United Kingdom 81: 125–172

Sullivan J M, Harken D E, Gorlin R 1968 Pharmologic control of thrombo-anabolic complication of cardiac valve replacement. New England Journal of Medicine 279: 576

Tricoulis DIM 1976 Treatment of Behcets disease with chlorambucil. British Journal of Ophthalmology 60: 55–59

Vannas S, Orma H 1957 Experience of treatment retinal venous occlusion with anticoagulants and anticlerosis therapy. Archives of Ophthalmology 58: 812–828

Whisnant, J P, Metsumoto N, Elveback L R 1973 The effect of anticoagulant treatment on the prognosis of patients with transient cerebral ischaemic attacks in a community. Mayo Clinic Proceedings 48: 844

Whitelocke R, Kearns M, Blach R K, Hamilton A M 1979 Diabetic maculopathy. Transactions of the Ophthalmological Society of the United Kingdom (in press)

Wilkinson I MS 1972 The vertebral artery: extracranial and intracranial structure. Archives of Neurology 27: 392

Wilkinson I M S, Russell R W R 1972 Arteries of the head and neck in giant cell arteritis. Archives of Neurology 27: 378

Williams B I, Peart W S 1978 Effect of posture on the intraocular pressure of patients with retinal vein obstruction. British Journal of Ophthalmology 62: 688–693

Wilson L A, Russell R W R 1977 Amaurosis fugax and carotid artery disease: indications for angiography. British Medical Journal ii: 435–437

Wilson L A 1977 Platelet survival in amaurosis fugax. In: Breddin K, Dorndorf W, Loew D, Marx R (eds) IV Colfarit-symposium, Berlin

Wilson L A, Russell R W R, Warlow C P 1979 Cardiovascular disease in patients with retinal artery occlusion. Lancet i: 292–294

17. Intravenous nutrition: indications, requirements and complications

H. F. Woods

Introduction

Attention to the nutritional needs of a patient ranks in importance with that given to the maintenance of normal cardiovascular, respiratory and renal function.

Parenteral nutrition is a form of therapy which has been gradually introduced during the last 25 years. It's development depended upon the accumulation of knowledge concerning the metabolic response to injury and disease together with accurate assessment of human nutritional requirements. Considerable impetus was provided by the work of Dudrick and his colleagues (Dudrick et al, 1968) who showed that total parenteral nutrition could provide sufficient nutrients to sustain normal growth and development in the mammal.

The concept underlying parenteral nutrition is simple and can be simply expressed in the form of an equation:

Normal nutrition via the gut ≡ Infusion of nutrients into the circulation

However, continued experience has greatly refined the technique and revealed that it is accompanied by considerable hazards and side effects, some of which show that the equation above is an over-simplification.

INDICATIONS

Within the general hospital it has been estimated that between one and five per cent of all acute hospital admissions will require parenteral nutrition as part of their management. The indications for its use can be deduced by reference to two main starting points. Firstly why was the technique developed and secondly to what extent does malnutrition exist within the hospital population and what are the consequences for the patient? Parenteral nutrition was developed in order to meet the nutritional needs of the patient when feeding via the gastrointestinal tract was not possible or was not indicated. It follows from this that the main indications stem from gastrointestinal disease particularly so called 'gastrointestinal failure' and gastrointestinal surgery. The conventional indications can be divided into three main groups as shown in Table 17.1. Although the list is long the individual indications must be considered in the light of one main criterion, namely that of efficacy. In many instances there is little proof of efficacy and it is valuable to review selected parts of the content of Table 17.1 in this light, together with a survey of the more general problem of the extent of malnutrition within the hospital population.

The nutritional status of hospital patients

The incidence of detectable nutritional deficiencies within medical and surgical inpatients has been shown to be high in surveys performed in this country and the United States (Bistrian et al, 1974, 1976; Bollet & Owens, 1973; Hill et al, 1977). In one of these studies (Hill et al, 1977) there was evidence that a deterioration of nutritional state continued during the hospital stay and that in many cases it was unrecognised and thus untreated.

Table 17.1   The indications for parenteral nutrition

General	Specific	Occasional
As a supplement to the oral route	Enterocutaneous fistulae	Schizophrenia
During prolonged postoperative starvation (over 4 days)	Inflammatory bowel disease	Anorexia nervosa
As an adjunct to tumour chemotherapy	Short bowel syndrome	
In conjunction with enteral feeding	Acute pancreatitis	
	Acute renal failure	
	Following severe burn injury	
	Hepatic coma	
	Congenital deformities of the upper gastrointestinal tract	

Some figures abstracted from the paper of Hill et al (1977) relating to surgical inpatients serve to illustrate this point (see Table 17.2). Similar figures have been obtained for medical inpatients, Bistrain et al (1976).

Table 17.2   Nutritional state of unselected surgical inpatients (This data has been abstracted from the paper of Hill et al, 1977)

Measurement	% of patients with a low value[*]
Weight/height ratio	21
Triceps skinfold thickness	56
Arm muscle circumference	48
Serum albumin	26
Haemoglobin	20
Plasma transferrin	41
Leukocyte ascorbic acid	34
Red cell — folate	24
vitamin B_{12}	20
vitamin B_6	6

[*] In all cases the patient was assigned to the low value group on the bases of either comparison with standard tables of values (anthropometric measurements) or with a control group.

Such measurements do not however in themselves necessarily justify the use of nutritional therapy to support the patient. The justification emerges when the consequences of malnutrition, particularly of protein are considered (Table 17.3). These are mainly the increased morbidity and mortality which ensue from the increased susceptibility to infection, impaired immune competence, delayed tissue repair and healing. These are, for the most part, the result of loss of body protein stores and occur irrespective of the underlying disease process be it severe trauma, burns, systemic disease or specific organ disease. In addition the individual patient

Table 17.3   The clinical consequences of protein malnutrition

Loss of weight
Impaired humoral and cellular immune competence
Increased susceptibility to infection
Increased risk of wound dehiscence
Oedema
Increased mortality

may have other nutritional deficiencies such as those of vitamins and in the elderly the very fact of increased age is accompanied by nutritional deficiencies.

If then it is accepted that the existence of malnutrition does render the individual to be 'at risk' particularly in relation to subsequent surgery or sepsis, can the use of parenteral nutrition improve the prognosis in that individual? This question returns us to the subject of efficacy and is best answered by discussion of certain indications included in Table 17.1.

A good example is that of inflammatory and granulomatous bowel disease particularly where the upper gastrointestinal tract is involved. In cases of ulcerative colitis or Crohn's disease parenteral nutrition may be indicated during an acute exacerbation or in relation to surgery either during the immediate preoperative period or postoperatively because of the development of complications such as fistulae.

For example Meng & Sandstead (1972) described five patients with inflammatory bowel disease who were successfully fed intravenously. These authors described one patient with Crohn's disease in detail. They were able to maintain this patient for 38 days using sources of nitrogen, calories and vitamins together with minerals infused continuously into a central vein. In this case there was true gain in weight and closure of an enterocutaneous fistula. Other similar cases are described by Dudrick et al (1969). Such cases illustrate the value of parenteral nutrition. Patients with inflammatory bowel disase may have a long history of poor food intake as a result of anorexia or frequent diarrhoea. Gross weight loss may have occurred with muscle wasting and low plasma protein concentrations are often found. In addition sepsis in the form of abscesses can occur.

Two main benefits thus accrue from parenteral nutrition, firstly the reversal of the nutritional deficit which is known to be associated with a poor prognosis and secondly the healing of fistulas. Before the use of parenteral nutrition the mortality amongst patients with upper gastrointestinal tract fistulae was high (approx. 40 per cent). The case cited above is an example of recent experience and it seems that 80 per cent of such fistulae close spontaneously and the mortality falls to below 10 per cent with the use of parenteral nutrition (MacFayden et al, 1973).

Some authorities suggest that parenteral nutrition is the treatment of choice when inflammatory bowel disease is complicated by severe diarrhoea or fistulae (Meng & Sandstead, 1972). It allows complete bypass of the bowel and thus what has been called 'physiological rest' to occur.

The presence of malignant disease is now an important indication. Until recently there had been fears that the tumour would grow at the expense of the host but experience has shown this not to be the case. The patient with cancer may have muscle wasting accompanied by a negative nitrogen balance and suppression of the immune response (Smythe et al, 1971). These effects and their influence on wound healing and resistance to infection are particularly important in the patient with cancer who is to have surgery, chemotherapy or radiotherapy or a combination of these treatments. The use of parenteral nutrition in such patients has been beneficial in allowing a better response to therapy (Copeland et al, 1974, 1978). However, as has been pointed out in a recent British Medical Journal Leading Article (British Medical Journal, 1979), judgement of efficacy is particularly difficult in such patients.

The final group in Table 17.1 lists conditions in which parenteral nutrition has been used but in no circumstances can these be considered as absolute indications and the hazards of the therapy may well outweigh any benefit in such cases.

Adherence to a list of suggested or proven indications is not ideal; the clinician should ask the question 'does the patient need nutritional therapy?' When this question has been asked there are a number of alternatives which range from simple measures such as altering the frequency and palatability of oral feeds and the use of so called elemental diets on the one hand to parenteral feeding on the other. It is useful to have a logical train of decision and the one reproduced in Figure 17.1 is based on that outlined by Lee (1979).

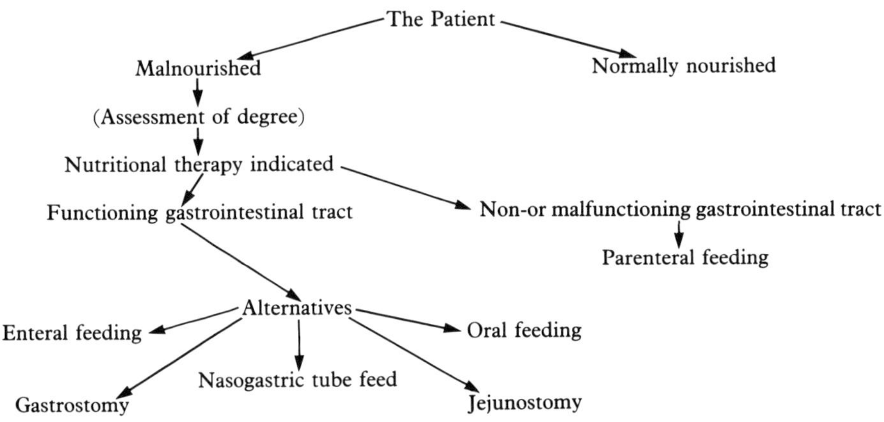

Fig. 17.1   Alternatives for nutritional support (After Lee, 1979, with permission.)

The availability of the newer enteral feeding methods using chemically defined diets has modified the use of parenteral nutrition as many patients who would have been fed intravenously are now managed by using these alternatives. Implicit in the scheme shown is the nutritional assessment of the patient. Such assessment is usually based on a combination of physical measurements of body constituents using anthropometric methods and chemical determinations of blood and urinary constituents. The apparatus needed for the anthropometric measurements is simple, being a tape measure, an accurate weighing machine and a pair of skinfold calipers. The chemical measurements combine those which are universally available and others which are only available in research laboratories. A method of measurement of malnutrition which uses a combination of such measurements is that formulated by Blackburn et al (1976). However, a simple universally acceptable way of quantitating nutritional status which can be applied in any hospital is not available and for the most part the assessment of malnutrition is related to the decision as to whether certain measurements are outside normal limits. Once a patient has been placed in the malnourished group it is less easy to grade the degree of malnutrition without recourse to technically complicated methods such as whole body potassium counting (Goode & Hawkins, 1978). The main indicators of nutritional state used by Blackburn et al (1976) are shown in Table 17.4.

Table 17.4 Indicators of nutritional depletion (After Blackburn et al, 1976)

Anthropometric	Chemical	Other
Percentage weight loss (over 10%)	Serum albumin (less than 35 g/l)	Skin anergy
Mid arm circumference (less than 23 cm male) (less than 22 cm female)	Serum transferrin (less than 2 g/l)	Lymphopaenia
Triceps skinfold thicknesss (less than 10 mm male) (less than 13 mm female)		

At present the most important markers of malnutrition are not known and we are still at the stage where the decision to use parenteral feeding is mainly clinical being based on a combination of clinical acumen and experience.

Ideally the measurements should be part of a pre-feeding assessment and can then be repeated at intervals to measure the response to treatment and possibly to detect complications. In this latter regard the existence of widespread abnormalities which may be relevant to subsequent adverse effects have been documented (Newton et al, 1979).

REQUIREMENTS

There are two main requirements for parenteral nutrition. The first is an access to the circulation in the form of a centrally placed venous catheter. A discussion of catheter placement technique and care is not indicated here but some factors are considered in the section describing complications. The second requirement is for the nutrients themselves which are listed in Table 17.5. This section will consider the size of the requirements and how these can be provided.

Table 17.5 Nutrient requirements for parenteral nutrition

Water and electrolytes
Energy
Nitrogen as amino acids
Trace nutrients
Vitamins

The requirements for energy and nitrogen are closely interrelated. The daily nitrogen need can be measured by estimating the urine nitrogen losses together with those occurring via fistulae. In practice the chemical estimation of total urinary nitrogen loss is not necessary because the urinary urea content has been shown to be a close approximation to the total nitrogen loss (e.g. Jourdan, 1977). A more general guide is given in Table 17.6 where the nitrogen requirements for groups of patients are listed. If weight loss is to be prevented and protein synthesis increased and hence muscle mass restored, adequate nitrogen must be provided. In general an increased nitrogen intake will result in a decrease in a net negative nitrogen balance up to a point where further increase in nitrogen intake is not accompanied by further improvement in nitrogen balance. This general relationship is however dependent upon the energy intake and it is not possible to achieve a positive nitrogen balance unless the energy input is equal to or in excess of the basal metabolic requirement for a particular individual. Many studies have also shown that when the nitrogen intake is adequate for an individual more positive nitrogen balance may be attained by providing energy greater than the basal requirement (e.g. Johnston et al, 1976). Reference to Table 17.6 makes it clear that in a catabolic patient who is in a net catabolic equilibrium with burns or renal failure the energy and nitrogen requirements may be very large. The general relationship has led to the rule that the nitrogen : energy ratio should be about 1 gram of nitrogen to 200 kcal (0.84 MJ).

Table 17.6 Nitrogen and energy requirements (After Woolfson, 1979)

| | | Clinical state | | |
Requirement	Non-catabolic	Normal active man	Intermediate	Catabolic
Energy (MJ/24 hours)	7–9	11–14	11–14	15–18
Nitrogen (g/24 hours)	7.5	8.5	14	25

Table 17.7 A comparison of oral and parenteral amino acid requirements in adults (After Munro, 1972)

| | Daily requirement (mg/kg) | | |
Route of administration	Total	Essential	Essential as % of total
Oral (observed)	425	80	19
Parenteral (observed)	less than 770	less than 140	less than 25%
Parenteral (recommended)			
(a) Normal	800–1600	200– 800	25–50%
(b) Postoperative	1000–2000	400–1000	25–50%

The ideal energy-providing substrate does not exist (Newton et al, 1978) and many alternatives have been used. Glucose and fat emulsions have emerged and are now the preferred energy sources. Their relative value has been the subject of controversy. In subjects who are not in a net catabolic state both substrates have an equal effect on nitrogen balance (Greenberg et al, 1976; Jeejeebhoy et al, 1976), but in the catabolic patient nitrogen balance is directly related to carbohydrate intake and not to fat intake. This suggests that carbohydrate may be the energy source of choice for sustaining nitrogen retention in catabolic patients. It may be however that this only applies in the short term in some patients who are unable to fully utilise infused fat because lipolysis is progressing at a maximal rate and the patient is fully adapted to having a high ketone body concentration and also utilising these compounds as energy sources at a maximal rate.

Fat emulsions offer the advantage of providing a small osmolar load to the patient and their safety has been established (Wretlind, 1974). There has been doubt as to whether the infused fats are utilised but the evidence now seems to indicate that they are indeed metabolised. However there have been reports of fat 'overload' with widespread lipid deposition in patients with reduced ability to utilise fat. The monitoring of fat usage can be carried out by measuring the serum triglyceride concentration. An alternative is to determine the fractional removal rate after stopping the fat infusion but a simple method is to see whether the plasma is turbid six hours after stopping infusion indicating retarded removal. It should also be remembered that many biochemical and haematological tests are invalidated by the presence of infused fat and all such measurements should be carried out using blood drawn after stopping the infusion of fat.

In the case of glucose the main problems are of hyperglycaemia and hyperosmolar states. In general the aim should be to keep the blood glucose concentration below 10 mmol/litre. This means frequent checks of blood glucose concentration and the adjustment of insulin dosage. Although recommendations have been made for the rate of insulin administration in relation to glucose the requirement is very variable and the dose may have to be very high at the start of therapy and then decline. The initial insulin resistance may be caused by high circulating catecholamine and cortisol levels reflecting the serious underlying illness.

These two substrates, fat and glucose, can both be administered in equal proportions to supply a large amount of energy in a low volume with a low osmolar load. Thus Lee (1978) has suggested an energy providing regimen consisting of 750 ml of 50 per cent (w/v) glucose and 750 ml of 20 per cent fat emulsion infused over 24 hours. This provides 3000 kcal (12.6 MJ) in a volume of 1.5 litres.

Other energy providing substrates such as fructose, sorbitol and xylitol do not offer any advantage over glucose and fat, particularly as their use has been accompanied by serious side effects (Woods, 1974).

Nitrogen requirements
There are two ways of providing nitrogen. A malnourished patient with low plasma protein concentrations can immediately be given plasma or purified plasma protein fraction to rapidly restore the plasma osmotic pressure until such time as there can be new synthesis of protein from infused amino acids, the second way of providing nitrogen. The requirements can be roughly estimated as in Table 17.6. More exact estimates can be assessed using the method of Lee & Hartley (1975). This summates the losses of urinary urea (calculated as grams of nitrogen), the urinary protein loss and a correction based on the rise in blood urea concentration. Normally nitrogen losses via the faeces and skin are small but in patients with severe diarrhoea or fistulas the loss of nitrogen from the gut may be large and have to be determined and added to the total.

Commercial amino acid solutions are either protein hydrolysates or mixtures of crystalline amino acids. The advantage of the latter lies in the way in which the composition can be varied to satisfy special requirements. The 'ideal' composition of amino acid mixtures has been the subject of much controversy and discussion. The protein and amino acid requirements of man are well documented (see Hegsted, 1964 for review) and the relative proportions of essential and non-essential amino acids as constituents of the total protein requirement for subjects of various ages are known.

The requirements for parenteral nutrition might be expected to differ from those for oral intake because the infused amino acids do not pass to the liver via the portal vein. There is evidence that the proportions of individual essential amino acids needed for parenteral feeding are different from those optimal for oral feeding. This is shown in Table 17.7 where oral and parenteral amino acid requirements for the adult are compared. The reader is referred to the review of Lee (1978) for a detailed comparison of the amino acid contents of the solutions currently available.

No solution can provide a suitable mixture for all patients and attempts are being made to formulate solutions which are suitable for particular conditions. For example the work of Fischer et al (1974), has shown an elevated concentration of phenylalanine, tryptophan and methionine in patients with hepatic failure. In addition the concentrations of the branch chain amino acids, leucine, isoleucine and valine are lowered. Thus it should be possible to design solutions with a composition reflecting these changes having less aromatic amino acids and more branched chain amino acids than standard mixtures. This would allow the adequate provision of nitrogen for protein synthesis without aggravating the amino acid abnormalities or the neurological symptoms in hepatic failure. Again each patient should be assessed carefully and an appropriate mixture used. In addition to the optimal energy requirements for nitrogen utilisation adequate amounts of potassium and magnesium are required: the ratios being 5 mmol potassium to 1 gram nitrogen and 1 mmol magnesium to 1 gram of nitrogen.

Nitrogen-sparing therapy with isotonic amino acids must be mentioned. The need for simultaneous energy provision with nitrogen is established, however Blackburn et al (1973) showed than an infusion of an isotonic 3 per cent (w/v) amino acid solution, without simultaneous extra energy provision, had a greater nitrogen sparing effect (judged on the basis of nitrogen losses) in surgical patients than has 5 per cent (w/v) glucose. This use of amino acids is said to depend on the metabolic adaptations seen after prolonged starvation. Thus Blackburn et al (1973) found raised blood ketone body and higher esterified fatty acid concentrations together with low insulin levels in their patients. They suggested that the release of lipid fuels from fat stores occurred because of the low insulin levels, and that this decreased muscle breakdown as a source of substrates for glucose synthesis. This work has been repeated with varying degrees of success but it is clear that the large nutritional needs of the severely catabolic patient will only be met by full parenteral feeding.

Water, electrolytes, minerals and vitamins
The calculations of water and electrolyte requirements for parenteral nutrition are no different from those used for other types of management. It should be remembered however that both water and electrolyte losses may be very large in patients with gastrointestinal disease and diarrhoea and fistulae. When calculating balances the electrolyte and water content of the nutrient solutions must be taken into account. These may be large particularly in terms of sodium content.

The complications due to specific deficiencies of certain minerals and vitamins during parenteral nutrition are well documented and some are discussed in the final section of this chapter. Although the nutritional requirements of normal man have been extensively investigated and are well documented so far as most trace elements and vitamins are concerned this does not apply to the patient about to be fed intravenously. Many patients have gross depletion of body stores of such nutrients before therapy and thus they require a loading dose before parenteral nutrition starts. In addition the daily requirement may be in excess of that usually recommended. The problems of administration have largely been removed by the commercial production of vitamin and trace element preparations for injection and infusion.

COMPLICATIONS

In common with all other types of therapy the use of parenteral nutrition is accompanied by complications. Their occurrence results from interactions between three factors:
1. The nature of the substances being infused
2. The method of their delivery to the patient
3. The nature of the underlying illness.

Some complications are relatively frequent and their incidence in series of patients is known. In most cases however no accurate estimate of incidence is available and it can reasonably be assumed that the serious nature of the underlying disease will, in many cases, mask the adverse event in such a way as to prevent it's recognition.

The list of complications is long (Table 17.8) but discussion of selected items can illustrate that the complications arise through the factors listed above.

Table 17.8 Complications of intravenous nutrition

Local	Adverse effects	Systemic
1. Thrombosis		1. Septicaemia
2. Extravasation necrosis		2. Jaundice
3. Sepsis		3. Metabolic
4. Mechanical complications of cannulation		4. Emboli
		5. Kinetic
		6. Toxicity of plastic materials
		7. Non-compatibility of constituents
		8. Miscellaneous

The local consequences of catheter placement
The need to have an access to the circulation in the form of a catheter means that the patient may suffer the local hazards of catheter placement. These are listed in Table 17.8 and do not require further discussion except to point out that the provision of a specialised nutritional team or unit within which a given individual has considerable experience of catheter insertion can minimise these risks. These may be considered as local hazards (Table 17.8). However, the largest group of complications is that which are systemic (Table 17.8). Within this group septicaemia and infections together with certain metabolic complications will be discussed below.

Septicaemia and infection

It is clear that the administration of parenteral nutrition is accompanied by a considerable incidence of infection. This risk was well reviewed by Allen (1978) and Table 17.9 shows the incidence of septicaemia during total parenteral nutrition in this author's series. However the information is difficult to assess because of the heterogeneity of the groups of patients studied. The incidence is much higher than that accompanying a peripheral fluid infusion and led to considerable criticism of parenteral nutrition on the basis that the risks outweighed benefits (Duma, 1971). There is some evidence that the incidence has decreased in recent years.

Table 17.9   The incidence of septicaemia during total parenteral nutrition (After Allen, 1978, with permission.)

Year	No. of series	Total no. of patients	Rate of Septicaemia Bacterial	Fungal	(%) Total
1969	4	79	1.7*	3*	7.8
1970	3	90	19.6	24.7	44.3
1971	1	49	11	16	27
1972	12	2837	6.7*	6.6*	11.3
1973	3	242	4.3	4.0	8.3
1974	8	754	6.1	4.3	10.4
1975	3	230	0*	0.5*	3.3
1976	4	625	6.3*	2.25*	18.0

The figures with asterisks are from series where the data are incomplete so far as the rates for both bacterial and fungal infections are concerned.

The factors involved in the causation of infection are numerous and illustrate the types of interaction described above. The presence of a catheter within the circulation is a major factor. Catheter sepsis is a systemic infection which is not secondary to a distant focus of infection and is cured after the removal of the catheter. Blood cultures are positive and the culture of the catheter tip is often positive. The majority of such infections are the result of the spread of organisms from the skin around the site of insertion to the fibrin sheath surrounding the intravascular part of the catheter. Alternatively the spread can be via the catheter lumen after contamination of the infusion line or infusion fluid. To prevent access via these routes the catheter should be inserted through skin at a distance from the venous insertion and may be tunnelled subcutaneously (Solassol & Joyeaux, 1976). Strict aseptic care of the insertion site is required. The presence of heavy skin contamination such as that found with fistulae and infected wounds is an added risk. The use of the input line for other infusions or injection should be avoided together with the placing of multiple junctions within the line. It is of interest that while many patients have active infection at a distant site spread via the blood is not common (Ryan et al, 1974).

The organisms involved differ in type from those causing septicaemia under other circumstances. In half the cases fungi have been isolated and these are mostly Candida species which make up 60 per cent of fungi isolated. Of the bacteria isolated the Gram-positive cocci *Staphylococcus aureus* and *Staph. albus* predominate; Gram-negative organisms are rearely found (Allen, 1978).

So far as the solutions are concerned, these provide a very favourable growth medium for fungi and bacteria because of their chemical composition (Gelbart et al, 1973). If a solution becomes infected it provides a reservoir for continuing reinfection. Such contamination is either intrinsic (infected during manufacture) or extrinsic (infected during use). Intrinsic contamination of intravenous solutions as a group has often been described. Duma (1976) has discussed this and revealed that in the 10-year period up to 1975, 43 million containers of parenteral products were withdrawn by manufacturers in the United States of America. In general the reason for withdrawal was microbial contamination and during the period studied there were 54 deaths and 410 other incidents thought to be caused by infection. However, it is clear that in most cases the contaminated solutions were not those used for parenteral nutrition and to the author's knowledge there has been no recorded evidence of intrinsic contamination of a solution specifically designed for parenteral nutrition.

On the other hand when a solution has been prepared and a cannula inserted numerous opportunities for extrinsic contamination exist. The rate of bacterial contamination of such solutions before infusion (i.e. once they have been mixed or prepared) is less than 3 per cent. It is clear that this does not explain the high incidence of infection during intravenous nutrition and moreover Maki et al (1974) found that the organism isolated from the blood was in many cases not the same as that isolated from the solution infused in cases of septicaemia.

It is now generally agreed that such cases represent extrinsic contamination. Once access to the circulation is established infection can be introduced at many sites (see Table 17.10). The availability of a parenteral nutrition team can markedly lower the incidence of sepsis. Such a group is responsible for the sterile preparation of the solutions together with the insertion of the cannula and it's subsequent care and that of the infusion line. An important rule is that no substances other than the prepared solutions should enter the circulation via the 'nutrition' line. Sanders & Sheldon (1976) have demonstrated the efficacy of this policy. They were able to lower the

Table 17.10 Sites for contamination of parenteral nutrition solutions

1. IN CONTAINER
    a. Defective containers
        punctures
        cracks
    b. Additives
    c. Container changes
    d. Container attachment
    e. Container air vents

2. IN LINE
    a. 'Piggyback' junctions
    b. Connections
    c. Venous pressure measurements in open systems
    d. Arterial pressure transducers
    e. Injections
    f. Infusions of blood or blood products
    g. In-line filters

3. AT CANNULA
    a. Insertion
    b. Cannula manipulation
    c. Infection at insertion site

overall septicaemia rate from 29 per cent to 8 per cent by the introduction of a team. Some help has been provided by the manufacturers who have introduced sterile welded infusion lines for use with so called 'big bag' contrainers thus removing the necessity for complex 'plumbing'.

The final factor contributing to infection is the state of the patient. The combination of poor immune responses, previous antimicrobial, corticosteroid or immunosuppressive therapy makes them more susceptible to infection.

Nutrient deficiencies

It might be expected that the infusion of pure dietary constituents in place of oral nutrition may lead to the gradual development of deficiencies of trace nutrients and vitamins. The widespread use of L-amino acid mixtures manufactured from pure crystalline acids as nitrogen sources rather than protein hydrolysates is an example. Included in the hydrolysate were the trace nutrients which were associated with or bound to the starting protein used in manufacture.

The so called trace metals provide an informative example. There have been several descriptions of a well defined clinical syndrome due to zinc deficiency which develops during parenteral nutrition in both children and adults. For example Arakawa et al (1976) described two infants who, while being fed intravenously, developed an illness consisting of hair loss, diarrhoea and a pustular rash in the oral and gluteal regions. This syndrome responsed to zinc administration and at diagnosis was accompanied by low zinc concentrations in blood. The condition closely resembles the syndrome of infant zinc deficiency known as acrodermatitis enteropathica.

In the adult urinary losses of zinc are large following trauma and during infection and muscle wasting. Fleming et al (1976) have decribed zinc deficiency in adult patients being fed intravenously. Those subjects with bowel fistulae or diarrhoea seem to be particularly at risk. Zinc is essential for protein synthesis and the experience of Fleming et al (1976) makes it clear that the clinical effects of zinc deficiency usually become apparent when the patient starts to gain muscle mass.

A further example which illustrates the contributory factors listed earlier in this paper is that of acute folate deficiency. This condition, accompanied by thrombocytopaenia and a low leukocyte count, has been described by Wardrop et al (1975) as occurring soon after the start of parenteral feeding (one to two weeks).

The first factor involved is the patients themselves. Many of those who require parenteral feeding have conditions such as Crohn's disease or gastric carcinoma which are known to be associated with folate deficiency. In other cases sepsis and a long history of poor dietary intake secondary to small bowel disease can lead to depleted folate stores. In a recent study Newton et al (1979) found that over half a group of patients who were about to be fed intravenously had a low plasma folate concentration before treatment was started.

The second factor concerns the nature of the solutions being infused. Wardrop et al (1975) found that the infusion of an amino acid-sorbitol-ethanol mixture for one day led to a fall in serum folate concentrations from their initial normal values. These authors suggested that the nutrient responsible was the ethanol. This is not the case because two further cases were later reported by Green (1977) and Smith et al (1978) were able to produce acute falls in serum folate concentration by the infusion of amino acid mixtures either infused alone or with a carbohydrate energy source.

Attention was thus drawn to the amino acid composition of the solutions infused. Folate derivatives are essential confactors in the metabolism of one carbon (1–C) units and a major source of such units is the amino acid methionine. The amino acid solutions currently available all have methionine as a constituent in many cases in large concentration. In view of its metabolic role in relation to folate the infusion of large quantities of methionine might be expected to alter the demand for folate. In normal man Connor et al (1978) were able to produce a signifcant fall in serum folate concentration by oral methionine supplementation of a normal diet. The dose used was 8 grams per day which if complete absorption from the gut lumen occurred, is almost identical to the dose given intravenously by Wardrop et al (1975). The plasma methionine concentrations achieved were close to those reported by Smits & Wells (1975) for patients receiving 7.2 grams methionine per day via the intravenous route.

These results suggest that the production of folate deficiency may result partly from the infusion of a normal nutrient in an excessive amount. The capacity of the normal subject to clear methionine from the plasma following an intravenous bolus of an amino acid mixture is far exceeded by an infusion of 7 to 8 grams per day (Burger, 1977).

These examples stress two important principles so far as the management of the patient is concerned. Firstly there is a need for comprehensive metabolic and nutritional screening before treatment is started. Secondly there is a need for frequent review of progress to detect complications early.

THE COST OF PARENTERAL NUTRITION

Parenteral nutrition is expensive and the question of cost versus benefit has to be considered. When the drug bill for a general hospital is examined it is often found that the total for parenteral nutrition ranks high in the list.

One way to quantitate this is to calculate the cost of regimens containing amounts of amino acid nitrogen close to those recommended in Table 17.6 for different groups of patients. These can be compared with the cost of providing the same amount of nitrogen by means of enteral feeding. Table 17.11 shows such a comparison for two daily nitrogen requirements excluding the cost of consumables such as tubing, cannulae and other solutions and additives. It is clear that the parenteral route is more

Table 17.11   A comparison of costs for enteral and parenteral nutrition.
The costs of two regimens containing comparable amounts of nitrogen have been calculated. In each case the amounts of nitrogen were chosen to match the requirements of a non-catabolic (I) and catabolic (II) subject as in Table 17.7. The table has been drawn up using data relating to commercially available preparations, and refers to treatment costs for one day. The energy source has been included to give an optimal energy : nitrogen ratio for the intravenous regimens.

Regimen No.	Amount of nitrogen (grams)	Cost per gram of nitrogen (£)	Total cost per day (£)
I { Enteral	8.19	1.13	8.90
I { Parenteral	8.0	1.59	12.75
II { Enteral	20.0	0.74	14.76
II { Parenteral	21.3	1.41	30.0

expensive than the enteral for a given nitrogen dose. In part this may reflect higher manufacturing costs for sterile solutions but the cost per gram of nitrogen in the L-amino acid solutions marketed in the United Kingdom varies from £0.84 to £1.90.

However, a cost-benefit analysis must include the value of any benefits. If, for example, feeding is followed by fewer postoperative complications, the resulting decrease in length of hospital stay may more than cover the cost of nutritional treatment.

FINAL CONCLUSIONS

The technique and 'art' of intravenous feeding has advanced considerably and the dangers inherent in the therapy are now recognised.

A measure of these advances can be obtained from the success of long-term home parenteral nutrition in patients who have undergone almost total gut resection. There are now many cases in whom nutritional and metabolic normality have been maintained over several years (e.g. Broviac & Scribner, 1974). A general benefit has been the stimulus parenteral feeding has given to human nutritional research and the information it has provided concerning the nutritional requirements of man.

REFERENCES

Allen J R 1978 The incidence of nosocomial infection in patients receiving total parenteral nutrition. In: Johnston I D A (ed) Advances in parenteral nutrition. MTP Press, Lancaster, p 339–378

Arakawa T, Tamura T, Igarashi Y, Suzuki H, Sandstead H H 1976 Zinc deficiency in two infants during total parenteral alimentation for diarrhoea. American Journal of Clinical Nutrition 29: 197–204

Bistrian B R, Blackburn G L, Hallowell E, Heddle R 1974 Protein status of general surgical patients. Journal of the American Medical Association 230: 858–860

Bistrain B R, Blackburn G L, Vitale J, Cochran D, Naylor J 1976 Prevalence of malnutrition in general medical patients. Journal of the American Medical Association 235: 1567–1570

Blackburn G L, Flatt, J P, Clowes G H A, O'Donnell T E, Hensak T W 1973 Protein sparing therapy during periods of starvation with sepsis or trauma. Annals of Surgery 177: 588–593

Blackburn G L, Bistrain B R, Maini B S, Benotti P, Bothe A, Gibbons G, Smith M F 1976 Manual for nutritional/metabolic assessment of the hospitalized patient. Nutrition Support Service, New England Deaconess Hospital, Harvard Medical School, Boston, Mass

Bollett A J, Owens S O 1973 Evaluation of nutritional status of selected hospitalized patients. American Journal of Clinical Nutrition 26: 931–935

Broviac J W, Scribner B H 1974 Prolonged parenteral nutrition in the home. Surgery, Gynaecology and Obstetrics 139: 24–31

Bürger Y 1977 Untersuchungen über die Verwertung parenteral zugeführter Aminosäuren bei gesunden Erwachsenen. Infusionstherapie 4: 273–278

Connor H, Newton D J, Preston F E, Woods H F 1978 Oral methionine loading as a cause of acute serum folate deficiency: it's relevance to parenteral nutrition. Postgraduate Medical Journal 54: 318–320

Copeland E M, MacFadyen B J, Dudrick S J 1974 Intravenous hyperalimentation in cancer patients. Journal of Surgical Research 16: 241–247

Copeland E M, Dudrick S J 1978 The importance of parenteral nutrition as an adjunct to cancer treatment. In: Johnston I D A (ed) Advances in parenteral nutrition. MTP Press, Lancaster, p 473–496

Dudrick S J, Wilmore D W, Vars H M, Rhoads J E 1968 Long term total parenteral nutrition with growth development and positive nitrogen balance. Surgery 64: 134–142

Dudrick S J, Wilmore D W, Vars H M, Rhoads J E 1969 Can intravenous feeding as the sole means of nutrition support growth in the child and restore weight in the adult? An affirmative answer. Annals of Surgery 169: 974–984

Duma R J 1971 First of all do no harm. New England Journal of Medicine 285: 1258–1259

Duma R J 1976 Thomas Latta, what have we done? — The hazards of intravenous therapy. New England Journal of Medicine 294: 1178–1180

Fischer J E, Voshimura N, James H, Cummings M G, Abbel R M, Deindoefer F 1974 Plasma amino acids in patients with hepatic encephalopathy. Effect of amino acid infusions. American Journal of Surgery 127: 40–45

Fleming C R, Hodges R E, Hurley L S 1976 A prospective study of serum copper and zinc levels in patients receiving total parenteral nutrition. American Journal of Clinical Nutrition 29: 70–77

Gelbart S M, Reinhardt G F, Greenlee H B 1973 Multiplication of nosocomial pathogens in intravenous feeding solutions. Applied Microbiology 26: 874–879

Goode A W, Hawkins T 1978 The use of ^{40}K counting and its relationship to other estimates of lean body mass. In: Johnston I D A (ed) Advances in parenteral nutrition. MTP Press, Lancaster, p 557–570

Green P J 1977 Folate deficiency and intravenous nutrition. Lancet 1: 814

Greenberg G R, Marliss E B, Anderson G H, Langer B, Spence W, Tovee E B, Jeejeebhoy K N 1976 Protein-sparing therapy in postoperative patients. Effects of added hypocaloric glucose or lipid. New England Journal of Medicine 294: 1411–1416

Hegsted P M 1964 Protein requirements. In: Munro H N, Allison J B (eds) Mammalian protein metabolism, Academic Press, New York vol II pp 135–171

Hill G L, Blackett R L, Pickford I, Burkinshaw L, Young G A, Warren J V, Schorath C J, Morgan D B 1977 Malnutrition in surgical patients. An unrecognized problem. Lancet 1: 689–692

Jeejeebhoy K N, Anderson G H, Nakhooda A F, Greenberg G R, Sanderson I, Marliss E B 1976 Metabolic studies in total nutrition with lipid in man. Journal of Clinical Investigation 57: 125–136

Jourdan M H 1977 Some aspects of protein nutrition and metabolism in postoperative surgical patients. In Baxter D H, Jackson G M (eds) Clinical parenteral nutrition. Geistlich Education, Chester, p 158–168

Johnston I D A, Tweedle D, Spivey J 1976 Intravenous feeding after surgical operation. In: Wilkinson A W (ed) Parenteral nutrition. Churchill Livingstone, Edinburgh, p 189–197

Leading Article 1979 Parenteral nutrition before surgery? British Medical Journal 2: 1529–1530

Lee H A, Hartley T F 1975 A method of determining daily nitrogen requirements. Postgraduate Medical Journal 51: 441–455

Lee H A 1978 Parenteral nutrition. In: Dickerson J W T, Lee H A (eds) Nutrition in the clinical management of disease. Edward Arnold, London, p 349–376

Lee H A 1979 Why enteral nutrition? In: Johnston I D A, Lee H A (eds) Developments in clinical nutrition. MCS Consultants, Tunbridge Wells, p 15–24

MacFadyen B V, Dudrick S J, Ruberg R L 1973 Management of gastrointestinal fistulae with parenteral hyperalimentation. Surgery 74: 100–105

Maki D G, Anderson R L, Shulman J A 1974 In-use contamination of intravenous infusion fluid. Applied Microbiology 28: 778–784

Meng H C, Sandstead H H 1972 Long-term total parenteral nutrition in patients with chronic inflammatory diseases of the intestine. In: Wilkinson A W (ed) Parenteral nutrition. Churchill Livingstone, Edinburgh, p 213–233

Newton D J, Clark R G, Woods H F, Connor H 1979 Metabolic abnormalities in patients prior to parenteral feeding. Proceedings of the Nutrition Society 38(2): A–74.

Newton D, Connor H, Woods H F 1978 Metabolic pathways for carbohydrates in parenteral nutrition. In: Johnston I D A (ed) Advances in parenteral nutrition. MTP Press, Lancaster, p 29–44

Ryan J A, Abel R M, Abbott W M, Hopkins C C, Chesney T. McC, Colley R, Phillips K, Fischer J F 1974 Catheter complications in total parenteral nutrition. A prospective study of 200 consecutive patients. New England Journal of Medicine 290: 757–761

Sanders R A, Sheldon G F 1976 Septic complications of total parenteral nutrition — a five-year experience. American Journal of Surgery 132: 214–220

Smith R C, Tennant G B, Williams R H P, Wardrop C A J, Hughes L F 1978 Acute depression of serum folate due to ethanol-free parenteral nutrition and surgical trauma. British Journal of Surgery 65: 364

Smits B J, Wells F E 1974 Preliminary studies on the utilization and metabolic effects of aminoplex 5. Clinical Trials Journal, Suppl. 1: 186–204

Smythe P M, Schonland M, Brereton-Stiles G G, Coovadia H M, Grace H J, Loening W E K, Mafoyane A, Parent M A, Vos G H 1971 Thymolymphatic deficiency and depression of cell-mediated immunity in protein calorie malnutrition. Lancet 2: 939–943

Solassol C, Joyeux H 1976 Ambulatory parenteral nutrition. In: Fischer J E (ed) Total parenteral nutrition. Little Brown & Co., Boston, p 285–301

Wardrop C A J, Heatley R V, Tennant G B, Hughes L E 1975 Acute folate deficiency in surgical patients on amino acid/ethanol intravenous nutrition. Lancet 2: 640–642

Woods H F 1974 Some metabolic aspects of parenteral feeding. In: Truelove S C, Trowell J (eds) Topics in gastroenterology no 2. Blackwell Scientific Publications, Oxford, p 191–207

Woolfson A M J 1978 Metabolic considerations in nutritional support. In: Johnston I D A, Lee H A, (eds) Developments in clinical nutrition. MCS Consultants, Tunbridge Wells, p 35–47

Wretlind A 1974 Fat emulsions. In: Lee H A (ed) Parenteral Nutrition in Acute Metabolic Illness. Academic Press, London & New York, p 77–95

Index